# ADDICTION

## Handbook & Resource Guide

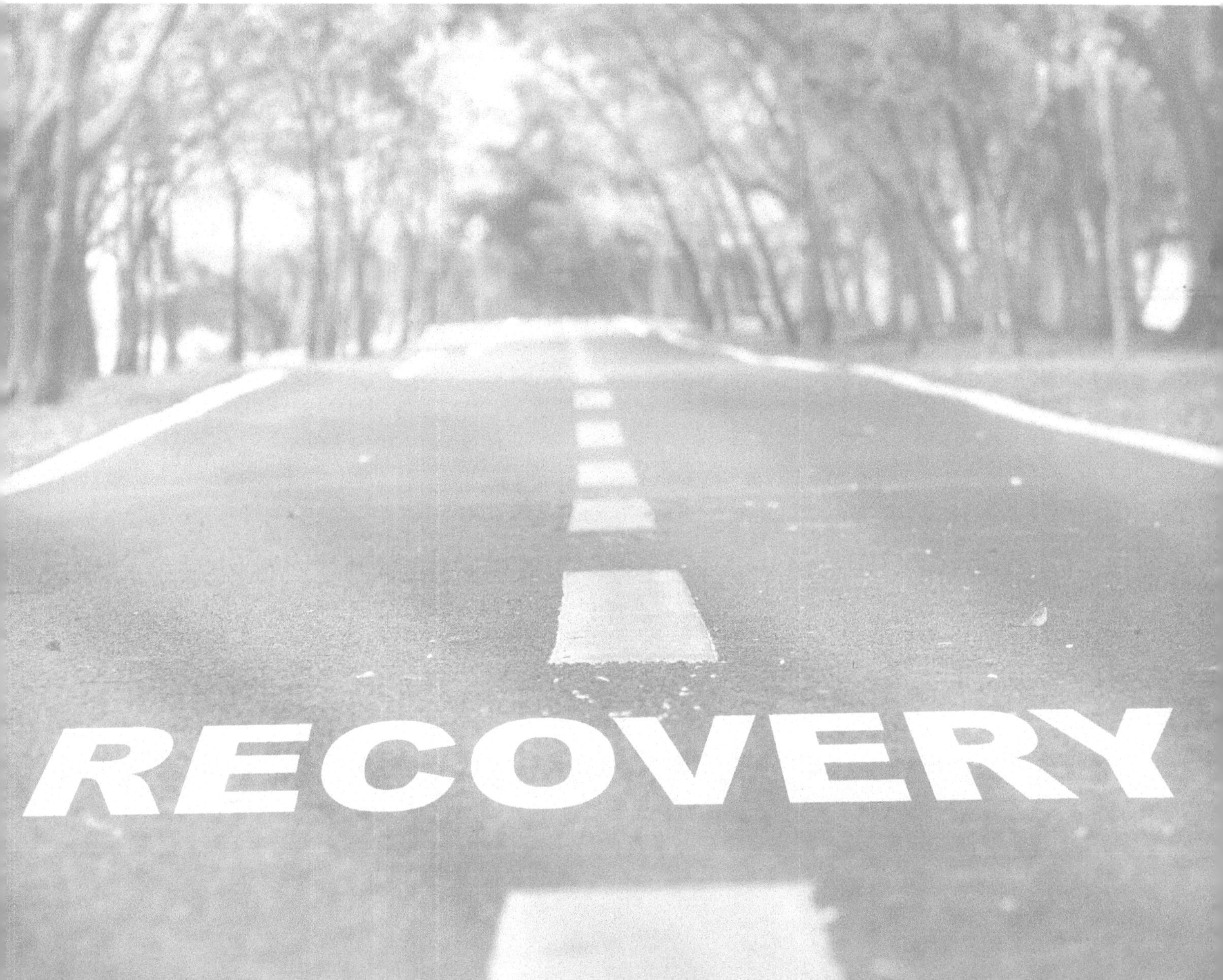

FIRST EDITION

# ADDICTION

## Handbook & Resource Guide

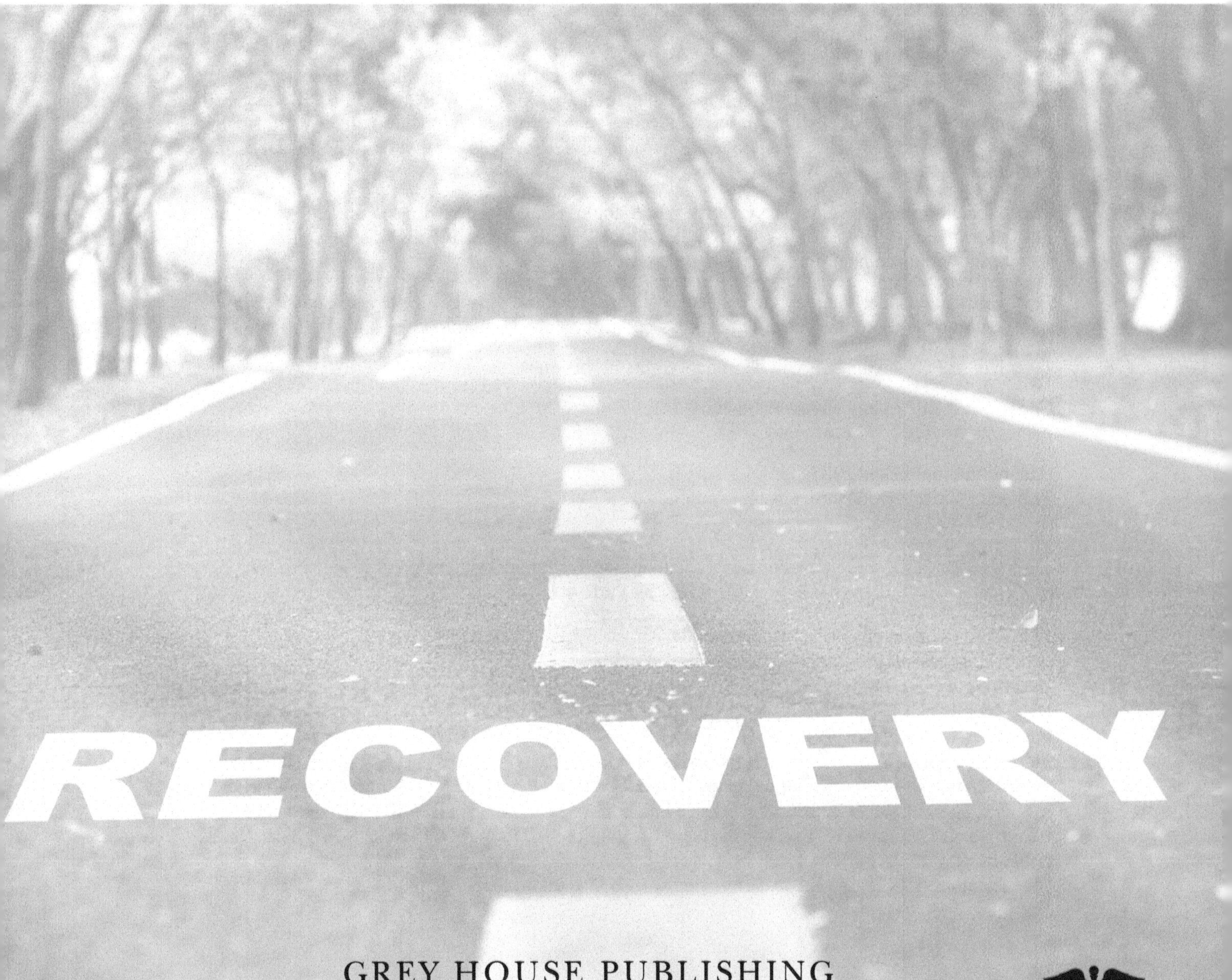


GREY HOUSE PUBLISHING

Grey House Health & Wellness Guides

PUBLISHER: Leslie Mackenzie
EDITORIAL DIRECTOR: Stuart Paterson
MARKETING DIRECTOR: Jessica Moody
EDITORIAL ASSISTANT: Margarita Vachenkova

Grey House Publishing, Inc.
4919 Route 22
Amenia, NY 12501
518.789.8700
Fax: 845.373.6390
www.greyhouse.com
books@greyhouse.com



First edition published 2023.
Printed in Canada by Marquis Book Printing.

Publisher's Cataloging-In-Publication Data
(Prepared by Parlew Associates)

Title: Addiction handbook & resource guide.
Other Titles: Addiction handbook and resource guide.
Description: First edition. | Amenia, NY : Grey House Publishing, 2023. | Series: [Grey House health & wellness guides ; 7] | Includes index. | Includes color illustrations.
Identifiers: ISBN 9781637005231 (hardback) | ISBN 9781637005248 (ebook)
Subjects: LCSH: Comorbidity — Handbooks, manuals, etc. | Compulsive behavior — Handbooks, manuals, etc. | Psychology, Pathological — Handbooks, manuals, etc. | Substance abuse — Handbooks, manuals, etc. | LCGFT: Reference works. | Handbooks and manuals. | BISAC: MEDICAL / Mental Health. | PSYCHOLOGY / Psychopathology / Addiction. | SOCIAL SCIENCE / Disease & Health Issues.
Classification: LCC RC533.A33 2023 (print) | RC533 (ebook) | DDC 616.86—dc23

# Table of Contents



## Section One: Studies & Statistics



## Section Two: Addiction & Mental Health Resources

## Section Three: Health Complications of Addiction

## Section Four: Appendixes & Indexes

# Publisher's Note

Grey House Publishing is pleased to announce the *Addiction Handbook & Resource Guide*—the seventh volume in a health series that supports our long-standing consumer health titles on such topics as mental health, older Americans, chronic illness, pediatric disorders, and people with disabilities. This title follows *Dementia Handbook & Resource Guide, Cardiovascular Disease Handbook & Resource Guide, Autoimmune Diseases Handbook & Resource Guide, Nutrition, Obesity & Eating Disorders Handbook & Resource Guide, Diabetes Handbook & Resource Guide*, and *Autism Spectrum Handbook & Resource Guide.*

This work covers addiction and related mental health conditions, and 18 common comorbidities, from AIDS/HIV to stroke.

The *Addiction Handbook & Resource Guide* combines valuable, easy-to-understand educational information for consumers, patients, and their families, with official reports and releases about substance misuse, addiction, mental health factors, and treatments and further resources for co-occurring conditions. This new volume is arranged in the following sections:

### Introduction

This detailed introduction to the book and to addiction specifically, written by health specialist Patricia S. Edens, PhD, RN, LFACHE, provides information on the types of addiction, recognizing symptoms, treatment options, health complications, and preventing addiction.

### Section One: Studies & Statistics

This robust, colorful section of 350 pages includes detailed reports, journal articles, fact sheets, infographics, and useable materials such as vaccination cards, from a number of sources including the U.S. Department of Health & Human Services, National Institute on Drug Abuse, Centers for Disease Control and Prevention, and Substance Abuse and Mental Health Services Administration. It begins with an annotated table of contents, followed by two detailed reports on addiction and substance misuse in America. From there, articles take readers through some of the most commonly misused substances, including alcohol, marijuana, and opioids, as well as addressing current mental health considerations such as the effects of the COVID-19 pandemic.

Following this are helpful backgrounders, facts, and treatment plans about the specific conditions related to addiction that are covered in Section Three, including AIDS/HIV, Alzheimer's disease/dementias, autoimmune diseases, cancer, cardiovascular diseases, chronic pain, depressive disorders, gastrointestinal (GI) disorders, hepatitis, impotence, infertility and pregnancy, kidney disease, liver disease, respiratory illnesses, sexually transmitted diseases (STDs), sleep disorders, and stroke.

### Section Two: Addiction & Mental Health Resources

This section details a variety of resources for individuals experiencing addiction, their families, and caregivers, including agencies and associations, foundations, libraries and resource centers, research centers, support groups and hotlines, print resources, digital resources, and web sites.

### Section Three: Risk Factors & Complications

This section includes 18 conditions that are considered to commonly co-occur with addiction. Overviews written by Patricia S. Edens detail the conditions themselves, how they relate to addiction, and both common and cutting-edge treatment options. Patient, family and caregiver resources follow.

Following that, users will find the following pieces of backmatter:

- **Glossary of Terms** lists major terms and concepts related to addiction, including terms to avoid, terms to use, and why.
- **Slang Terms and Code Words** presents an exhaustive list of common and uncommon alternate expressions to describe illicit drugs.
- **Entry Index** lists all directory entries alphabetically.
- **Geographic Index** organizes listings alphabetically by state.

The *Addiction Spectrum Handbook & Resource Guide* is a necessary reference for public and academic libraries, as well as education and health care collections, providing information crucial to individuals with addiction issues, their broader support network, caseworkers, social workers, and other education and health care providers.

# Introduction

When you hear the term addiction, you might automatically think of drug addiction. However, addiction is so much more. Considered a chronic medical disease, addiction involves a complex interplay of circuits in the brain, genetics, environment and experiences of life. Research has redefined the discussion surrounding addiction. Addiction is now defined as a disease that affects the brain and not as a choice or personal failing. Regardless of the type of addiction, it is treatable with early recognition of the disease and appropriate interventions. Individuals with addiction use substances or engage in behaviors that may be compulsive and lead to harmful consequences. The impact of addiction on family and friends must never be underestimated. Emotional or physical abuse of family members, including children, and the financial drain on families as the individual supports an addiction, have long-term consequences often equated to a truck hitting the entire family. Efforts toward prevention and treatment are often as successful as those for any chronic disease. There is a stigma associated with any addiction diagnosis. Understanding the disease, risk factors, prevention and treatment options, and the role of health and wellness is critical to management, remission and recovery.

## Types of Addiction

The types of addiction may be experienced singularly or in combination. Addictions involving substance use, referred to as chemical addiction, create a physical dependence on a drug or chemical agent. Substance addictions can involve prescription drugs such as opioids, illegal drugs such as cocaine or methamphetamines, and easily accessible chemicals such as alcohol and nicotine. There is confusion about chemical addiction. Is it substance misuse, dependency or addiction? The most recent edition of the *Diagnostic and Statistical Manual of Mental Disorders* (DSM-5) prefers the term "substance use disorder" and allows providers to further define the diagnosis as mild, moderate or severe. Moving away from the term "abuse" also may help destigmatize addiction as a disease.

Behavioral addictions occur when individuals lose control of their actions to engage in behaviors that may bring temporary feelings of happiness, even if they offer no long-term benefit. Addictions to food, sex, the internet, video games, shopping, exercise and gambling are just a few common behavioral addictions. While substance addictions are easily understood, many people struggle to understand behavioral addictions as these behaviors are normal in moderation or when they are not done to excess. Compulsive behaviors often occur with impulse control disorders and may lead to severe addictions.

Behavioral addictions recognized by the DSM-5 include gambling addiction and internet gaming disorder, but other activities may still be categorized as a behavioral addiction requiring intervention. Mental health issues and mental disorders may cause both a substance addiction and a behavioral addiction. Medical experts agree that certain behaviors may become problems over time but are still debating when behaviors become addictions and what specific behaviors can become addictive. The issue is that scientific, peer-reviewed evidence is not sufficient to name, for example, shopping, sex or exercise as addictions, while still agreeing that these addictive behaviors exist. Social media addictions, such as to Facebook and other platforms, while often considered a problem, may not rise to the medical diagnosis of addiction.

## Understanding Addiction

Understanding and recognizing symptoms of addiction are the beginning points of addressing the issue. Addiction interferes with normal brain function related to a process known as the reward system. Dopamine, a neurotransmitter, and other chemicals are released by the brain in response to something that the individual finds enjoyable. Shopping with a friend, sharing a meal or glass of wine, or using cocaine, triggers the reward system to release chemicals. While these chemicals do not create the feelings of pleasure or euphoria, they do reinforce the brain's association between activities and feelings of pleasure, encouraging the individual to seek the pleasure-inducing feelings in the future.

Wanting to experience these pleasant feelings or euphoria can trigger cravings, especially when exposed to cues, such as a party where people are drinking, a visit to a casino, or shopping with a friend. With every exposure, the amount of dopamine release is increased until the brain realizes there is sufficient dopamine and decreases the production level. Eventually, the individual needs more dopamine than the brain is producing to create the same "high" feeling resulting in what is defined as tolerance. Complicating matters is that the brain decreases dopamine production in response to natural triggers like having sex or enjoying a hobby. To overcome this tolerance, individuals engage in increasingly risky behaviors to attempt to increase dopamine production by the brain. Stopping these behaviors is extremely difficult without professional help involving medications, counseling or other therapies.

**Recognizing Symptoms**

Recognizing the common symptoms of substance use disorder include:

- Having cravings so intense it affects the ability to think about other things
- Discomfort if you can't easily access the substance
- An increasing need to use more of the substance to get the same feeling
- Risky use of the substance such as at work or while driving
- Spending less time on previous activities or with family and friends
- An inability to carry out activities of daily living such as work, school or managing home
- An inability to stop the substance and withdrawal symptoms if you try to quit

Recognizing the common symptoms of behavior addictions, including the two DSM-5 defined addictions of gambling and internet gaming disorder, include:

- Excessive time spent in a behavior
- The urge to participate in a behavior to the detriment of daily life, including work and relationships
- Depending on the behavior to manage unwanted emotions
- Difficulty avoiding the behavior and lying to other people about the time spent on the behavior
- Restlessness, irritability, depression, anxiety and other withdrawal symptoms if attempting to quit
- Feeling compelled to continue the behavior even when it causes distress

**Treatment**

Seeking professional help based on any of the above defined symptoms is crucial. With substance use disorder, medically supervised detoxification may be indicated. While detox, as it's often referred to, will not treat the underlying condition of addiction, it does help the individual get through the withdrawal process safely. Residential treatment, outpatient treatment, psychotherapy, medication to help reduce cravings and support groups such as Alcoholics Anonymous or Narcotics Anonymous may aid in recovery. For behavioral addictions, cognitive behavioral therapy (CBT) that focuses on thoughts and emotions and reframing them in the moment combined with more productive coping skills is critical. Self-help groups combined with therapy may deliver better outcomes. Recent studies have shown that some antidepressants may be beneficial to address addictive behaviors.

Newer strategies, including the availability of on-line or telephonic therapy sessions, may also be useful. There are a variety of substance abuse and behavioral addiction hotlines that are resources of note, including the Suicide Prevention Hotline, Gambling Addiction Hotlines, and others.

### Health Complications of Addiction

People with addiction often have other health issues such as heart and lung problems, stroke, cancer or mental health issues. Diagnostic tests often show the damage caused by long-term substance abuse. Tobacco smoke and vaping can cause cancers, and vaping has been shown to destroy lung tissue. Dental issues, or meth mouth, result from methamphetamine abuse. Inhalants may destroy tissue and nerve cells, including in the brain and nasal cavities. Motor vehicle accidents and unsafe decisions as a result of substance use disorder may result in brain, orthopedic and other injuries. Drug use may trigger or worsen mental health conditions. Abusing substances during pregnancy can cause neonatal abstinence syndrome (NAS), and babies will exhibit withdrawal symptoms at birth. Some drug-exposed children will have developmental problems, seizures, and thinking problems. Substances are passed to the infant from breast milk generating more long-term effects for the child.

Substance abuse disorder may also encourage risky health behaviors leading to disease and spread of infectious disease such as AIDS and hepatitis. There is a documented increased risk of motor vehicle accidents with the use of illicit drugs or misuse of prescription drugs. Behavioral addictions may also contribute to health-related complications as risky behaviors to achieve the euphoria evident in addiction may occur.

### Preventing Addiction

Preventing early use of alcohol and drugs decreases the chance of addiction. In teenagers, life changes such as moving, family divorce or changing schools may increase risks. In adults, a divorce or job loss may increase the risk of drug use. Living independent of family support may also create an ease of access to addictive substances and behaviors.

Behavioral addictions, such as compulsive gambling, can stimulate the brain just as drugs and alcohol can. Gambling is often used to escape problems or relieve feelings of helplessness or depression. If money problems occur, the individual may see gambling as a way to get money. Internet gaming disorder is evident if there is reduced control over gaming habits leading to negative impacts on activities of daily living. While other behavioral addictions may not be formally recognized with a DSM-5 code, excessive shopping when money is tight, sex addiction exhibited by multiple risky partners and other risky behaviors should be addressed at first evidence.

Taking action at the first sign of risky behaviors that could lead to addiction is key to preventing addiction.

### Summary

Understanding addiction is the first step to preventing or managing the condition. Asking for help if symptoms present is crucial. Seeking assistance from health professionals and treatment facilities will enhance the road to recovery. Gathering information is important to better understand a personalized approach to addiction prevention and care.

*—Patricia S. Edens, PhD, RN, LFACHE*

# SECTION ONE: STUDIES & STATISTICS

This first section of the *Addiction Handbook & Resource Guide* includes the most current research on how addiction relates to the featured health conditions, with data, fact sheets, reports, and studies from the U.S. Department of Health & Human Services, National Institute on Drug Abuse, Centers for Disease Control and Prevention, U.S. Administration on Aging, National Istitute of Environmental Health Sciences, Substance Abuse and Mental Health Services Administration, U.S. Food and Drug Administration, and more. Totaling 350 pages, Studies & Statistics comprises over 25 detailed reports, summaries, journal articles, and fact sheets, with easy to understand graphics. Colorful photos, graphs, charts, and maps help to visualize the data.

# FACING ADDICTION IN AMERICA

*The Surgeon General's Report on Alcohol, Drugs, and Health*

U.S. Department of Health & Human Services

# CHAPTER 1.
# INTRODUCTION AND OVERVIEW OF THE REPORT

## Chapter 1 Preview

The United States has a serious substance misuse problem. Substance misuse is the use of alcohol or drugs in a manner, situation, amount, or frequency that could cause harm to the user or to those around them. Alcohol and drug misuse and related substance use disorders affect millions of Americans and impose enormous costs on our society. In 2015, 66.7 million people in the United States reported binge drinking in the past month and 27.1 million people were current users of illicit drugs or misused prescription drugs.[3] The accumulated costs to the individual, the family, and the community are staggering and arise as a consequence of many direct and indirect effects, including compromised physical and mental health, increased spread of infectious disease, loss of productivity, reduced quality of life, increased crime and violence, increased motor vehicle crashes, abuse and neglect of children, and health care costs.

The most devastating consequences are seen in the tens of thousands of lives that are lost each year as a result of substance misuse. Alcohol misuse contributes to 88,000 deaths in the United States each year; 1 in 10 deaths among working adults are due to alcohol misuse.[6] In addition, in 2014 there were 47,055 drug overdose deaths including 28,647 people who died from a drug overdose involving some type of opioid, including prescription pain relievers and heroin—more than in any previous year on record.[7]

Even though the United States spends more than any other country on health care, it ranks 27th in life expectancy, which has plateaued or decreased for some segments of the population at a time when life expectancy continues to increase in other developed countries—and the difference is largely due to substance misuse and associated physical and mental health problems. For example, recent research has shown an unprecedented increase in mortality among middle-aged White Americans between 1999 and 2014 that was largely driven by alcohol and drug misuse and suicides, although this trend was not seen within other racial and ethnic populations such as Blacks and Hispanics.[8] An analysis from the Centers for Disease Control and Prevention (CDC) demonstrated that alcohol and drug misuse accounted for a roughly 4-month decline in life expectancy among White Americans; no other cause of death had a larger negative impact in this population.[9]

Substance misuse and substance use disorders also have serious economic consequences, costing more than $400 billion annually in crime, health, and lost productivity.[10,11] These costs are of a similar order of magnitude to those associated with other serious health problems such as diabetes, which is estimated to cost the United States $245 billion each year.[12] Alcohol misuse and alcohol use disorders alone costs the United States approximately $249 billion in lost productivity, health care expenses, law enforcement, and other criminal justice costs.[10] The costs associated with drug use disorders and use of illegal drugs and non-prescribed medications were estimated to be more than $193 billion in 2007.[11]

Despite decades of expense and effort focused on a criminal justice–based model for addressing substance use-related problems, substance misuse remains a national public health crisis that continues to rob the United States of its most valuable asset: its people. In fact, high annual rates of past-month illicit drug use and binge drinking among people aged 12 years and older from 2002 through 2014 (Figure 1.1) emphasize the importance of implementing evidence-based public-health-focused strategies to prevent and treat alcohol and drug problems in the United States.[13]A public health approach seeks to improve the health and safety of the population by addressing underlying social, environmental, and economic determinants of substance misuse and its consequences, to improve the health, safety, and well-being of the entire population.

Figure 1.1: Past Month Rates of Substance Use Among People Aged 12 or Older: Percentages, 2002-2014, 2014 National Survey on Drug Use and Health (NSDUH)

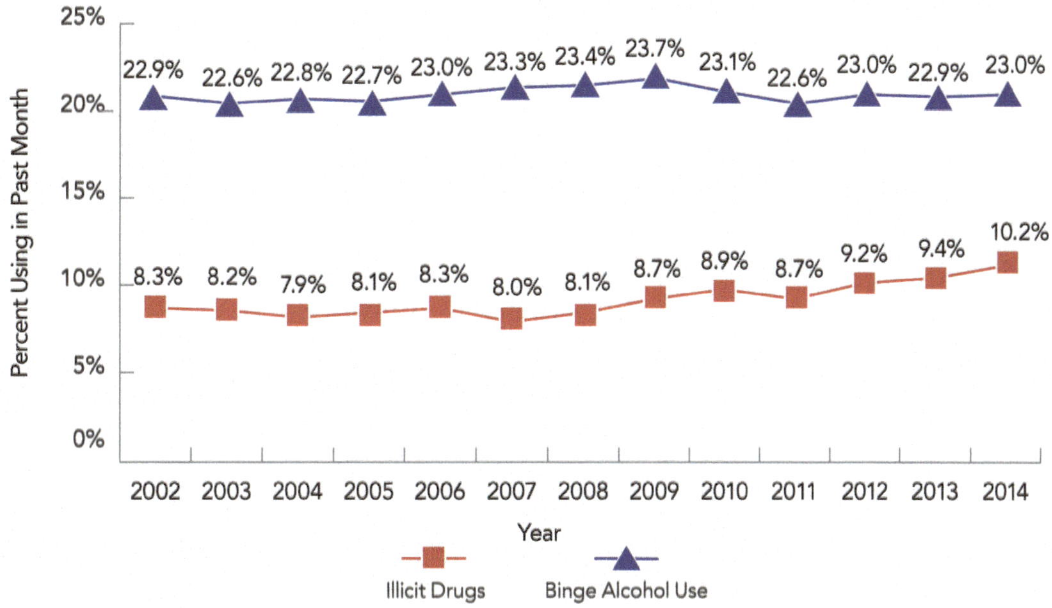


Notes: *The National Survey on Drug Use and Health* (NSDUH) obtains information on nine categories of illicit drugs: marijuana (including hashish), cocaine (including crack), heroin, hallucinogens, and inhalants, as well as the nonmedical use of prescription-type pain relievers, tranquilizers, stimulants, and sedatives; see the section on nonmedical use of psychotherapeutic drugs for the definition of nonmedical use. Estimates of "illicit drug use" reported from NSDUH reflect the use of these nine drug categories. Difference between the Illicit Drug Use estimate for 2002-2013 and the 2014 estimate is statistically significant at the .05 level for all years against 2014. Binge drinking for NSDUH data collected in 2014 is defined as five or more drinks on the same occasion on at least one day in the past 30 days. There was no significant difference between 2002-2013 against 2014. In 2015, changes were made to the NSDUH questionnaire and data collection procedures that do not allow comparisons between 2015 and previous years for a number of outcomes.

Source: Center for Behavioral Health Statistics and Quality, (2015).[13]

This *Surgeon General's Report* has been created because of the important health and social problems associated with alcohol and drug misuse in America. As described in this *Report,* a comprehensive approach is needed to address substance use problems in the United States that includes several key components:

- Enhanced public education to improve awareness about substance use problems and demand for more effective policies and practices to address them;
- Widespread implementation of evidence-based prevention policies and programs to prevent substance misuse and related harms;
- Improved access to evidence-based treatment services, integrated with mainstream health care, for those at risk for or affected by substance use disorders;
- Recovery support services (RSS) to assist individuals in maintaining remission and preventing relapse; and
- Research-informed public policies and financing strategies to ensure that substance misuse and use disorder services are accessible, compassionate, efficient, and sustainable.

Recognizing these needs, the *Report* explains the neurobiological basis for substance use disorders and provides the biological, psychological, and social frameworks for improving diagnosis, prevention, and treatment of alcohol and drug misuse. It also describes evidence-based prevention strategies, such as public policies that can reduce substance misuse problems (e.g., driving under the influence [DUI]); effective treatment strategies, including medications and behavioral therapies for treating substance use disorders; and RSS for people who have completed treatment. Additionally, the *Report* describes recent changes in health care financing, including changes in health insurance regulations, which support the integration of clinical prevention and treatment services for substance use disorders into mainstream health care practice, and defines a research agenda for addressing alcohol and drug misuse as medical conditions.

Thus, this first *Surgeon General's Report on Alcohol, Drugs, an‹ Health* is not issued simply because of the prevalence of substance misuse or even the related devastating harms and costs, but also to help inform policymakers, health care professionals, and the general public about effective, practical, and sustainable strategies to address these problems. These strategies have the potential to substantially reduce substance misuse and related problems; promote early intervention for substance misuse and substance use disorders; and improve the availability of high-quality treatment and RSS for persons with substance use disorders.

### KEY TERMS

**The Public Health System**. The Public Health System is defined as "all public, private, and voluntary entities that contribute to the delivery of essential public health services within a jurisdiction" and includes state and local public health agencies, public safety agencies, health care providers, human service and charity organizations, recreation and arts-related organizations, economic and philanthropic organizations, and education and youth development organizations.[2]

**The Health Care System**. The World Health Organization defines a health care system as (1) all the activities whose primary purpose is to promote, restore, and/or maintain health, and (2) the people, institutions, and resources, arranged together in accordance with established policies, to improve the health of the population they serve. The health care system is made up of diverse health care organizations ranging from primary care, specialty substance use disorder treatment (including residential and outpatient settings), mental health care, infectious disease clinics, school clinics, community health centers, hospitals, emergency departments, and others.[5]

## A Public Health Model for Addressing Substance Misuse and Related Consequences

A public health systems approach to substance misuse and its consequences, including substance use disorders, aims to:

- Define the problem through the systematic collection of data on the scope, characteristics, and consequences of substance misuse;
- Identify the risk and protective factors that increase or decrease the risk for substance misuse and its consequences, and the factors that could be modified through interventions;
- Work across the public and private sector to develop and test interventions that address social, environmental, or economic determinants of substance misuse and related health consequences;
- Support broad implementation of effective prevention and treatment interventions and recovery supports in a wide range of settings; and
- Monitor the impact of these interventions on substance misuse and related problems as well as on risk and protective factors.

A healthy community is one with not just a strong health care system but also a strong public health educational system, safe streets, effective public transportation and affordable, high quality food and housing – where all individuals have opportunities to thrive. Thus, community leaders should work together to mobilize the capacities of health care organizations, social service organizations, educational systems, community-based organizations, government health agencies, religious institutions, law enforcement, local businesses, researchers, and other public, private, and voluntary entities that can contribute to the above aims. Everyone has a role to play in addressing substance misuse and its consequences and thereby improving the public health.

# Substances Discussed in this Report

This *Report* defines a **substance** as a psychoactive compound with the potential to cause health and social problems, including substance use disorders (and their most severe manifestation, addiction). These substances can be divided into three major categories: Alcohol, Illicit Drugs (a category that includes prescription drugs used nonmedically), and Over-the-Counter Drugs. Some specific examples of the substances included in each of these categories are included in Table 1.1. Over-the-Counter Drugs are not discussed in this *Report*, but are included in Appendix D – Important Facts about Alcohol and Drugs.

Although different in many respects, the substances discussed in this *Report* share three features that make them important to public health and safety. *First, many people use an• misuse these substances:* 66.7 million individuals in the United States aged 12 or older admitted to binge drinking in the past month and 27.1 million people aged 12 or older used an illicit drug in the past month.[3]

### Table 1.1: Categories and Examples of Substances

| Substance Category | Representative Examples |
|---|---|
| Alcohol | • Beer<br>• Wine<br>• Malt liquor<br>• Distilled spirits |
| Illicit Drugs | • Cocaine, including crack<br>• Heroin<br>• Hallucinogens, including LSD, PCP, ecstasy, peyote, mescaline, psilocybin<br>• Methamphetamines, including crystal meth<br>• Marijuana, including hashish*<br>• Synthetic drugs, including K2, Spice, and "bath salts"**<br>• Prescription-type medications that are used for nonmedical purposes<br>  o Pain Relievers - Synthetic, semi-synthetic, and non-synthetic opioid medications, including fentanyl, codeine, oxycodone, hydrocodone, and tramadol products<br>  o Tranquilizers, including benzodiazepines, meprobamate products, and muscle relaxants<br>  o Stimulants and Methamphetamine, including amphetamine, dextroamphetamine, and phentermine products; mazindol products; and methylphenidate or dexmethylphenidate products<br>  o Sedatives, including temazepam, flurazepam, or triazolam and any barbiturates |
| Over-the-Counter Drugs and Other Substances | • Cough and cold medicines**<br>• Inhalants, including amyl nitrite, cleaning fluids, gasoline and lighter gases, anesthetics, solvents, spray paint, nitrous oxide |

Notes: The *Report* discusses the substances known to have a significant public health impact. These substances are also included in NSDUH. Additionally, NSDUH includes tobacco products (cigarettes, smokeless tobacco, cigars, and pipe tobacco); however, tobacco products are not discussed in this *Report* at length because they have been covered extensively in other Surgeon General's Reports.[14-17]

* As of June 2016, 25 states and the District of Columbia have legalized medical marijuana use, four states have legalized retail marijuana sales, and the District of Columbia has legalized personal use and home cultivation (both medical and recreational). It should be noted that none of the permitted uses under state laws alter the status of marijuana and its constituent compounds as illicit drugs under Schedule I of the federal Controlled Substances Act. See the section on Marijuana: A Changing Legal and Research Environment later in this chapter for more detail on this issue.

** These substances are not included in NSDUH and are not discussed in this *Report*. However, important facts about these drugs are included in Appendix D - Important Facts about Alcohol and Drugs.

*Secon•, in•ivi•uals can use these substances in a manner that causes harm to the user or those aroun• them.* This is called **substance misuse** and often results in health or social problems, referred to in this *Report* as **substance misuse problems.** Misuse can be of low severity and temporary, but it can also result in serious, enduring, and costly consequences due to motor vehicle crashes,[18,19] intimate partner and sexual violence,[20] child abuse and neglect,[21] suicide attempts and fatalities,[22] overdose deaths,[23] various forms of cancer[24] (e.g., breast cancer in women),[25] heart and liver diseases,[26] HIV/AIDS,[27] and problems related to drinking or using drugs during pregnancy, such as fetal alcohol spectrum disorders (FASDs) or neonatal abstinence syndrome (NAS).[28]

*Thir•, prolonge•, repeate• misuse of any of these substances can pro•uce changes to the brain that can lea• to a* ***substance use disorder****, an in•epen•ent illness that significantly impairs health an• function an• may require specialty treatment.* Disorders can range from mild to severe. Severe and chronic substance use disorders are commonly referred to as **addictions.**

**i FOR MORE ON THIS TOPIC**

See the section on *Diagnosing a Substance Use Disorder* later in this chapter.

## Key Terms Used in the Report

**Addiction:** The most severe form of substance use disorder, associated with compulsive or uncontrolled use of one or more substances. Addiction is a chronic brain disease that has the potential for both recurrence (relapse) and recovery.

**Substance:** A psychoactive compound with the potential to cause health and social problems, including substance use disorders (and their most severe manifestation, addiction). For a list of substance categories included in this *Report* see Table 1.1. Note: Cigarettes and other tobacco products are only briefly discussed here due to extensive coverage in prior Surgeon General's Reports.[14-17]

**Substance Use:** The use—even one time—of any of the substances in this *Report*.

**Substance Misuse:** The use of any substance in a manner, situation, amount, or frequency that can cause harm to users or to those around them. For some substances or individuals, any use would constitute misuse (e.g., underage drinking, injection drug use).

**Binge Drinking:** Binge drinking for men is drinking 5 or more standard alcoholic drinks, and for women, 4 or more standard alcoholic drinks on the same occasion on at least 1 day in the past 30 days.

**Heavy Drinking:** Defined by the CDC as consuming 8 or more drinks per week for women, and 15 or more drinks per week for men, and by the Substance Abuse and Mental Health Services Administration (SAMHSA), for research purposes, as binge drinking on 5 or more days in the past 30 days.

**Standard Drink:** Based on the *2015-2020 Dietary Guidelines for Americans*, a standard drink is defined as shown in the graphic below. All of these drinks contain 14 grams (0.6 ounces) of pure alcohol.

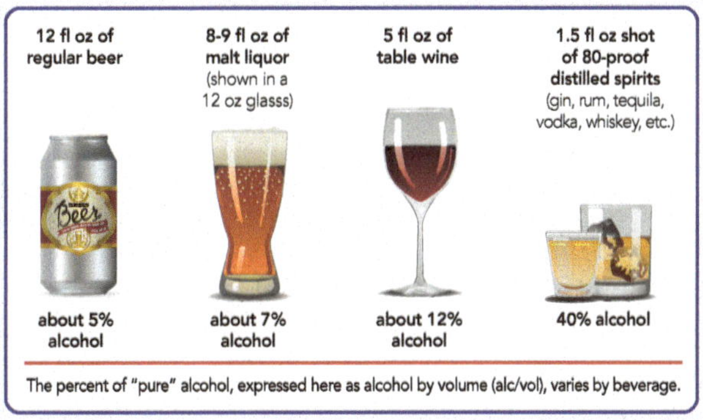


Source: U.S. Department of Health and Human Services and U.S. Department of Agriculture, (2015).[29]

**Substance Misuse Problems or Consequences:** Any health or social problem that results from substance misuse. Substance misuse problems or consequences may affect the substance user or those around them, and they may be acute (e.g., an argument or fight, a motor vehicle crash, an overdose) or chronic (e.g., a long-term substance-related medical, family, or employment problem, or chronic medical condition, such as various cancers, heart disease, and liver disease). These problems may occur at any age and are more likely to occur with greater frequency of substance misuse.

**Substance Use Disorder:** A medical illness caused by repeated misuse of a substance or substances. According to the Fifth Edition of the *Diagnostic and Statistical Manual of Mental Disorders* (DSM-5),[30] substance use disorders are characterized by clinically significant impairments in health, social function, and impaired control over substance use and are diagnosed through assessing cognitive, behavioral, and psychological symptoms. Substance use disorders range from mild to severe and from temporary to chronic. They typically develop gradually over time with repeated misuse, leading to changes in brain circuits governing incentive salience (the ability of substance-associated cues to trigger substance seeking), reward, stress, and executive functions like decision making and self-control. Multiple factors influence whether and how rapidly a person will develop a substance use disorder. These factors include the substance itself; the genetic vulnerability of the user; and the amount, frequency, and duration of the misuse. Note: A severe substance use disorder is commonly called an addiction.

**Relapse:** The return to drug use after a significant period of abstinence.

**Recovery:** A process of change through which individuals improve their health and wellness, live a self-directed life, and strive to reach their full potential. Even individuals with severe and chronic substance use disorders can, with help, overcome their substance use disorder and regain health and social function. This is called remission. When those positive changes and values become part of a voluntarily adopted lifestyle, that is called "being in recovery." Although abstinence from all substance misuse is a cardinal feature of a recovery lifestyle, it is not the only healthy, pro-social feature.

## Prevalence of Substance Use, Misuse Problems, and Disorders

How widespread are substance use, misuse, and substance use disorders in the United States? The annual *National Survey on Drug Use an• Health* (NSDUH) gathers data on the scope and prevalence of substance use, misuse, and related disorders, as well as utilization of substance use disorder treatment, among Americans aged 12 and older, representing more than 265 million people. Table 1.2 provides selected findings from the 2015 NSDUH. The table provides only general statistics for the United States as a whole; readers are urged to consult NSDUH's detailed tables[3] for subpopulation estimates.

Over 175 million persons aged 12 and older (65.7 percent of this population) reported alcohol use in the past year, with over 66 million (24.9 percent) reporting binge drinking in the past month (Table 1.2). More than 36 million (13.5 percent) reported using marijuana in the past year, 12.5 million reported misusing prescription pain relievers, and over 300,000 reported using heroin in the past year. Almost 8 percent of the population met diagnostic criteria for a substance use disorder for alcohol or illicit drugs, and another 1 percent met diagnostic criteria for both an alcohol and illicit drug use disorder. Although 20.8 million people (7.8 percent of the population) met the diagnostic criteria for a substance use disorder in 2015, only 2.2 million individuals (10.4 percent) received any type of treatment. Of those treated, 63.7 percent received treatment in specialty substance use disorder treatment programs.[3]

**KEY TERMS**

**Prevalence**. The proportion of a population who have (or had) a specific characteristic—for example, an illness, condition, behavior, or risk factor— in a given time period.

Several specific findings shown in Table 1.2 bear emphasis. Past year misuse of prescription psychotherapeutic drugs was reported by 18.9 million individuals in 2015 (7.1 percent of the population).[3] Within this category, prescribed opioid pain relievers (e.g., OxyContin®, Vicodin®, Lortab®) accounted for 12.5 million people, followed by tranquilizers, such as Xanax®, reported by 6.1 million people; stimulants, such as Adderall® or Ritalin®, reported by 5.3 million people; and sedatives, such as Valium®, reported by 1.5 million people.[3]

### Substance Use Disorder Treatment Programs

Historically, treatment services were designed for people with severe substance use disorders (addictions), and programs were generally referred to as "specialty addiction treatment programs." Today, individuals with mild to severe substance use disorders may receive treatment. These treatments are delivered by specialty programs, as well as by more generalist providers (e.g., primary care and general mental health providers). Not everyone with a substance use disorder will need ongoing treatment; many will require only a brief intervention and monitoring. Because treatments vary substantially in level of specialization, content, duration, and setting, and because those receiving services may differ substantially in the severity, duration, and complexity of their substance use disorder, this *Report* uses the phrase "substance use disorder treatment" as the generic term to capture the broad spectrum of advice, therapies, services, and monitoring provided to the group of individuals with mild to severe substance use disorders. The programs and services that provide specialty treatment are referred to as "substance use disorder treatment programs or services."

The prevalence of past 30-day use of "any illicit drugs" (a broad category including marijuana/hashish, cocaine/crack, heroin, hallucinogens, inhalants, and prescription psychotherapeutic medications used nonmedically) rose from 9.4 percent in 2013 to 10.2 percent in 2014 among persons aged 12 and older (Figure 1.2). This 2014 prevalence rate for illicit drugs is significantly higher than it was in any year from 2002 to 2013. However, no significant changes were observed that year specifically in the use of prescription psychotherapeutic drugs, cocaine, or hallucinogens, suggesting that the observed increase was primarily related to increased use of marijuana. Marijuana was the most frequently used illicit drug (35.1 million past year users).[31] The rate for past month marijuana use in 2014 was significantly higher than it was in any year from 2002 to 2013, with the prevalence of past 30-day marijuana use rising from 7.5 percent in 2013 to 8.4 percent in 2014.[13] (Note: In 2015, changes were made to the NSDUH questionnaire and data collection procedures that do not allow for the presentation of trend data beyond 2014. For more information, see *Summary of the Effects of the 2015 NSDUH Questionnaire Re•esign: Implications for Data Users.*[32])

## Demographics of Substance Use

Table 1.3 and Table 1.4 show substance use by demographic characteristics. Prevalence of substance misuse and substance use disorders differs by race and ethnicity and gender, and these factors can also influence access to health care and substance use disorder treatment. Past year alcohol use for men was 68.6 percent and for women it was 62.9 percent. Past month binge alcohol use was 29.6 percent for men and 20.5 percent for women. The prevalence of past month binge alcohol use was 24.1 percent for American Indians or Alaska Natives, 25.7 percent for Hispanics or Latinos, and 26.0 for Whites. Prevalence of an alcohol use disorder was 7.8 percent for men and 4.1 percent for women. The prevalence of an illicit drug use disorder was 3.8 percent for men and 2.0 percent for women.

Table 1.2: Past Year Substance Use, Past Year Initiation of Substance Use, and Met Diagnostic Criteria for a Substance Use Disorder in the Past Year Among Persons Aged 12 Years or Older for Specific Substances: Numbers in Millions and Percentages, 2015 National Survey on Drug Use and Health (NSDUH)

| Substance | Past Year Use or Misuse[v] | | Past Year Initiation Among Total Population[vi] | | Met Diagnostic Criteria for a Substance Use Disorder[vi,vii] | |
|---|---|---|---|---|---|---|
| | # | % | # | % | # | % |
| Alcohol | 175.8 | 65.7 | 4.8 | 1.8 | 15.7 | 5.9 |
| Drinking Pattern | | | | | | |
| Binge Drinking[i] | 66.7 | 24.9 | da | da | da | da |
| Heavy Drinking[i] | 17.3 | 6.5 | da | da | da | da |
| Any Illicit Drug[ii] | 47.7 | 17.8 | nr | nr | 7.7 | 2.9 |
| Cocaine/Crack | 36.0 | 1.8 | 1.0 | 0.4 | 0.9 | 0.3 |
| Heroin | 0.8 | 0.3 | 0.1 | 0.1 | 0.6 | 0.2 |
| Hallucinogens | 4.7 | 1.8 | 1.2 | 0.4 | 0.3 | 0.1 |
| Marijuana[iii] | 36.0 | 13.5 | 2.6 | 1.0 | 4.0 | 1.5 |
| Inhalants | 1.8 | 0.7 | 0.6 | 0.2 | 0.1 | 0.0 |
| Misuse of Psychotherapeutics[iv] | 18.9 | 7.1 | nr | nr | 2.7 | 1.0 |
| Pain Relievers | 12.5 | 4.7 | 2.1 | 0.8 | 2.0 | 0.8 |
| Tranquilizers | 6.1 | 2.3 | 1.4 | 0.5 | 0.7 | 0.3 |
| Stimulants | 5.3 | 2.0 | 1.3 | 0.5 | 0.4 | 0.2 |
| Sedatives | 1.5 | 0.6 | 0.4 | 0.2 | 0.2 | 0.1 |
| Alcohol or Any Illicit Drugs[ii] | 182.3 | 68.1 | nr | nr | 20.8 | 7.8 |
| Alcohol and Any Illicit Drugs[ii] | 41.3 | 15.4 | nr | nr | 2.7 | 1.0 |

Notes: Past year initiates are defined as persons who used the substance(s) for the first time in the 12 months before the date of interview. The "nr = not reported due to measurement issues" notation indicates that the estimate could be calculated based on available data but is not calculated due to potential measurement issues. The "da" indication means does not apply.

i. Binge and heavy drinking, as defined by SAMHSA, are reported only for the period of 30 days before the interview date. SAMHSA defines binge use of alcohol for males and females as "drinking five (males)/four (females) or more drinks on the same occasion (i.e., at the same time or within a couple of hours of each other) on at least 1 day in the past 30 days" and heavy use of alcohol for both males and females as "binge drinking on each of 5 or more days in the past 30 days."

ii. Illicit drug use includes the misuse of prescription psychotherapeutics or the use of marijuana, cocaine (including crack), heroin, hallucinogens, inhalants, or methamphetamine.

iii. As of June 2016, 25 states and the District of Columbia have legalized medical marijuana use. Four states have legalized retail marijuana sales; the District of Columbia has legalized personal use and home cultivation (both medical and recreational). It should be noted that none of the permitted uses under state laws alter the status of marijuana and its constituent compounds as illicit drugs under Schedule I of the federal Controlled Substances Act.

iv. Misuse of prescription-type psychotherapeutics includes the nonmedical use of pain relievers, tranquilizers, stimulants, or sedatives and does not include over-the-counter drugs.

v. Estimates of misuse of psychotherapeutics and stimulants include data from new methamphetamine items added in 2005 and 2006 and are not comparable with estimates presented in NSDUH reports before 2007. See Section B.4.8 in Appendix B of the Results from the 2008 NSDUH.

vi. Estimates of misuse of psychotherapeutics and stimulants do not include data from new methamphetamine items added in 2005 and 2006.

vii. Diagnostic criteria for a substance use disorder is based on definitions found in the Fourth Edition of the *Diagnostic and Statistical Manual of Mental Disorders* (DSM-IV).

Source: Center for Behavioral Health Statistics and Quality, (2016).[3]

Figure 1.2: Trends in Binge Drinking and Past 30-Day Use of Illicit Drugs among Persons Aged 12 Years or Older, 2014 National Survey on Drug Use and Health (NSDUH)

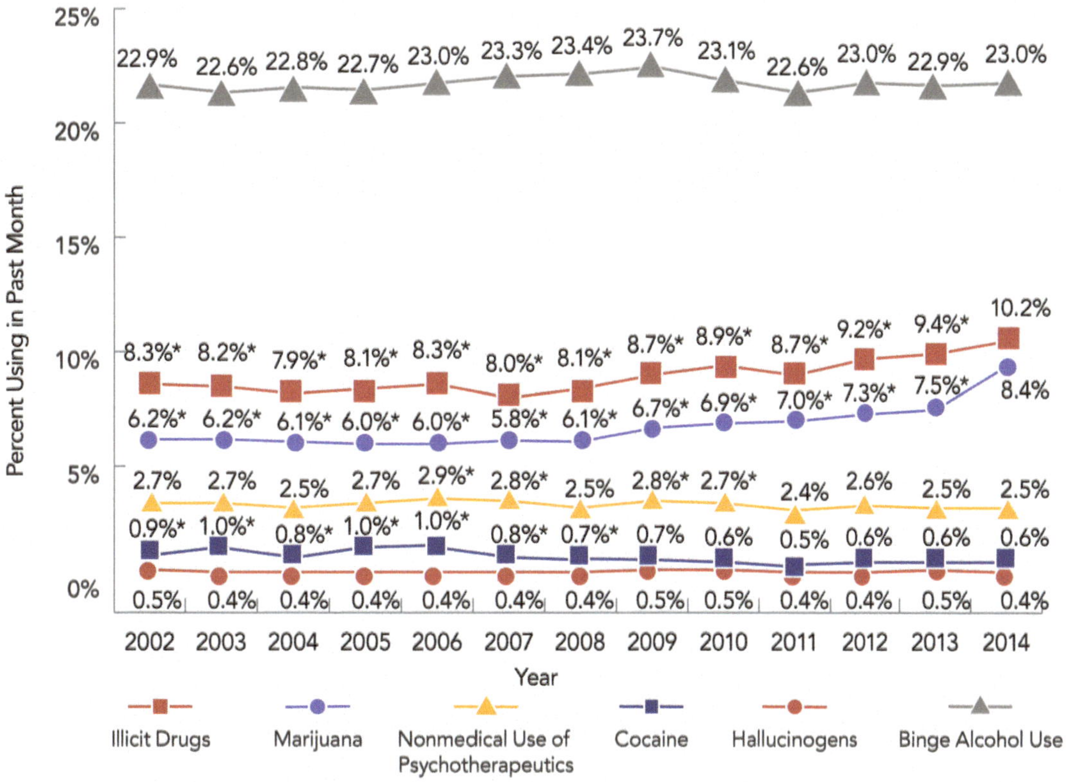


Notes: *Difference between this estimate and the 2014 estimate is statistically significant at the .05 level. Illicit drugs include marijuana/hashish, cocaine (including crack), heroin, hallucinogens, inhalants, or prescription psychotherapeutics used non-medically. Nonmedical use of prescription psychotherapeutics includes the nonmedical use of pain relievers, tranquilizers, stimulants, or sedatives. In 2015, changes were made to the NSDUH questionnaire and data collection procedures that do not allow comparisons between 2015 and previous years for a number of outcomes.

Source: Center for Behavioral Health Statistics and Quality, (2015).[13]

## Relevance of Substance Use and Misuse

It is sometimes thought that concern over substance use and misuse should be secondary to the *real* issue of substance use disorders and especially their severest manifestation, addiction, which has captured media headlines and has been linked to many health and social problems. This is an important misconception. Individuals with substance use disorders have elevated rates of substance misuse–related health and social problems and costs, but as shown in the last columns of Table 1.2, Table 1.3, and Table 1.4, many people who misuse substances do not meet the diagnostic criteria for a substance use disorder. For example, binge drinking at least once during the past month was self-reported by over 66 million individuals. By definition, those episodes have the potential for producing harm to the user and/or to those around them, through increases in motor vehicle crashes, violence, and alcohol-poisonings.[33] Similarly, in 2015, 12.5 million individuals misused a pain reliever in the past year—setting the stage for a potential overdose—but only 2.9 million met diagnostic criteria for a prescription medication disorder.[3]

Table 1.3: Past Year Alcohol Use, Past Month Binge Alcohol Use, and Met Diagnostic Criteria for a Substance Use Disorder in the Past Year Among Persons Aged 12 Years or Older: Numbers in Millions and Percentages, 2015 National Survey on Drug Use and Health (NSDUH)

| Demographic Group | Past Year Alcohol Use | | Past Month Binge Alcohol Use[ii] | | Met Diagnostic Criteria for a Substance Use Disorder in Past Year[i] | |
|---|---|---|---|---|---|---|
| | # | % | # | % | # | % |
| Alcohol | | | | | | |
| Male | 89.0 | 68.6 | 38.4 | 29.6 | 10.1 | 7.8 |
| Female | 86.9 | 62.9 | 28.3 | 20.5 | 5.6 | 4.1 |
| White | 119.9 | 70.3 | 44.4 | 26.0 | 10.4 | 6.1 |
| Black or African American | 18.6 | 58.0 | 7.5 | 23.4 | 1.6 | 4.9 |
| American Indian or Alaska Native | 0.7 | 51.4 | 0.3 | 24.1 | 0.1 | 9.7 |
| Native Hawaiian or Other Pacific Islander | 0.4 | 51.1 | 0.1 | 17.8 | 0.04 | 5.4 |
| Asian | 7.8 | 53.1 | 2.1 | 14.0 | 0.5 | 3.2 |
| Two or More Races | 2.7 | 57.8 | 1.1 | 22.9 | 0.3 | 6.2 |
| Hispanic or Latino | 25.7 | 59.0 | 11.2 | 25.7 | 2.8 | 6.4 |

Table 1.4: Past Year Substance Use, Past 30-Day Illicit Drug Use, and Met Diagnostic Criteria for a Substance Use Disorder in the Past Year Among Persons Aged 12 Years or Older: Numbers in Millions and Percentages, 2015 National Survey on Drug Use and Health (NSDUH)

| Demographic Group | Past Year Use | | Past 30-Day Illicit Drug Use | | Met Diagnostic Criteria for a Substance Use Disorder in Past Year[i] | |
|---|---|---|---|---|---|---|
| | # | % | # | % | # | % |
| Any Illicit Drug[iii] | | | | | | |
| Male | 26.6 | 20.5 | 16.2 | 12.5 | 5.0 | 3.8 |
| Female | 21.2 | 15.3 | 10.9 | 7.9 | 2.8 | 2.0 |
| White | 30.5 | 17.9 | 17.4 | 10.2 | 4.8 | 2.8 |
| Black or African American | 6.6 | 20.7 | 4.0 | 12.5 | 1.1 | 3.5 |
| American Indian or Alaska Native | 0.3 | 22.9 | 0.2 | 14.2 | 0.06 | 4.1 |
| Native Hawaiian or Other Pacific Islander | 0.1 | 20.5 | 0.07 | 9.8 | 0.03 | 4.5 |
| Asian | 1.4 | 9.2 | 0.6 | 4.0 | 0.2 | 1.2 |
| Two or More Races | 1.3 | 27.1 | 0.8 | 17.2 | 0.2 | 4.9 |
| Hispanic or Latino | 7.4 | 17.2 | 4.0 | 9.2 | 1.3 | 3.0 |

i. Diagnostic criteria for a substance use disorder is based on definitions found in the Fourth Edition of the *Diagnostic and Statistical Manual of Mental Disorders* (DSM-IV).

ii. Binge drinking, as defined by SAMHSA, are reported only for the period of 30 days before the interview date. SAMHSA defines binge use of alcohol for males and females as "drinking five (males)/four (females) or more drinks on the same occasion (i.e., at the same time or within a couple of hours of each other) on at least 1 day in the past 30 days.

iii. Illicit drugs include marijuana/hashish, cocaine (including crack), heroin, hallucinogens, inhalants, or misuse of prescription-type psychotherapeutics, including data from original methamphetamine questions but not including new methamphetamine items added in 2005 and 2006.

Source: Center for Behavioral Health Statistics and Quality, (2016).[3]

The clear implications of these data are that a comprehensive approach to reducing the misuse of alcohol and drugs—one that includes the implementation of effective prevention programs and policy strategies as well as high-quality treatment services—is needed to reduce the problems and costs of substance misuse in the United States. In fact, greater impact is likely to be achieved by reducing substance misuse in the general population—that is, among people who are *not* addicted—than among those with severe substance use problems. Of course, efforts to reduce general population rates of substance use and misuse are also likely to reduce rates of substance use disorders, because substance use disorders typically develop over time following repeated episodes of misuse (often at escalating rates) that result in the progressive changes to brain circuitry that underlie addiction.

i FOR MORE ON THIS TOPIC

See Chapter 2 - *The Neurobiology of Substance Use, Misuse, and Addiction.*

## Costs and Impact of Substance Use and Misuse

Alcohol misuse, illicit drug use, misuse of medications, and substance use disorders are estimated to cost the United States more than $400 billion in lost workplace productivity (in part, due to premature mortality), health care expenses, law enforcement and other criminal justice costs (e.g., drug-related crimes), and losses from motor vehicle crashes.[10,11] Furthermore, about three quarters of the costs associated with alcohol use were due to binge drinking, and about 40 percent of those costs were paid by government, emphasizing the huge cost of alcohol misuse to taxpayers.[34]

These costs are not unique to the United States. A 2010 study examined the global burden of disability attributable to substance misuse problems and disorders, focusing particularly on lost ability to work and years of life lost to premature mortality. Costs were calculated for 20 age groups and both sexes in 187 countries.[35] Mental and substance use disorders were the leading causes of years lived with disability worldwide, largely because these problems strike individuals early in their lives and can continue—especially if untreated—for long periods.

In addition to the costs to society, substance misuse can have many direct and indirect health and personal consequences for individuals. The direct effects on the user depend on the specific substances used, how much and how often they are used, how they are taken (e.g., orally vs. injected), and other factors. Acute effects can range from changes in mood and basic body functions, such as heart rate or blood pressure, to overdose and death. Alcohol misuse and drug use can also have long-term effects on physical and mental health and can lead to substance use disorders. For example, drug use is associated with chronic pain conditions and cardiovascular and cardiopulmonary diseases.[36,37] Alcohol misuse is associated with liver and pancreatic diseases, hypertension, reproductive system disorders, trauma, stroke, FASD, and cancers of the oral cavity, esophagus, larynx, pharynx, liver, colon, and rectum.[26,28] For breast cancer, studies have shown that even moderate drinking may increase the risk.[25]Although alcohol consumption is associated with adverse health effects as noted above, the *2015-2020 Dietary Gui•elines for*

*Americans* indicate that moderate alcohol use can be part of a healthy diet, but only when used by adults of legal drinking age.[i]

In addition, alcohol and drug use by pregnant women can have profound effects on the developing fetus. Alcohol use during pregnancy can lead to a wide range of disabilities in children, the most severe of which is FASD, characterized by intellectual disabilities, speech and language delays, poor social skills, and sometimes facial deformities. Use of drugs, such as opioids during pregnancy, can result in NAS, a drug-withdrawal syndrome requiring medical intervention and extended hospital stay for newborns. Use of some drugs, such as cocaine, during pregnancy may also lead to premature birth or miscarriage. In addition, substance use during pregnancy may interfere with a child's brain development and result in later consequences for mental functioning and behavior.

Substance misuse also can affect a user's nutrition and sleep, as well as increase the risk for trauma, violence, injury, and contraction of communicable diseases, such as HIV/AIDS and Hepatitis C. These consequences can all contribute to the spectrum of public health consequences of substance misuse and need to be considered both independently and collectively when developing and implementing clinical and public health interventions.

Substance misuse problems can also result in other serious and sometimes fatal health problems and extraordinary costs; they may also lead to unexpected death from other causes. Three examples of these serious, sometimes lethal, problems related to substance misuse are highlighted below.

## Driving Under the Influence

In 2014, 9,967 people were killed in motor vehicle crashes while driving under the influence of alcohol, representing nearly one third (31 percent) of all traffic-related fatalities in the United States.[38] DUI continues to be among the most frequent causes for arrests every year.[39] But at approximately 1.3 million per year, these arrests represent only about 1 percent of the actual alcohol-impaired driving incidents reported in national surveys, suggesting that there are many more people who drive while impaired that have not been arrested, putting themselves and others at high risk of being harmed.[18,40] In addition to the deaths that result from DUI, the National Highway Traffic Safety Administration (NHTSA) estimates that DUI costs the United States more than $44 billion each year in prosecution, higher insurance rates, higher taxes, medical claims, and property damage.[41]

As important as they are, these statistics account for only alcohol-related driving impairment and fail to measure other impairing substances. A study by NHTSA tested oral fluid and blood specimens from a random sample of drivers at the roadside (during daytime on Friday or nighttime Friday to Sunday) and

i Moderate alcohol use is defined by the *2015-2020 Dietary Guidelines for Americans* as up to 1 drink per day for women and up to 2 drinks per day for men—and only by adults of legal drinking age. Many individuals should not consume alcohol, including individuals who are taking certain over-the-counter or prescription medications or who have certain medical conditions, those who are recovering from an alcohol use disorder or are unable to control the amount they drink, and anyone younger than age 21 years. In addition, drinking during pregnancy may result in negative behavioral or neurological consequences in the offspring.

found 12 to 15 percent had used one or more illegal substances.[42] Drivers tested positive for drugs in approximately 16 percent of all motor vehicle crashes.[43]

## Overdose Deaths

Overdose deaths are typically caused by consuming substances at high intensity and/or by consuming combinations of substances such as alcohol, sedatives, tranquilizers, and opioid pain relievers to the point where critical areas in the brain that control breathing, heart rate, and body temperature stop functioning.

### *Alcohol Overdose (Alcohol Poisoning)*

The CDC reports more than 2,200 alcohol overdose deaths in the United States each year—an average of six deaths every day.[44] More than three quarters (76 percent) of alcohol overdose deaths occur among adults between ages 35 and 64, and 76 percent of those who die from alcohol overdose are men.

### *Drug Overdose (Illicit and Prescription Drugs)*

Opioid analgesic pain relievers are now the most prescribed class of medications in the United States, with more than 289 million prescriptions written each year.[45,46] The increase in prescriptions of opioid pain relievers has been accompanied by dramatic increases in misuse (Table 1.1) and by a more than 200 percent increase in the number of emergency department visits from 2005 to 2011.[47] In 2014, 47,055 drug overdose deaths occurred in the United States, and 61 percent of these deaths were the result of opioid use, including prescription opioids and heroin.[7] Heroin overdoses have more than tripled from 2010 to 2014.[7] Heroin overdoses were more than five times higher in 2014 (10,574) then ten years before in 2004 (1,878). Additionally, rates of cocaine overdose were higher in 2014 than in the previous six years (5,415 deaths from cocaine overdose). In 2014, there were 17,465 overdoses from illicit drugs and 25,760 overdoses from prescription drugs.[48] Drug overdose deaths also occur as a result of the illicit manufacturing and distribution of synthetic opioids, such as fentanyl, and the illegal diversion of prescription opioids. Illicit fentanyl, for example, is often combined with heroin or counterfeit prescription drugs or sold as heroin, and may be contributing to recent increases in drug overdose deaths.[7,49]

**KEY CONCEPT**

**The Opioid Crisis.** Over-prescription of powerful opioid pain relievers beginning in the 1990s led to a rapid escalation of use and misuse of these substances by a broad demographic of men and women across the country.[1] This led to a resurgence of heroin use, as some users transitioned to using this cheaper street cousin of expensive prescription opioids. As a result, the number of people dying from opioid overdoses soared—increasing nearly four-fold between 1999 and 2014.[4]

## Intimate Partner Violence, Sexual Assault, and Rape

Intimate partner violence, sexual assault, and rape are crimes with long-lasting effects on victims and great cost to society.[50,51] These crimes happen to both women and men and are often associated with substance use. A recent national survey found that 22 percent of women and 14 percent of men reported experiencing severe physical violence from an intimate partner in their lifetimes.[52] In this survey, 19.3 percent of women and 1.7 percent of men reported being raped in their lifetimes, while 43.9 percent of women and 23.4 percent of men reported some other form of sexual violence in their lifetimes.[52] Substance misuse is often related to these crimes.

Numerous studies have found a high correlation between substance use and intimate partner violence,[53-56] although this does not mean that substance use causes intimate partner violence. In addition to evidence from the criminal justice arena, recent systematic reviews have found that substance use is both a risk factor for and a consequence of intimate partner violence.[57-59]

A recent survey of sexual assault and sexual misconduct on college campuses found that use of alcohol and drugs are important risk factors for nonconsensual sexual contact among undergraduate, graduate, and professional students.[20] It is clear that substance use and intimate partner violence and sexual assault are closely linked; however, more research is needed on the nature of the relationship between substance use and these forms of violence to determine how substance use contributes to the perpetration of violence and victimization and how violence contributes to subsequent substance use among both perpetrators and victims.

# Vulnerability to Substance Misuse Problems and Disorders

## Risk and Protective Factors: Keys to Vulnerability

Substance misuse problems and substance use disorders are not inevitable. An individual's vulnerability may be partly predicted by assessing the nature and number of their community, caregiver/family, and individual-level risk and protective factors.

> **i FOR MORE ON THIS TOPIC**
>
> See Chapter 3 - *Prevention Programs and Policies.*

Significant community-level risk factors for substance misuse and use disorders include easy access to inexpensive alcohol and other substances. Caregiver/family-level risk factors include low parental monitoring, a family history of substance use or mental disorders, and high levels of family conflict or violence. At the individual level, major risk factors include current mental disorders, low involvement in school, a history of abuse and neglect, and a history of substance use during adolescence, among others.[60]

Community-level protective factors include higher cost for alcohol and other drugs (often achieved by increasing taxes on these products); regulating the number and concentration of retailers selling various substances (e.g., density of alcohol outlets or marijuana dispensaries); preventing illegal alcohol and other drug sales by enforcing existing laws and holding retailers accountable for harms caused by illegal sales (e.g., commercial host [dram shop] liability); availability of healthy recreational and social activities; and other population-level policies and their enforcement.[61] Caregiver/family-level protective factors include support and regular monitoring by parents.[60] Some important individual-level protective factors include involvement in school, engagement in healthy recreational and social activities, and good coping skills.[60]

Three important points about vulnerability should be highlighted. First, no single individual or community-level factor determines whether an individual will develop a substance misuse problem or disorder. Second, most risk and protective factors can be modified through preventive programs and policies to reduce vulnerability. Third, although substance misuse problems and disorders may occur at any age, adolescence and young adulthood are particularly critical at-risk periods. Research now indicates that the majority of those who meet criteria for a substance use disorder in their lifetime started using substances during adolescence and met the criteria by age 20 to 25.[62-64] One likely reason for this vulnerability in adolescence and young adulthood is that alcohol and other substances have particularly potent effects on developing brain circuits, and recent scientific findings indicate that brain development is not complete until approximately age 21 to 23 in women and 23 to 25 in men.[65-67] Among the last brain regions to reach maturity is the prefrontal cortex, the brain region primarily responsible for "adult" abilities, such as delay of reward, extended reasoning, and impulse control. This area of the brain is one of the most affected regions in a substance use disorder.

> **i FOR MORE ON THIS TOPIC**
>
> See Chapter 2 - *The Neurobiology of Substance Use, Misuse, and Addiction.*

Substance misuse can begin at any age. Therefore, it is important to focus on prevention of substance misuse across the lifespan as well as the prevention of substance use disorders.

# Diagnosing a Substance Use Disorder

## Changes in Understanding and Diagnosis of Substance Use Disorders

Repeated, regular misuse of any of the substances listed in Figure 1.2 may lead to the development of a substance use disorder. Severe substance use disorders are characterized by compulsive use of substance(s) and impaired control of substance use. Substance use disorder diagnoses are based on criteria specified in the American Psychiatric Association's *Diagnostic and Statistical Manual of Mental Disorders* (DSM). Much of the substance use disorder data included in this *Report* is based on definitions included in the DSM-IV, which described two distinct disorders: substance abuse and substance dependence, with specific diagnostic criteria for each. Anyone meeting one or more of the abuse criteria—which focused largely on the negative consequences associated with substance misuse, such as being unable to fulfill family or work obligations, experiencing legal trouble, or engaging in hazardous behavior as a result of drug use—would receive the "abuse" diagnosis. Anyone with three or more of the dependence criteria, which included symptoms of drug tolerance, withdrawal, escalating and uncontrolled substance use, and the use of the substance to the exclusion of other activities, would receive the "dependence" diagnosis. Notably, addiction is not listed as a formal diagnosis in the DSM. However, substance

> **KEY CONCEPT**
>
> **Misuse versus Abuse**. This *Report* uses the term substance misuse, a term that is roughly equivalent to substance *abuse*. Substance abuse, an older diagnostic term, was defined as use that is unsafe (e.g., drunk or drugged driving), use that leads a person to fail to fulfill responsibilities or gets them in legal trouble, or use that continues despite causing persistent interpersonal problems like fights with a spouse.
>
> However, "substance abuse" is increasingly avoided by professionals because it can be shaming. Instead, substance misuse is now the preferred term. Although misuse is not a diagnostic term, it generally suggests use in a manner that could cause harm to the user or those around them.

dependence was often used interchangeably with addiction, and tolerance and withdrawal were considered, by many, cardinal features of addiction.

The DSM-5, which is the fifth and current version of the DSM, integrates the two DSM-IV disorders, substance abuse and substance dependence, into a single disorder called *substance use disorder* with *mild*, *moderate*, and *severe* sub-classifications. Individuals are evaluated for a substance use disorder based on 10 or 11 (depending on the substance) equally weighted diagnostic criteria (Table 1.5). Most of these overlap with those used to diagnose DSM-IV dependence and abuse. Individuals exhibiting fewer than two of the symptoms are not considered to have a substance use disorder. Those exhibiting two or three symptoms are considered to have a "mild" disorder, four or five symptoms constitutes a "moderate" disorder, and six or more symptoms is considered a "severe" substance use disorder.[30] In this *Report*, addiction is used to refer to substance use disorders at the severe end of the spectrum and are characterized by compulsive substance use and impaired control over use.

**KEY TERMS**

**Tolerance**. Alteration of the body's responsiveness to alcohol or a drug such that higher doses are required to produce the same effect achieved during initial use.

**Withdrawal**. A set of symptoms that are experienced when discontinuing use of a substance to which a person has become dependent or addicted, which can include negative emotions such as stress, anxiety, or depression, as well as physical effects such as nausea, vomiting, muscle aches, and cramping, among others. Withdrawal symptoms often lead a person to use the substance again.

### Table 1.5: Criteria for Diagnosing Substance Use Disorders

| Diagnostic Criteria for Substance Use Disorders |
|---|
| Using in larger amounts or for longer than intended |
| Wanting to cut down or stop using, but not managing to |
| Spending a lot of time to get, use, or recover from use |
| Craving |
| Inability to manage commitments due to use |
| Continuing to use, even when it causes problems in relationships |
| Giving up important activities because of use |
| Continuing to use, even when it puts you in danger |
| Continuing to use, even when physical or psychological problems may be made worse by use |
| Increasing tolerance |
| Withdrawal symptoms |

Notes: Fewer than 2 symptoms = no disorder; 2-3 = mild disorder; 4-5 = moderate disorder; 6 or more = severe disorder.

Source: American Psychiatric Association, (2013).[30]

## Implications of the New Diagnostic Criteria

The new diagnostic criteria are likely to reduce the "all or nothing" thinking that has characterized the substance use field. Tolerance and withdrawal remain major clinical symptoms, but they are no longer the deciding factor in whether an individual "has an addiction." Substance use disorders, including addiction, can occur with *all* substances listed in Table 1.1, *not* just those that are able to produce

## What is an Intervention?

Intervention here and throughout this *Report* means a professionally delivered program, service, or policy designed to prevent substance misuse or treat an individual's substance use disorder. It does not refer to an arranged meeting or confrontation intended to persuade a friend or loved one to quit their substance misuse or enter treatment—the type of "intervention" sometimes depicted on television. Planned surprise confrontations of the latter variety—a model developed in the 1960s, sometimes called the "Johnson Intervention"—have not been demonstrated to be an effective way to engage people in treatment.[68] Confrontational approaches in general, though once the norm even in many behavioral treatment settings, have not been found effective and may backfire by heightening resistance and diminishing self-esteem on the part of the targeted individual.[69]

tolerance and withdrawal. It is also important to understand that substance use disorders do not occur immediately but over time, with repeated misuse and development of more symptoms. This means that it is both possible and highly advisable to identify emerging substance use disorders, and to use evidence-based early interventions to stop the addiction process before the disorder becomes more chronic, complex, and difficult to treat.

This type of proactive clinical monitoring and management is already done within general health care settings to address other potentially progressive illnesses that are brought about by unhealthy behaviors.[70] For example, patients with high blood pressure may be told to adjust their activity and stress in order to reduce the progression of hypertension. Typically, these individuals are also clinically monitored for key symptoms to ensure that symptoms do not worsen.

**i FOR MORE ON THIS TOPIC**

See Chapter 6 - *Health Care Systems and Substance Use Disorders.*

There are compelling reasons to apply similar procedures in emerging cases of substance misuse. Routine screening for alcohol and other substance use should be conducted in primary care settings to identify early symptoms of a substance use disorder (especially among those with known risk and few protective factors). This should be followed by informed clinical guidance on reducing the frequency and amount of substance use, family education to support lifestyle changes, and regular monitoring.

Research has shown that substance use disorders are similar in course, management, and outcome to other chronic illnesses, such as hypertension, diabetes, and asthma.[71] Unfortunately, substance use disorders have not been treated, monitored, or managed like other chronic illnesses, nor has care for these conditions been covered by insurance to the same degree. Nonetheless, it is possible to adopt the same type of chronic care management approach to the treatment of substance use disorders as is now used to manage most other chronic illnesses.[70-72] Evidence-based behavioral interventions, medications, social support services, clinical monitoring, and RSS make this type of chronic care management possible, often by the same health care teams that currently treat other chronic illnesses.

**i FOR MORE ON THIS TOPIC**

See Chapter 4 - *Early Intervention, Treatment, and Management of Substance Use Disorders* and Chapter 6 - *Health Care Systems and Substance Use Disorders.*

Evidence also shows that such an approach will improve the effectiveness of treatments for substance use disorders. Remission of substance use and even full recovery can now be achieved if evidence-based care is provided for adequate periods of time, by properly trained health care professionals, and augmented by supportive monitoring, RSS, and social services. This fact is supported by a national survey showing that there are more than 25 million individuals who once had a problem with alcohol or drugs who no longer do.[73]

## The Separation of Substance Use Treatment and General Health Care

Until quite recently, substance misuse problems and substance use disorders were viewed as social problems, best managed at the individual and family levels, and sometimes through the existing social infrastructure—such as schools and places of worship, and, when necessary, through civil and criminal justice interventions.[74] In the 1970s, when rates of substance misuse increased, including by college students and Vietnam War veterans, most families and traditional social services were not prepared to handle this problem.[75] Despite a compelling national need for treatment, the existing health care system was neither trained to care for nor especially eager to accept patients with substance use disorders.

For these reasons, a new system of substance use disorder treatment programs was created, but with administration, regulation, and financing placed outside mainstream health care.[74,75] This meant that with the exception of detoxification in hospital-based settings, virtually all treatment was delivered by programs that were geographically, financially, culturally, and organizationally separate from mainstream health care. Of equal historical importance was the decision to focus treatment only on addiction. This left few provisions for detecting or intervening clinically with the far more prevalent cases of early-onset, mild, or moderate substance use disorders.

Creating this system of substance use disorder treatment programs was a critical element in addressing the burgeoning substance use disorder problems in our nation. However, that separation also created unintended and enduring impediments to the quality and range of care options. For example, separate systems for substance use disorder treatment and other health care needs may have exacerbated the negative public attitudes toward people with substance use disorders. Additionally, the pharmaceutical industry was hesitant to invest in the development of new medications for individuals with substance use disorders, because they were not convinced that a market for these medications existed. Consequently, until the 1990s, few U.S. Food and Drug Administration (FDA) approved medications were available to treat addictions.[76,77]

Meanwhile, despite numerous research studies documenting high prevalence rates of substance use disorders among patients in emergency departments, hospitals, and general medical care settings, mainstream health care generally failed to recognize or address substance use disorders.[78] In fact, a recent study by the CDC found that in 2011, only 1 in 6 United States adults and 1 in 4 binge drinkers had *ever* been asked by a health professional about their drinking behavior.[79] Furthermore, the percent of adult binge drinkers who had been asked about their drinking had not changed since 1997, reflecting the challenges involved in fostering implementation of screening and counseling services for alcohol misuse in clinical settings. This has been a costly mistake, with often deadly consequences. A recent study showed that the presence of a substance use disorder often doubles the odds for the subsequent development of chronic and expensive medical illnesses, such as arthritis, chronic pain, heart disease, stroke, hypertension, diabetes, and asthma.[80]

In this regard, fatal medication errors due to unforeseen interactions between a prescribed medication for a diagnosed medical condition and unscreened, unaddressed patient substance use increased ten-fold over the past 20 years.[81] To address this problem, researchers suggested "...(1) screening patients for use...of alcohol and/or street drugs; (2) taking extra precautions when prescribing medicines with known dangerous interactions with alcohol and/or street drugs; and (3) teaching the patient the risks of mixing medicines with alcohol and/or street drugs."[81] Similar recommendations focusing on prescribed opioids have been issued by the CDC to curb the rise in opioid overdose deaths.[82] Again, screening for substance use and substance use disorders before and during the course of opioid prescribing, combined with patient education, are recommended.[82]

Yet despite these and other indications of extreme threats to health care quality, safety, effectiveness, and cost containment, as of this writing, few general health care organizations screen for, or offer services for, the early identification and treatment of substance use disorders. Moreover, few medical, nursing, dental, or pharmacy schools teach their students about substance use disorders;[83-86] and, until recently, few insurers offered adequate reimbursement for treatment of substance use disorders.[87,88]

## Recent Changes in Health Care Policy and Law

> **i FOR MORE ON THIS TOPIC**
>
> See Chapter 6 - *Health Care Systems and Substance Use Disorders.*

The longstanding separation of substance use disorders from the rest of health care began to change with enactment of the Paul Wellstone and Pete Domenici Mental Health Parity and Addiction Equity Act of 2008 (MHPAEA) and the Affordable Care Act in 2010.[89,90] MHPAEA requires that the financial requirements and treatment limitations imposed by health plans and insurers for substance use disorders be no more restrictive than the financial requirements and treatment limitations they impose for medical and surgical conditions. The Affordable Care Act requires the majority of United States health plans and insurers to offer prevention, screening, brief interventions, and other forms of treatment for substance use disorders.[89]

It is difficult to overstate the importance of these two Acts for creating a public health-oriented approach to reducing substance misuse and related disorders. These laws and related changes in health care financing are creating incentives for health care organizations to integrate substance use disorder treatment with general health care. Many questions remain, but those questions are no longer *whether* but *how* this much-needed integration will occur. These changes combine to create a new, challenging but exceptionally promising era for the prevention and treatment of substance use disorders and set the context for this *Report.*

# Marijuana: A Changing Legal and Research Environment

Although this *Report* does not examine the issue of marijuana legalization, its continually evolving legal status is worth mentioning because of implications for both research and policy. As mentioned elsewhere, marijuana is the most commonly used illicit drug in the United States, with 22.2 million people aged 12 or older using it in the past month.[3] In recent years marijuana use has become more socially acceptable among both adults and youth, while perceptions of risk among adolescents of the drug's harms have been declining over the past 13 years.[91]

As use of marijuana and its constituent components and derivatives becomes more widely accepted, it is critical to strengthen understanding of the effects and consequences for individual users and for public health and safety. Conducting such research can be complex as laws and policies vary significantly from state to state. For example, some states use a decriminalization model, which means production and sale of marijuana are still illegal and no legal marijuana farms, distributors, companies, stores, or advertising are permitted. Through ballot initiatives, other states have "legalized" marijuana use, which means they allow the production and sales of marijuana for personal use. Additionally, some states have legalized marijuana for medical purposes, and this group includes a wide variety of different models dictating how therapeutic marijuana is dispensed. The impacts of state laws regarding therapeutic and recreational marijuana are still being evaluated, although the differences make comparisons between states challenging.[92]

As of June 2016, 25 states and the District of Columbia have legalized medical marijuana use. Four states have legalized retail sales; the District of Columbia has legalized personal use and home cultivation (both medical and recreational), with more states expecting to do so. None of the permitted uses under state laws alters the status of marijuana and its constituent compounds as illicit drugs under Schedule I of the federal Controlled Substances Act.[93] It should also be noted that use for recreational purposes has not been legalized by any jurisdiction for people under age 21, and few jurisdictions have legalized medical marijuana for young people. While laws are changing, so too is the drug itself with average potency more than doubling over the past decade (1998 to 2008).[94] The ways marijuana is used are also changing – in addition to smoking, consuming edible forms like baked goods and candies, using vaporizing devices, and using high-potency extracts and oils (e.g., "dabbing") are becoming increasingly common.[95] Because these products and methods are unregulated even in states that have legalized marijuana use, users may not have accurate information about dosage or potency, which can lead and has led to serious consequences such as hospitalizations for psychosis and other overdose-related symptoms.[95] Marijuana use can also impair driving skills and, while estimates vary, is linked to a roughly two-fold increase in accident risk.[96-98] The risk is compounded when marijuana is used with alcohol.[96,99]

There is a growing body of research suggesting the potential therapeutic value of marijuana's constituent cannabinoid chemicals in numerous health conditions including pain, nausea, epilepsy, obesity, wasting disease, addiction, autoimmune disorders, and other conditions. Given the possibilities around therapeutic use, it is necessary to continue to explore ways of easing existing barriers to research. Marijuana has more than 100 constituent cannabinoid compounds, with cannabidiol (CBD) and tetrahydrocannabinol (THC, the chemical responsible for most of marijuana's intoxicating effects) being the most well-studied. Evidence collected so far in clinical investigations of the marijuana plant is still insufficient to meet

FDA standards for a finding of safety and efficacy for any therapeutic indications. However, the FDA has approved three medications containing synthetically derived cannabinoids: Marinol capsules and Syndros oral solution (both containing dronabinol, which is identical in chemical structure to THC), and Cesamet capsules (containing nabilone, which is similar in structure to THC) for severe nausea and wasting in certain circumstances, for instance in AIDS patients. Recognizing the potential therapeutic importance of compounds found in marijuana, the FDA has granted Fast Track designation to four development programs of products that contain marijuana constituents or their synthetic equivalents. The therapeutic areas in which products are being developed granted Fast Track by FDA include the treatment of pain in patients with advanced cancer; treatment of Dravet syndrome (two programs), a rare and catastrophic treatment-resistant form of childhood epilepsy; and treatment of neonatal hypoxic ischemic encephalopathy, brain injury resulting from oxygen deprivation during birth.

Additionally, there are clinical investigations for the treatment of refractory seizure syndromes, including Lennox Gastaut Syndrome, and for treatment of post-traumatic stress disorder (PTSD). However, further exploration of these issues always requires consideration of the serious health and safety risks associated with marijuana use. Research shows that risks can include respiratory illnesses, dependence, mental health-related problems, and other issues affecting public health such as impaired driving. Within this context of changing marijuana policies at the state level, research is needed on the impact of different models of legalization and how to minimize harm based on what has been learned from legal substances subject to misuse, such as alcohol and tobacco. Continued assessment of barriers to research and surveillance will help build the best scientific foundation to support good public policy while also protecting the public health.

# Purpose, Focus, and Format of the *Report*

## The Audience

This *Report* is intended for individuals, families, community members, educators, health care professionals, public health practitioners, advocates, public policymakers, and researchers who are looking for effective, sustainable solutions to the problems created by alcohol and other substances. To meet those needs, the *Report* reviews and synthesizes the most important and reliable scientific findings in key topic areas and distills those findings into recommendations for:

- Improving public awareness of substance misuse and related problems;
- Reducing negative attitudes related to substance use disorders;
- Closing the gap between what is known to reduce substance misuse at the population level and within specific subgroups, and the implementation of these effective programs, policies, and environmental strategies at the federal, state, and community levels;
- Understanding the need for and effectiveness of programs for high-risk populations;
- Expanding the capacity of health care systems to deliver evidence-based substance use disorder treatment;
- Integrating financing and health care system models to facilitate access and affordability of care for substance use disorders;

- Continuing to build the science base of effective prevention, treatment, and recovery practices and policies; and
- Engaging stakeholders in reducing substance use and misuse problems and protecting the health of all individuals across the lifespan.

Because of the broad audience, the *Report* is purposely written in accessible language without excessive scientific jargon. The *Report* also focuses on current issues and practical questions that trouble so many people:

- What are the health and social impacts of alcohol and drug use and misuse in the United States? What key factors influence these behaviors?
- What are the major substance misuse problems facing the United States?
- What causes substance use disorders and why do they change people so dramatically?
- Can substance misuse problems and disorders be prevented? How?
- What constitutes effective treatment?
- Can addicted individuals recover? What will it take to manage their disorders and sustain recovery?

## Topics Covered in the *Report*

Individual chapters in the *Report* review the science associated with the major substance use, misuse, and disorder issues for specific topics. Tobacco, also an addictive substance, is mentioned only briefly, because problems associated with tobacco use and nicotine addiction have been covered extensively in other Surgeon General's Reports.[14-16,100-103]

Because of the broad audience and the practical emphasis, the *Report* is intentionally selective rather than exhaustive, emphasizing findings that have the potential for the greatest public health impact and the greatest potential for action. For readers wanting greater scientific detail or more specific information, detailed research reports, as well as supplemental resource materials, are supplied in references, in the Appendices, and in special emphasis boxes throughout the *Report.*

## Scientific Standards Used to Develop the *Report*

Findings cited in all of the chapters came from electronic database searches of research articles published in English. Within those searches, priority was given to systematic literature reviews and to findings that were replicated by multiple controlled trials. However, many important issues in prevention, treatment, recovery, and health care systems have not yet been examined in rigorous controlled trials, or are not appropriate for such research designs. In these cases, the best available evidence was cited and labeled according to the reporting conventions published by the CDC:[104]

- *Well-supported*: Evidence derived from multiple controlled trials or large-scale population studies.
- *Supported*: Evidence derived from rigorous but fewer or smaller trials or restricted samples.
- *Promising*: Findings that do not derive from rigorously controlled studies but that nonetheless make practical or clinical sense and are widely practiced.

In cases in which evidence was based on findings of neurobiological research, the CDC standards were adapted.

A summary of the key findings appears at the beginning of each chapter. The key findings highlight what is currently known from available research about the chapter topic, as well as the strength of the evidence. As with the rest of the *Report,* the key findings are not intended to be exhaustive, but are instead considered the important "take-aways" from each chapter. Readers interested in a fuller discussion of the topics are encouraged to read the chapters in their entirety.

## Addressing Substance Use in Specific Populations

As indicated, the chapters are designed to prioritize best available research findings that apply most broadly across different substances and across various subgroups, while also identifying program and policy interventions that have strong evidence for particular substances (e.g., alcohol), when available. The rationale for this decision is that the available research suggests that the genetic, neurobiological, and environmental processes underlying substance use, misuse, and disorders are largely similar across most known substances and unrelated to the age, sex, race and ethnicity, gender identity, or culture of the individual. The available research also clearly indicates that many of the interventions, including population-level policies, focused programs, behavioral therapies, medications, and social services shown to be effective in one subgroup are *generally* effective for other subgroups. Put differently, it is reasonable to assume that the findings presented in this *Report* are relevant for many substance use types and patterns; for most age, gender, racial and ethnic, and cultural subgroups; and for many special needs subgroups (e.g., those with co-occurring mental or physical illnesses; those involved with the criminal justice system).

However, this general statement has some important caveats. First, the statement depends heavily on the phrase "available research." There is insufficient research examining subgroup differences in the neurobiology of substance use disorders and in interventions aimed at preventing, treating, and promoting recovery from substance use disorders. Additional research designed to examine these differences and to test interventions in specific populations is needed.

A second caveat is that individual variability in response to standard prevention, treatment, and recovery support interventions is common throughout health care. Individuals with the same disease often react quite differently to the same medicine or behavioral intervention. Accordingly, general health care has moved toward "personalized medicine," an individualized treatment regimen derived from specific information about the individual's genetics and stage of illness, as well as lifestyle, language, culture, and personal preferences. Personalized care is not common in the substance use disorder field because many prevention, treatment, and recovery regimens were created as standardized "programs" rather than individualized protocols.

The third caveat to the statement on general research findings is that even if research has shown that certain medications, therapies, or recovery support services are likely to be *effective,* this does not mean that they will be *a•equate,* especially for groups with specific needs. For example, a medication that is effective in blocking the rewarding effects of opioid use will not fully address the multiple, complex problems of those with opioid use disorders, nor address any co-occurring health conditions such as depression or HIV/AIDS.

Recognizing these limitations to the generalizability of research findings, each chapter has a dedicated section on Specific Populations that focuses particularly on age, racial and ethnic subgroups, and individuals with co-occurring mental and physical illnesses. Findings relevant to other important groups (e.g., military veterans; lesbian, gay, bisexual, and transgender [LGBT] populations; those with criminal justice involvement; those in rural areas) are referred to throughout the *Report* when available.

## The Organization of the Report

This *Report* is divided into Chapters, highlighting the key issues and most important research findings in those topics. The final chapter concludes with recommendations for key stakeholders, including implications for practice and policy.

This Chapter 1 - Introduction and Overview describes the overall rationale for the *Report*, defines key terms used throughout the *Report*, introduces the major issues covered in the topical chapters, and describes the organization, format, and the scientific standards that dictated content and emphasis within the *Report*.

Chapter 2 - The Neurobiology of Substance Use, Misuse, and Addiction reviews brain research on the neurobiological processes that turn casual substance use into a compulsive disorder.

Chapter 3 - Prevention Program and Policies reviews the scientific evidence on preventing substance misuse, substance use-related problems, and substance use disorders.

Chapter 4 - Early Intervention, Treatment, and Management of Substance Use Disorders describes the goals, settings, and stages of treatment, and reviews the effectiveness of the major components of early intervention and treatment approaches, including behavioral therapies, medications, and social services.

Chapter 5 - Recovery: The Many Paths to Wellness discusses perspectives on remission and recovery from substance use disorders and reviews the types and effectiveness of RSS.

Chapter 6 - Health Care Systems and Substance Use Disorders reviews ongoing changes in organization, delivery, and financing of care for substance use disorders in both specialty treatment programs and in mainstream health care settings.

Chapter 7 - Vision for the Future: A Public Health Approach presents a realistic vision for a comprehensive, effective, and humane public health approach to addressing substance misuse and substance use disorders in our country, including actionable recommendations for parents, families, communities, health care organizations, educators, researchers, and policymakers.

The **Appendices** provide additional detail about the topics covered in this *Report*. Appendix A - Review Process for Prevention Programs details the review process for the prevention programs included in Chapter 3 and the evidence on these programs; Appendix B - Evidence-Based Prevention Programs and Policies provides detail on scientific evidence grounding the programs and policies discussed in Chapter 3; Appendix C - Resource Guide provides resources specific to those seeking information on preventing and treating substance misuse or substance use disorders; and Appendix D - Important Facts about Alcohol and Drugs contains facts about alcohol and specific drugs, including descriptions, uses and possible health effects, treatment options, and statistics as of 2015.

# References


1. Kolodny, A., Courtwright, D. T., Hwang, C. S., Kreiner, P., Eadie, J. L., Clark, T. W., & Alexander, G. C. (2015). The prescription opioid and heroin crisis: A public health approach to an epidemic of addiction. *Annual Review of Public Health, 36,* 559-574.

2. Centers for Disease Control and Prevention. (2014). The public health system and the 10 essential public health services. Retrieved from http://www.cdc.gov/nphpsp/essentialservices.html. Accessed on August 16, 2016.

3. Center for Behavioral Health Statistics and Quality. (2016). *Results from the 2015 National Survey on Drug Use an• Health: Detaile• tables.* Rockville, MD: Substance Abuse and Mental Health Services Administration.

4. Volkow, N. D. (2014). *America's a••iction to opioi•s: Heroin an• prescription •rug abuse.* Senate Caucus on International Narcotics Control: National Institute on Drug Abuse. Retrieved from https://www.drugabuse.gov/about-nida/legislative-activities/testimony-to-congress/2015/americas-addiction-to-opioids-heroin-prescription-drug-abuse. Accessed on February 16, 2016.

5. World Health Organization. (2015). Health systems strengthening glossary, G-H. *Health Systems.* Retrieved from http://www.who.int/healthsystems/hss_glossary/en/index5.html. Accessed on August 16, 2016.

6. Stahre, M., Roeber, J., Kanny, D., Brewer , R. D., & Zhang, X. (2014). Contribution of excessive alcohol consumption to deaths and years of potential life lost in the United States. *Preventing Chronic Disease, 11*(E109).

7. Rudd, R. A., Aleshire, N., Zibbel, J. E., & Gladden, R. M. (2016). Increases in drug and opioid overdose deaths — United States, 2000–2014. *MMWR, 64*(50), 1378-1382.

8. Case, A., & Deaton, A. (2015). Rising morbidity and mortality in midlife among white non-Hispanic Americans in the 21st century. *Procee•ings of the National Aca•emy of Sciences, 112*(49), 15078-15083.

9. Kochanek, K. D., Arias, E., & Bastian, B. A. (2016). *The effect of changes in selecte• age-specific causes of •eath on non-Hispanic white life expectancy between 2000 an• 2014.* (NCHS Data Brief No. 250). Atlanta, GA: Centers for Disease Control and Prevention.

10. Sacks, J. J., Gonzales, K. R., Bouchery, E. E., Tomedi, L. E., & Brewer, R. D. (2015). 2010 national and state costs of excessive alcohol consumption. *American Journal of Preventive Me•icine, 49*(5), e73-e79.

11. National Drug Intelligence Center. (2011). *National •rug threat assessment.* Washington, DC: U.S. Department of Justice.

12. Centers for Disease Control and Prevention. (2014). *National Diabetes Statistics Report: Estimates of •iabetes an• its bur•en in the Unite• States, 2014.* Atlanta, GA: U.S. Department of Health and Human Services.

13. Center for Behavioral Health Statistics and Quality. (2015). *Behavioral health tren•s in the Unite• States: Results from the 2014 National Survey on Drug Use an• Health.* (HHS Publication No. SMA 15-4927 NSDUH Series H-50). Rockville, MD: Substance Abuse and Mental Health Services Administration.

14. U.S. Department of Health and Human Services. (2000). *Re•ucing tobacco use: A report of the Surgeon General.* Atlanta, GA: U.S. Department of Health and Human Services, Centers for Disease Control and Prevention, National Center for Chronic Disease Prevention and Health Promotion, Office on Smoking and Health.

15. U.S. Department of Health and Human Services. (2004). *The health consequences of smoking: A report of the Surgeon General.* Atlanta, GA: U.S. Department of Health and Human Services, Centers for Disease Control and Prevention, National Center for Chronic Disease Prevention and Health Promotion, Office on Smoking and Health.

16. U.S. Department of Health and Human Services. (2014). *The health consequences of smoking: 50 years of progress. A Report of the Surgeon General.* Atlanta, GA: U.S. Department of Health and Human Services, Centers for Disease Control and Prevention, National Center for Chronic Disease Prevention and Health Promotion, Office on Smoking and Health.

17. U.S. Department of Health and Human Services. (2012). *Preventing tobacco use among youth an• young a•ults: A report of the Surgeon General.* Atlanta, GA: Centers for Disease Control and Prevention, National Center for Chronic Disease Prevention and Health Promotion, Office on Smoking and Health.

18. Jewett, A., Shults, R. A., Banerjee, T., & Bergen, G. (2015). Alcohol-impaired driving among adults—United States, 2012. *MMWR, 64*(30), 814-817.

19. McMillan, G. P., & Lapham, S. (2006). Effectiveness of bans and laws in reducing traffic deaths: Legalized Sunday packaged alcohol sales and alcohol-related traffic crashes and crash fatalities in New Mexico. *American Journal of Public Health, 96*(11), 1944-1948.

20. Cantor, D., Fisher, B., Chibnall, S., Townsend, R., Lee, H., Bruce, C., & Thomas, C. (2015). *Report on the AAU campus climate survey on sexual assault an• sexual miscon•uct assault an• sexual miscon•uct.* Rockville, MD: The Association of American Universities.

21. Runyan, D., Wattam, C., Ikeda, R., Hassan, F., & Ramiro, L. (2002). Child abuse and neglect by parents and other caregivers. In E. Krug, L. L. Dahlberg, J. A. Mercy, A. B. Zwi, & R. Lozano (Eds.), *Worl• report on violence an• health.* (pp. 59-86). Geneva, Switzerland: World Health Organization.

22. U.S. Department of Health and Human Services, Office of the Surgeon General, & National Action Alliance for Suicide Prevention. (2012). *2012 National strategy for suici•e prevention: Goals an• objectives for action.* Washington, DC: U.S. Department of Health and Human Services.

23. Paulozzi, L. J., Kilbourne, E. M., & Desai, H. A. (2011). Prescription drug monitoring programs and death rates from drug overdose. *Pain Me•icine, 12*(5), 747-754.

24. Bagnardi, V., Rota, M., Botteri, E., Tramacere, I., Islami, F., Fedirko, V., . . . Pasquali, E. (2015). Alcohol consumption and site-specific cancer risk: A comprehensive dose–response meta-analysis. *British Journal of Cancer, 112*(3), 580-593.

25. Jung, S., Wang, M., Anderson, K., Baglietto, L., Bergkvist, L., Bernstein, L., . . . Eliassen, A. H. (2015). Alcohol consumption and breast cancer risk by estrogen receptor status: In a pooled analysis of 20 studies. *International Journal of Epi•emiology.*

26. Rehm, J., Mathers, C., Popova, S., Thavorncharoensap, M., Teerawattananon, Y., & Patra, J. (2009). Global burden of disease and injury and economic cost attributable to alcohol use and alcohol-use disorders. *The Lancet, 373*(9682), 2223-2233.

27. Baliunas, D., Rehm, J., Irving, H., & Shuper, P. (2010). Alcohol consumption and risk of incident human immunodeficiency virus infection: A meta-analysis. *International Journal of Public Health, 55*(3), 159-166.

28. Sokol, R. J., Delaney-Black, V., & Nordstrom, B. (2003). Fetal alcohol spectrum disorder. *JAMA, 290*(22), 2996-2999.

29. U.S. Department of Health and Human Services, & U.S. Department of Agriculture. (2015). 2015–2020 Dietary Guidelines for Americans: Appendix 9. Alcohol. *Dietary gui•elines for Americans, 2015-2020.* (8th ed.).

30. American Psychiatric Association. (2013). *Diagnostic an• statistical manual of mental •isor•ers (DSM-5)* (5th ed.). Arlington, VA: American Psychiatric Publishing.

31. Center for Behavioral Health Statistics and Quality. (2015). *Results from the 2014 National Survey on Drug Use an• Health: Detaile• tables.* Rockville, MD: Substance Abuse and Mental Health Services Administration.

32. Center for Behavioral Health Statistics and Quality. (2016). *Summary of the effects of the 2015 NSDUH questionnaire re•esign: Implications for •ata users.* Rockville, MD: Substance Abuse and Mental Health Services Administration.

33. Centers for Disease Control and Prevention. (n.d.). Alcohol and public health: Alcohol-related disease impact (ARDI). Retrieved from https://nccd.cdc.gov/DPH_ARDI/Default/Default.aspx. Accessed on July 9, 2016.

34. Centers for Disease Control and Prevention. (2016). Excessive drinking is draining the U.S. economy. Retrieved from http://www.cdc.gov/features/costsofdrinking/. Accessed on July 5, 2016.

35. Whiteford, H. A., Degenhardt, L., Rehm, J., Baxter, A. J., Ferrari, A. J., Erskine, H. E., . . . Vos, T. (2013). Global burden of disease attributable to mental and substance use disorders: Findings from the Global Burden of Disease Study 2010. *The Lancet, 382*(9904), 1575-1586.

36. Lange, R. A., & Hillis, L. D. (2001). Cardiovascular complications of cocaine use. *New Englan• Journal of Me•icine, 345*(5), 351-358.

37. Degenhardt, L., & Hall, W. (2012). Extent of illicit drug use and dependence, and their contribution to the global burden of disease. *The Lancet, 379,* 55-70.

38. National Highway Traffic Safety Administration. (2015). *Traffic safety facts 2014 •ata: Alcohol-impaire• •riving.* (DOT HS 812 231). Washington, DC: U.S. Department of Transportation.

39. National Highway Traffic Safety Administration (NHTSA). (2014). *Traffic safety facts 2013 •ata: Alcohol-impaire• •riving.* (DOT HS 812 102). Washington, DC: U.S. Department of Transportation.

40. Federal Bureau of Investigation (FBI). (2012). Estimated number of arrests: United States, 2012 *Crime in the Unite• States 2012: Uniform crime reports.* Retrieved from https://www.fbi.gov/about-us/cjis/ucr/crime-in-the-u.s/2012/crime-in-the-u.s.-2012/tables/29tabledatadecpdf. Accessed on April 11, 2016.

41. Blincoe, L., Miller, T. R., Zaloshnja, E., & Lawrence, B. A. (2015). *The economic an• societal impact of motor vehicle crashes, 2010 (Revise•).* (DOT HS 812 013). Washington, DC: National Highway Traffic Safety Administration.

42. Berning, A., Compton, R., & Wochinger, K. (2015). *Results of the 2013–2014 National Roa•si•e Survey of Alcohol an• Drug Use by •rivers.* (DOT HS 812 118). Washington, DC: National Highway Traffic Safety Administration.

43. Compton, R. P., & Berning, A. (2015). *Drug an• alcohol crash risk.* (DOT HS 812 117). Washington, DC: National Highway Traffic Safety Administration.

44. Centers for Disease Control and Prevention. (2015). Alcohol poisoning deaths. Vital signs: Alcohol poisoning kills six people each day. Retrieved from http://www.cdc.gov/media/dpk/2015/dpk-vs-alcohol-poisoning.html. Accessed on April 6, 2016.

45. Levy, B., Paulozzi, L., Mack, K. A., & Jones, C. M. (2015). Trends in opioid analgesic–prescribing rates by specialty, US, 2007–2012. *American Journal of Preventive Me•icine, 49*(3), 409-413.

46. Volkow, N. D., McLellan, T. A., Cotto, J. H., Karithanom, M., & Weiss, S. R. B. (2011). Characteristics of opioid prescriptions in 2009. *JAMA, 305*(13), 1299-1301.

47. Crane, E. H. (2013). *The CBHSQ Report: Emergency •epartment visits involving narcotic pain relievers.* Rockville, MD: Substance Abuse and Mental Health Services Administration, Center for Behavioral Health Statistics and Quality.

48. Centers for Disease Control and Prevention. (2016). CDC Wonder: Multiple cause of death 1999 - 2014. Retrieved from http://wonder.cdc.gov/wonder/help/mcd.html. Accessed on May 17, 2016.

49. Drug Enforcement Administration. (2016). DEA Report: Counterfeit pills fueling U.S. fentanyl and opioid crisis: Problems resulting from abuse of opioid drugs continue to grow. Retrieved from https://www.dea.gov/divisions/hq/2016/hq072216.shtml. Accessed on August 16, 2016.

50. McCollister, K. E., French, M. T., & Fang, H. (2010). The cost of crime to society: New crime-specific estimates for policy and program evaluation. *Drug an• Alcohol Depen•ence, 108*(1-2), 98-109.

51. National Center for Injury Prevention and Control. (2003). *Costs of intimate partner violence against women in the Unite• States.* Atlanta, GA: Centers for Disease Control and Prevention.

52. Breiding, M. J. (2014). Prevalence and characteristics of sexual violence, stalking, and intimate partner violence victimization—National Intimate Partner and Sexual Violence Survey, United States, 2011. *MMWR, 63*(8), 1-18.

53. Klein, A. R. (2009). *Practical implications of current •omestic violence research: For law enforcement, prosecutors an• ju•ges.* (NCJ 225722). Washington, DC: U.S. Department of Justice, Office of Justice Programs.

54. Friday, P. C., Lord, V. B., Exum, M. L., & Hartman, J. L. (2006). *Evaluating the impact of a specialize• •omestic violence police unit. Final report for National Institute of Justice.* (215916). Washington, DC: U.S. Department of Justice, National Institute of Justice.

55. Brookoff, D. (1997). *Drugs, alcohol, an• •omestic violence in Memphis.* Washington, DC: U.S. Department of Justice, National Institute of Justice.

56. Smith, P. H., Homish, G. G., Leonard, K. E., & Cornelius, J. R. (2012). Intimate partner violence and specific substance use disorders: Findings from the National Epidemiologic Survey on Alcohol and Related Conditions. *Psychology of A••ictive Behaviors, 26*(2), 236-245.

57. Vagi, K. J., Rothman, E. F., Latzman, N. E., Tharp, A. T., Hall, D. M., & Breiding, M. J. (2013). Beyond correlates: A review of risk and protective factors for adolescent dating violence perpetration. *Journal of Youth an• A•olescence, 42*(4), 633-649.

58. Stith, S. M., Smith, D. B., Penn, C. E., Ward, D. B., & Tritt, D. (2004). Intimate partner physical abuse perpetration and victimization risk factors: A meta-analytic review. *Aggression an• Violent Behavior, 10*(1), 65-98.

59. Exner-Cortens, D., Eckenrode, J., & Rothman, E. (2013). Longitudinal associations between teen dating violence victimization and adverse health outcomes. *Pe•iatrics, 131*(1), 71-78.

60. Stone, A. L., Becker, L. G., Huber, A. M., & Catalano, R. F. (2012). Review of risk and protective factors of substance use and problem use in emerging adulthood. *A••ictive Behaviors, 37*(7), 747-775.

61. Elder, R. W., Lawrence, B., Ferguson, A., Naimi, T. S., Brewer, R. D., Chattopadhyay, S. K., . . . Task Force on Community Preventive Services. (2010). The effectiveness of tax policy interventions for reducing excessive alcohol consumption and related harms. *American Journal of Preventive Me•icine, 38*(2), 217-229.

62. Kessler, R. C., Berglund, P., Demler, O., Jin, R., Merikangas, K. R., & Walters, E. E. (2005). Lifetime prevalence and age-of-onset distributions of DSM-IV disorders in the National Comorbidity Survey Replication. *Archives of General Psychiatry, 62*(6), 593-602.

63. Compton, W. M., Thomas, Y. F., Stinson, F. S., & Grant, B. F. (2007). Prevalence, correlates, disability, and comorbidity of DSM-IV drug abuse and dependence in the United States: Results from the national epidemiologic survey on alcohol and related conditions. *Archives of General Psychiatry, 64*(5), 566-576.

64. Hasin, D. S., Stinson, F. S., Ogburn, E., & Grant, B. F. (2007). Prevalence, correlates, disability, and comorbidity of DSM-IV alcohol abuse and dependence in the United States: Results from the National Epidemiologic Survey on Alcohol and Related Conditions. *Archives of General Psychiatry, 64*(7), 830-842.

65. Hanson, K. L., Medina, K. L., Padula, C. B., Tapert, S. F., & Brown, S. A. (2011). Impact of adolescent alcohol and drug use on neuropsychological functioning in young adulthood: 10-year outcomes. *Journal of Chil• an• A•olescent Substance Abuse, 20*(2), 135-154.

66. Giedd, J. N., Blumenthal, J., Jeffries, N. O., Castellanos, F. X., Liu, H., Zijdenbos, A., . . . Rapoport, J. L. (1999). Brain development during childhood and adolescence: A longitudinal MRI study. *Nature Neuroscience, 2*(10), 861-863.

67. Squeglia, L. M., Tapert, S. F., Sullivan, E. V., Jacobus, J., Meloy, M. J., Rolfing, T., & Pfefferbaum, A. (2015). Brain development in heavy-drinking adolescents. *American Journal of Psychiatry, 172*(6), 532-542.

68. Miller, W. R., Meyers, R. J., & Tonigan, J. S. (1999). Engaging the unmotivated in treatment for alcohol problems: A comparison of three strategies for intervention through family members. *Journal of Consulting an• Clinical Psychology, 67*(5), 688-697.

69. White, W. L., & Miller, W. R. (2007). The use of confrontation in addiction treatment: History, science and time for change. *Counselor, 8*(4), 12-30.

70. Bodenheimer, T., Wagner, E. H., & Grumbach, K. (2002). Improving primary care for patients with chronic illness: The chronic care model, Part 2. *JAMA, 288*(15), 1909-1914.

71. McLellan, A. T., Lewis, D. C., O'Brien, C. P., & Kleber, H. D. (2000). Drug dependence, a chronic medical illness: Implications for treatment, insurance, and outcomes evaluation. *JAMA, 284*(13), 1689-1695.

72. McLellan, A. T., Starrels, J. L., Tai, B., Gordon, A. J., Brown, R., Ghitza, U., . . . Horton, T. (2014). Can substance use disorders be managed using the chronic care model? Review and recommendations from a NIDA Consensus Group. *Public Health Reviews, 35*(2), 1-14.

73. Feliz, J. (2012). Survey: Ten percent of American adults report being in recovery from substance abuse or addiction. Retrieved from http://www.drugfree.org/newsroom/survey-ten-percent-of-american-adults-report-being-in-recovery-from-substance-abuse-or-addiction/. Accessed on April 12, 2016.

74. White, W. (2014). *Slaying the •ragon: The history of a••iction treatment an• recovery in America* (2nd Ed.). Bloomington, IL: Chestnut Health Systems.

75. Musto, D. F. (1987). *The American •isease: Origins of narcotic control* (Expanded ed.). New York, NY: Oxford University Press.

76. Rettig, R. A., Yarmolinsky, A., & Institute of Medicine (US) Committee on Federal Regulation of Methadone Treatment (Eds.). (1995). *Fe•eral regulation of metha•one treatment.* Washington, DC: National Academies Press.

77. Ries, R. K., Fielen, D. A., Miller, S. C., & Saltz, R. (Eds.). (2014). *The ASAM principles of a••iction me•icine* (5th ed.): Wolters Kluwer.

78. Institute of Medicine, & Committee on Crossing the Quality Chasm. (2006). *Improving the quality of health care for mental an• substance-use con•itions.* Washington, DC: National Academies Press.

79. McKnight-Eily, L. R., Liu, Y., Brewer, R. D., Kanny, D., Lu, H., Denny, C. H., . . . Centers for Disease Control and Prevention. (2014). Vital signs: Communication between health professionals and their patients about alcohol use - 44 states and the District of Columbia, 2011. *MMWR, 63*(1), 16-22.

80. Scott, K. M., Lim, C., Al-Hamzawi, A., Alonso, J., Bruffaerts, R., Caldas-de-Almeida, J. M., . . . de Jonge, P. (2016). Association of mental disorders with subsequent chronic physical conditions: World mental health surveys from 17 countries. *JAMA Psychiatry, 73*(2), 150-158.

81. Phillips, D. P., Barker, G. E., & Eguchi, M. M. (2008). A steep increase in domestic fatal medication errors with use of alcohol and/or street drugs. *Archives of Internal Me•icine, 168*(14), 1561-1566.

82. Dowell, D., Haegerich, T. M., & R., C. (2016). CDC guideline for prescribing opioids for chronic pain - United States. *MMWR, 65*(1), 1-49.

83. Parish, C. L., Pereyra, M. R., Pollack, H. A., Cardenas, G., Castellon, P. C., Abel, S. N., . . . Metsch, L. R. (2015). Screening for substance misuse in the dental care setting: Findings from a nationally representative survey of dentists. *A••iction, 110*(9), 1516-1523.

84. Denisco, R. C., Kenna, G. A., O'Neil, M. G., Kulich, R. J., Moore, P. A., Kane, W. T., . . . Katz, N. P. (2011). Prevention of prescription opioid abuse: The role of the dentist. *The Journal of the American Dental Association, 142*(7), 800-810.

85. Krause, M., Vainio, L., Zwetchkenbaum, S., & Inglehart, M. R. (2010). Dental education about patients with special needs: A survey of US and Canadian dental schools. *Journal of Dental Education, 74*(11), 1179-1189.

86. Tommasello, A. C. (2004). Substance abuse and pharmacy practice: What the community pharmacist needs to know about drug abuse and dependence. *Harm Reduction Journal, 1*(3), 1-15.

87. Barry, C. L., & Huskamp, H. A. (2011). Moving beyond parity—mental health and addiction care under the ACA. *New England Journal of Medicine, 365*(11), 973-975.

88. McLellan, A. T., & Meyers, K. (2004). Contemporary addiction treatment: A review of systems problems for adults and adolescents. *Biological Psychiatry, 56*(10), 764-770.

89. Patient Protection and Affordable Care Act, 42 U.S.C. § 18001, H.R. 3590, Public Law No. 111–148, 124 Stat. 119 Stat. (2010).

90. Paul Wellstone and Pete Domenici Mental Health Parity and Addiction Equity Act of 2008, H.R. 6983 (2008).

91. Miech, R. A., Johnston, L. D., O'Malley, P. M., Bachman, J. G., & Schulenberg, J. E. (2016). *Monitoring the Future national survey results on drug use, 1975-2015: Volume I, secondary school students.* Ann Arbor, MI: Institute for Social Research, The University of Michigan.

92. Pacula, R. L., Powell, D., Heaton, P., & Sevigny, E. L. (2015). Assessing the effects of medical marijuana laws on marijuana use: The devil is in the details. *Journal of Policy Analysis and Management, 34*(1), 7-31.

93. Office of National Drug Control Policy. (n.d.). Answers to frequently asked questions about marijuana. Retrieved from https://www.whitehouse.gov/ondcp/frequently-asked-questions-and-facts-about-marijuana. Accessed on June 27, 2016.

94. Mehmedic, Z., Chandra, S., Slade, D., Denham, H., Foster, S., Patel, A. S., . . . ElSohly, M. A. (2010). Potency trends of 9-THC and other cannabinoids in confiscated cannabis preparations from 1993 to 2008. *Journal of Forensic Sciences, 55*(5), 1209-1217.

95. National Institute on Drug Abuse. (2016). DrugFacts: Marijuana. Retrieved from https://www.drugabuse.gov/publications/drugfacts/marijuana. Accessed on June 20, 2016.

96. Ramaekers, J. G., Berghaus, G., van Laar, M., & Drummer, O. H. (2004). Dose related risk of motor vehicle crashes after cannabis use. *Drug and Alcohol Dependence, 73*(2), 109-119.

97. Li, M.-C., Brady, J. E., DiMaggio, C. J., Lusardi, A. R., Tzong, K. Y., & Li, G. (2012). Marijuana use and motor vehicle crashes. *Epidemiologic Reviews, 34*(1), 65-72.

98. Asbridge, M., Hayden, J. A., & Cartwright, J. L. (2012). Acute cannabis consumption and motor vehicle collision risk: Systematic review of observational studies and meta-analysis. *BMJ, 344*, e536.

99. Hartman, R. L., & Huestis, M. A. (2013). Cannabis effects on driving skills. *Clinical Chemistry, 59*(3), 478-492.

100. U.S. Department of Health, Education, and Welfare. (1964). *Smoking and health: Report of the advisory committee to the Surgeon General of the Public Health Service.* Washington, DC: U.S. Public Health Service, Office of the Surgeon General.

101. U.S. Department of Health and Human Services. (1986). *The health consequences of using smokeless tobacco: A report of the A•visory Committee to the Surgeon General.* Washington, DC: U.S. Department of Health and Human Services.

102. U.S. Department of Health and Human Services. (1994). *Preventing tobacco use among young people: A report of the Surgeon General.* Atlanta, GA: U.S. Department of Health and Human Services, Centers for Disease Control and Prevention, National Center for Chronic Disease Prevention and Health Promotion, Office on Smoking and Health.

103. U.S. Department of Health and Human Services. (2010). *How tobacco smoke causes •isease: The biology an• behavioral basis for smoking-attributable •isease: A report of the Surgeon General.* Atlanta, GA: U.S. Department of Health and Human Services, Centers for Disease Control and Prevention, National Center for Chronic Disease Prevention and Health Promotion, Office on Smoking and Health.

104. Puddy, R. W., & Wilkins, N. (2011). *Un•erstan•ing evi•ence Part 1: Best available research evi•ence. A gui•e to the continuum of evi•ence of effectiveness.* Atlanta, GA: Centers for Disease Control and Prevention.

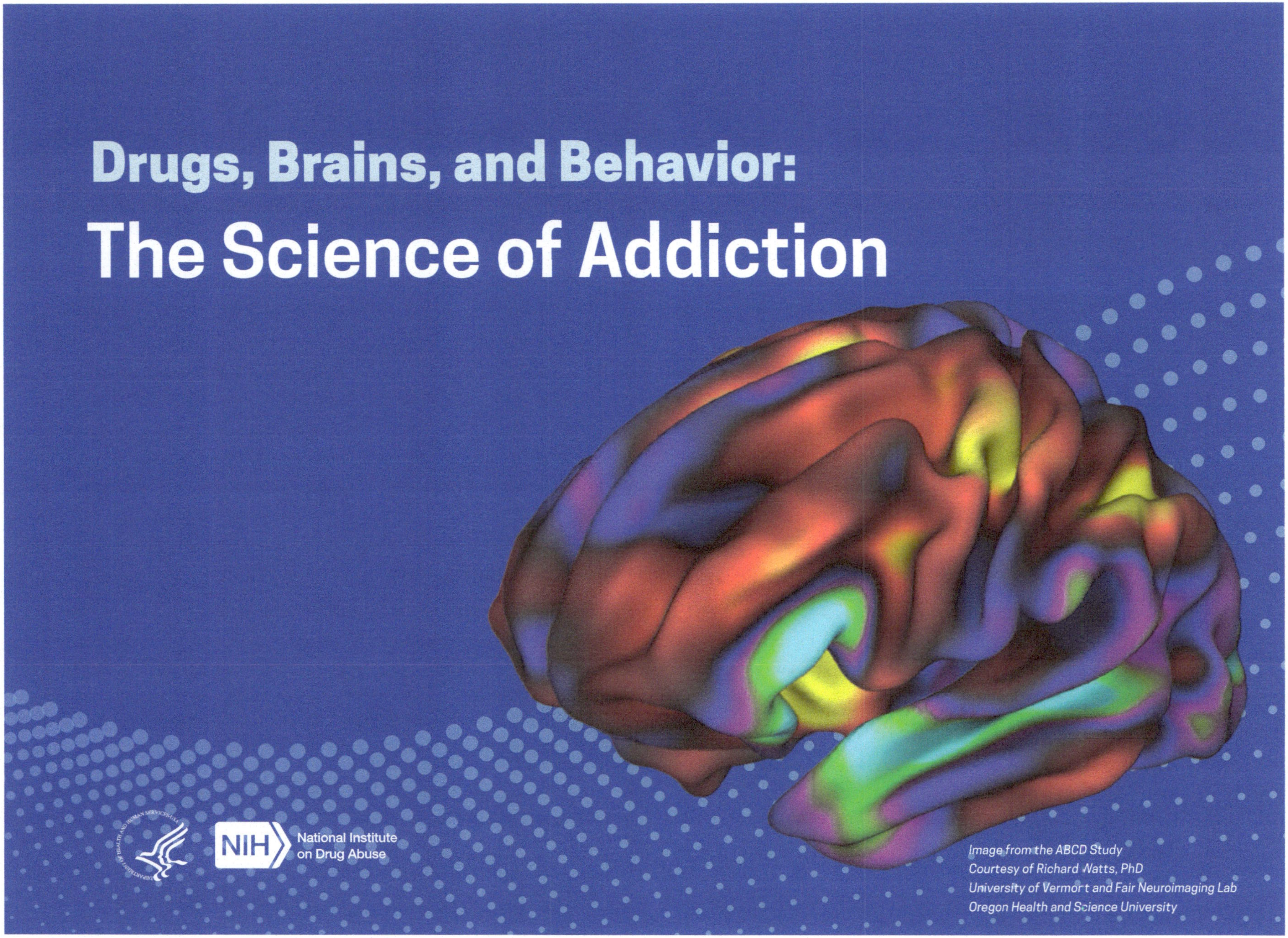
Drugs, Brains, and Behavior:
The Science of Addiction
National Institute on Drug Abuse
NIH
Image from the ABCD Study
Courtesy of Richard Watts, PhD
University of Vermont and Fair Neuroimaging Lab
Oregon Health and Science University

# INTRODUCTION

Why study

## DRUG USE AND ADDICTION?

Use and misuse of alcohol, nicotine, and illicit drugs, and misuse of prescription drugs cost Americans more than $700 billion a year in increased health care costs, crime, and lost productivity.[1,2,3] Every year, illicit and prescription drug overdoses cause tens of thousands of deaths (nearly 70,000 in 2018), alcohol contributes to the death of more than 90,000 Americans, while tobacco is linked to an estimated 480,000 deaths per year.[4,5] (Hereafter, unless otherwise specified, *drugs* refers to all of these substances.)

**People of all ages suffer the harmful consequences of drug use and addiction:**

- **Teens** who use drugs may act out and may do poorly in school or drop out.[6] Using drugs when the brain is still developing may cause lasting brain changes and put the user at increased risk of dependence.[7]
- **Adults** who use drugs can have problems thinking clearly, remembering, and paying attention. They may develop poor social behaviors as a result of their drug use, and their work performance and personal relationships suffer.
- **Parents'** drug use can mean chaotic, stress-filled homes, as well as child abuse and neglect.[8] Such conditions harm the well-being and development of children in the home and may set the stage for drug use in the next generation.[9]
- **Babies** exposed to drugs in the womb may be born premature and underweight. This exposure can slow the child's ability to learn and affect behavior later in life.[10] They may also become dependent on opioids or other drugs used by the mother during pregnancy, a condition called neonatal abstinence syndrome (NAS).

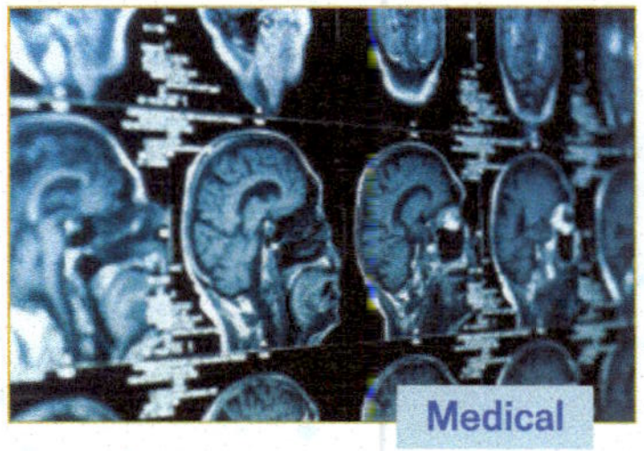


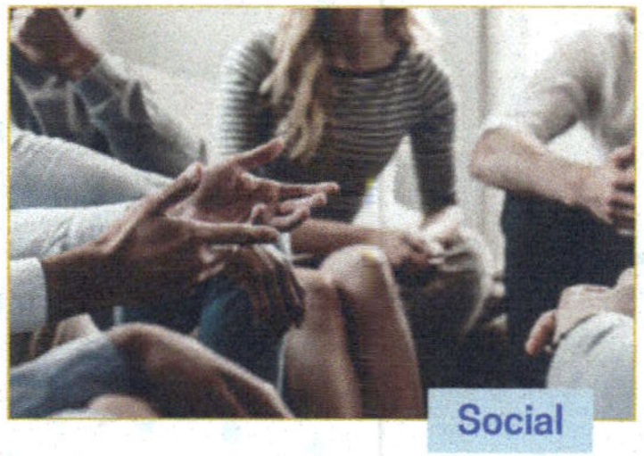


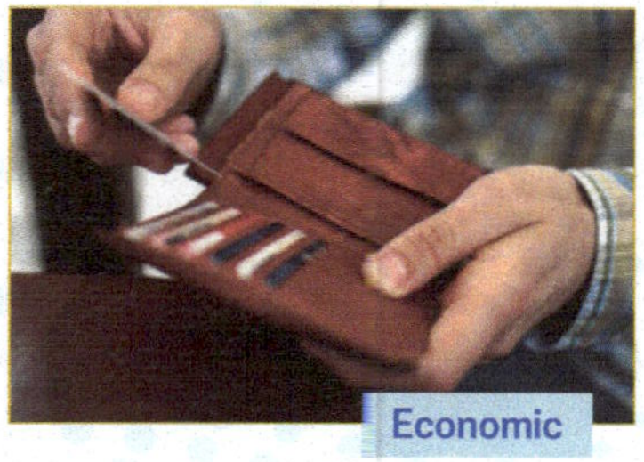


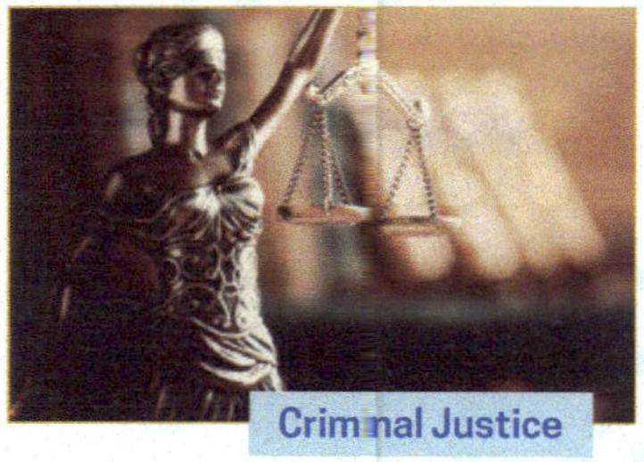


### How does science provide solutions for drug use and addiction?

Scientists study the effects drugs have on the brain and behavior. They use this information to develop programs for preventing drug use and for helping people recover from addiction. Further research helps transfer these ideas into practice in the community.

The consequences of drug use are vast and varied and affect people of all ages.

# Drug Misuse and Addiction

## What is DRUG ADDICTION?

Addiction is defined as a chronic, relapsing disorder characterized by compulsive drug seeking and use despite adverse consequences.† It is considered a brain disorder, because it involves functional changes to brain circuits involved in reward, stress, and self-control. Those changes may last a long time after a person has stopped taking drugs.[11]

Addiction is a lot like other diseases, such as heart disease. Both disrupt the normal, healthy functioning of an organ in the body, both have serious harmful effects, and both are, in many cases, preventable and treatable. If left untreated, they can last a lifetime and may lead to death.

Comparison Subject | 1 Month After Last Cocaine Use | 4 Months After Last Cocaine Use

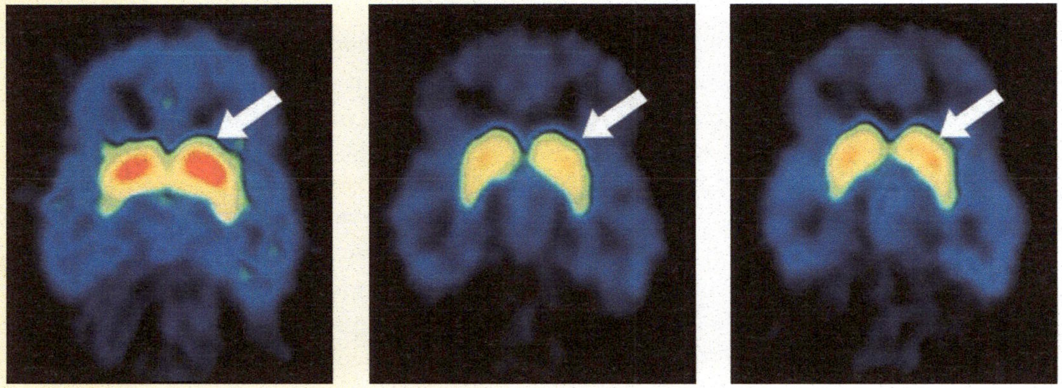

Low dopamine D2 receptors may contribute to the loss of control in cocaine users.

*Source: Facing Addiction in America: The Surgeon General's Report on Alcohol, Drugs, and Health*

*Modified with permission from Volkow et al. 1993*

*Note: These PET scans compare the brain of an individual with a history of cocaine use disorder (middle and right) to the brain of an individual without a history of cocaine use (left). The person who has had a cocaine use disorder has lower levels of the D2 dopamine receptor (depicted in red) in the striatum one month (middle) and four months (right) after stopping cocaine use compared to the non-user. The level of dopamine receptors in the brain of the cocaine user are higher at the 4-month mark (right), but have not returned to the levels observed in the non-user (left).*

*†The term addiction as used in this booklet is equivalent to a severe substance use disorder as defined by the Diagnostic and Statistical Manual of Mental Disorders, Fifth Edition (DSM-5, 2013).*

Why do

## PEOPLE TAKE DRUGS?

In general, people take drugs for a few reasons:

- **To feel good.** Drugs can produce intense feelings of pleasure. This initial euphoria is followed by other effects, which differ with the type of drug used. For example, with stimulants such as cocaine, the high is followed by feelings of power, self-confidence, and increased energy. In contrast, the euphoria caused by opioids such as heroin is followed by feelings of relaxation and satisfaction.
- **To feel better.** Some people who suffer from social anxiety, stress, and depression start using drugs to try to feel less anxious. Stress can play a major role in starting and continuing drug use as well as relapse (return to drug use) in patients recovering from addiction.
- **To do better.** Some people feel pressure to improve their focus in school or at work or their abilities in sports. This can play a role in trying or continuing to use drugs, such as prescription stimulants or cocaine.
- **Curiosity and social pressure.** In this respect, teens are particularly at risk because peer pressure can be very strong. Adolescence is a developmental period during which the presence of risk factors, such as peers who use drugs, may lead to substance use.

If taking drugs makes people feel good or better,

## WHAT'S THE PROBLEM?

When they first use a drug, people may perceive what seem to be positive effects. They also may believe they can control their use. But drugs can quickly take over a person's life. Over time, if drug use continues, other pleasurable activities become less pleasurable, and the person has to take the drug just to feel "normal." They have a hard time controlling their need to take drugs even though it causes many problems for themselves and their loved ones. Some people may start to feel the need to take more of a drug or take it more often, even in the early stages of their drug use. These are the signs of an addiction.

Even relatively moderate drug use poses dangers. Consider how a social drinker can become intoxicated, get behind the wheel of a car, and quickly turn a pleasurable activity into a tragedy that affects many lives. Occasional drug use, such as misusing an opioid to get high, can have similarly disastrous effects, including impaired driving and overdose.

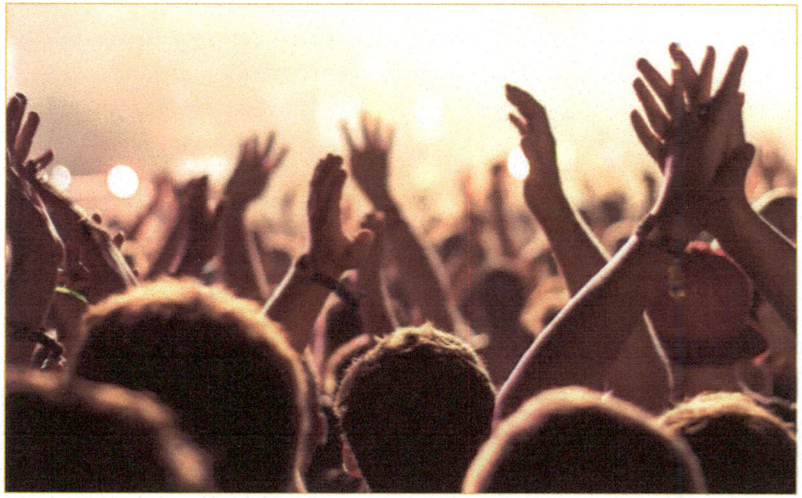

Do people choose to

## KEEP USING DRUGS?

The initial decision to take drugs is typically voluntary. But with continued use, a person's ability to exert self-control can become seriously impaired. This impairment in self-control is the hallmark of addiction.

Brain imaging studies of people with addiction show physical changes in areas of the brain that are critical to judgment, decision-making, learning and memory, and behavior control.[12] These changes help explain the compulsive nature of addiction.

Why do some people become addicted to drugs,

## WHILE OTHERS DO NOT?

As with other diseases and disorders, the likelihood of developing an addiction differs from person to person, and no single factor determines whether a person will become addicted to drugs. In general, the more *risk factors* a person has, the greater the chance that taking drugs will lead to drug use and addiction. *Protective factors,* on the other hand, reduce a person's risk. Risk and protective factors may be either environmental or biological.

*No single factor determines whether a person will become addicted to drugs.*

## Risk and Protective Factors for Drug Use, Misuse, and Addiction

| RISK FACTORS | PROTECTIVE FACTORS |
|---|---|
| Aggressive behavior in childhood[13,14] | Self-efficacy (belief in self-control)[15] |
| Lack of parental supervision[14,16] | Parental monitoring and support[16–18] |
| Low peer refusal skills[13,17,18] | Positive relationships[17,19] |
| Drug experimentation[14,20,21] | Extracurricular Activities[17,22] |
| Availability of drugs at school[21,23] | School anti-drug policies[17] |
| Community poverty[24,25] | Neighborhood resources[26] |

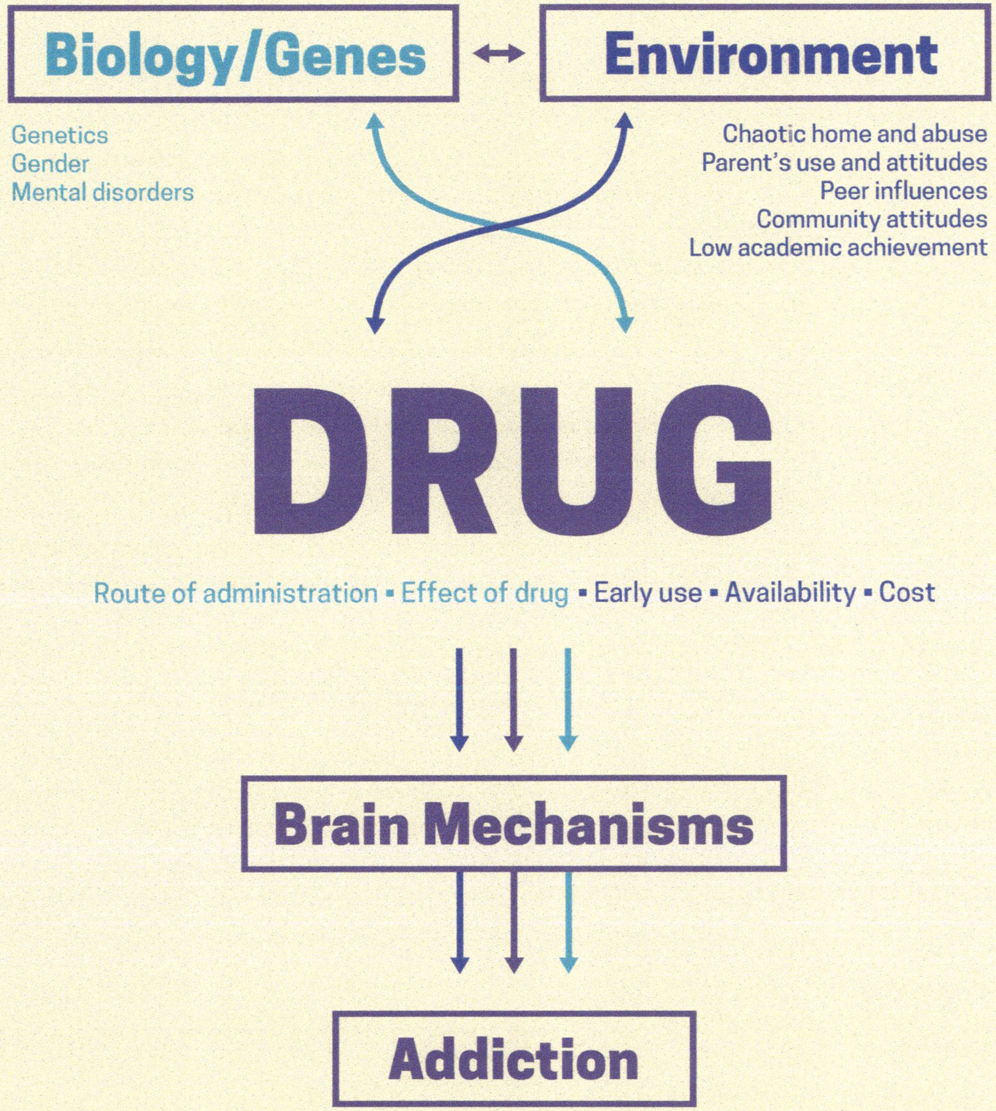


*Children's earliest interactions within the family are crucial to their healthy development and risk for drug use.*

## WHAT BIOLOGICAL FACTORS
### increase the risk of addiction?

Biological factors that can affect a person's risk of addiction include their genes, stage of development, and even gender or ethnicity. Scientists estimate that genes, including the effects environmental factors have on a person's gene expression, called epigenetics, account for between 40 and 60 percent of a person's risk of addiction.[27] Also, teens and people with mental disorders are at greater risk of drug use and addiction than others.[28]

## WHAT ENVIRONMENTAL FACTORS
### increase the risk of addiction?

Environmental factors are those related to the family, school, and neighborhood. Factors that can increase a person's risk include the following:

- **Home and family.** The home environment, especially during childhood, is a very important factor. Parents or older family members who use drugs or misuse alcohol, or who break the law, can increase children's risk of future drug problems.[29]
- **Peers and school.** Friends and other peers can have an increasingly strong influence during the teen years. Teens who use drugs can sway even those without risk factors to try drugs for the first time. Struggling in school or having poor social skills can put a child at further risk for using or becoming addicted to drugs.[30]

### What other factors increase the
## RISK OF ADDICTION?

- **Early use.** Although taking drugs at any age can lead to addiction, research shows that the earlier people begin to use drugs, the more likely they are to develop serious problems.[31] This may be due to the harmful effect that drugs can have on the developing brain.[32] It also may result from a mix of early social and biological risk factors, including lack of a stable home or family, exposure to physical or sexual abuse, genes, or mental illness. Still, the fact remains that early use is a strong indicator of problems ahead, including addiction.
- **How the drug is taken.** Smoking a drug or injecting it into a vein increases its addictive potential.[33,34] Both smoked and injected drugs enter the brain within seconds, producing a powerful rush of pleasure. However, this intense high can fade within a few minutes. Scientists believe this powerful contrast drives some people to repeatedly use drugs to recapture the fleeting pleasurable state.

### Images of Brain Development in Healthy Children and Teens (Ages 5–20)

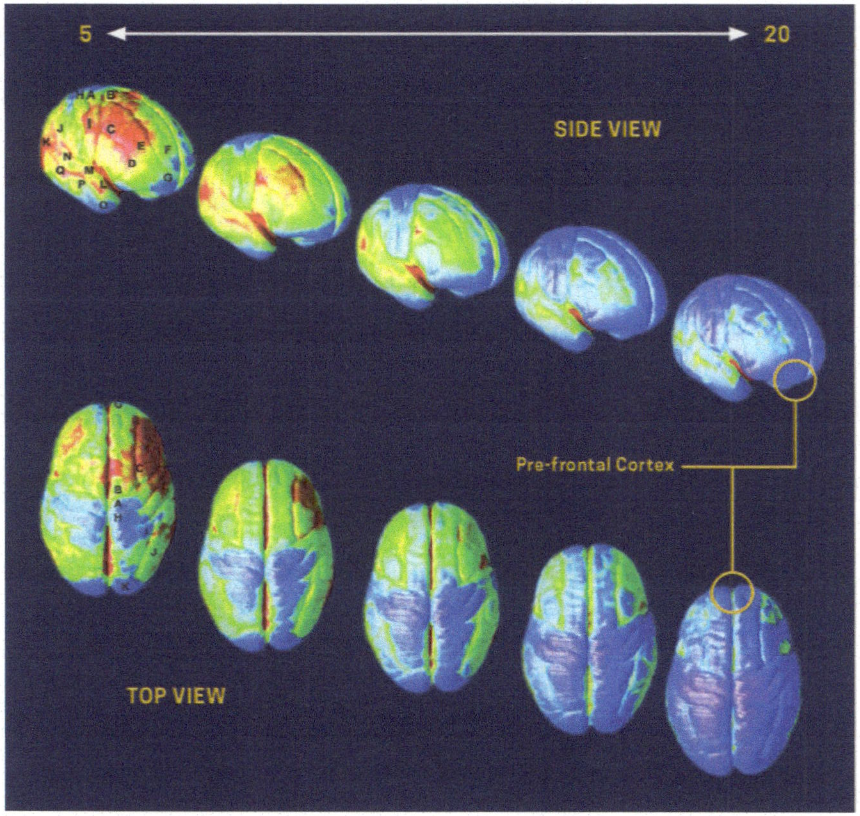


Source: PNAS 101:8174–8179, 2004.

*As the brain matures, experiences prune excess neural connections while strengthening those that are used more often. Many scientists think that this process contributes to the steady reduction in gray matter volume seen during adolescence (depicted as the yellow to blue transition in the figure). As environmental forces help determine which connections will wither and which will thrive, the brain circuits that emerge become more efficient. However, this is a process that can cut both ways because not all patterns of behavior are desirable or healthy. The environment is like an artist who creates a sculpture by chipping away excess marble; and just like bad artists can produce bad art, environments with negative factors (like drugs, malnutrition, bullying, or sleep deprivation) can lead to efficient but potentially harmful circuits that conspire against a person's well-being.*

The brain continues to develop into adulthood and undergoes

## DRAMATIC CHANGES DURING ADOLESCENCE

One of the brain areas still maturing during adolescence is the prefrontal cortex — the part of the brain that allows people to assess situations, make sound decisions, and keep emotions and desires under control. The fact that this critical part of a teen's brain is still a work in progress puts them at increased risk for trying drugs or continuing to take them. Introducing drugs during this period of development may cause brain changes that have profound and long-lasting consequences.

# Preventing Drug Misuse and Addiction: The Best Strategy

## Why is adolescence a critical time for PREVENTING DRUG ADDICTION?

As noted previously, early use of drugs increases a person's chances of becoming addicted. Remember, drugs change the brain—and this can lead to addiction and other serious problems. So, preventing early use of drugs or alcohol may go a long way in reducing these risks.

Risk of drug use increases greatly during times of transition. For an adult, a divorce or loss of a job may increase the risk of drug use. For a teenager, risky times include moving, family divorce, or changing schools.[35] When children advance from elementary through middle school, they face new and challenging social, family, and academic situations. Often during this period, children are exposed to substances such as cigarettes and alcohol for the first time. When they enter high school, teens may encounter greater availability of drugs, drug use by older teens, and social activities where drugs are used. When individuals leave high school and live more independently, either in college or as an employed adult, they may find themselves exposed to drug use while separated from the protective structure provided by family and school.

A certain amount of risk-taking is a normal part of adolescent development. The desire to try new things and become more independent is healthy, but it may also increase teens' tendencies to experiment with drugs. The parts of the brain that control judgment and decision-making do not fully develop until people are in their early or mid-20s. This limits a teen's ability to accurately assess the risks of drug experimentation and makes young people more vulnerable to peer pressure.[36]

Because the brain is still developing, using drugs at this age has more potential to disrupt brain function in areas critical to motivation, memory, learning, judgment, and behavior control.[12]

### Can research-based programs prevent
## DRUG ADDICTION IN YOUTH?

**Yes.** The term research-based or evidence-based means that these programs have been designed based on current scientific evidence, thoroughly tested, and shown to produce positive results. Scientists have developed a broad range of programs that positively alter the balance between risk and protective factors for drug use in families, schools, and communities. Studies have shown that research-based programs, such as described in NIDA's *Principles of Substance Abuse Prevention for Early Childhood: A Research-Based Guide* and *Preventing Drug Use among Children and Adolescents: A Research-Based Guide for Parents, Educators, and Community Leaders*, can significantly reduce early use of tobacco, alcohol, and other drugs.[37] Also, while many social and cultural factors affect drug use trends, when young people perceive drug use as harmful, they often reduce their level of use.[38]

### How do research-based
## PREVENTION PROGRAMS WORK?

These prevention programs work to boost protective factors and eliminate or reduce risk factors for drug use. The programs are designed for various ages and can be used in individual or group settings, such as the school and home. There are three types of programs:

- **Universal programs** address risk and protective factors common to all children in a given setting, such as a school or community.
- **Selective programs** are for groups of children and teens who have specific factors that put them at increased risk of drug use.
- **Indicated programs** are designed for youth who have already started using drugs.

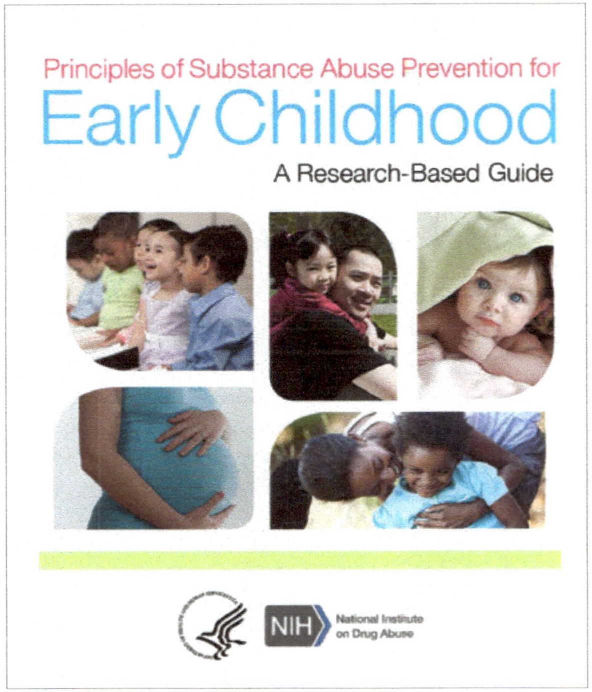


*National drug use surveys indicate some children are already using drugs by age 12 or 13.*

*Prevention is the best strategy.*

## Young Brains Under Study

Using cutting-edge imaging technology, scientists from the NIDA's Adolescent Brain Cognitive Development (ABCD) Study will look at how childhood experiences, including use of any drugs, interact with each other and with a child's changing biology to affect brain development and social, behavioral, academic, health, and other outcomes. As the only study of its kind, the ABCD study will yield critical insights into the foundational aspects of adolescence that shape a person's future.

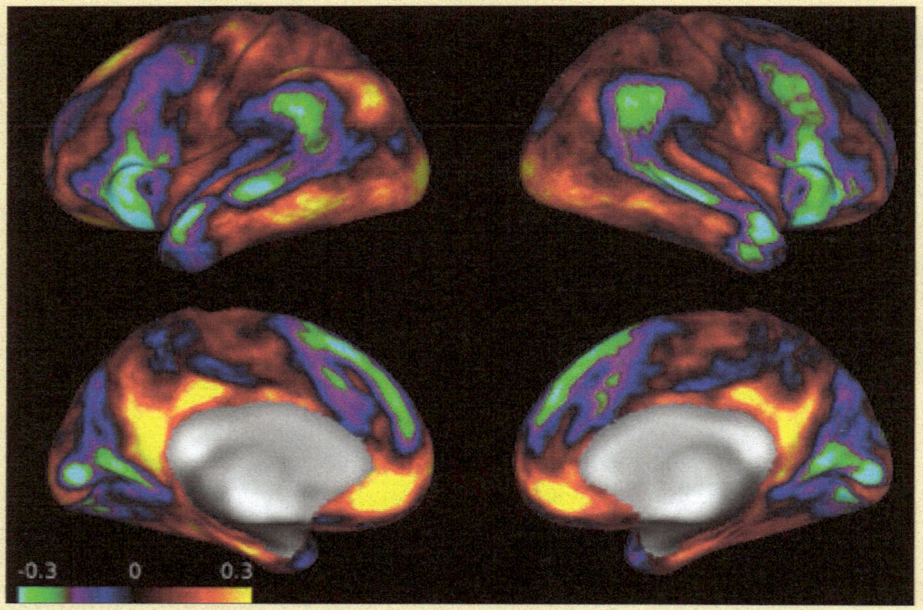


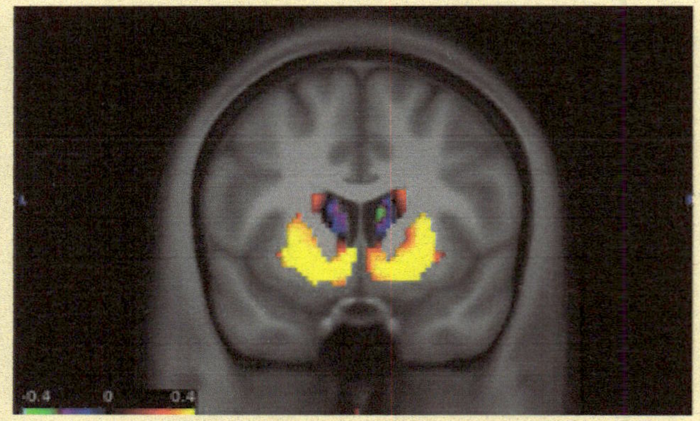


*These brain images show the reward-related circuitry in the cortical and subcortical regions of the brain that tend to be more active when a child is successful at achieving a reward. While all of the images show the regions of the brain that are active to reward, the regions in yellow and red are the most active.*

*Courtesy of the ABCD Study. Adapted from Casey et al., 2018 https://doi.org/10.1016/j.dcn.2018.03.001*

### Economics of Prevention

**Evidence-based interventions for substance use can save society money in medical costs and help individuals remain productive members of society. Such programs can return anywhere from very little to $65 per every dollar invested in prevention.[39]**

# Drugs and the Brain

Introducing the

## HUMAN BRAIN

The human brain is the most complex organ in the body. This three-pound mass of gray and white matter sits at the center of all human activity—you need it to drive a car, to enjoy a meal, to breathe, to create an artistic masterpiece, and to enjoy everyday activities. The brain regulates your body's basic functions, enables you to interpret and respond to everything you experience, and shapes your behavior. In short, *your brain is you* — everything you think and feel, and who you are.

How does the

## BRAIN WORK?

The brain is often likened to an incredibly complex and intricate computer. Instead of electrical circuits on the silicon chips that control our electronic devices, the brain consists of billions of cells, called *neurons,* which are organized into circuits and networks. Each neuron acts as a switch controlling the flow of information. If a neuron receives enough signals from other neurons that it is connected to, it fires, sending its own signal on to other neurons in the circuit.

**Here's how people communicate.**

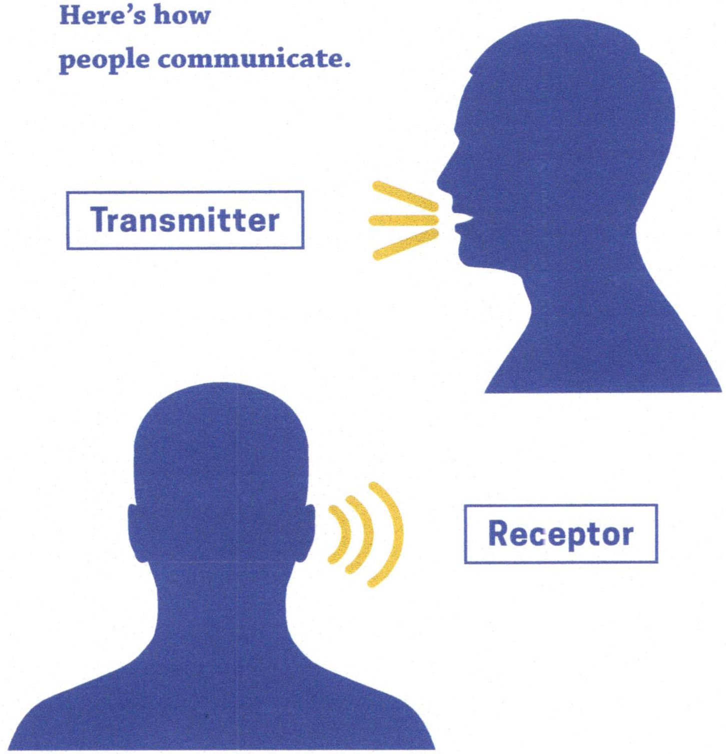

The brain is made up of many parts with interconnected circuits that all work together as a team. Different brain circuits are responsible for coordinating and performing specific functions. Networks of neurons send signals back and forth to each other and among different parts of the brain, the spinal cord, and nerves in the rest of the body (the peripheral nervous system).

To send a message, a neuron releases a *neurotransmitter* into the gap (or *synapse)* between it and the next cell. The neurotransmitter crosses the synapse and attaches to receptors on the receiving neuron, like a key into a lock. This causes changes in the receiving cell. Other molecules called *transporters* recycle neurotransmitters (that is, bring them back into the neuron that released them), thereby limiting or shutting off the signal between neurons.

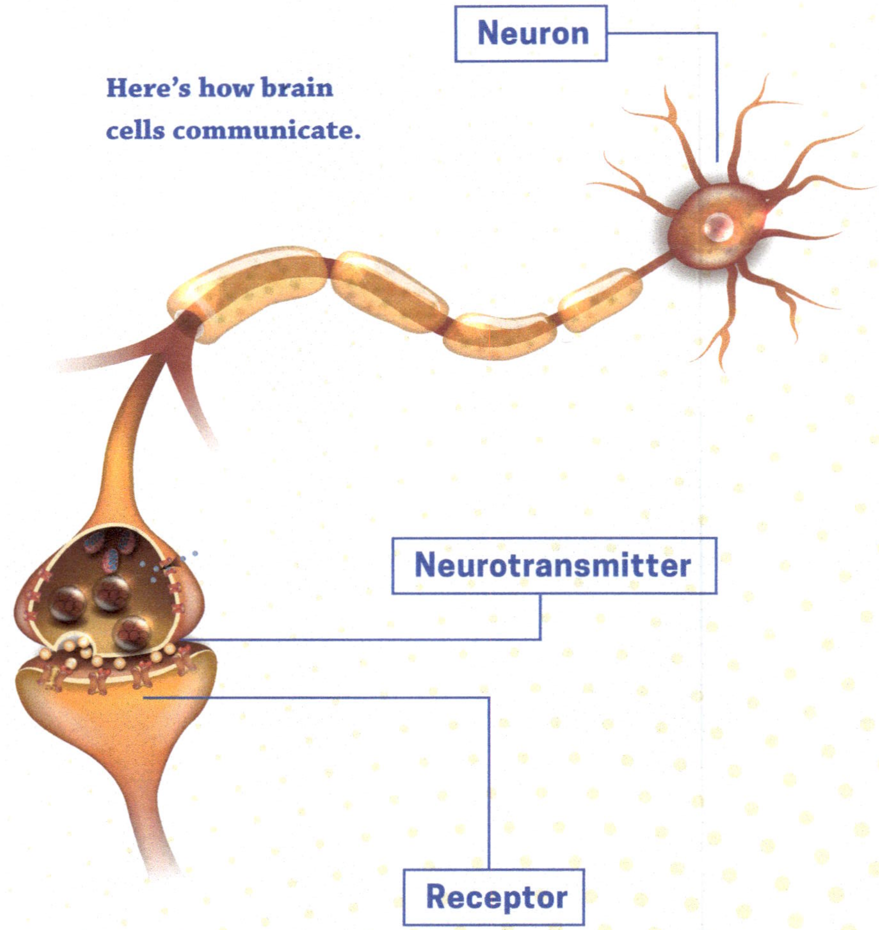


Here's how brain cells communicate.

## How do drugs WORK IN THE BRAIN?

Drugs interfere with the way neurons send, receive, and process signals via neurotransmitters. Some drugs, such as marijuana and heroin, can activate neurons because their chemical structure mimics that of a natural neurotransmitter in the body. This allows the drugs to attach onto and activate the neurons. Although these drugs mimic the brain's own chemicals, they don't activate neurons in the same way as a natural neurotransmitter, and they lead to abnormal messages being sent through the network.

Other drugs, such as amphetamine or cocaine, can cause the neurons to release abnormally large amounts of natural neurotransmitters or prevent the normal recycling of these brain chemicals by interfering with transporters. This too amplifies or disrupts the normal communication between neurons.

What parts of the brain are

## AFFECTED BY DRUG USE?

Drugs can alter important brain areas that are necessary for life-sustaining functions and can drive the compulsive drug use that marks addiction. Brain areas affected by drug use include:

- *The basal ganglia,* which play an important role in positive forms of motivation, including the pleasurable effects of healthy activities like eating, socializing, and sex, and are also involved in the formation of habits and routines. These areas form a key node of what is sometimes called the brain's "reward circuit." Drugs over-activate this circuit, producing the euphoria of the drug high. But with repeated exposure, the circuit adapts to the presence of the drug, diminishing its sensitivity and making it hard to feel pleasure from anything besides the drug.
- *The extended amygdala* plays a role in stressful feelings like anxiety, irritability, and unease, which characterize withdrawal after the drug high fades and thus motivates the person to seek the drug again. This circuit becomes increasingly sensitive with increased drug use. Over time, a person with substance use disorder uses drugs to get temporary relief from this discomfort rather than to get high.
- *The prefrontal cortex* powers the ability to think, plan, solve problems, make decisions, and exert self-control over impulses. This is also the last part of the brain to mature, making teens most vulnerable. Shifting balance between this circuit and the circuits of the basal ganglia and extended amygdala make a person with a substance use disorder seek the drug compulsively with reduced impulse control.

Some drugs like opioids also disrupt other parts of the brain, such as the brain stem, which controls basic functions critical to life, including heart rate, breathing, and sleeping. This interference explains why overdoses can cause depressed breathing and death.

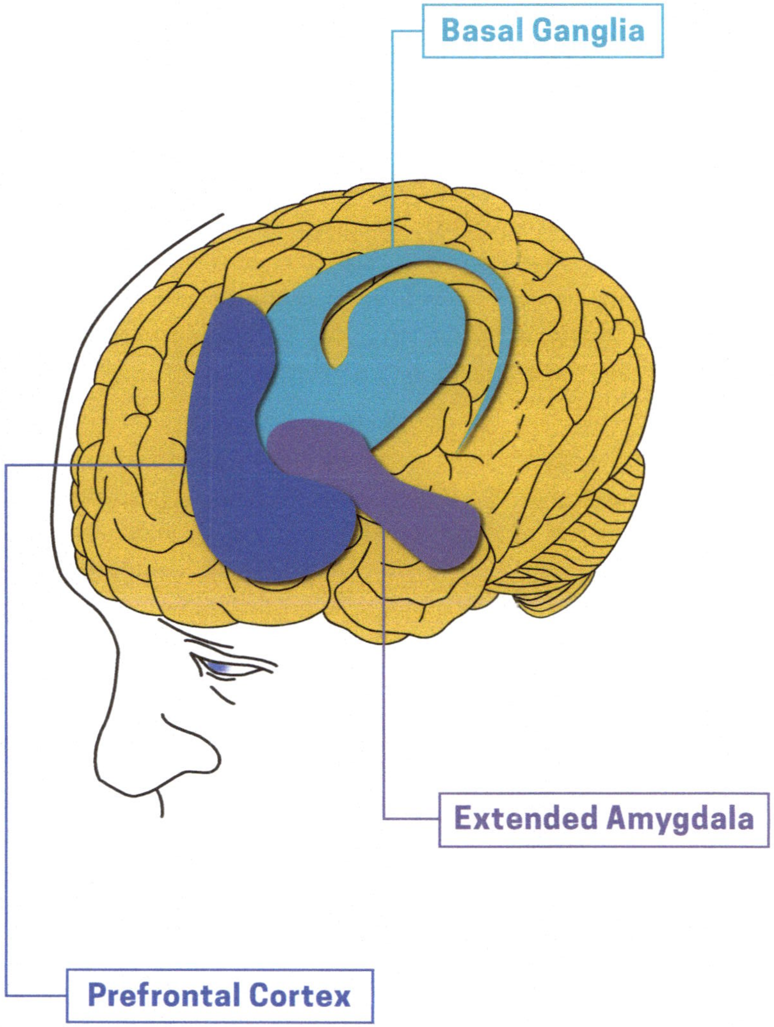


*Source: Facing Addiction in America: The Surgeon General's Report on Alcohol, Drugs, and Health*

## How do DRUGS PRODUCE PLEASURE?

Pleasure or euphoria — the high from drugs — is still poorly understood, but probably involves surges of chemical signaling compounds including the body's natural opioids (endorphins) and other neurotransmitters in parts of the basal ganglia (the reward circuit). When some drugs are taken, they can cause surges of these neurotransmitters much greater than the smaller bursts naturally produced in association with healthy rewards like eating, hearing or playing music, creative pursuits, or social interaction.

It was once thought that surges of the neurotransmitter *dopamine* produced by drugs directly caused the euphoria, but scientists now think dopamine has more to do with getting us to repeat pleasurable activities (reinforcement) than with producing pleasure directly.

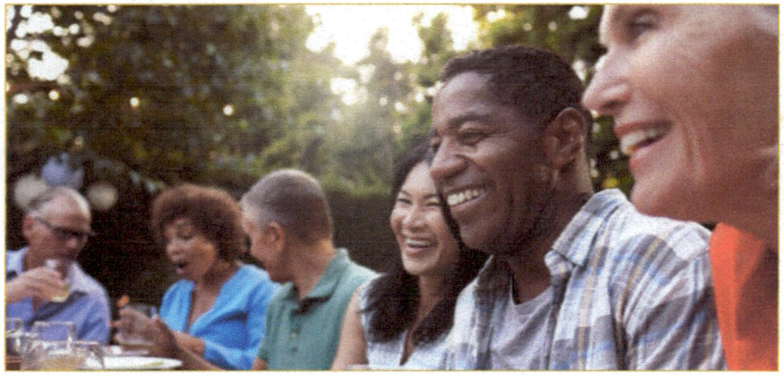

*Simple activities in everyday life can produce small bursts of neurotransmitters in the brain bringing pleasurable feelings. Drugs can hijack that process.*

## How does DOPAMINE REINFORCE DRUG USE?

The feeling of pleasure is how a healthy brain identifies and reinforces beneficial behaviors, such as eating, socializing, and sex. Our brains are wired to increase the odds that we will repeat pleasurable activities. The neurotransmitter dopamine is central to this. Whenever the reward circuit is activated by a healthy, pleasurable experience, a burst of dopamine signals that something important is happening that needs to be remembered. This dopamine signal causes changes in neural connectivity that make it easier to repeat the activity again and again without thinking about it, leading to the formation of habits.

Just as drugs produce intense euphoria, they also produce much larger surges of dopamine, powerfully reinforcing the connection between consumption of the drug, the resulting pleasure, and all the external cues linked to the experience. Large surges of dopamine "teach" the brain to seek drugs at the expense of other, healthier goals and activities.

Cues in a person's daily routine or environment that have become linked with drug use because of changes to the reward circuit can trigger uncontrollable cravings whenever the person is exposed to these cues, even if the drug itself is not available. This learned "reflex" can last a long time, even in people who haven't used drugs in many years. For example, people who have been drug free for a decade can experience cravings when returning to an old neighborhood or house where they used drugs. Like riding a bike, the brain remembers.

Why are drugs more addictive than

## NATURAL REWARDS?

For the brain, the difference between normal rewards and drug rewards can be likened to the difference between someone whispering into your ear and someone shouting into a microphone. Just as we turn down the volume on a radio that is too loud, the brain of someone who misuses drugs adjusts by producing fewer neurotransmitters in the reward circuit, or by reducing the number of receptors that can receive signals. As a result, the person's ability to experience pleasure from naturally rewarding (i.e., reinforcing) activities is also reduced.

This is why a person who misuses drugs eventually feels flat, without motivation, lifeless, and/or depressed, and is unable to enjoy things that were previously pleasurable. Now, the person needs to keep taking drugs to experience even a normal level of reward — which only makes the problem worse, like a vicious cycle. Also, the person will often need to take larger amounts of the drug to produce the familiar high — an effect known as *tolerance*.

### Some drugs target the brain's pleasure center

**Brain reward (dopamine pathways)**

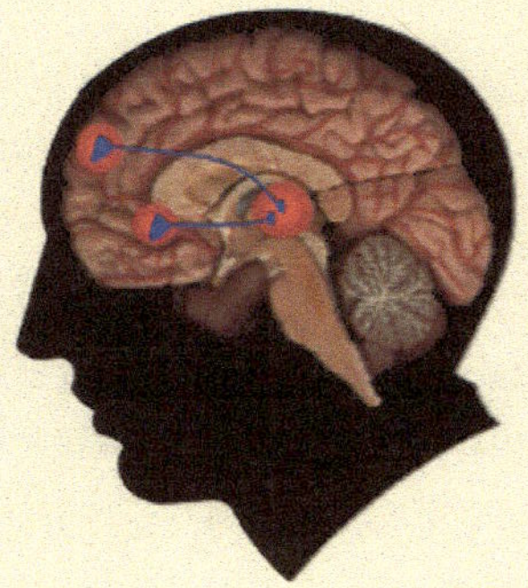

*These brain circuits are important for natural rewards such as food, music, and sex.*

**How drugs can increase dopamine**

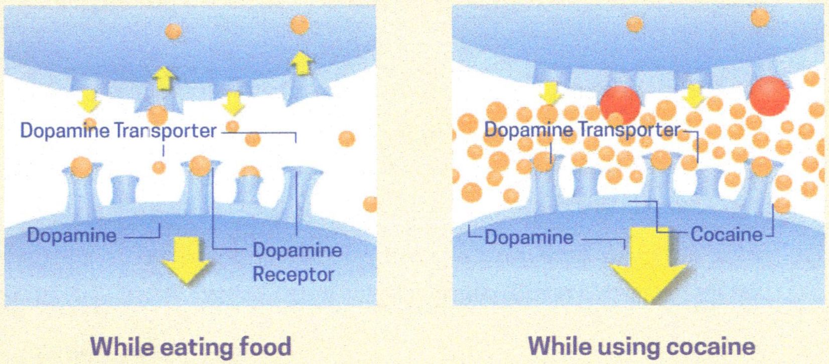


*Typically, dopamine increases in response to natural rewards such as food. When cocaine is taken, dopamine increases are exaggerated, and communication is denied.*

## *Long-term drug use impairs brain functioning.*

For more information on drugs and the brain, order NIDA's *Teaching Addiction Science* series or the *Mind Matters* series at *www.drugabuse.gov/parent-teacher.html*. These items and others are available to the public free of charge.

# Addiction and Health

## What are the other health CONSEQUENCES OF DRUG ADDICTION?

People with addiction often have one or more associated health issues, which could include lung or heart disease, stroke, cancer, or mental health conditions. Imaging scans, chest X-rays, and blood tests can show the damaging effects of long-term drug use throughout the body.

For example, it is now well-known that tobacco smoke can cause many cancers, methamphetamine can cause severe dental problems, known as meth mouth, and that opioids can lead to overdose and death. In addition, some drugs, such as inhalants, may damage or destroy nerve cells, either in the brain or the peripheral nervous system (the nervous system outside the brain and spinal cord).

Drug use can also increase the risk of contracting infections. HIV and hepatitis C (a serious liver disease) can occur from sharing injection equipment or from unsafe practices such as condom-less sex.[40,41] Infection of the heart and its valves (endocarditis) and skin infection (cellulitis) can occur after exposure to bacteria by injection drug use.[42]

## Does drug use cause OTHER MENTAL DISORDERS OR VICE VERSA?

Drug use and other mental disorders often co-exist. In some cases, mental disorders such as anxiety, depression, or schizophrenia may come before addiction. In other cases, drug use may trigger or worsen those mental health conditions, particularly in people with specific vulnerabilities.[43,44]

Some people with disorders like anxiety or depression may use drugs in an attempt to alleviate psychiatric symptoms. This may exacerbate their mental disorder in the long run, as well as increase the risk of developing addiction.[43,44] Treatment for all conditions should happen concurrently.

*Addiction and HIV/AIDS are intertwined health conditions.*

How can addiction
## HARM OTHER PEOPLE?

Beyond the harmful consequences for the person with the addiction, drug use can cause serious health problems for others. Some of the more severe consequences of addiction are:

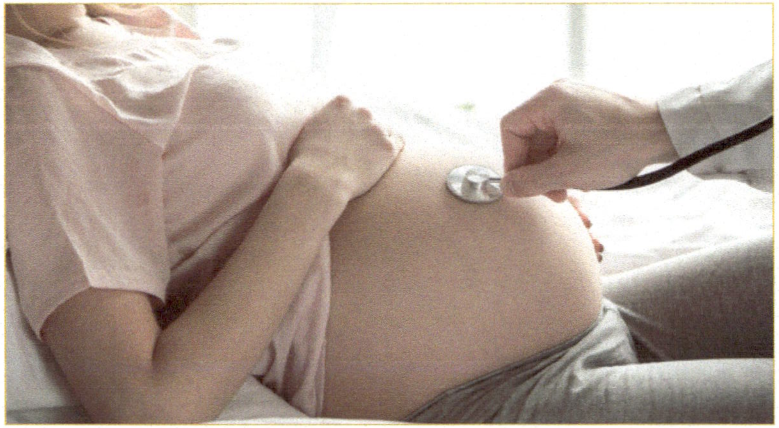

- **Negative effects of drug use while pregnant or breastfeeding** A mother's substance or medication use during pregnancy can cause her baby to go into withdrawal after it's born, which is called neonatal abstinence syndrome (NAS). Symptoms will differ depending on the substance used, but may include tremors, problems with sleeping and feeding, and even seizures.[45] Some drug-exposed children will have developmental problems with behavior, attention, and thinking. Ongoing research is exploring if these effects on the brain and behavior extend into the teen years, causing continued developmental problems. In addition, some substances can make their way into a mother's breast milk. Scientists are still learning about long-term effects on a child who is exposed to drugs through breastfeeding.

THE IMPACT OF ADDICTION CAN BE
## FAR-REACHING

- Heart disease
- Stroke
- Cancer
- HIV/AIDS
- Hepatitis B and C
- Endocarditis
- Cellulitis
- Lung disease
- Mental health conditions

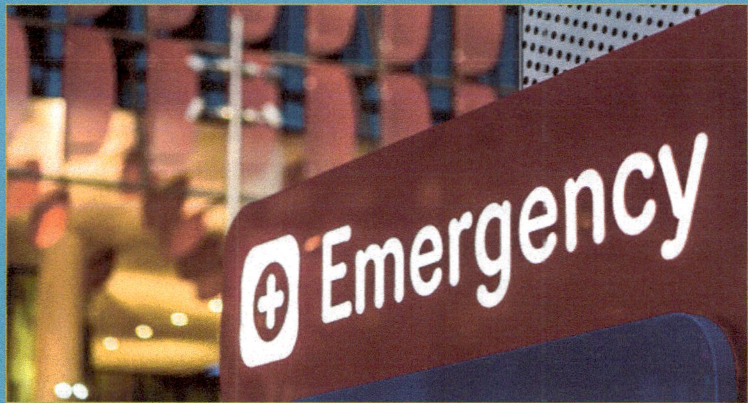

- **Negative effects of secondhand smoke**
  Secondhand tobacco smoke exposes bystanders to at least 250 chemicals that are known to be harmful, particularly to children.[46] Involuntary exposure to secondhand smoke increases the risks of heart disease and lung cancer in people who have never smoked.[5] Additionally, the known health risks of secondhand exposure to tobacco smoke raise questions about whether secondhand exposure to marijuana smoke poses similar risks. At this point, little research on this question has been conducted. However, a study found that some nonsmoking participants exposed for an hour to high-THC marijuana in an unventilated room reported mild effects of the drug, and another study showed positive urine tests in the hours directly following exposure.[47,48] If you inhale secondhand marijuana smoke, it's unlikely you would fail a drug test, but it is possible.

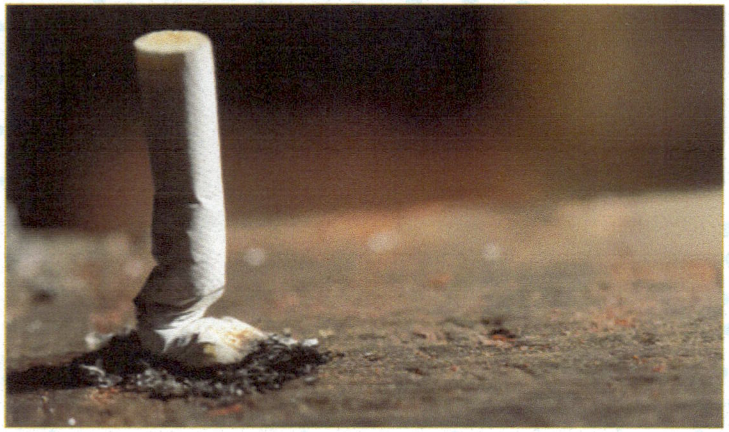

- **Increased spread of infectious diseases**
  Injection of drugs accounts for 1 in 10 of cases of HIV. Injection drug use is also a major factor in the spread of hepatitis C,[49] and can be the cause of endocarditis and cellulitis. Injection drug use is not the only way that drug use contributes to the spread of infectious diseases. Drugs that are misused can cause intoxication, which hinders judgment and increases the chance of risky sexual behaviors such as condom-less sex.
- **Increased risk of motor vehicle accidents**
  Use of illicit drugs or misuse of prescription drugs can make driving a car unsafe—just like driving after drinking alcohol. Drugged driving puts the driver, passengers, and others who share the road at risk. In 2016, almost 12 million people ages 16 or older reported driving under the influence of illicit drugs, including marijuana.[50] After alcohol, marijuana is the drug most often linked to impaired driving. Research studies have shown negative effects of marijuana on drivers, including an increase in lane weaving, poor reaction time, and altered attention to the road.

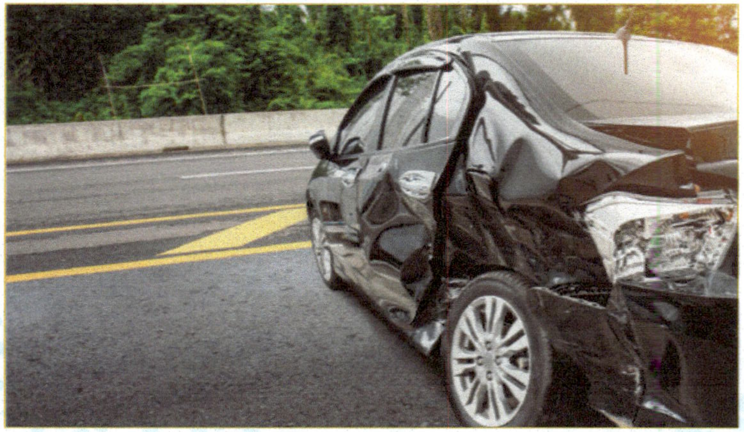

# Treatment and Recovery

## Can addiction be TREATED SUCCESSFULLY?

**Yes,** addiction is a treatable disorder. Research on the science of addiction and the treatment of substance use disorders has led to the development of research-based methods that help people to stop using drugs and resume productive lives, also known as being in *recovery*.

**Brain Recovery with Prolonged Abstinence**

Healthy Person

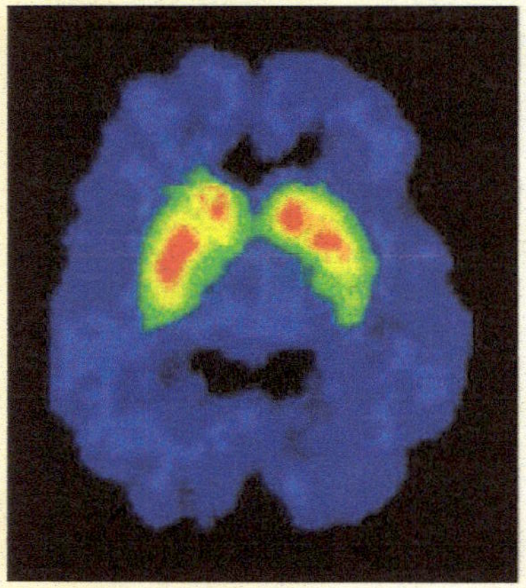

Meth User: 1 month abstinence

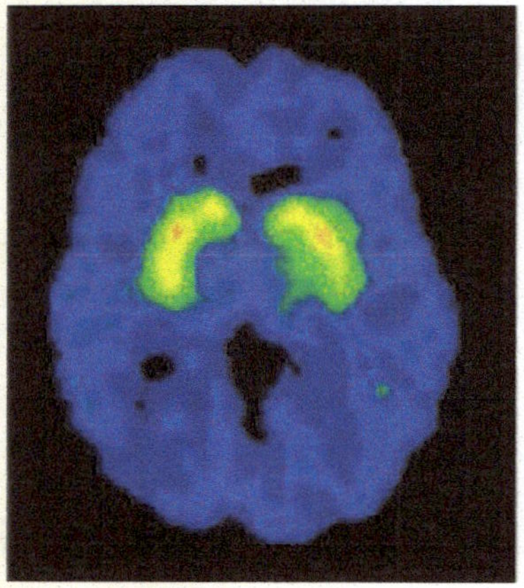

Meth User: 14 months abstinence

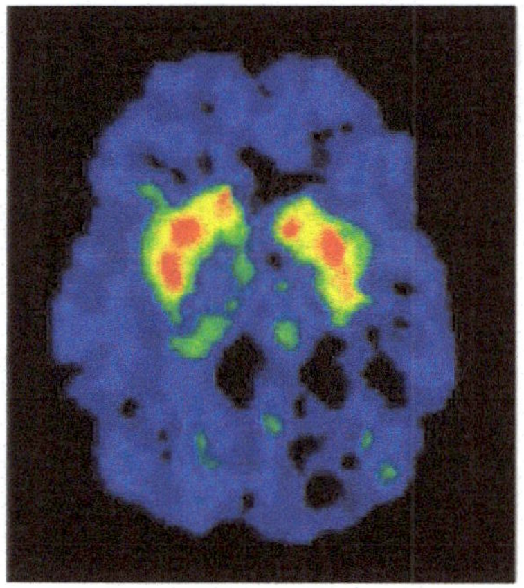

These images showing the density of dopamine transporters in the brain illustrate the brain's remarkable ability to recover, at least in part, after a long abstinence from drugs — in this case, methamphetamine.[51]

*Source: The Journal of Neuroscience, 21(23):9414-9418. 2001*

## Can addiction be CURED?

Like other chronic diseases such as heart disease or asthma, treatment for drug addiction usually isn't a cure. But addiction *can* be managed successfully. Treatment enables people to counteract addiction's disruptive effects on their brain and behavior and regain control of their lives.

Does relapse to drug use mean

## TREATMENT HAS FAILED?

**No.** The chronic nature of addiction means that for some people *relapse,* or a return to drug use after an attempt to stop, can be part of the process, but newer treatments are designed to help with relapse prevention. Relapse rates for drug use are similar to rates for other chronic medical illnesses. If people stop following their medical treatment plan, they are likely to relapse.

Treatment of chronic diseases involves changing deeply rooted behaviors, and relapse doesn't mean treatment has failed. When a person recovering from an addiction relapses, it indicates that the person needs to speak with their doctor to resume treatment, modify it, or try another treatment.[52]

**Comparison of Relapse Rates Between Substance Use Disorders and Other Chronic Illnesses**

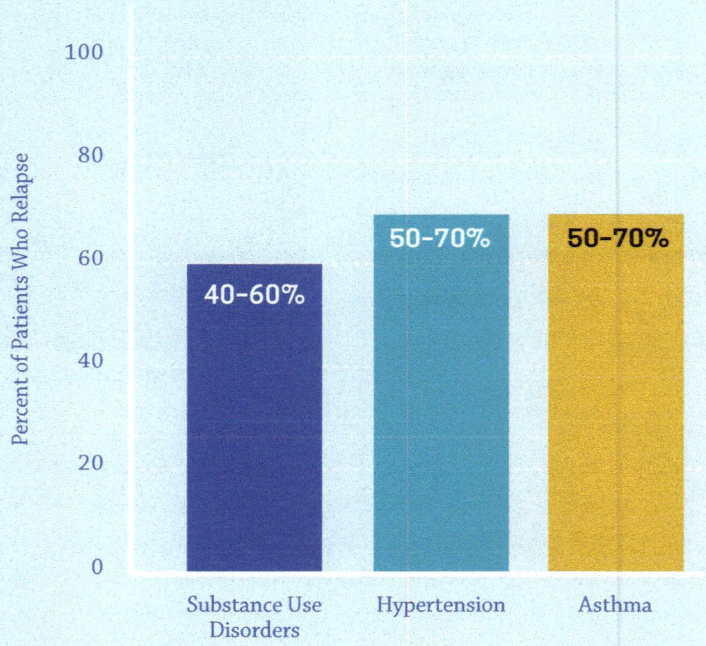


*Source: JAMA, 284:1689-1695, 2000*

*Relapse rates for people treated for substance use disorders are compared with those for people treated for high blood pressure and asthma. Relapse is common and similar across these illnesses. Therefore, substance use disorders should be treated like any other chronic illness. Relapse serves as a sign for resumed, modified, or new treatment.*

*While relapse is a normal part of recovery, for some drugs, it can be very dangerous — even deadly. If a person uses as much of the drug as they did before quitting, they can easily overdose because their bodies are no longer adapted to their previous level of drug exposure. An overdose happens when the person uses enough of a drug to produce uncomfortable feelings, life-threatening symptoms, or death.*

What are the principles of

## EFFECTIVE TREATMENT?

Research shows that when treating addictions to opioids (prescription pain relievers or drugs like heroin or fentanyl), medication should be the first line of treatment, usually combined with some form of behavioral therapy or counseling. Medications are also available to help treat addiction to alcohol and nicotine.

Additionally, medications are used to help people detoxify from drugs, although detoxification is not the same as treatment and is not sufficient to help a person recover. Detoxification alone without subsequent treatment generally leads to resumption of drug use.

For people with addictions to drugs like stimulants or cannabis, no medications are currently available to assist in treatment, so treatment consists of behavioral therapies. Treatment should be tailored to address each patient's drug use patterns and drug-related medical, mental, and social problems.

*Discoveries in science lead to breakthroughs in drug use treatment.*

What medications and devices help

## TREAT DRUG ADDICTION?

Different types of medications and devices may be useful at different stages of treatment to help a patient stop using drugs, stay in treatment, and avoid relapse.

- **Treating withdrawal.** When patients first stop using drugs, they can experience various physical and emotional symptoms, including restlessness or sleeplessness, as well as depression, anxiety, and other mental health conditions. Certain treatment medications and devices reduce these symptoms, which makes it easier to stop the drug use.
- **Staying in treatment.** Some treatment medications and mobile applications are used to help the brain adapt gradually to the absence of the drug. These treatments act slowly to help prevent drug cravings and have a calming effect on body systems. They can help patients focus on counseling and other psychotherapies related to their drug treatment.
- **Preventing relapse.** Science has taught us that stress cues linked to the drug use (such as people, places, things, and moods), and contact with drugs are the most common triggers for relapse. Scientists have been developing therapies to interfere with these triggers to help patients stay in recovery.

## COMMON MEDICATIONS USED TO TREAT DRUG ADDICTION AND WITHDRAWAL

### Opioid

- Methadone
- Buprenorphine
- Extended-release naltrexone
- Lofexidine

### Nicotine

- Nicotine replacement therapies (available as a patch, inhaler, or gum)
- Bupropion
- Varenicline

### Alcohol

- Naltrexone
- Disulfiram
- Acamprosate

How do behavioral therapies

## TREAT DRUG ADDICTION?

Behavioral therapies help people in drug addiction treatment modify their attitudes and behaviors related to drug use. As a result, patients are able to handle stressful situations and various triggers that might cause another relapse. Behavioral therapies can also enhance the effectiveness of medications and help people remain in treatment longer.

- **Cognitive-behavioral therapy** seeks to help patients recognize, avoid, and cope with the situations in which they're most likely to use drugs.
- **Contingency management** uses positive reinforcement such as providing rewards or privileges for remaining drug-free, for attending and participating in counseling sessions, or for taking treatment medications as prescribed.
- **Motivational enhancement therapy** uses strategies to make the most of people's readiness to change their behavior and enter treatment.
- **Family therapy** helps people (especially young people) with drug use problems, as well as their families, address influences on drug use patterns and improve overall family functioning.
- **Twelve-step facilitation (TSF)** is an individual therapy typically delivered in 12 weekly session to prepare people to become engaged in 12-step mutual support programs. 12-step programs, like Alcoholic Anonymous, are not medical treatments, but provide social and complementary support to those treatments. TSF follows the 12-step themes of acceptance, surrender, and active involvement in recovery.

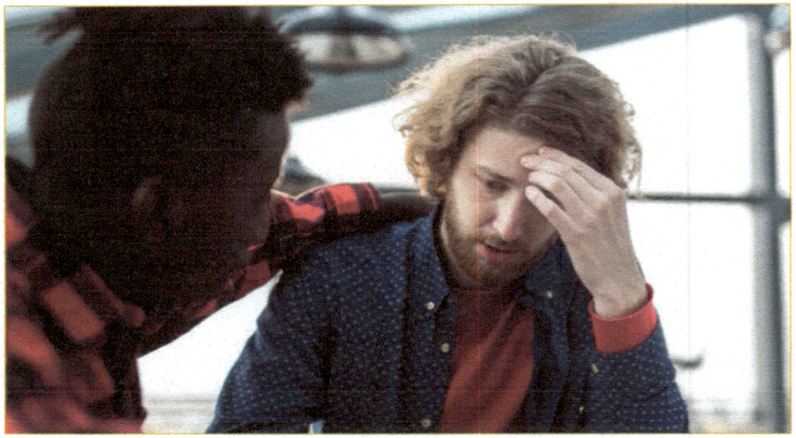

How do quality treatment programs help patients

## RECOVER FROM ADDICTION?

Stopping drug use is just one part of a long and complex recovery process. When people enter treatment, addiction has often caused serious consequences in their lives, possibly disrupting their health and how they function in their family lives, at work, and in the community.

Because addiction can affect so many aspects of a person's life, treatment should address the needs of the whole person to be successful. Counselors may select from a menu of services that meet the specific medical, mental, social, occupational, family, and legal needs of their patients to help in their recovery.

For more information on drug treatment, see *Principles of Drug Addiction Treatment: A Research-Based Guide*, and *Principles of Adolescent Substance Use Disorder Treatment: A Research-Based Guide.*

*Treatment must address the whole person.*

# Citations


1. National Drug Intelligence Center. *The economic impact of illicit drug use on American society.* Washington, DC: United States Department of Justice, 2011.
2. Rehm J, Mathers C, Popova S, Thavorncharoensap M, Teerawattananon Y, Patra J. Global burden of disease and injury and economic cost attributable to alcohol use and alcohol-use disorders. Lancet 373(9682):2223-2233, 2009.
3. Centers for Disease Control and Prevention. *Best Practices for Comprehensive Tobacco Control Programs* — 2014. Atlanta: U.S. Department of Health and Human Services, Centers for Disease Control and Prevention, National Center for Chronic Disease Prevention and Health Promotion, Office on Smoking and Health, 2014.
4. Centers for Disease Control and Prevention. (2020, March 20). Drug and Opioid-Involved Overdose Deaths — United States, 2017–2018. *Morbidity and Mortality Weekly Reports.* Retrieved from https://www.cdc.gov/mmwr/volumes/69/wr/mm6911a4.htm
5. U.S. Department of Health and Human Services. *The Health Consequences of Smoking—50 Years of Progress: A Report of the Surgeon General.* Atlanta, GA: U.S. Department of Health and Human Services, Centers for Disease Control and Prevention, National Center for Chronic Disease Prevention and Health Promotion, Office on Smoking and Health, 2014.
6. Tice P, Lipari R, van Horn S. *Substance Use among 12th Grade Aged Youths, by Dropout Status.* Rockville, MD: Center for Health Statistics and Quality, Substance Abuse and Mental Health Administration; 2017. https://www.samhsa.gov/data/sites/default/files/report_3196/ShortReport-3196.pdf. Accessed June 4, 2018.
7. Chen C-Y, Storr CL, Anthony JC. Early-onset drug use and risk for drug dependence problems. *Addict Behav.* 2009;34(3):319-322. doi:10.1016/j.addbeh.2008.10.021
8. Lander L, Howsare J, Byrne M. The impact of substance use disorders on families and children: from theory to practice. *Soc Work Public Health.* 2013;28(0):194-205. doi:10.1080/19371918.2013.759005
9. Simmons LA, Havens JR, Whiting JB, Holz JL, Bada H. Illicit drug use among women with children in the United States: 2002–2003. *Ann Epidemiol.* 2009;19(3):187-193. doi:10.1016/j.annepidem.2008.12.007
10. Shankaran S, Lester BM, Das A, Bauer CR, Bada HS, Lagasse L, Higgins R. Impact of maternal substance use during pregnancy on childhood outcome. *Semin Fetal Neonatal Med* 12(2):143-150, 2007.
11. Goldstein RZ, Volkow ND. Dysfunction of the prefrontal cortex in addiction: neuroimaging findings and clinical implications. *Nat Rev Neurosci.* 2011;12(11):652-669. doi:10.1038/nrn3119
12. Fowler JS, Volkow ND, Kassed CA, Chang L. Imaging the addicted human brain. *Sci Pract Perspect* 3(2):4-16, 2007.
13. Grant B, S Stinson F, Harford T. Grant BF, Stinson FS, Harford TC. Age at onset of alcohol use and DSM-IV alcohol abuse and dependence: a 12-year follow-up. *J Subst Abuse.* 2001;13:493-504. doi:10.1016/S0899-3289(01)00096-7
14. Zucker RA, Donovan JE, Masten AS, Mattson ME, Moss HB. Early developmental processes and the continuity of risk for underage drinking and problem drinking. *Pediatrics.* 2008;121 Suppl 4:S252-S272. doi:10.1542/peds.2007-2243B

15. DiClemente CC, Fairhurst SK, Piotrowski NA. Self-efficacy and addictive behaviors. In: *Self-Efficacy, Adaptation, and Adjustment: Theory, Research, and Application*. The Plenum series in social/clinical psychology. New York, NY, US: Plenum Press; 1995:109-141.

16. Hill KG, Hawkins JD, Catalano RF, Abbott RD, Guo J. Family influences on the risk of daily smoking initiation. *J Adolesc Health Off Publ Soc Adolesc Med*. 2005;37(3):202-210. doi:10.1016/j.jadohealth.2004.08.014

17. Guo J, Hawkins JD, Hill KG, Abbott RD. Childhood and adolescent predictors of alcohol abuse and dependence in young adulthood. *J Stud Alcohol*. 2001;62(6):754-762.

18. Brook JS, Brook DW, Gordon AS, Whiteman M, Cohen P. The psychosocial etiology of adolescent drug use: a family interactional approach. *Genet Soc Gen Psychol Monogr*. 1990;116(2):111-267.

19. Duncan GJ, Wilkerson B, England P. Cleaning up their act: The effects of marriage and cohabitation on licit and illicit drug use. *Demography*. 2006;43(4):691-710. doi:10.1353/dem.2006.0032

20. Chassin L, Pitts SC, Prost J. Binge drinking trajectories from adolescence to emerging adulthood in a high-risk sample: predictors and substance abuse outcomes. *J Consult Clin Psychol*. 2002;70(1):67-78.

21. Sher KJ, Rutledge PC. Heavy drinking across the transition to college: predicting first-semester heavy drinking from precollege variables. *Addict Behav*. 2007;32(4):819-835. doi:10.1016/j.addbeh.2006.06.024

22. National Institute on Drug Abuse. *Preventing Drug Use Among Children and Adolescents, A Research-Based Guide for Parents, Educators and Community Leaders* Second Edition, 2003. Bethesda, MD: U.S. Department of Health and Human Services, National Institutes of Health, National Institute on Drug Abuse, 2003.

23. Brook JS, Kessler RC, Cohen P. The onset of marijuana use from preadolescence and early adolescence to young adulthood. *Dev Psychopathol*. 1999;11(4):901-914.

24. Herting JR, Guest AM. Components of satisfaction with local areas in the metropolis. *Sociol Q*. 1985;26(1):99-116. doi:10.1111/j.1533-8525.1985.tb00218.x

25. Hawkins JD, Arthur MW, Catalano RF. Preventing substance abuse. *Crime Justice*. 1995;19:343-427. doi:10.1086/449234

26. Chalk R, Phillips DA. *Youth Development and Neighborhood Influences: Challenges and Opportunities*. National Academies Press; 1997.

27. Bevilacqua L, Goldman D. Genes and addictions. *Clin Pharmacol Ther*. 2009;85(4):359-361. doi:10.1038/clpt.2009.6

28. Substance Abuse and Mental Health Services Administration. *Mental and Substance Use Disorders*. https://www.samhsa.gov/disorders. Published June 20, 2014. Accessed June 4, 2018.

29. Biederman J, Faraone SV, Monuteaux MC, Feighner JA. Patterns of alcohol and drug use in adolescents can be predicted by parental substance use disorders. *Pediatrics*. 2000;106(4):792-797.

30. Whitesell M, Bachand A, Peel J, Brown M. Familial, social, and individual factors contributing to risk for adolescent substance use. *Journal of Addiction*. https://www.hindawi.com/journals/jad/2013/579310/. Published 2013. Accessed June 4, 2018.

31. Substance Abuse and Mental Health Services Administration. *Mental and Substance Use Disorders*. https://www.samhsa.gov/disorders. Published June 20, 2014. Accessed June 4, 2018.

32. Lynskey MT, Heath AC, Bucholz KK, Slutske WS, Madden PAF, Nelson EC, Statham DJ, Martin NG. Escalation of drug use in early-onset cannabis users vs co-twin controls. *JAMA* 289: 427-33, 2003.

33. Squeglia LM, Jacobus J, Tapert SF. The influence of substance use on adolescent brain development. *Clin Neurosci Soc ENCS*. 2009;40(1):31-38.

34. Verebey K, Gold MS. From coca leaves to crack: the effects of dose and routes of administration in abuse liability. *Psychiatr Annals* 18:513–520, 1988.

35. Hatsukami DK, Fischman MW. Crack cocaine and cocaine hydrochloride: Are the differences myth or reality. *JAMA* 276:1580-1588, 1996.

36. Krohn MD, Lizotte AJ, Perez CM. The interrelationship between substance use and precocious transitions to adult statuses. *J Health Soc Behav* 38(1):87-103, 1997.

37. Gogtay N, Giedd JN, Lusk L, Hayashi KM, Greenstein D, Vaituzis AC, Nugent TF 3rd, Herman DH, Clasen LS, Toga AW, Rapoport JL, Thompson PM. Dynamic mapping of human cortical development during childhood through early adulthood. *Proc Natl Acad Sci* 101(21):8174-8179, 2004.

38. National Institute on Drug Abuse. *Preventing Drug Abuse among Children and Adolescents: A Research-Based Guide for Parents, Educators, and Community Leaders (Second Edition)* (NIH Publication No. 04-4212[A]). Rockville, MD, 2003.

39. Johnston, LD, O'Malley, PM, Miech, RA, Bachman, JG, & Schulenberg, JE (2014). *Monitoring the Future national survey results on drug use: 1975-2013: Overview, key findings on adolescent drug use.* Ann Arbor: Institute for Social Research, The University of Michigan.

40. Washington State Institute for Public Policy. (2017). Benefit-cost results. Retrieved from http://www.wsipp.wa.gov/BenefitCost?topicId=. Accessed on June 14, 2018.

41. El-Bassel N, Shaw SA, Dasgupta A, Strathdee SA. Drug use as a driver of HIV risks: re-emerging and emerging issues. *Curr Opin HIV AIDS*. 2014;9(2):150-155. doi:10.1097/COH.0000000000000035

42. Klevens RM, Hu DJ, Jiles R, Holmberg SD. Evolving epidemiology of hepatitis C virus in the United States. *Clin Infect Dis Off Publ Infect Dis Soc Am*. 2012;55 Suppl 1:S3-S9. doi:10.1093/cid/cis393

43. Moss R, Munt B. Injection drug use and right sided endocarditis. *Heart*. 2003;89(5):577-581.

44. Kelly TM, Daley DC. Integrated treatment of substance use and psychiatric disorders. *Soc Work Public Health*. 2013;28(0):388-406. doi:10.1080/19371918.2013.774673

45. Ross S, Peselow E. Co-occurring psychotic and addictive disorders: neurobiology and diagnosis. *Clin Neuropharmacol*. 2012;35(5):235-243. doi:10.1097/WNF.0b013e318261e193

46. Ko JY, Wolicki S, Barfield WD, et al. CDC Grand Rounds: public health strategies to prevent neonatal abstinence syndrome. *MMWR Morb Mortal Wkly Rep*. 2017;66. doi:10.15585/mmwr.mm6609a2

47. National Cancer Institute. *Secondhand Smoke and Cancer.* National Cancer Institute. https://www.cancer.gov/about-cancer/causes-prevention/risk/tobacco/second-hand-smoke-fact-sheet. Published January 12, 2011. Accessed June 4, 2018.

48. Röhrich J, Schimmel I, Zörntlein S, et al. Concentrations of delta9-tetrahydrocannabinol and 11-nor-9-carboxytetrahydrocannabinol in blood and urine after passive exposure to Cannabis smoke in a coffee shop. *J Anal Toxicol*. 2010;34(4):196-203.

49. Cone EJ, Bigelow GE, Herrmann ES, et al. Non-smoker exposure to secondhand cannabis smoke. I. Urine screening and confirmation results. *J Anal Toxicol*. 2015;39(1):1-12. doi:10.1093/jat/bku116

50. Zibbell JE, Asher AK, Patel RC, et al. Increases in acute hepatitis C virus infection related to a growing opioid epidemic and associated injection drug use, United States, 2004 to 2014. Am J Public Health. 2018;108(2). https://ajph.aphapublications.org/doi/10.2105/AJPH.2017.304132. Accessed June 4, 2018.

51. Center for Behavioral Health Statistics and Quality. *Results from the 2016 National Survey on Drug Use and Health: Detailed Tables.* Rockville, MD: Substance Abuse and Mental Health Services Administration; 2017.

52. Volkow ND, Chang L, Wang GJ, Fowler JS, Franceschi D, Sedler M, Gatley SJ, Miller E, Hitzemann R, Ding YS, Logan J. Loss of dopamine transporters in methamphetamine abusers recovers with protracted abstinence. *J Neurosci* 21(23):9414-9418, 2001.

53. McLellan AT, Lewis DC, O'Brien CP, Kleber HD. Drug dependence, a chronic medical illness: implications for treatment, insurance, and outcomes evaluation. *JAMA* 284(13):1689-1695, 2000.

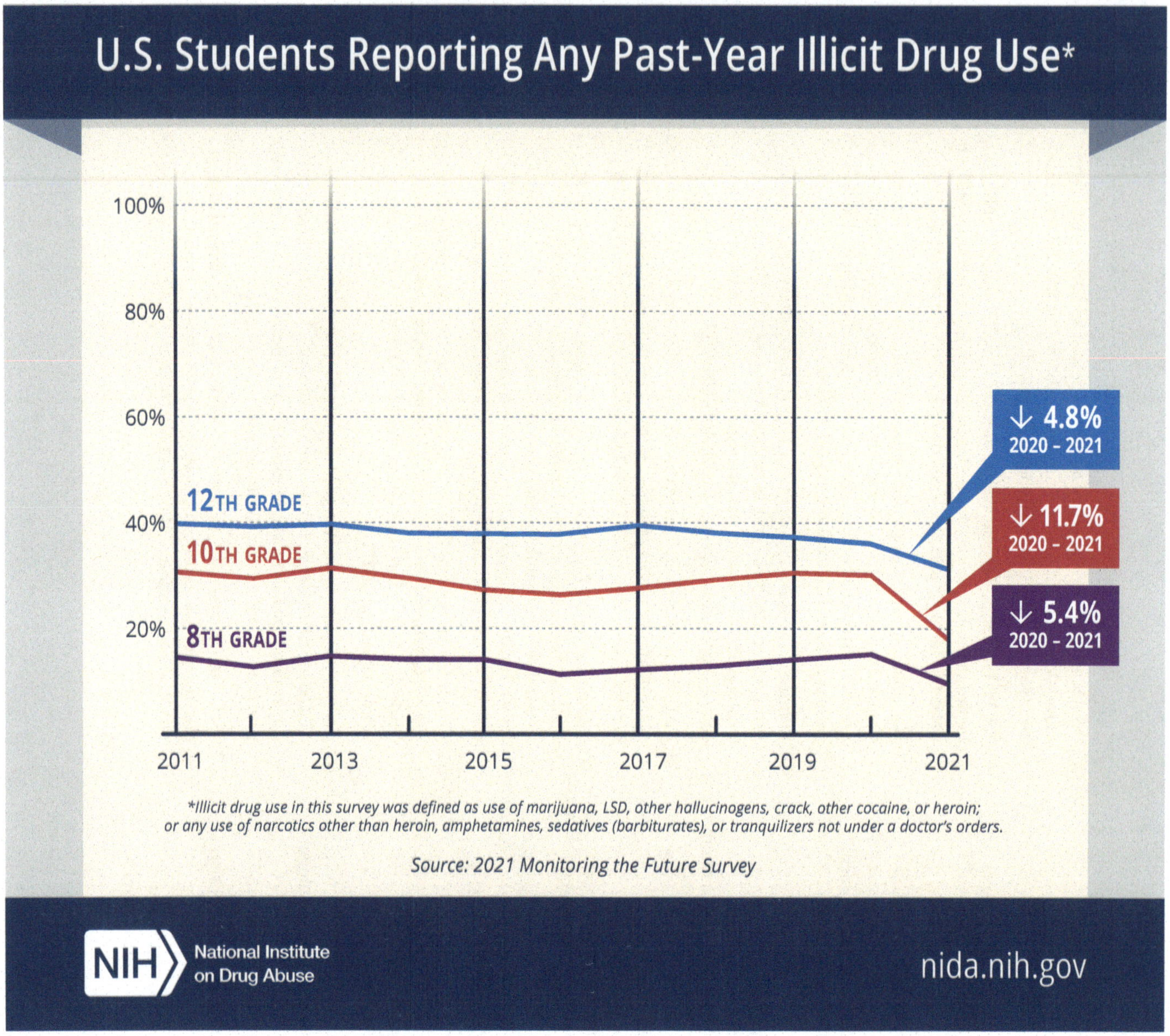
U.S. Students Reporting Any Past-Year Illicit Drug Use*
100%
80%
60%
40%
20%
12TH GRADE
10TH GRADE
8TH GRADE
2011
2013
2015
2017
2019
2021
↓ 4.8%
2020 - 2021
↓ 11.7%
2020 - 2021
↓ 5.4%
2020 - 2021
*Illicit drug use in this survey was defined as use of marijuana, LSD, other hallucinogens, crack, other cocaine, or heroin; or any use of narcotics other than heroin, amphetamines, sedatives (barbiturates), or tranquilizers not under a doctor's orders.
Source: 2021 Monitoring the Future Survey
NIH
National Institute
on Drug Abuse
nida.nih.gov

THE SURGEON GENERAL'S CALL TO ACTION

# TO PREVENT AND REDUCE UNDERAGE DRINKING

## What It Means to **YOU**

***A Guide to Action for Families***

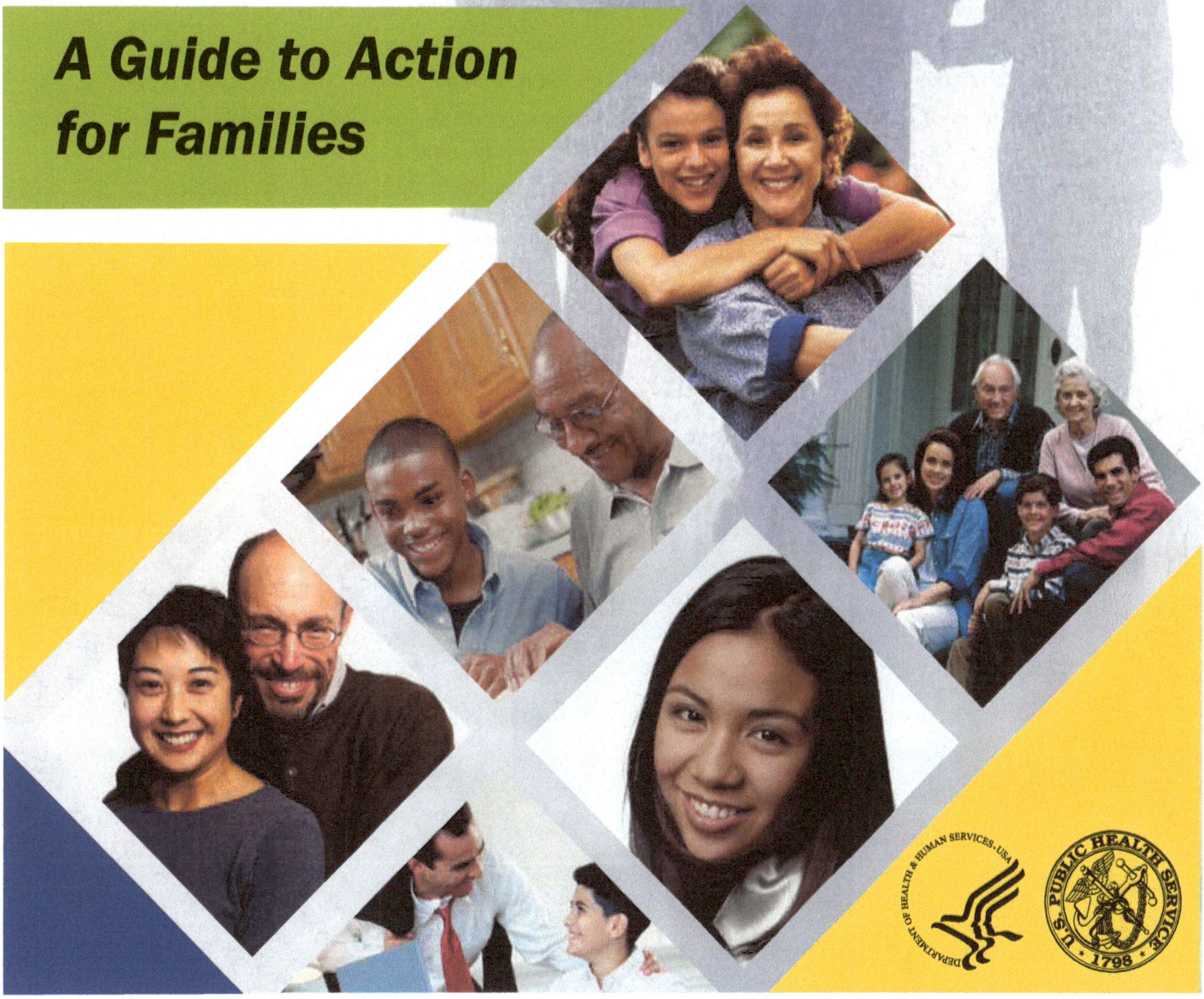

# TODAY, NEARLY 10.8 MILLION YOUTH, AGES 12-20, ARE UNDERAGE DRINKERS

Drinking alcohol can harm the growing body and brain. That's why it's important for young people to grow up alcohol-free. And it takes everyone to help young people choose not to drink alcohol. It takes you.

## What Is Underage Drinking?

When anyone under age 21 drinks alcohol, we call it underage drinking. And underage drinking is against the law, except in special cases, such as when it is part of a religious ceremony. Underage drinking is also dangerous. It can harm the mind and body of a growing teen in ways many people don't realize.

Yet, children and teens still drink, even though it can harm them. Underage drinking is a serious problem, with roots deep in our culture. It is time to change that picture. It's time to take action. It's time to stop looking the other way. It's time to tell children and teens that underage drinking is not okay. It will take a lot of work over time to change how people think about underage drinking. It's a long-term project for parents, schools, local groups, community leaders, and other concerned adults. And it's a project that should start when children are young and continue through the teen years.

- In any month, more youth are drinking than are smoking cigarettes or using marijuana.

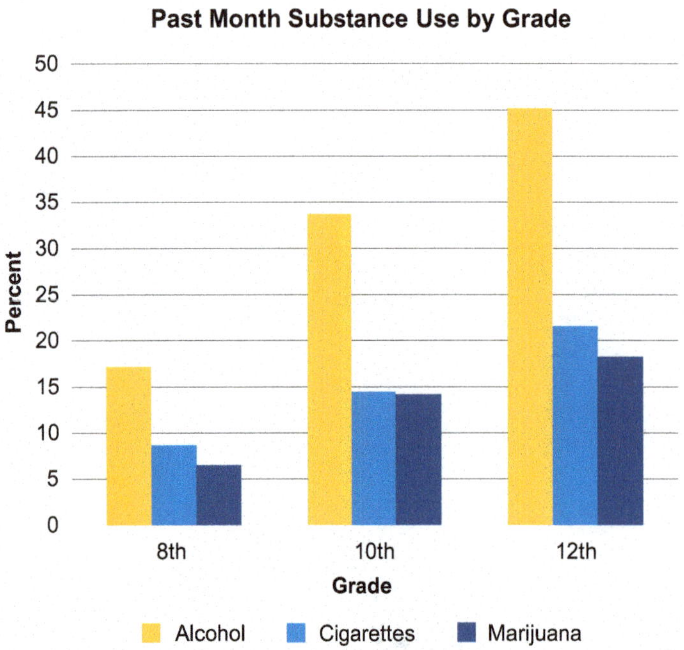


—Johnston, et al. *2006 Monitoring the Future National Survey Results on Drug Use.*

**More teens drink alcohol than smoke or use drugs.**

# THE FACTS

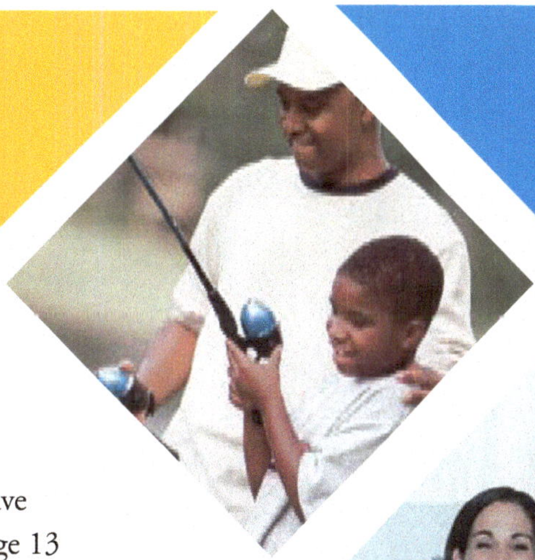

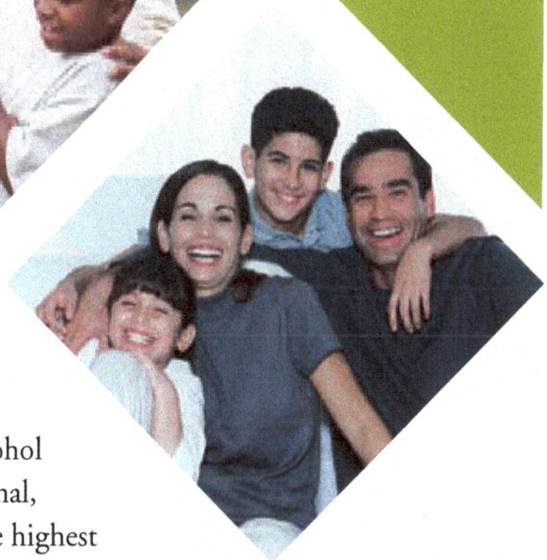

- As they grow older, the chance that young people will use alcohol grows. Approximately 10% of 12-year-olds say they have used alcohol at least once. By age 13 that number doubles. And by age 15, approximately 50% have had at least one drink.
- Alcohol dependence is a term doctors use when people have trouble controlling their drinking, and when their consumption of, or preoccupation with, alcohol occurs to the extent that it interferes with normal personal, family, social, or work life. Alcohol dependence rates are highest among young people between ages 18 and 20. And they're not even old enough to drink legally.

## Did You Know?

- The greatest influence on young people's decisions to begin drinking is the world they live in, which includes their families, friends, schools, the larger community, and society as a whole.
- Alcohol use by young people often is made possible by adults. After all, teens can't legally get alcohol on their own.

### FAST FACT

Most young people who start drinking before age 21 do so when they are about 13-14 years old. That's why it's important to start talking early and keep talking about underage drinking. And that's why ALL adults working with young people should send the same message that underage drinking is not okay.

# WHAT IS "A DRINK," ANYWAY?

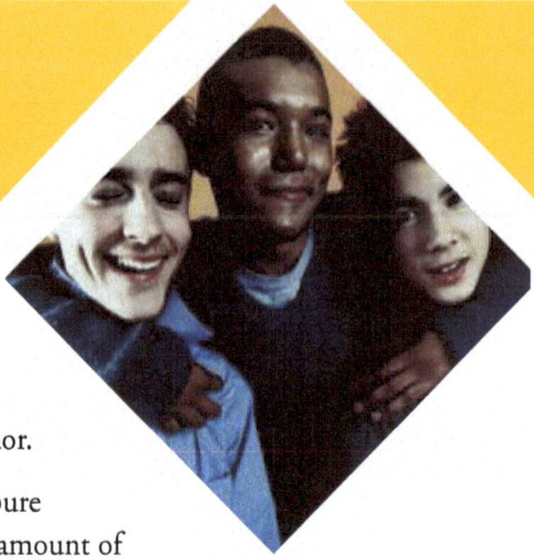

A drink can come in many forms. It can be a shot of hard liquor or a mixed drink containing vodka, rum, tequila, gin, scotch, etc. It can also be wine, a wine cooler, beer, or malt liquor.

A standard drink is any drink that contains about 14 grams of pure alcohol (about 0.6 fluid ounces or 1.2 tablespoons). This is the amount of alcohol usually found in—

- One 12-ounce beer
- One 4- to 5-ounce glass of wine
- One 1.5-ounce shot of 80 proof liquor

## What's a Standard Drink?

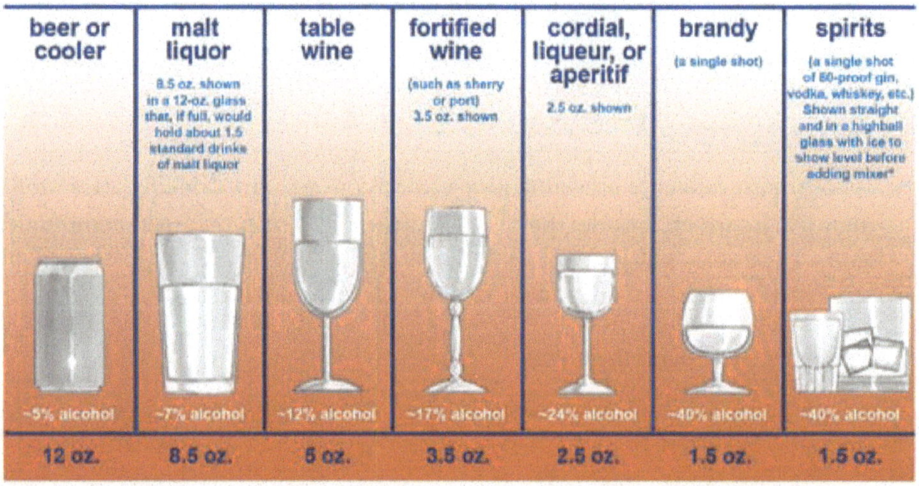


*Note: It can be difficult to estimate the number of standard drinks served in a single mixed drink made with hard liquor. Depending on factors, such as type of spirits and the recipe, one mixed drink can contain from one to three or more standard drinks.

But not all drinks are standard drinks. In fact, different drinks often have different amounts of alcohol. Mixed drinks may contain more than one shot of liquor, and different beers or wines may not have the same amount of alcohol in them, even when the drinks are the same size. For example, some beers and beer products, like "ice" beers, and malt liquors, and some wines, have more alcohol than others.

**Remember, the legal drinking age is 21 and underage drinking can be a threat to health and development.**

# WHY IS UNDERAGE DRINKING A PROBLEM?

**So many young people drink.** Many more young people use alcohol than tobacco or illegal drugs. By age 18, more than 70% of teens have had at least one drink.

**When young people drink, they drink a lot at one time.** Teens drink less often than adults. But when teens do drink, they drink more than adults. On average, young people have about 5 drinks on a single occasion. This is called binge drinking, a very dangerous way of drinking that can lead to serious problems and even death.

**Early drinking can cause later alcohol problems.** Of adults who started drinking before age 15, around 40% say they have the signs of alcohol dependence. That rate is four times higher than for adults who didn't drink until they were age 21.

**Percent of Youth Who Have Used Alcohol by Age and Gender**

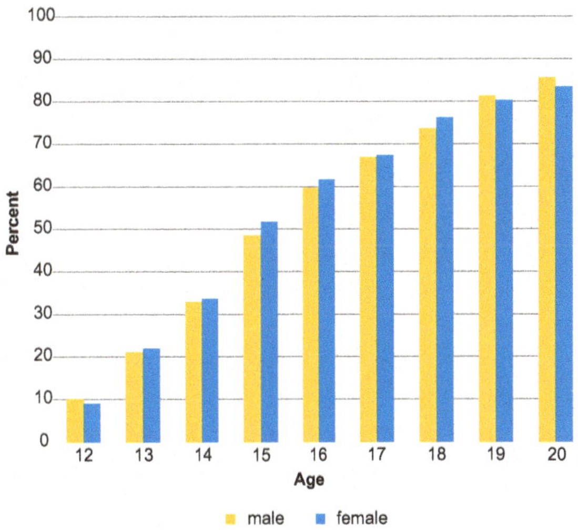


—SAMHSA, *2005 National Survey on Drug Use & Health (NSDUH)*

**FAST FACT**

Rates of death and injury nearly triple between the early teen years and early adult life. Dangerous activities like underage drinking play a large role. That's why ending teen alcohol use can help save lives.

**Alcohol may have a special appeal for young people.** The teen years are a time of adventure, challenges, and taking risks. Alcohol is often one of the risks young people take. But most people don't know how alcohol affects a teen's body and behavior. They don't realize that alcohol can affect young people in different ways from adults. And they don't realize that underage drinkers can also harm people other than themselves.

# THE RESULTS OF UNDERAGE DRINKING CAN BE GRAVE

## Many people don't know that underage alcohol use—

- **Is a major cause of death from injuries among young people.** Each year, approximately 5,000 people under the age of 21 die as a result of underage drinking; this includes about 1,900 deaths from motor vehicle crashes, 1,600 as a result of homicides, 300 from suicide, as well as hundreds from other injuries such as falls, burns, and drownings.
- **Increases the risk of carrying out, or being a victim of, a physical or sexual assault.**
- **Can affect the body in many ways.** The effects of alcohol range from hangovers to death from alcohol poisoning.
- **Can lead to other problems.** These may include bad grades in school, run-ins with the law, and drug use.
- **Affects how well a young person judges risk and makes sound decisions.** For example, after drinking, a teen may see nothing wrong with driving a car or riding with a driver who has been drinking.
- **Plays a role in risky sexual activity.** This can increase the chance of teen pregnancy and sexually transmitted diseases (STDs), including HIV, the virus that causes AIDS.
- **Can harm the growing brain, especially when teens drink a lot.** Today we know that the brain continues to develop from birth through the teen years into the mid-20s.

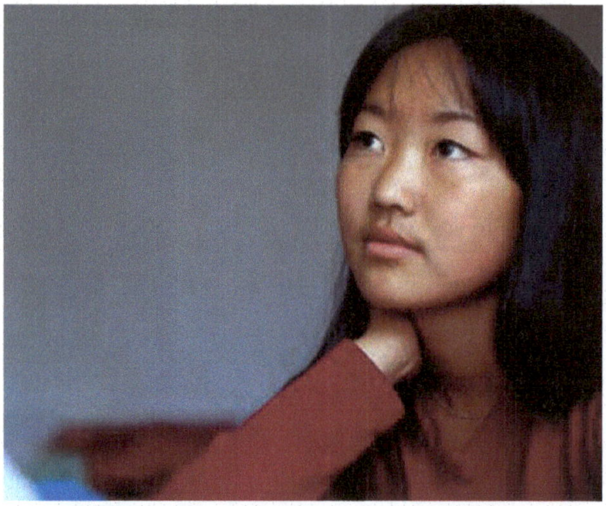

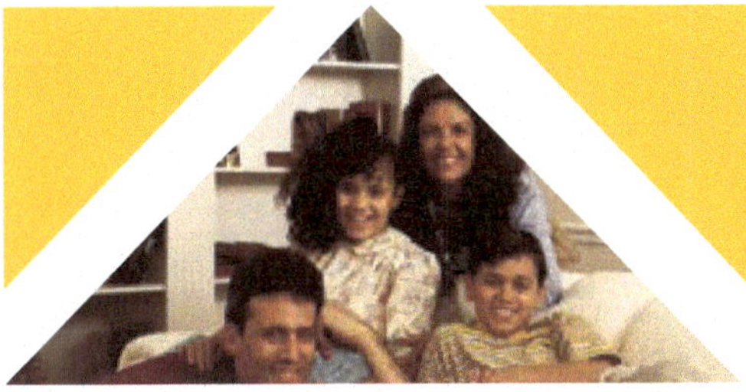

## The Teen Years Are a Time of Many Changes

- Boys physically become young men and girls become young women.
- Young people move from elementary to middle to high school. Responsibilities increase. For example, teens learn to drive, may get a job, and have more chores and more homework.
- Teens spend less time with their parents. They spend more time alone or with friends. They also like to stay up later and sleep in.
- Teens search for who they really are and who they want to be. They worry about friendships and social groups. And they have growing romantic and sexual interests.
- The desire for adventure, excitement, and action increases. That's why many young people want to take more chances, try new things, and be more independent.

These changes are important steps on the road to adult life. However, these changes also increase the chance that some young people may turn to alcohol.

## Did You Know?

**The different "worlds" teens live in can have a big effect on their drinking.** Some young people are more involved with family than others. Others turn to their friends first. Still others turn to social groups like sports teams and clubs, faith-based groups, or groups of like-minded youth. The Internet, media, music, and videos are also an important part of the world of most teens. All of these affect a young person's choices about using alcohol.

**FAST FACT**

Factors in an adolescent's environment affect both the appeal of alcohol and its availability. Among these factors are the social systems within which teens function and with which they interact. Examples of these social systems are parents, friends, family, schools, and the community. The media and the larger social culture, including how alcohol is marketed and portrayed, also contribute to alcohol's appeal to young people.

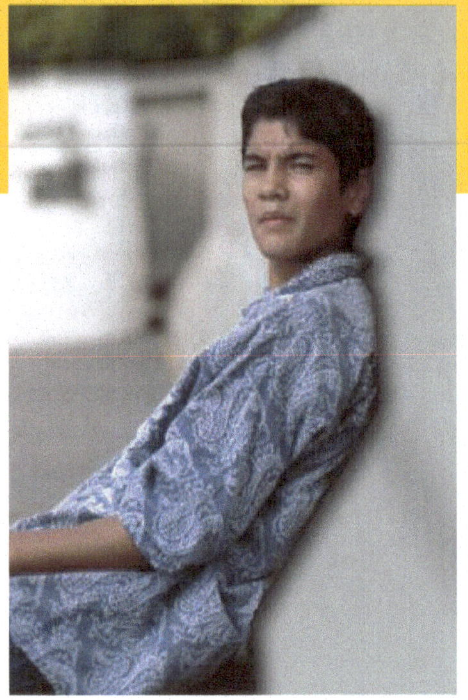

## Why Teens May Choose to Drink

Many things affect a young person's decisions about drinking—

- The different "worlds" in which teens live, including family, friends, school, and community
- A greater desire to take risks
- Less connection to parents and more independence
- More time spent with friends and by themselves
- Increased stress
- Greater attention to what teens see and hear about alcohol

## Did You Know?

Teens with behavior or family problems are at higher risk for alcohol use. And if anyone in the family has a drinking problem, it can affect the entire family. It also may affect a teen's choices about drinking.

**FAST FACT**

Youth with histories of behavior problems (for example, delinquent activity, impulsive actions, and difficulty controlling responses) are more likely to use alcohol than are other young people. The same is true for youth who have an unusually strong desire for new experiences and sensations, and for those with histories of family conflict and stress, and/or alcohol problems.

# UNDERAGE DRINKING IS EVERYONE'S PROBLEM

## Underage drinking can affect anyone, including people who don't drink.

- Underage alcohol use can lead to dangerous behavior, property damage, and violence.
- The results can be injury and even death for the drinker, and for other people nearby.
- About 45% of people who die in car crashes involving a drinking driver under age 21 are people other than the driver.

The effects of underage drinking can be felt by everyone. That makes underage alcohol use everyone's problem.

### FAST FACT

Most 6-year-olds know that alcohol is only for adults. Between ages 9 and 13, youth begin to think that alcohol use is okay. That's why it's never too early to start talking with young people about the dangers of underage drinking.

Teens say that they rely on adults in their lives more than anyone else to help them make tough decisions and to provide good advice.

# ENDING UNDERAGE DRINKING IS EVERYONE'S JOB

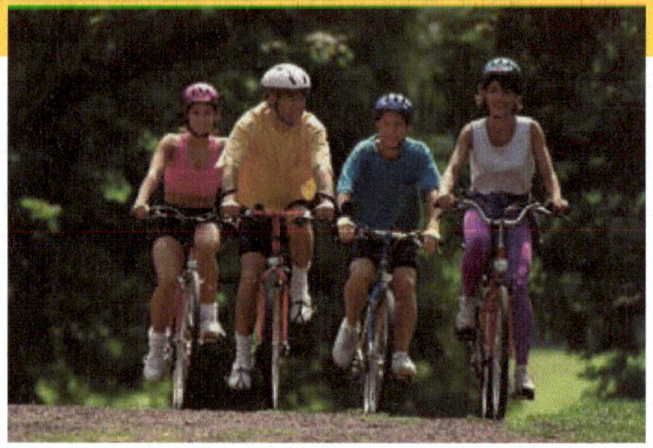

## There is a role for everyone.

- Everyone can work together to create a community where young people can grow up and feel good about themselves without drinking.
- Everyone in the community should deliver the message that underage drinking is not okay. The message should be the same whether youth hear it in school, at home, in places of worship, on the sports field, in youth programs, or in other places where young people gather.
- It is important for families to pay attention to what's happening with their teens.
- Young people can learn about the dangers of alcohol use. They can change how they and others think about drinking.

**It's time to change how we all think, talk, and act when it comes to underage drinking. We need to stop accepting it and to start discouraging it. It's time to help young people understand that it is not okay for them to drink alcohol. The discussion needs to start long before youth start thinking about drinking.**

# WHAT FAMILIES CAN DO ABOUT UNDERAGE ALCOHOL USE

**While many teens drink alcohol, underage alcohol use is not inevitable.** Families are not helpless to prevent it. Focus your efforts on the factors that protect teens from alcohol use. At the same time, you can work to reduce the factors that increase the chance that they will drink.

## Support your teens and give them space to grow.

- Be involved in your teens' lives. Be loving and caring.
- Encourage your teens' growing independence, but set appropriate limits.
- Make it easy for your teens to share information about their lives.
- Know where your teens are, what they're doing, who they're with, and who their friends are.
- Find ways for your teens to be involved in family life, such as doing chores or caring for a younger brother or sister.
- Set clear rules, including rules about alcohol use. Enforce the rules you set.

## Talk with your teens about alcohol use.

- When you talk with your teens about drinking, listen to them and respect what they say.
- Make clear your expectation that your teens will not drink.
- Teach your children about the dangers of underage drinking.
- Discuss laws about underage drinking, including the age 21 law.

## Help your teens make good decisions about alcohol.

- Help your teens know how to resist alcohol.
- Help them find ways to have fun without alcohol.
- Do not give alcohol to your teens. Tell them that any alcohol in your home is off limits to them and to their friends.
- Don't let your teens attend parties where alcohol is served. Make sure alcohol isn't available at teen parties in your own home.
- Set clear rules about not drinking and enforce them consistently.
- Help your teens avoid dangerous situations such as riding in a car driven by someone who has been drinking.
- Help your teens get professional help if you're worried about their involvement with alcohol.

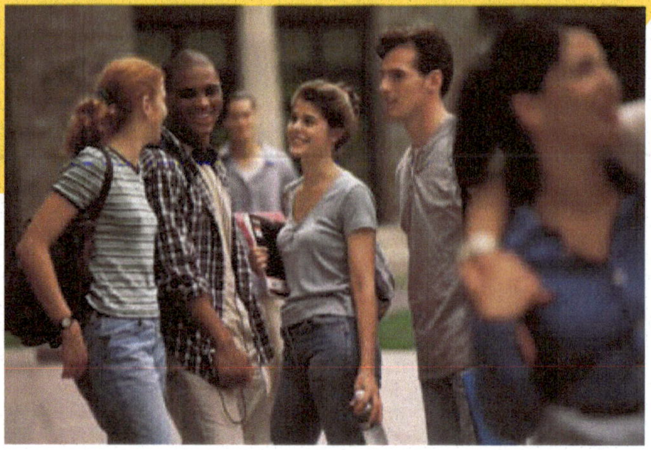

**Be aware of factors that may increase the risk of teen alcohol use.**

- Significant social transitions such as graduating to middle or high school, or getting a driver's license
- A history of conduct problems
- Depression and other serious emotional problems
- A family history of alcoholism
- Contact with peers involved in deviant activities

**Be a positive adult role model.**

- If you drink yourself, drink responsibly. That means not drinking too much or too often.
- Stay away from alcohol in high-risk situations. For example, don't drive or go boating when you've been drinking.
- Get help if you think you have an alcohol-related problem.

**Work with others.**

No matter how close you and your teens are, it may not be enough to prevent them from drinking. It's hard for families to do this alone. It's important to reach out to schools, communities, and government. You can help protect teens from underage alcohol use by working to see to it that—

- Schools and the community support and reward young people's decisions not to drink.
- Rules about underage drinking are in place at home, at school, and in your community. Penalties for breaking the rules are well known. Rules are enforced the same way for everyone.
- All laws about underage alcohol use are well known and enforced.
- Parties and social events at home and elsewhere don't permit underage drinking.

HOW CAN I TELL IF MY CHILD HAS BEEN USING MARIJUANA?

CAN A PERSON BECOME ADDICTED TO MARIJUANA?

WHAT ARE THE SHORT-TERM EFFECTS OF MARIJUANA USE?

HOW DOES MARIJUANA AFFECT DRIVING?

HOW LONG DOES MARIJUANA STAY IN THE BODY?

DOES MARIJUANA LEAD TO THE USE OF OTHER DRUGS?

HOW MANY TEENS USE MARIJUANA?

CAN MARIJUANA AFFECT MY CHILD'S GRADES?

CAN A PERSON WHO USES MARIJUANA HAVE A BAD REACTION?

WHAT ARE THE EFFECTS OF MARIJUANA?

ARE THERE TREATMENTS FOR PEOPLE ADDICTED TO MARIJUANA?

# MARIJUANA: FACTS PARENTS NEED TO KNOW

*Revised*

HOW CAN I PREVENT MY CHILD FROM GETTING INVOLVED WITH MARIJUANA?

WHAT ABOUT EFFECTS ON PREGNANCY?

IS MARIJUANA USE LINKED TO LOSS OF MOTIVATION?

HOW IS MARIJUANA USED?

WHAT ARE THE LONG-TERM EFFECTS OF MARIJUANA USE?

WHAT DOES MARIJUANA DO TO THE BRAIN?

IS MARIJUANA MEDICINE?

National Institute on Drug Abuse
National Institutes of Health

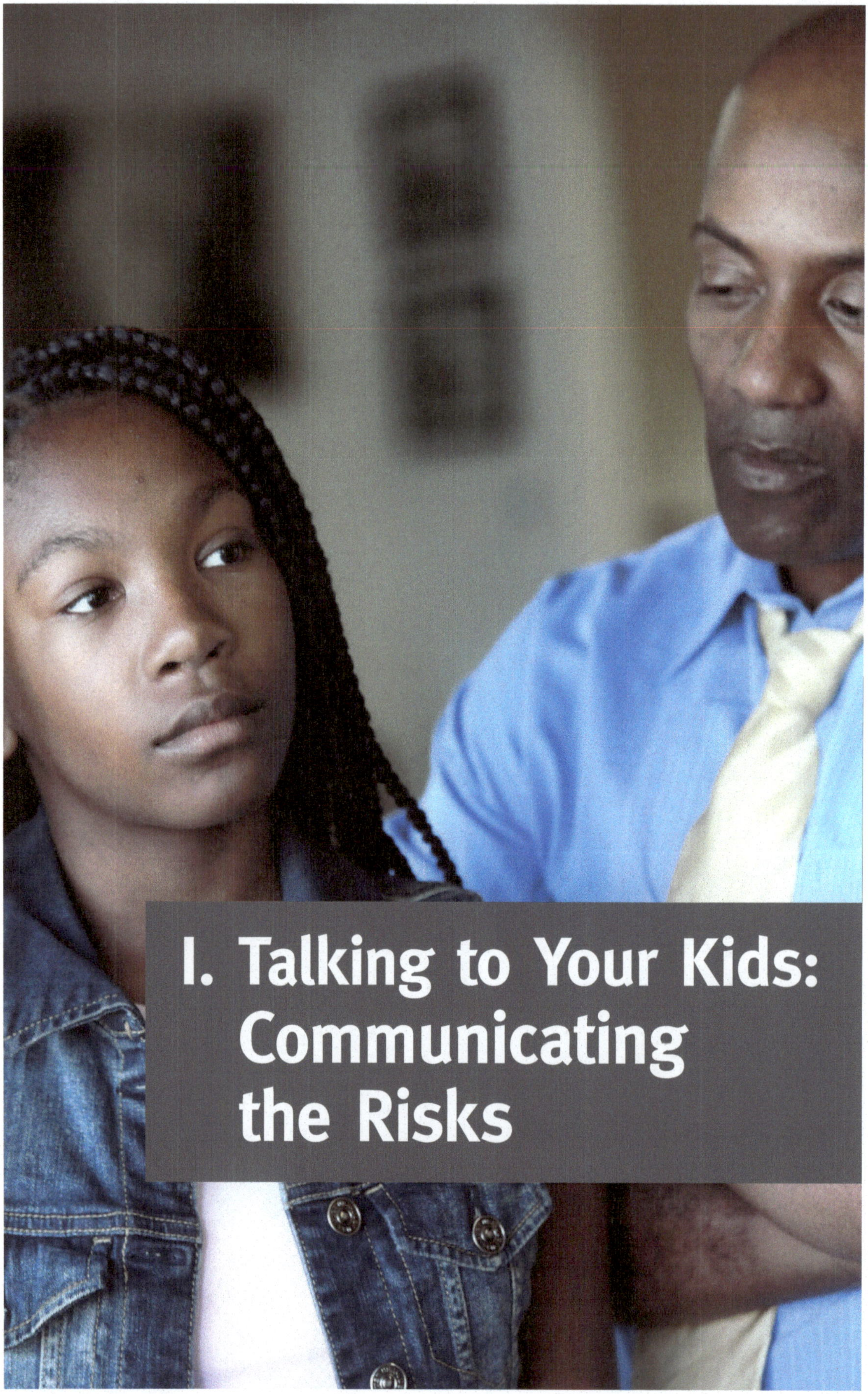

# I. Talking to Your Kids: Communicating the Risks

## Introduction

**Why do young people use marijuana?** Young people start using marijuana for many reasons. Curiosity, peer pressure, and the desire to fit in with friends are common ones. Those who have already begun to smoke cigarettes or use alcohol, or who have untreated mental health conditions (such as depression, anxiety, or ADHD), or who have experienced trauma are at increased risk for marijuana use.

For some, drug use begins as a means of coping with anxiety, anger, depression, or boredom. But, in fact, being high can be a way of simply avoiding the problems and challenges of growing up. Parents, grandparents, and older siblings are models that children follow, and research suggests that family members' use of alcohol and drugs plays a strong role in whether a young person starts using drugs.

Indeed, all aspects of a teen's environment—home, school, and community—can influence if he or she will try drugs.

## How can I prevent my child from using marijuana?

There is no quick or simple solution for preventing teen drug use. But research shows parents have a big influence on their teens, even when it doesn't seem that way. Talk openly with your children and stay actively engaged in their lives.

To help you get started, the next section provides some key points about marijuana research findings that you can share with your kids to help them sort out fact from myth and help them make the best decisions they can. These key points address the types of questions and comments that we receive from teens every day on our NIDA for Teens website and Drugs and Health blog. Following that brief section, the FAQs and additional resources will equip you with even more information.

## Did you know?

**Marijuana can be addictive.** Despite common belief, repeated marijuana use can lead to addiction, which means that people can have trouble quitting, even if it is having a negative impact on their lives. Research suggests that about 30 percent of people who use marijuana have some level of marijuana use disorder even if they are not yet addicted.[1] People who begin using marijuana before the age of 18 are more likely to develop a marijuana use disorder than adults.[2] Among youth receiving substance use disorder treatment, marijuana accounts for the largest percentage of admissions—almost 50 percent among those 12 to 17 years old.[3]

**Marijuana is unsafe if you're behind the wheel.** Marijuana impairs judgment and many other skills needed for safe driving: alertness, concentration, coordination, and reaction time. Marijuana use makes it difficult to judge distances and react to signals and sounds on the road. Marijuana is the most commonly identified illegal drug in deadly crashes, sometimes in combination with alcohol or other drugs. By itself, marijuana is thought to roughly double a driver's chances of being in a crash, and the combination of marijuana and even small amounts of alcohol is even more dangerous[4,5]—more so than either substance alone.[6]

---

1 Hasin DS, Saha TD, Kerridge BT, et al. Prevalence of Marijuana Use Disorders in the United States Between 2001-2002 and 2012-2013. *JAMA Psychiatry.* 2015;72(12):1235-1242. doi:10.1001/jamapsychiatry.2015.1858.

2 Winters KC, Lee C-YS. Likelihood of developing an alcohol and cannabis use disorder during youth: association with recent use and age. *Drug Alcohol Depend.* 2008;92(1-3):239-247. doi:10.1016/j.drugalcdep.2007.08.005.

3 Center for Behavioral Health Statistics and Quality. (2017). 2016 National Survey on Drug Use and Health: Detailed Tables. Substance Abuse and Mental Health Services Administration, Rockville, MD.

4 Biecheler M-B, Peytavin J-F, Sam Group, Facy F, Martineau H. SAM survey on "drugs and fatal accidents": search of substances consumed and comparison between drivers involved under the influence of alcohol or cannabis. *Traffic Inj Prev.* 2008;9(1):11-21. doi:10.1080/15389580701737561.

5 DRUID Final Report: Work Performed, Main Results and Recommendations. EU DRUID Programme; 2012. http://www.roadsafetyobservatory.com/Evidence/Details/10940.

6 Hartman RL, Huestis MA. Cannabis effects on driving skills. *Clin Chem.* 2013;59(3):478-492. doi:10.1373/clinchem.2012.194381.

**Marijuana is linked to school failure, lower income, and poorer quality of life.** Marijuana has negative effects on attention, motivation, memory, and learning that can persist after the drug's immediate effects wear off—especially in people who use regularly. Someone who uses marijuana daily may be functioning at a reduced intellectual level most or all of the time. Compared with their nonsmoking peers, students who use marijuana are more likely to drop out of high school.[7] People who use marijuana regularly for a long time report decreased overall life satisfaction, including poorer mental and physical health, memory and relationship problems, lower salaries, and less career success.[8]

**Marijuana is linked to some mental illnesses.** Although scientists don't yet fully understand how the use of marijuana might impact the development of mental illness, high doses can bring on a panic attack or even acute *psychosis*—thinking that is detached from reality, sometimes including hallucinations. In people who already have the severe mental illness *schizophrenia* (involving symptoms such as hallucinations, paranoia, and disorganized thinking), marijuana use can worsen its symptoms. Also, evidence suggests that early marijuana use may increase the risk of psychotic disorders among those at higher genetic risk for these disorders.

---

[7] Macleod J, Oakes R, Copello A, et al. Psychological and social sequelae of cannabis and other illicit drug use by young people: a systematic review of longitudinal, general population studies. *Lancet Lond Engl.* 2004;363(9421):1579-1588. doi:10.1016/S0140-6736(04)16200-4.

[8] Zwerling C, Ryan J, Orav EJ. The efficacy of preemployment drug screening for marijuana and cocaine in predicting employment outcome. *JAMA.* 1990;264(20):2639-2643.

Marijuana has negative effects on attention, motivation, memory, and learning that can persist after the drug's immediate effects wear off—especially in people who use regularly.

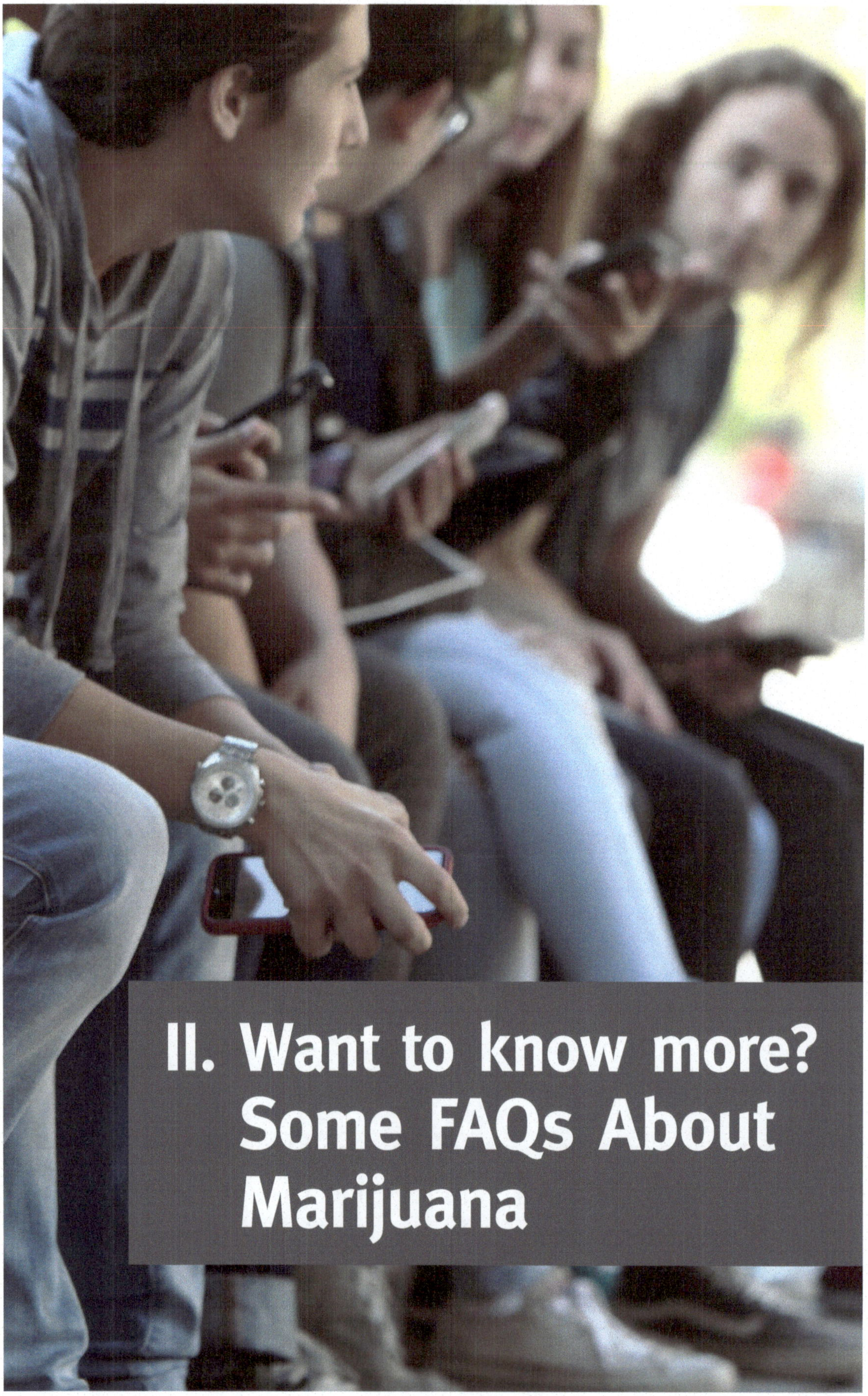

# II. Want to know more? Some FAQs About Marijuana

## What is marijuana? What is cannabis?

Marijuana refers to the dried leaves, flowers, stems, and seeds from the *Cannabis sativa* or *Cannabis indica* plant. The terms cannabis and marijuana are often used interchangeably. Extracts from the plant can be made into hash oil or wax. Cannabis products contain the mind-altering chemical *delta-9-tetrahydrocannabinol* (THC). They can also contain more than 400 other chemicals.

## How do people use marijuana?

People who use marijuana may roll loose marijuana leaves into a cigarette (called a joint) or smoke it in a pipe or a water pipe, often referred to as a bong. Some people mix marijuana into foods (called edibles) or use it to brew a tea. Another method is to slice open a cigar and replace some or all of the tobacco with marijuana, creating what is known as a blunt. Some people are vaping—using electronic vaporizers (called e-vaporizers or vapes) that allow people to inhale vapor and not smoke. Another popular method on the rise is vaping THC-rich resins extracted from the marijuana plant, an often dangerous practice called dabbing.

## How many teens use marijuana?

NIDA's annual Monitoring the Future survey reports that marijuana use has remained stable over the past few years among 8th, 10th, and 12th grade students. About 10 percent of 8th graders, 26 percent of 10th graders, and 37 percent of 12th graders reported using marijuana in the last year. At the same time, teens are developing more positive attitudes about using marijuana, with 71 percent of high school seniors saying they do not view regular marijuana smoking as very harmful.[9]

Researchers have found that the use of marijuana and other drugs usually peaks in the late teens and early twenties, then declines in later years. Therefore, marijuana use among young people remains a natural concern for parents and is the focus of continuing research, particularly regarding its impact on brain development, which continues into a person's early twenties. Researchers are studying how long marijuana's effects last and if the changes could be permanent.

---

[9] Miech RA, Schulenberg JE, Johnston LD, et al. *National adolescent drug trends in 2017: Findings released* [Press release]. Ann Arbor, MI. December 2017. Available at: http://www.monitoringthefuture.org/.

## How does marijuana produce the high?

When people smoke marijuana, they feel its effects almost immediately. The psychoactive chemical THC spreads to every organ in the body, including the brain, and attaches to specific receptors on nerve cells. This affects the areas of the brain that control pleasure, memory, thinking, concentration, movement, coordination, appetite, pain, and sensory and time perception.

THC is structurally similar to chemicals produced naturally by the body, called *endocannabinoids,* which play a role in normal brain development and function. Because of the endocannabinoid system's wide-ranging influence over many critical functions, marijuana can have multiple effects—not just on the brain, but on a person's general health. Some of these effects last only as long as marijuana is in the body while others may build up over time to cause longer-lasting problems, including addiction.

Although detectable amounts of THC can remain in the body for days or even weeks after use, the noticeable effects of smoked marijuana usually last from 1 to 3 hours. If consumed in foods, the effects come on slower and can last for many hours.

## What are marijuana's effects on the brain, body, and behavior?

**Short-term effects (while using or right after using)**

- learning, attention, and memory problems
- distorted perception (sights, sounds, time, touch)
- poor coordination and motor skills
- increased heart rate
- anxiety, paranoia
- psychosis (not common)

**Effects that last longer than the short term (a few days) but may not be permanent**

- learning and memory problems
- sleep problems

## DAILY MARIJUANA USE

**is more common among 12th graders than daily cigarette use.**

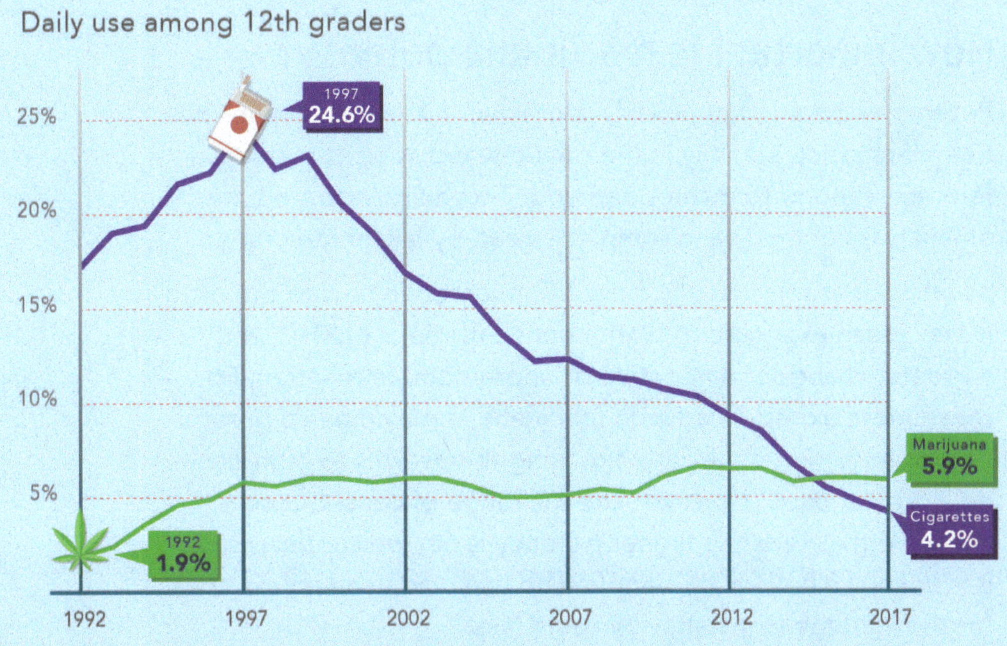


*Source: Monitoring the Future national survey results on drug use: 1975–2017: Overview, key findings on adolescent drug use. Ann Arbor: Institute for Social Research, The University of Michigan.*

**Long-term effects (effects of repeated use)**

- risk of marijuana addiction
- long-term learning and memory problems if heavy use begins during youth
- risk for chronic cough, bronchitis
- risk of schizophrenia in some people with higher genetic risk
- in rare cases, risk of recurrent episodes of severe nausea and vomiting

## What determines how marijuana affects an individual?

Like any other drug, marijuana's effects on a person depends on many factors, including the person's previous experience with the drug or other drugs, biology (e.g., genes), how the drug is taken, and the drug's potency (its strength).

## How important is marijuana potency?

Potency—the amount of THC contained in the marijuana—has been increasing steadily in the past few decades as marijuana farmers respond to market demand. These findings are based on analyses of marijuana samples seized by law enforcement.

So what does this actually mean? For someone new to the drug, it may mean exposure to higher concentrations of THC, with a greater chance of a negative or unpredictable reaction. For those more experienced with marijuana, it may mean a greater risk for addiction if they are exposing themselves to high doses on a regular basis. However, the full range of consequences linked with marijuana's higher potency is not well understood. It is unknown how much people who use marijuana adjust for the increase in potency by using less.

## Does using marijuana lead to other drug use?

The majority of people who use marijuana do not go on to use other "harder" substances, like cocaine or heroin. However, some research shows that people often try marijuana before trying other substances.[10] We also know from animal studies that rats given repeated doses of THC show heightened behavioral responses and altered brain activation not only when further exposed to THC, but also when exposed to other drugs such as morphine.[11] Researchers are now looking at the possibility that exposure to marijuana as a teen can cause changes in

---

[10] Secades-Villa R, Garcia-Rodríguez O, Jin CJ, Wang S, Blanco C. Probability and predictors of the cannabis gateway effect: a national study. *Int J Drug Policy.* 2015;26(2):135-142. doi:10.1016/j.drugpo.2014.07.011.

[11] Cadoni C, Pisanu A, Solinas M, Acquas E, Di Chiara G. Behavioural sensitization after repeated exposure to Delta 9-tetrahydrocannabinol and cross-sensitization with morphine. *Psychopharmacology (Berl).* 2001;158(3):259-266. doi:10.1007/s002130100875.

the brain that make a person more likely to get addicted to marijuana or other drugs, such as alcohol, opioids, or cocaine.

It is important to point out, however, that research has not fully explained any of these observations, which are complex and likely to involve a combination of biological, social, and psychological factors.

## Does smoking marijuana cause lung cancer?

Studies have not found an increased risk of lung cancer in marijuana smokers compared with nonsmokers. However, marijuana smoke does irritate the lungs and increases the likelihood of other lung and breathing problems.[12,13] Moreover, many people who smoke marijuana also smoke cigarettes, which do cause cancer, and research suggests that quitting tobacco can be harder if the person uses marijuana.

## Can marijuana produce withdrawal symptoms when someone quits?

Yes. Many people who use the drug long-term and then stop have symptoms that are similar to those of nicotine withdrawal—irritability, sleep problems, anxiety, decreased appetite and various forms of physical discomfort—which may prompt relapse (a return to drug use). Withdrawal symptoms are generally mild and peak a few days after use has stopped. They gradually disappear within about 2 weeks.[14,15] While these symptoms do not pose an immediate threat to health, they can make it hard for someone to stop using the drug. Because withdrawal is not as obvious or as painful as withdrawal symptoms from some other drugs such as opioids, many people do not realize that stopping marijuana use can cause withdrawal symptoms.

---

12 Tashkin DP. Effects of marijuana smoking on the lung. *Ann Am Thorac Soc.* 2013;10(3):239-247. doi:10.1513/AnnalsATS.201212-127FR.

13 Owen KP, Sutter ME, Albertson TE. Marijuana: respiratory tract effects. *Clin Rev Allergy Immunol.* 2014;46(1):65-81. doi:10.1007/s12016-013-8374-y.

14 Budney AJ, Hughes JR. The cannabis withdrawal syndrome. *Curr Opin Psychiatry.* 2006; 19(3):233-238. doi:10.1097/01.yco.0000218592.00689.e5.

15 Gorelick DA, Levin KH, Copersino ML, et al. Diagnostic Criteria for Cannabis Withdrawal Syndrome. *Drug Alcohol Depend.* 2012;123(1-3):141-147. doi:10.1016/j.drugalcdep.2011.11.007.

## How harmful is K2/Spice (or "synthetic cannabinoids")?

Synthetic cannabinoids, which are sometimes also called K2 or Spice, consist of many human-made mind-altering chemicals that are either sprayed on dried, shredded plant material to be smoked, or sold as liquids to be inhaled in e-vaporizers. These chemicals are called cannabinoids because they have chemicals that act on the same brain cell receptors as THC, but are often much more powerful and unpredictable. Because of this similarity, synthetic cannabinoids are sometimes misleadingly called "synthetic marijuana" (or "fake weed"), and are often labeled "not fit for human consumption." Many are now illegal, but their manufacturers are constantly creating new chemical compounds to sidestep legal restrictions. Their effects, like the ingredients, often vary, but emergency rooms report large numbers of young people appearing with rapid heart rates, vomiting, and negative mental responses including hallucinations after using these substances. Some states are reporting an increased number of overdose cases involving synthetic cannabinoid products where users are experiencing severe bleeding, likely due to product contamination.

## Are there treatments for people addicted to marijuana?

Behavioral therapies are available and are similar to those used for treating other drug or alcohol addictions. These include motivational enhancement therapies to develop people's own motivation to stay in treatment; cognitive behavioral therapies to teach strategies for avoiding drug use and its triggers (and for effectively managing stress); and motivational incentives, which provide vouchers or small cash rewards for showing up for treatment and staying drug free.

There are currently no medications approved by the U.S. Food and Drug Administration (FDA) for treating marijuana addiction, although promising research is under way to find medications to treat withdrawal symptoms and ease craving and other effects of marijuana.

## What are other risks related to marijuana that my child should know?

Many parents and teens may not have thought about some of these risks:

- As with many misused drugs, marijuana use interferes with judgment, which can lead to risky behaviors. For example, someone using marijuana might drive under the influence or ride with someone else who is intoxicated and get into a car crash, or might engage in risky sexual behavior and contract a sexually transmitted infection.
- Regular marijuana use has been linked with increased risk for several mental problems, including depression, anxiety, suicidal thoughts, personality disturbances, and psychosis. Whether or not marijuana causes these problems, or is a response to them, is still unknown. More research is needed to confirm and better understand these links.
- Research suggests that marijuana use during pregnancy may be linked to future developmental and hyperactivity disorders.[16–19] However, the fact that pregnant women who use marijuana are also more likely to smoke cigarettes or drink alcohol makes it difficult to determine exactly how much of these effects are due to marijuana. In addition, some research suggests that after pregnancy, THC passes into the breast milk of nursing mothers in moderate amounts.[20] More research is needed to learn how this affects the baby's developing brain. The American College of Obstetricians and Gynecologists recommends against using marijuana during pregnancy.

---

[16] Campolongo P, Trezza V, Ratano P, Palmery M, Cuomo V. Developmental consequences of perinatal cannabis exposure: behavioral and neuroendocrine effects in adult rodents. *Psychopharmacology (Berl).* 2011;214(1):5-15. doi:10.1007/s00213-010-1892-x.

[17] Fried PA, Watkinson B, Gray R. A follow-up study of attentional behavior in 6-year-old children exposed prenatally to marihuana, cigarettes, and alcohol. *Neurotoxicol Teratol.* 1992;14(5):299-311.

[18] Goldschmidt L, Day NL, Richardson GA. Effects of prenatal marijuana exposure on child behavior problems at age 10. *Neurotoxicol Teratol.* 2000;22(3):325-336.

[19] Fried PA, Smith AM. A literature review of the consequences of prenatal marihuana exposure. An emerging theme of a deficiency in aspects of executive function. *Neurotoxicol Teratol.* 2001;23(1):1-11.

[20] Hayatbakhsh MR, Flenady VJ, Gibbons KS, et al. Birth outcomes associated with cannabis use before and during pregnancy. *Pediatr Res.* 2012;71(2):215-219. doi:10.1038/pr.2011.25.

## Is marijuana medicine?

Research shows that some chemicals in marijuana, THC as well as cannabidiol (CBD), could have medical uses. The FDA has approved some THC-based medications to treat nausea in patients undergoing chemotherapy and to help patients with AIDS gain an appetite. However, these medications are not smoked. The FDA has also approved a CBD oil-based medication to treat rare and severe forms of epilepsy. Additional clinical trials are being conducted to develop medications that contain THC and/or CBD for pain relief and seizure disorders.

## How can I tell if my child has been using marijuana?

Parents should be aware of changes in their child's behavior, such as not brushing hair or teeth, skipping showers, changes in mood, and challenging relationships with family members, and a change in friends. In addition, changes in grades, skipping classes or missing school, loss of interest in sports or other favorite activities, changes in eating or sleeping habits, and getting in trouble in school or with law enforcement could all be related to drug use—or may indicate other problems. See the list of specific warning signs for marijuana use below.

**If your child is using marijuana, he or she might:**

- seem unusually giggly and/or uncoordinated
- have very red, bloodshot eyes or use eye drops often
- have a hard time remembering things that just happened
- have drugs or drug paraphernalia—drug-related items including pipes and rolling papers—possibly claiming they belong to a friend if confronted
- have strangely smelling clothes or bedroom
- use incense and other deodorizers
- wear clothing or jewelry or have posters that promote drug use
- have unexplained lack of money or extra cash on hand

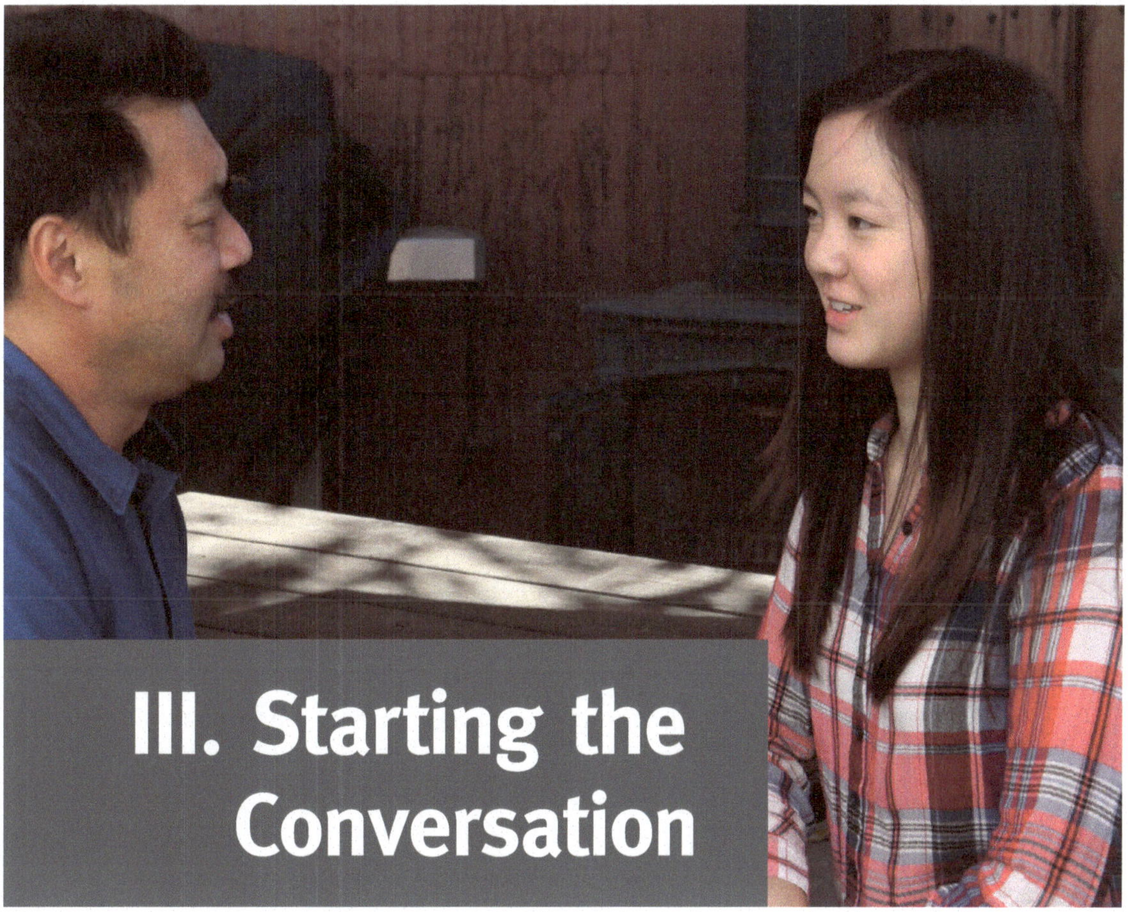

# III. Starting the Conversation

## Tips for Parents

- Be a good listener.
- Set clear expectations about drug and alcohol use, including real consequences for not following family rules.
- Help your child deal with peer pressure to use drugs.
- Get to know your child's friends and their parents.
- Monitor your child's whereabouts.
- Supervise teen activities.
- Talk to your child often.

**As this guide has shown, marijuana use can affect the health and well-being of children and teens at a critical point in their lives—when they are growing, learning, maturing, and laying the foundation for their adult years.**

As a parent, your children look to you for help and guidance in working out problems and in making decisions, including the decision not to use drugs. Even if you have used drugs in the past, you can have an open conversation about the dangers. Whether or not you tell your child about your past drug use is a personal decision. But experience can better equip us to teach others by drawing on the value of past mistakes. You can explain that marijuana is significantly more potent now and that we now know a lot more about the potential harmful effects of marijuana on the developing brain.

Greater acceptance of marijuana use, compared with use of other illegal drugs, continues to be the basis of differing opinions about its dangers, legal status, and potential value. Whether or not marijuana is legal for adult use or allowed for medical use in your state, it can be harmful for teens and can alter the course of a young life, preventing a person from reaching his or her full potential. That's reason enough to have this sometimes difficult conversation with your children. Be certain the discussion focuses on how much you care about your child's health.

We hope this guide encourages and helps parents to begin the dialogue and, more importantly, to keep the channels of communication open.

Want to become involved? Consider coordinating an event during National Drug and Alcohol Facts Week using free NIDA materials or contact us at **drugfacts@nida.nih.gov.** See **https://teens.drugabuse.gov/national-drug-facts-week.**

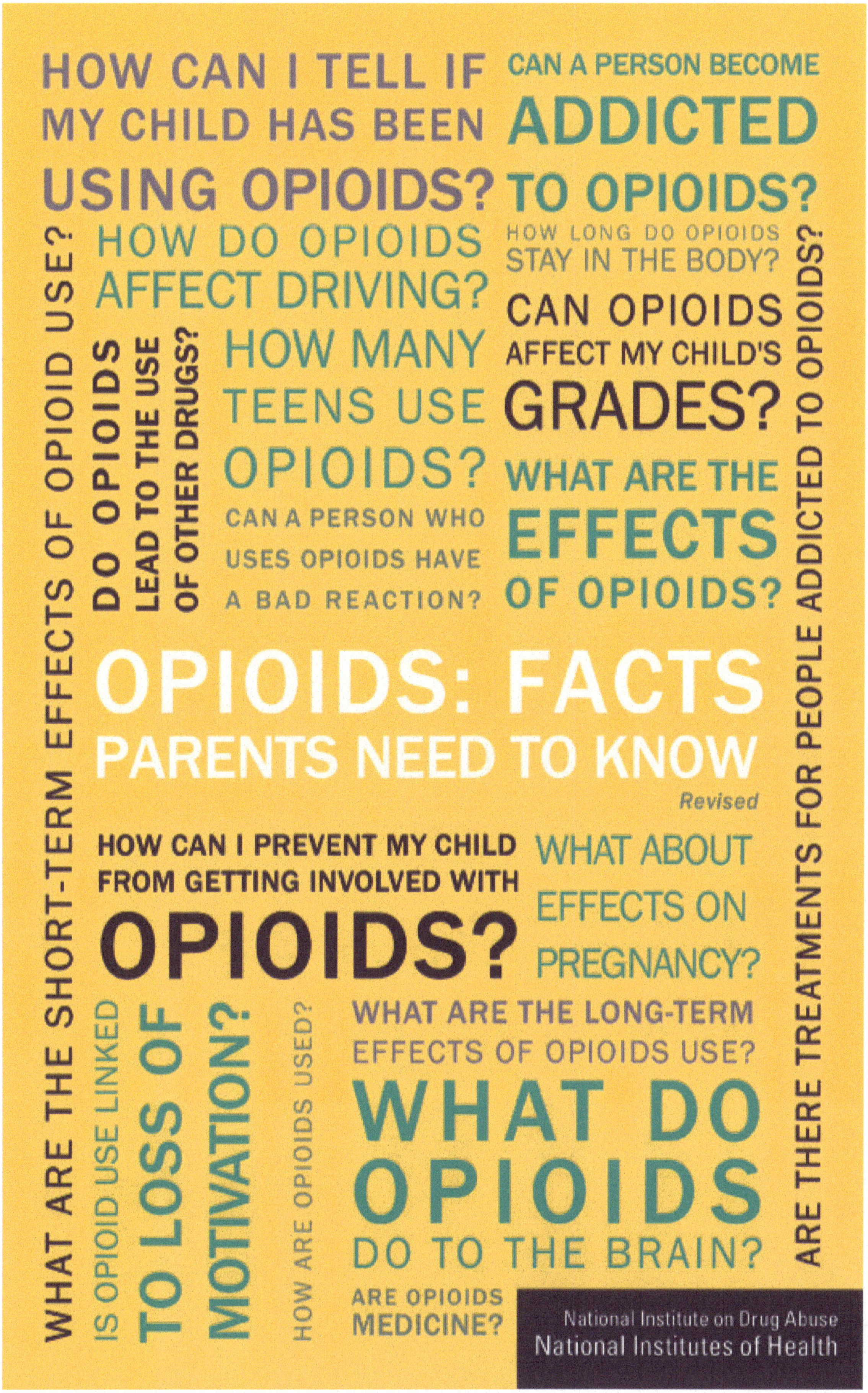
HOW CAN I TELL IF MY CHILD HAS BEEN USING OPIOIDS?
CAN A PERSON BECOME ADDICTED TO OPIOIDS?
WHAT ARE THE SHORT-TERM EFFECTS OF OPIOID USE?
HOW DO OPIOIDS AFFECT DRIVING?
HOW LONG DO OPIOIDS STAY IN THE BODY?
ARE THERE TREATMENTS FOR PEOPLE ADDICTED TO OPIOIDS?
DO OPIOIDS LEAD TO THE USE OF OTHER DRUGS?
HOW MANY TEENS USE OPIOIDS?
CAN OPIOIDS AFFECT MY CHILD'S GRADES?
CAN A PERSON WHO USES OPIOIDS HAVE A BAD REACTION?
WHAT ARE THE EFFECTS OF OPIOIDS?
OPIOIDS: FACTS PARENTS NEED TO KNOW
Revised
HOW CAN I PREVENT MY CHILD FROM GETTING INVOLVED WITH OPIOIDS?
WHAT ABOUT EFFECTS ON PREGNANCY?
IS OPIOID USE LINKED TO LOSS OF MOTIVATION?
HOW ARE OPIOIDS USED?
WHAT ARE THE LONG-TERM EFFECTS OF OPIOIDS USE?
WHAT DO OPIOIDS DO TO THE BRAIN?
ARE OPIOIDS MEDICINE?
National Institute on Drug Abuse
National Institutes of Health

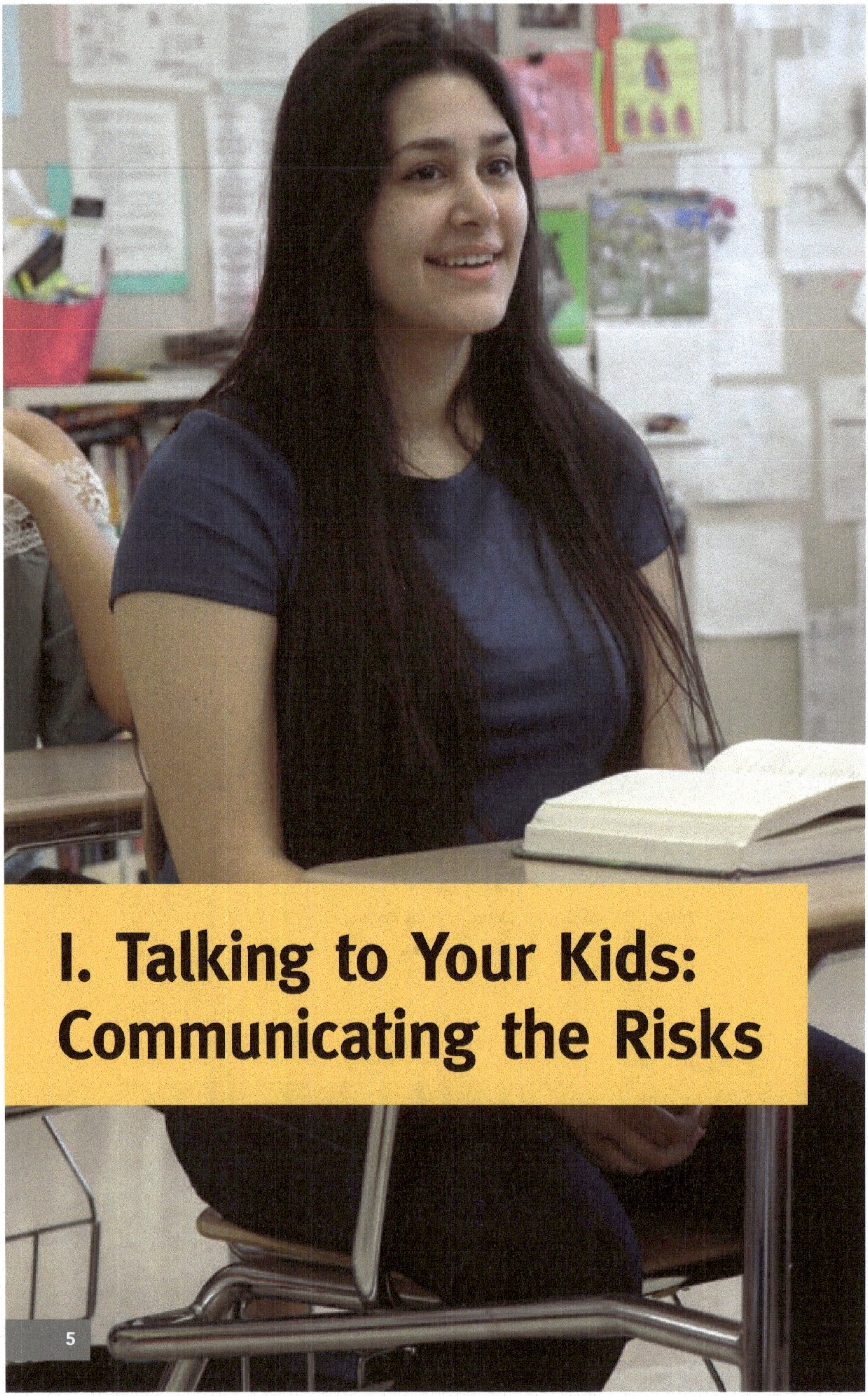
I. Talking to Your Kids:
Communicating the Risks
5

## Did you know?

**Opioid misuse can have lasting effects.** When opioids are misused, they can have harmful effects on your brain, like slowed breathing. Slowed breathing can then lead to short-and long-term health effects, including coma, brain damage, and death. Some studies have shown that repeated opioid misuse also can affect people's behavior, decision-making, and responses to stressful situations. So, it's important to be aware of any changes in your teen's behavior.

**Opioids can be addictive.** Opioids are among the most addictive drugs. Over time, opioids can change the brain, which leads to addiction. People who are addicted to opioids can feel a strong need to take the drug again and again. They may also experience severe withdrawal symptoms in the absence of the drug. These negative withdrawal symptoms, coupled with the strong desire to use opioids, are why some people continue to use opioids, despite negative consequences to their health and well-being.

**Opioid use can affect every area of your teen's life.** Using drugs early in life can lead to poor grades and bad relationships with friends and family. Opioid use can alter judgment and make it more likely your teen could make risky decisions like having unprotected sex or driving under the influence.[1–3]

---

[1] Dahl RE. Adolescent brain development: a period of vulnerabilities and opportunities. Keynote address. Ann N Y Acad Sci. 2004;1021:1-22. doi:10.1196/annals.1308.001

[2] Kessler RC, Berglund P, Demler O, Jin R, Merikangas KR, Walters EE. Lifetime prevalence and age-of-onset distributions of DSM-IV disorders in the National Comorbidity Survey Replication. Arch Gen Psychiatry. 2005;62(6):593-602. doi:10.1001/archpsyc.62.6.593

[3] Thornberry TP, Krohn MD, eds. Taking Stock of Delinquency - An Overview of Findings. New York, NY: Springer Science & Business Media; 2006. //www.springer.com/us/book/9780306473647. Accessed November 7, 2017.

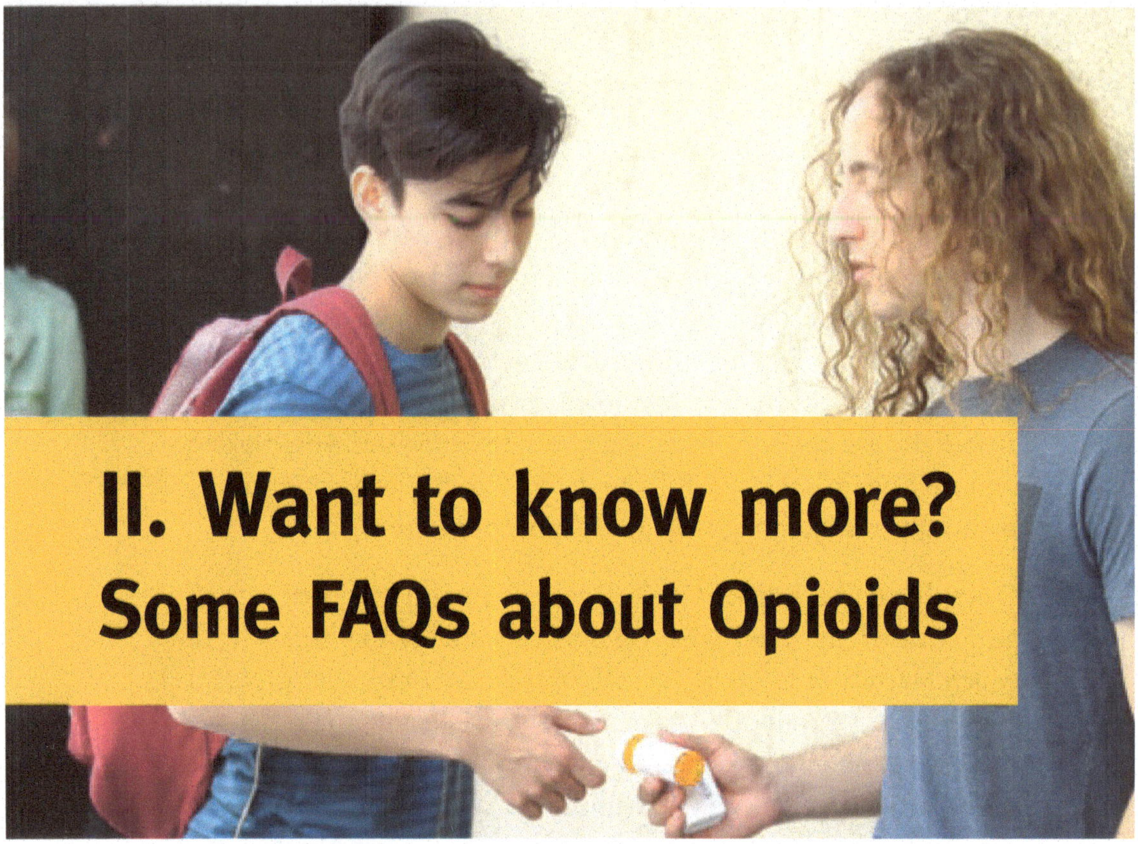

# II. Want to know more? Some FAQs about Opioids

### What are opioids?

There are legal opioids like prescription pain relievers and illegal opioids like heroin and illicit fentanyl.

Prescription opioids are powerful pain-reducing medications. Some prescription opioids are made directly from the opium poppy plant. Others are made by scientists in a laboratory although they have similar chemical structures.

## Heroin is an Opioid

### What is heroin?

Heroin is an addictive illegal drug made from morphine, a natural substance that is found in the seed pod of opium poppy plants in Southeast and Southwest Asia, Mexico, and Colombia. It is a type of opioid. Heroin can come in powder form or as a black sticky substance. Heroin can be injected, sniffed, snorted, or smoked.

Heroin may have many street names including Big H, Black Tar, Chiva, Hell Dust, Horse, Negra, Smack, and Thunder.

## What is the connection between prescription opioids and heroin?

Prescription pain relievers and heroin are chemically similar and produce similar effects. You can become addicted to both and overdose on both. Some people get addicted to prescription opioids and then switch to heroin. Others simply start using heroin.

In some communities, heroin is cheaper and potentially easier to get than prescription opioids, which is why some people who are addicted to prescription opioids sometimes switch. Data from 2011 showed that an estimated 4 to 6 percent who misuse prescription opioids switch to heroin[4–6] and about 80 percent of people who used heroin first misused prescription opioids.[4–6]

More recent data suggest that heroin is frequently the first opioid people use. In a study of those entering treatment for opioid use disorder, approximately one-third reported heroin as the first opioid they used regularly to get high.[7]

## What are the effects of heroin on the brain, body, and behavior?

Just like other opioids, heroin binds to the opioid receptors in the brain and body, causing euphoria and relieving pain. This means that the short-term and long-term effects will be similar to those experienced from prescription opioids. However, people who inject heroin can also experience collapsed veins.

Additionally, people who inject drugs increase their risk of getting HIV or hepatitis C. These diseases are passed from person to person through blood and other bodily fluids. When people share needles or other drug equipment, they can come into contact with these fluids. HIV, and less often hepatitis C, can also be spread through unprotected sex.

---

[4] Muhuri PK, Gfroerer JC, Davies MC. Associations of Nonmedical Pain Reliever Use and Initiation of Heroin Use in the United States. CBHSQ Data Rev. August 2013.

[5] Cicero TJ, Ellis MS, Surratt HL, Kurtz SP. The Changing Face of Heroin Use in the United States: A Retrospective Analysis of the Past 50 Years. JAMA Psychiatry. 2014;71(7):821-826. doi:10.1001/jamapsychiatry.2014.366.

[6] Carlson RG, Nahhas RW, Martins SS, Daniulaityte R. Predictors of transition to heroin use among initially non-opioid dependent illicit pharmaceutical opioid users: A natural history study. Drug Alcohol Depend. 2016;160:127-134. doi:10.1016/j.drugalcdep.2015.12.026.

[7] Cicero TJ, Ellis MS, Kasper ZA. Increased use of heroin as an initiating opioid of abuse. Addict Behav. 2017 Nov;74:63-66. doi: 10.1016/j.addbeh.2017.05.030. Epub 2017 May 23. PubMed PMID: 28582659. https://www.ncbi.nlm.nih.gov/pubmed/28582659

## What are the most commonly used prescription opioids?

Common opioid medicines include:

- hydrocodone (Vicodin®)
- oxycodone (OxyContin,® Percocet®)
- oxymorphone
- morphine (Kadian,® Avinza®)
- codeine
- fentanyl

## How do opioids affect the brain and make people feel high?

Opioids attach to and activate opioid receptors located in many areas of the brain, spinal cord, and other organs in the body, especially those involved in feelings of pain and pleasure.

When opioids attach to these receptors, they block pain signals sent from the brain to the body and release large amounts of dopamine in the brain's reward regions. Dopamine is the chemical responsible for motivating our actions and repeating pleasurable experiences. This release can strongly reinforce the act of taking the drug, making the user want to take the drug again and again despite negative consequences.

## What are the health effects of opioids?

In the short-term, opioids can relieve pain and make people feel relaxed. However, opioids can also have harmful effects, including:

- extreme drowsiness
- confusion
- nausea
- constipation
- slowed breathing

Over time, opioid use and misuse can lead to insomnia, muscle pain, heart problems, pneumonia, and addiction.

## How do people use opioids?

Prescription opioids are prescribed by doctors to treat pain and other health issues, such as controlling coughs and diarrhea. When used as prescribed and for a short time, opioids are relatively safe. But when they are misused, they can be dangerous.

**People misuse opioids by:**

- taking a prescription in ways other than instructed, like taking more than prescribed or taking it more often
- getting and using prescription pills from a friend or family member, even if it's for a real medical condition
- taking prescription drugs to get high
- mixing prescription opioids with alcohol or other drugs
- crushing pills or opening capsules, dissolving the powder in water, and injecting the liquid into a vein, or snorting the powder.

Some opioids, like heroin, aren't available by prescription. People use these drugs just to get high.

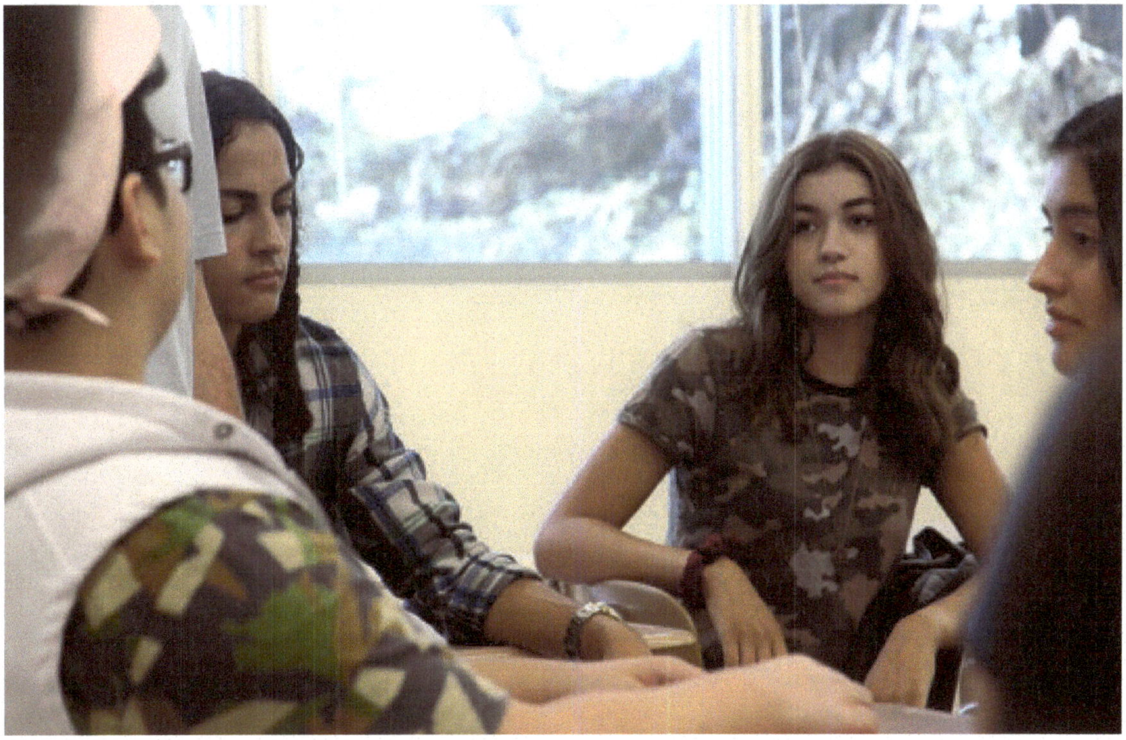

## Past-Year Misuse of Prescription/ Over-The-Counter vs. Illicit Drugs

*Among 12th graders in 2018*

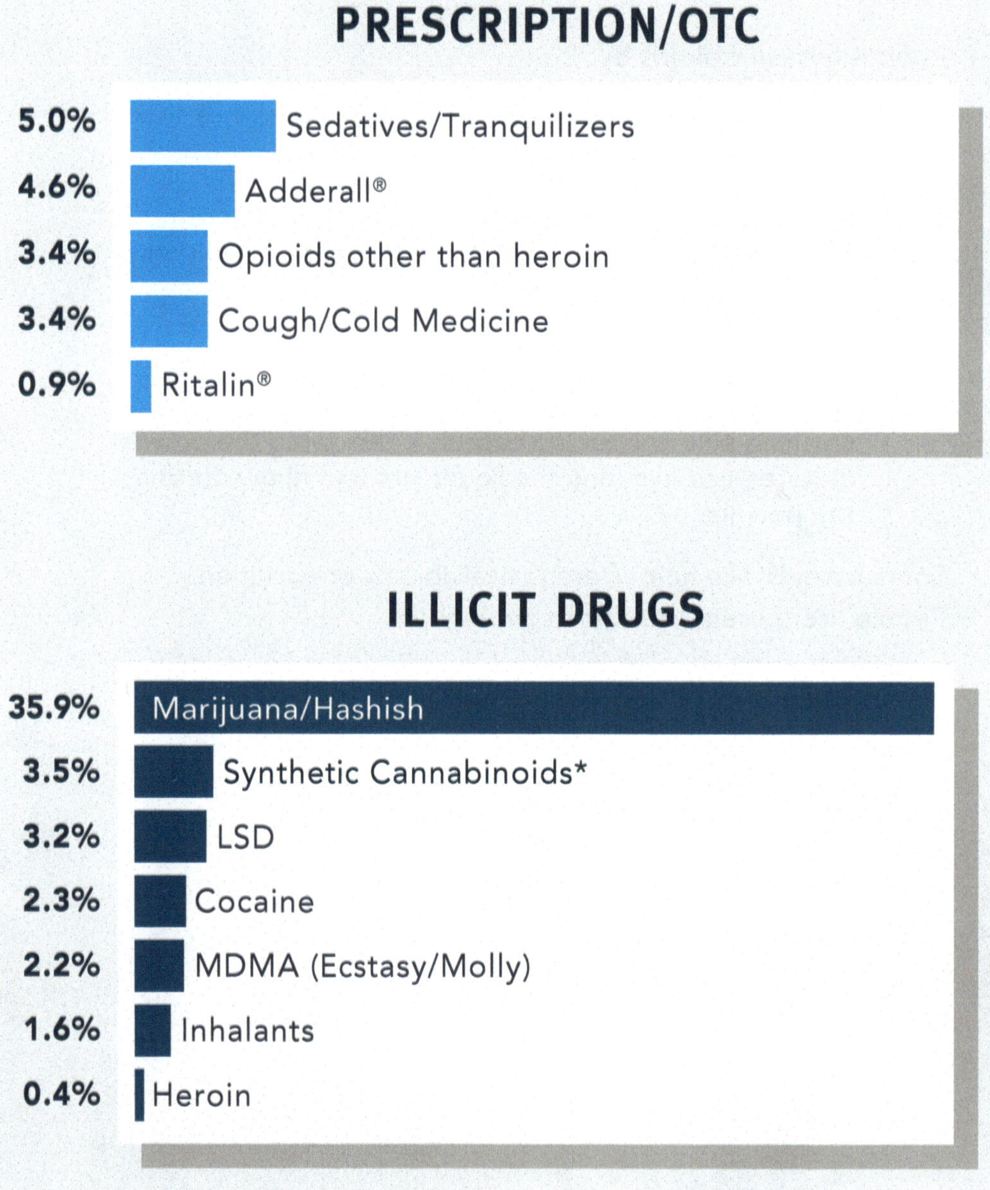


*Synthetic Cannabinoids are called Synthetic Marijuana in the survey.*

## VICODIN® AND OXYCONTIN®

**Past-year misuse of Vicodin® and OxyContin® among 12th graders has dropped dramatically in the past 15 years.**

**KEY**

**Vicodin®** **OxyContin®**

*Source: Monitoring the Future National Survey Results on Drug Use: 1975-2018: Overview, Key Findings on Adolescent Drug Use.*

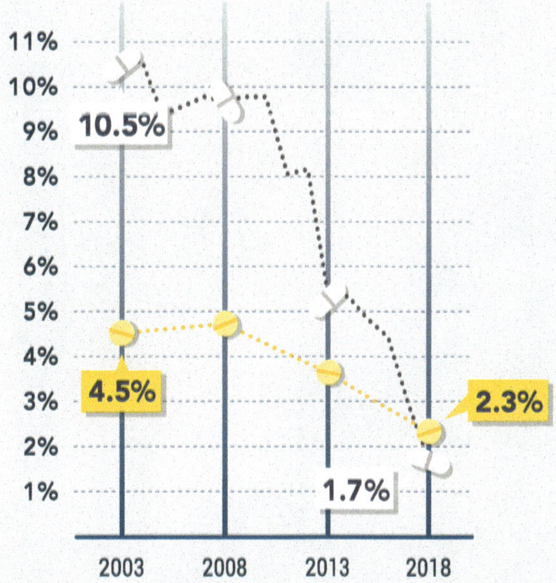


## How many teens misuse opioids?

According to NIDA's annual Monitoring the Future Survey of 8th, 10th, and 12th graders, the use of one popular prescription opioid, Vicodin®, has been decreasing since 2009.[8] In 2018, 1.7 percent of 12th graders misused Vicodin. These declining numbers likely reflect the hard work of parents and local community public health experts. However, opioid misuse rates increase after the age of 18, so it is critical to talk with teens early and frequently, to reinforce these health messages as they prepare to leave home and start their adult lives. For more information, please visit NIDA's **Drug and Alcohol Use in College-Age Adults in 2017** infographic.

[8] Johnston, L. D., Miech, R. A., O'Malley, P. M., Bachman, J. G., Schulenberg, J. E., & Patrick, M. E. (2019). Monitoring the Future national survey results on drug use, 1975-2018: Overview, key findings on adolescent drug use. Ann Arbor: Institute for Social Research, The University of Michigan

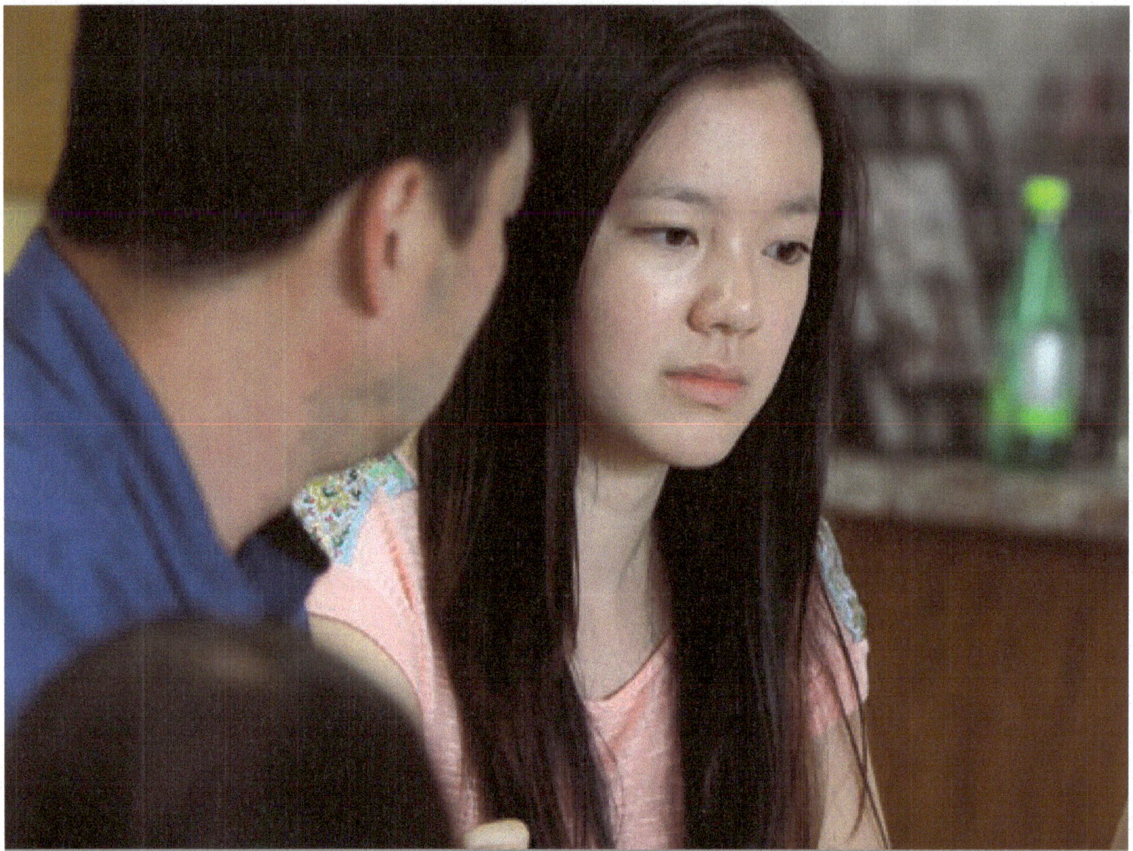

## Why do young people use opioids?

Curiosity, peer pressure, and the desire to fit in with friends are common reasons that preteens and teens start misusing opioids. For some, opioid use begins as a way of coping with anxiety, anger, depression, or boredom. Preteens, and teens in particular, may struggle with depression and anxiety but do not recognize it or want to talk about it. Parents often assume there is nothing wrong if their children do not discuss their feelings. Being high can be a way of simply avoiding the problems and challenges of growing up. Parents, grandparents, and older siblings are models who children follow, and research suggests that family members' use of alcohol and drugs plays a strong role in whether a young person starts using drugs, such as opioids.

Addiction means a person continues to seek and take the drug despite negative consequences. All aspects of the teen environment—home, school, and community—can influence if they will try, or even become addicted to drugs.

## How can I prevent my child from misusing opioids?

There is no quick or simple solution to prevent teens from misusing opioids. However, it can be done. Research shows that parents have a big influence on their teens. So, talk openly about the effects of opioids and other drugs with your children and stay actively engaged in their lives.

To help you get started, the next section provides some key points about opioids that you can share with your kids to help them make the best decisions to avoid opioid misuse. These key points address the types of questions and comments that we receive daily from our ***NIDA for Teens*** website and ***Drugs and Health Blog.*** Following that section, all the facts, questions, and listed resources will help equip you with even more information to talk about with your teen.

## Can my teen take someone else's prescription opioids if he or she is injured?

No. It is dangerous to give your child someone else's medication, even if he or she is in real pain. You should never give your children opioids that were not prescribed for them. Doctors prescribe opioids specifically based on a person's physical and medical history, such as weight, other medical conditions, or how opioids interact with other medicines your child might be taking. Without talking to a doctor, you won't know how the opioids will affect your child or what dose should be safely given. If your child is prescribed opioids, make sure you monitor their use carefully.

## I've heard of something called fentanyl. What is that?

Fentanyl is another type of opioid that is similar to morphine. It is 50 times stronger than heroin. As a prescription, it's used to treat severe pain and is also used in surgeries. But fentanyl is also made and used illegally. It is sometimes added to heroin or to other drugs, like cocaine and methamphetamine, causing potent and unpredictable drug combinations that can lead to fatal overdose.

## How can I tell if my child has been misusing opioids?

Changes in your child's behavior—such as not brushing their hair or teeth, skipping showers, changes in mood, and challenging relationships with friends and family—can be signs that your child is misusing opioids or other drugs. It's also important to look out for changes in grades, skipping classes or missing school, loss of interest in activities or friends that used to bring enjoyment, changes in sleeping and eating habits, and getting in trouble at school or with law enforcement. These changes could all be related to drug use—or may indicate other problems.

## Can my child use opioids if she is pregnant?

Even when taken as prescribed, opioid use during pregnancy may increase the risk of miscarriage or low birth weight. It can also cause neonatal abstinence syndrome, a medical condition where the baby is born dependent on opioids and has withdrawal symptoms after being born.

If a pregnant woman tries to stop taking opioids without medical help, she can put the baby at risk. It is important for pregnant women to tell their doctor about all the medications and other drugs they are taking, or planning to take, so that the baby has a greater chance of being born healthy. If a pregnant woman is misusing opioids, there are treatments that can help her.

## What is dependence and how is it different from addiction?

Many people who take prescription opioids for pain become dependent, but that is not the same as being addicted. Dependence occurs when your body has gotten used to the drug for pain, but then you feel really sick when you stop taking the drug. If your child is prescribed opioids, you should talk with his or her doctor about how to safely stop using them.

Addiction means a person continues to seek and take the drug despite negative consequences. It is possible to become dependent on opioids without being addicted, but dependence can lead to addiction in some cases.

## Can opioid addiction be treated?

Quitting opioids can be hard, but it is possible. You can work with your child's doctor to develop customized treatment plans that can include medications and therapy. There are three FDA-approved medicines to treat opioid addiction and reduce cravings, offering options to meet individual needs. Buprenorphine and methadone are medicines that bind to the same receptors in the brain as opioids, called opioid agonists or partial agonists. Naltrexone is another medication that treats opioid addiction, but it is called an antagonist, preventing opioids from having an effect on the brain. Additionally, the Food and Drug Administration recently approved a medicine called lofexidine to help make withdrawal symptoms easier for people who are trying to stop using opioids.

While many treatment centers do not offer medication, the National Academy of Sciences recently issued a scientific report stating that opioid agonists or partial agonists are especially effective, save lives, and have better long-term outcomes than other medications or no medications at all.[9] A combination of medication with behavioral therapy can reinforce treatment goals, rebuild relationships with friends and family, and build healthy life skills.

## Can you overdose on opioids?

Yes. Opioid overdose can cause slowed breathing, which can cause hypoxia—too little oxygen reaching the brain. Hypoxia can have psychological and neurological effects, including coma, permanent brain damage, or death.

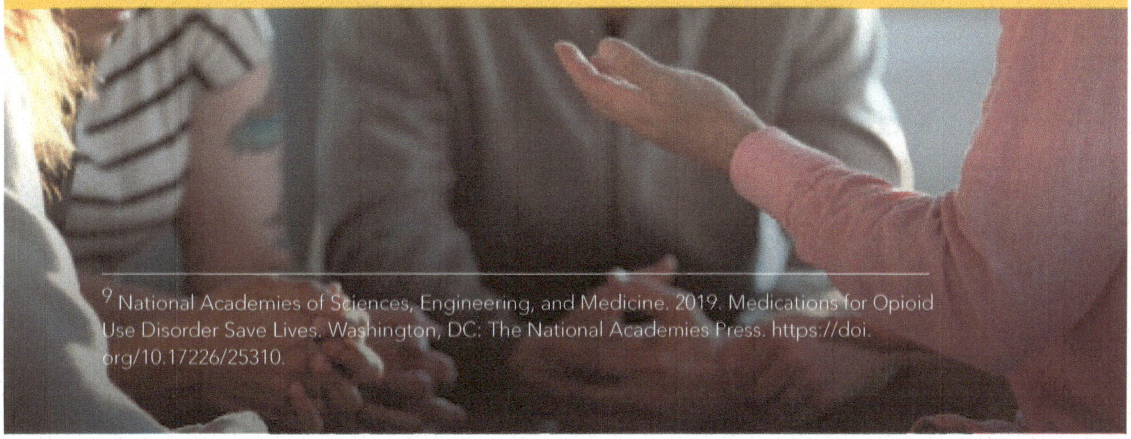

[9] National Academies of Sciences, Engineering, and Medicine. 2019. Medications for Opioid Use Disorder Save Lives. Washington, DC: The National Academies Press. https://doi.org/10.17226/25310.

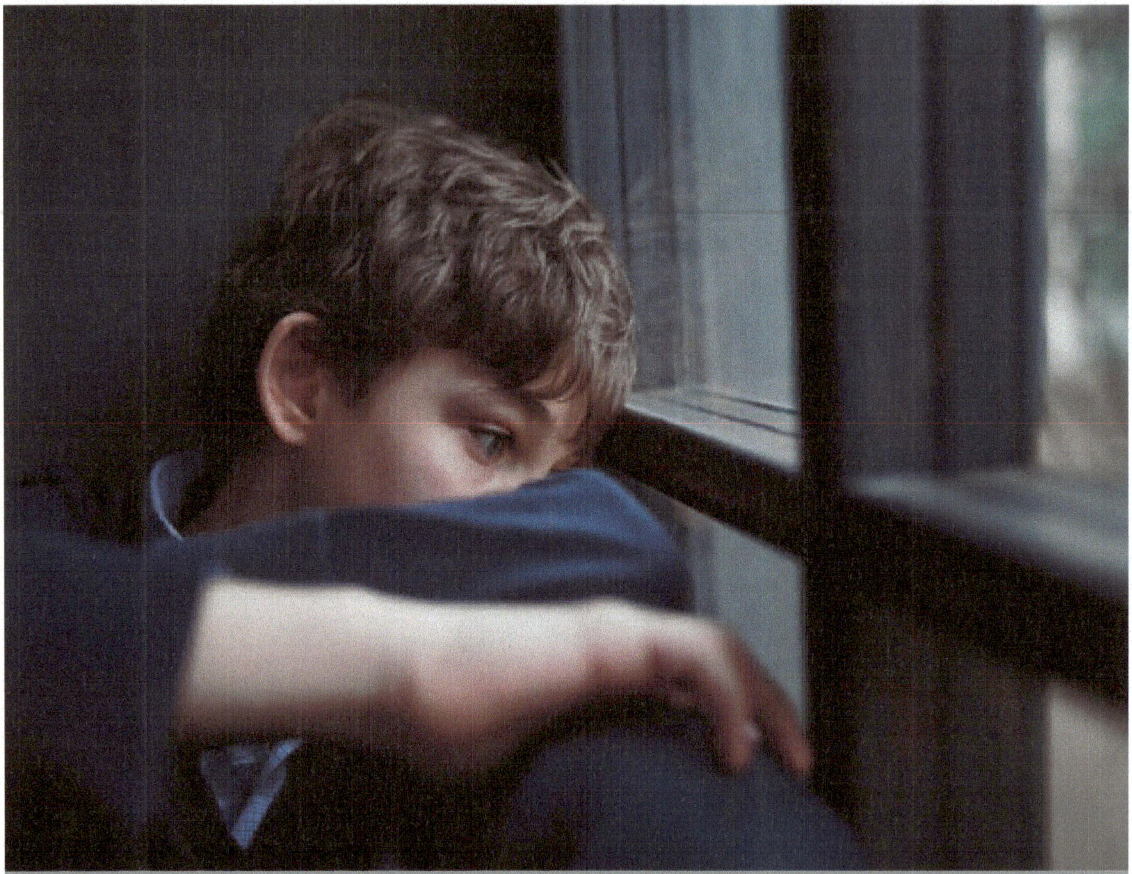

## Withdrawal Symptoms

Withdrawal symptoms from opioids can begin as early as a few hours after the drug was last taken and can include:

- muscle and bone pain
- sleep problems
- diarrhea and vomiting
- cold flashes with goose bumps
- uncontrollable leg movements
- severe cravings for the drug

Some people confuse withdrawal pain as the actual pain they started taking the drug for. Only a doctor can help evaluate the best approach to reducing the pain or discomfort during withdrawal.

## Can you stop an opioid overdose as it is happening?

Yes, with quick action. If you think your child has overdosed on opioids, the most important thing to do is call 911. When medical personnel arrive, they will likely administer naloxone — an FDA-approved medicine that can block the effects of opioids and rapidly reverse an overdose. Naloxone is available as an injectable liquid solution, an auto-injector, and an FDA-approved nasal spray.

Some states require doctors to write a prescription for naloxone, while others have passed laws that allow pharmacies to sell it without a personal prescription. This allows friends, family, and people in the community to keep naloxone on hand to save someone who is overdosing.

However, it is important to remember that naloxone doesn't take the place of medical care. It only works to reverse an opioid overdose in the body for 30 to 90 minutes, so it is possible for a person to still experience the effects of an overdose after naloxone wears off. Also, some opioids are stronger and might require multiple doses. Therefore, it is critical to call 911 so the patient can receive immediate attention.

People given naloxone should be observed constantly until emergency care arrives and they should be monitored for another two hours after the last naloxone dose is given to make sure breathing does not slow or stop. An overdose reversal is a key time for patients with opioid addiction to be connected with treatment for their addiction.

## What is being done to address the opioid overdose crisis?

Federal, state, and local governments, as well as advocacy organizations, researchers, and health professionals are working together to tackle this public health crisis from every angle.

**Such strategies include:**

- improving access to treatment and recovery services
- promoting the use of naloxone by first responders and bystanders
- strengthening our understanding of the crisis through better public health monitoring
- developing safe and effective medications and strategies for pain management
- improving medications to treat people who are addicted to opioids
- improving prevention strategies

Researchers funded by the National Institutes of Health (NIH) are exploring better ways to prevent and treat opioid misuse. They are looking at how opioids work on brain pathways so they can develop safer opioid medications that do not have the risk of addiction. Read about the NIH HEAL℠ (Helping to End Addiction Long-Term) Initiative here: **https://www.drugabuse.gov/drugs-abuse/opioids/nidas-role-in-nih-heal-initiative.**

Scientists are also developing better ways to deliver medications to the body. This includes long-lasting and implantable formulations that can deliver medication to treat opioid addiction for weeks or months, instead of having to take a pill daily or every other day.

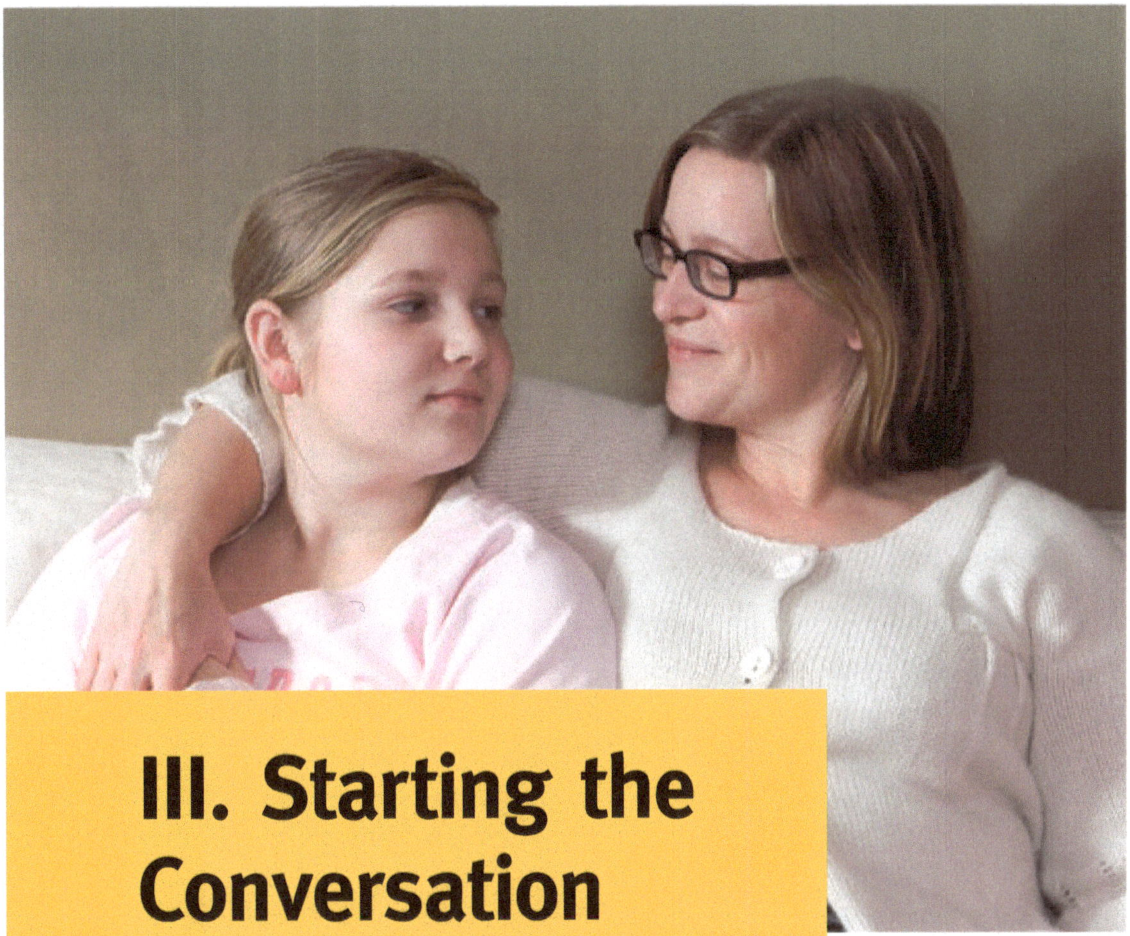

# III. Starting the Conversation

As this guide has shown, opioid misuse can affect the health and well-being of children and teens at a critical point in their lives — when they are growing, learning, maturing, and laying the foundation for their adult years.

As a parent, your children look to you for help and guidance in working out problems and in making decisions, including the decision not to use drugs. Even if you have used drugs in the past, you can have an open conversation about the dangers. Whether or not you tell your child about your past drug use is a personal decision. But experience can better equip us to teach others by drawing on the value of past mistakes. You can explain that there is an opioid crisis in the country and that misusing opioids can have potentially harmful effects on the developing brain.

**Tips for Parents**

- Be a good listener.
- Set clear expectations about drug and alcohol use, including real consequences for not following family rules.
- Help your child deal with peer pressure to use drugs.
- Get to know your child's friends and their parents.
- If concerned, have your child evaluated for mental health issues such as depression or anxiety.
- Monitor your child's whereabouts.
- Carefully monitor your child's medications.
- Do not leave unused opioids in accessible places in your home.
- Supervise teen activities.
- Talk to your child often.
- Do not ignore signs that your child is changing in negative ways.

Because opioids are available by prescription, many children and teens don't understand their danger, and even fewer recognize that heroin is an opioid. Many also do not realize that dangerous fentanyl is added to many street drugs. Misusing opioids can be harmful and can alter the course of young peoples' lives, preventing them from reaching their full potential. That's reason enough to have this difficult conversation with your children. Be certain that the discussion focuses on how much you care about your child's health.

We hope this guide encourages and helps parents to begin the dialogue and, more importantly, to keep open the channels of communication.

Want to become involved? Consider coordinating an event during National Drug and Alcohol Facts Week using free NIDA materials or contact us at **drugfacts@nida.nih.gov.** See **https://teens.drugabuse.gov/national-drug-facts-week.**

# IV. Other Useful Resources

There are numerous resources available, many right in your own community, where you can get information to help you talk to your children about drugs.

Some helpful sources to get such information are your local library, school, or community service organization. You may also contact the government organizations listed below.

**National Institute on Drug Abuse (NIDA)**

NIDA, as part of the National Institutes of Health, offers a wide variety of free publications, education materials, and videos to help parents talk to their children about drug use.

**Free resources include:**

- **Family Checkup,** (online or hard copy) that provides parents with research-based skills, such as videos with conversation tips on how to help their children make good personal choices
- **Drugs: Shatter the Myths,** a booklet that parents can give to their teens to help answer frequently asked questions about drugs and drug misuse
- **Step-by-Step Guide,** an online guide that offers guidance on what parents can do if their teen appears to be misusing drugs
- **Principles of Substance Abuse Prevention for Early Childhood,** an online report that addresses early interventions and their positive effects on development

Visit our **Parents & Educators** page for a list of other materials.

NIDA has more information about opioids and other drugs on both our **main website (https://www.drugabuse.gov/)** and our **NIDA for Teens (https://teens.drugabuse.gov/)** site. To order this and other hard copy NIDA publications, please visit **drugpubs.drugabuse.gov.**

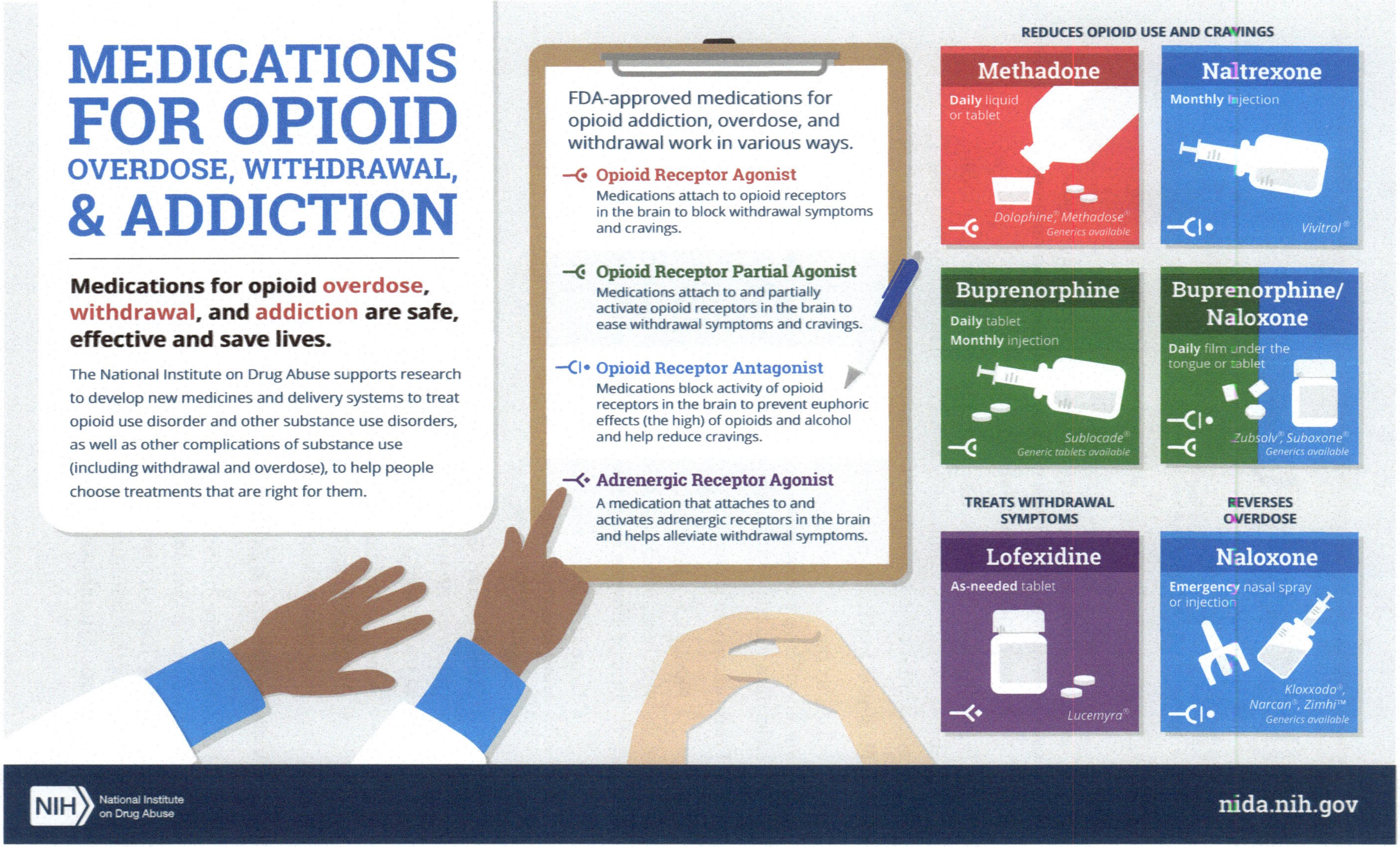
MEDICATIONS FOR OPIOID OVERDOSE, WITHDRAWAL, & ADDICTION
Medications for opioid overdose, withdrawal, and addiction are safe, effective and save lives.
The National Institute on Drug Abuse supports research to develop new medicines and delivery systems to treat opioid use disorder and other substance use disorders, as well as other complications of substance use (including withdrawal and overdose), to help people choose treatments that are right for them.
FDA-approved medications for opioid addiction, overdose, and withdrawal work in various ways.
Opioid Receptor Agonist
Medications attach to opioid receptors in the brain to block withdrawal symptoms and cravings.
Opioid Receptor Partial Agonist
Medications attach to and partially activate opioid receptors in the brain to ease withdrawal symptoms and cravings.
Opioid Receptor Antagonist
Medications block activity of opioid receptors in the brain to prevent euphoric effects (the high) of opioids and alcohol and help reduce cravings.
Adrenergic Receptor Agonist
A medication that attaches to and activates adrenergic receptors in the brain and helps alleviate withdrawal symptoms.
REDUCES OPIOID USE AND CRAVINGS
Methadone
Daily liquid or tablet
Dolophine®, Methadose®
Generics available
Naltrexone
Monthly injection
Vivitrol®
Buprenorphine
Daily tablet
Monthly injection
Sublocade®
Generic tablets available
Buprenorphine/ Naloxone
Daily film under the tongue or tablet
Zubsolv®, Suboxone®
Generics available
TREATS WITHDRAWAL SYMPTOMS
Lofexidine
As-needed tablet
Lucemyra®
REVERSES OVERDOSE
Naloxone
Emergency nasal spray or injection
Kloxxodo®, Narcan®, Zimhi™
Generics available
NIH National Institute on Drug Abuse
nida.nih.gov

## WHAT IS **FENTANYL?**

# Fentanyl is a synthetic opioid that is approximately 50X MORE POTENT THAN MORPHINE[1]

Many people are exposed to fentanyl without knowledge while others use it intentionally because of its potency.

**OVERDOSE DEATHS IN THE UNITED STATES EXCEEDED 100,000 IN A 12-MONTH PERIOD FOR THE FIRST TIME!**

64% of these deaths involved synthetic opioids, mainly illicitly manufactured fentanyls (IMFs) (May 2020-April 2021)[2]

This is up from the more than 91,000 overdose deaths that occurred the previous year. (December 2019-December 2020)[3]

**Although the northeast region continues to suffer the highest overdose deaths, several regions of the country showed sharp increases in IMF related deaths.**[2]

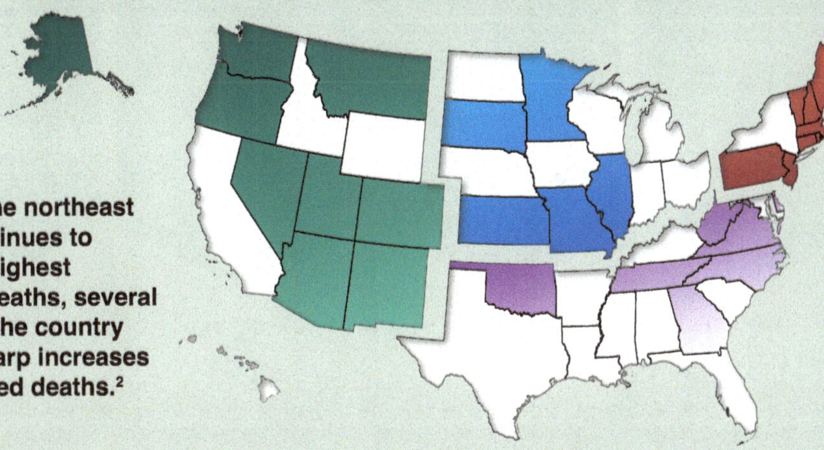

**Northeast**
3.5% increase; 5,194 deaths

**Midwest**
33.1% increase; 2,010 deaths

**South**
64.7% increase; 4,342 deaths

**West**
93.9% increase; 1,852 deaths

*In jurisdictions participating in State Unintentional Drug Overdose Reporting System (SUDORS).

## FENTANYL IS IMPACTING MINORITIES AT AN ALARMING RATE!

Non-Hispanic Blacks had the highest mortality rate due to synthetic opioids other than methadone in 2020. In addition, from 2013-2020, the highest changes in this rate were for: non-Hispanic Blacks, Hispanics, non-Hispanic Whites.[4]

**47.6X**

Overdose deaths involving IMF rose 47.6-fold among Non-Hispanic Blacks.[4]

**35.7X**

Overdose deaths involving IMF rose 35.7-fold among Hispanics.[4]

**15.9X**

Overdose deaths involving IMF rose 15.9-fold among Non-Hispanic Whites.[4]

## YOU CAN HELP SAVE LIVES - **CARRY NALOXONE!**

**AN OVERDOSE CAN HAPPEN ANYWHERE.**

If you suspect an opioid overdose, administer NALOXONE and get emergency medical assistance right away. NALOXONE is a small, easy to carry medicine that rapidly reverses an opioid overdose.

**Looking for NALOXONE?**

Visit: www.naloxoneforall.org

## HOW TO RECOGNIZE THE **SIGNS OF AN OVERDOSE.**

- UNRESPONSIVE
- IRREGULAR BREATHING
- GRAY, BLUE, OR PALE SKIN COLOR
- VERY SMALL PUPILS

## HOW TO **REVERSE AN OVERDOSE.**

Immediate action saves lives! Good Samaritan Laws protect you when you are trying to help someone in need.

**CALL 911 IMMEDIATELY**

Call 911, or direct someone nearby to call and say that you are supporting a suspected overdose.

**ADMINISTER NALOXONE**

Even though the person is unresponsive, 1) Announce that you are going to give naloxone 2) Spray the naloxone in the person's nose.

**ADMINISTER CPR**

Tilt the individual's head back to make sure their airways are open.

Apply chest compressions.

**GIVE NALOXONE AGAIN**

Administer additional Naloxone if the person does not regain color or breathing, otherwise continue chest compressions, until help arrives.

**REMAIN CALM & COMFORTING**

If the person is revived, remain calm and compassionate and encourage them to accept help or stay in a public place.

Harm reduction is all about keeping people safe in a practical way. **Simple tips are to:**

**CARRY NALOXONE | NEVER USE ALONE | GO SLOW | TEST YOUR DRUGS**

## **TEST YOUR DRUGS** FOR FENTANYL.

POSITIVE FOR FENTANYL

USE CAUTION

FENTANYL TEST STRIPS CAN BE USED TO DETERMINE THE PRESENCE OF FENTANYL IN YOUR SUBSTANCE.[5]

Even if your drugs test negative for fentanyl, use caution and remember the harm reduction steps to take.

1. Centers for Disease Control and Prevention. (n.d.). *Other Drugs*. Retrieved June 16, 2021, from https://www.cdc.gov/drugoverdose/data/otherdrugs.html.
2. O'Donnell J, Tanz LJ, Gladden RM, Davis NL, Bitting J. (2021). *Trends in and Characteristics of Drug Overdose Deaths Involving Illicitly Manufactured Fentanyls* –United States, 2019-2020. Morbidity Mortal Weekly Report, 70(1740-1746). DOI: http://dx.doi.org/10/.15585/mmwr.mm7050e3
3. Hedegaard H, Minino AM, Spencer MR, Warner M. (2021). *Drug overdose deaths in the United States*, 1999-2020. NCHS Data Brief, no 428. Hyattsville, MD:National Center for Health Statistics. DOI: https://dx.doi.org/10.15620/cdc:112340.
4. Agency for Healthcare Research and Quality. (n.d.). *Blacks Experiencing Fast-Rising Rates of Overdose Deaths Involving Synthetic Opioids Other than Methadone*. Retrieved June 16, 2021, from https://www.ahrq.gov/sites/default/files/wysiwyg/research/findings/nhqrdr/dataspotlight-opioid.pdf
5. How to Test Your Drugs Using Fentanyl Test Strips. [Brochure]. (n.d.) N.P. Retrieved April 6, 2022, from https://www1.nyc.gov/assets/doh/downloads/pdf/basas/fentanyl-test-strips-brochure.pdf.
6. Centers for Disease Control and Prevention. (2021). *Federal grantees may now use funds to purchase fentanyl test strips.* Retrieved September 14, 2021, from https://www.cdc.gov/media/releases/2021/p0407-Fentanyl-Test-Strips.html
7. CDC Health Advisory - https://emergency.cdc.gov/han/2020/han00438.asp

Disclaimer: This resource was funded in part with federal funds from the National Institute on Drug Abuse, Center for the Clinical Trials Network Dissemination Initiative (contract # 75N95020C00028RFP). The content was developed by experts and researchers and does not necessarily reflect the official position of the National Institute on Drug Abuse, National Institutes of Health, Department of Health and Human Services; nor does mention of trade names, commercial practices, or organizations imply endorsement by the U.S. government. This information should not be considered a substitute for legal counsel or individualized patient care and treatment decisions.

National Institute on Drug Abuse (NIDA)
Clinical Trials Network (CTN) Dissemination Initiative

Center *for* Addiction Medicine *and* Policy

Centers for Disease Control and Prevention

MMWR

Morbidity and Mortality Weekly Report

Weekly / Vol. 69 / No. 32

August 14, 2020

# Mental Health, Substance Use, and Suicidal Ideation During the COVID-19 Pandemic — United States, June 24–30, 2020

Mark É. Czeisler[1,2]; Rashon I. Lane MA[3]; Emiko Petrosky, MD[3]; Joshua F. Wiley, PhD[1]; Aleta Christensen, MPH[3]; Rashid Njai, PhD[3]; Matthew D. Weaver, PhD[1,4,5]; Rebecca Robbins, PhD[4,5]; Elise R. Facer-Childs, PhD[1]; Laura K. Barger, PhD[4,5]; Charles A. Czeisler, MD, PhD[1,4,5]; Mark E. Howard, MBBS, PhD[1,2,6]; Shantha M.W. Rajaratnam, PhD[1,4,5]

The coronavirus disease 2019 (COVID-19) pandemic has been associated with mental health challenges related to the morbidity and mortality caused by the disease and to mitigation activities, including the impact of physical distancing and stay-at-home orders.* Symptoms of anxiety disorder and depressive disorder increased considerably in the United States during April–June of 2020, compared with the same period in 2019 (*1,2*). To assess mental health, substance use, and suicidal ideation during the pandemic, representative panel surveys were conducted among adults aged ≥18 years across the United States during June 24–30, 2020. Overall, 40.9% of respondents reported at least one adverse mental or behavioral health condition, including symptoms of anxiety disorder or depressive disorder (30.9%), symptoms of a trauma- and stressor-related disorder (TSRD) related to the pandemic† (26.3%), and having started or increased substance use to cope with stress or emotions related to COVID-19 (13.3%). The percentage of respondents who reported having seriously considered suicide in the 30 days before completing the survey (10.7%) was significantly higher among respondents aged 18–24 years (25.5%), minority racial/ethnic groups (Hispanic respondents [18.6%], non-Hispanic black [black] respondents [15.1%]), self-reported unpaid caregivers for adults§ (30.7%), and essential workers¶ (21.7%).

* https://www.medrxiv.org/content/10.1101/2020.04.22.20076141v1.

† Disorders classified as TSRDs in the *Diagnostic and Statistical Manual of Mental Disorders* (DSM–5) include posttraumatic stress disorder (PTSD), acute stress disorder (ASD), and adjustment disorders (ADs), among others.

§ Unpaid adult caregiver status was self-reported. The definition of an unpaid caregiver for adults was a person who had provided unpaid care to a relative or friend aged ≥18 years to help them take care of themselves at any time in the last 3 months. Examples provided included helping with personal needs, household chores, health care tasks, managing a person's finances, taking them to a doctor's appointment, arranging for outside services, and visiting regularly to see how they are doing.

¶ Essential worker status was self-reported. The comparison was between employed respondents (n = 3,431) who identified as essential versus nonessential. For this analysis, students who were not separately employed as essential workers were considered nonessential workers.

INSIDE



**Continuing Education** examination available at https://www.cdc.gov/mmwr/mmwr_continuingEducation.html

**U.S. Department of Health and Human Services**
Centers for Disease Control and Prevention

Community-level intervention and prevention efforts, including health communication strategies, designed to reach these groups could help address various mental health conditions associated with the COVID-19 pandemic.

During June 24–30, 2020, a total of 5,412 (54.7%) of 9,896 eligible invited adults** completed web-based surveys†† administered by Qualtrics.§§ The Monash University Human Research Ethics Committee of Monash University (Melbourne, Australia) reviewed and approved the study protocol on human subjects research. Respondents were informed of the study purposes and provided electronic consent before commencement, and investigators received anonymized responses. Participants included 3,683 (68.1%) first-time respondents and 1,729 (31.9%) respondents who had completed a related survey during April 2–8, May 5–12, 2020, or both intervals; 1,497 (27.7%) respondents participated during all three intervals (*2,3*). Quota sampling and survey weighting were employed to improve cohort representativeness of the U.S. population by gender, age, and race/ethnicity.¶¶ Symptoms of anxiety disorder and depressive disorder were assessed using the four-item Patient Health Questionnaire*** (*4*), and symptoms of a COVID-19–related TSRD were assessed using the six-item Impact of Event Scale††† (*5*). Respondents also reported

** A minimum age of 18 years and residence within the United States as of April 2–8, 2020, were required for eligibility for the longitudinal cohort to complete a survey during June 24–30, 2020. Residence was reassessed during June 24–30, 2020, and one respondent who had moved from the United States was excluded from the analysis. A minimum age of 18 years and residence within the United States were required for eligibility for newly recruited respondents included in the cross-sectional analysis. For both the longitudinal cohort and newly recruited respondents, respondents were required to provide informed consent before enrollment into the study. All surveys underwent data quality screening procedures including algorithmic and keystroke analysis for attention patterns, click-through behavior, duplicate responses, machine responses, and inattentiveness. Country-specific geolocation verification via IP address mapping was used to ensure respondents were from the United States. Respondents who failed an attention or speed check, along with any responses identified by the data-scrubbing algorithms, were excluded from analysis.

†† The surveys contained 101 items for first-time respondents and 86 items for respondents who also participated in later surveys, with the 15 additional items for first-time respondents consisting of questions on demographics. The survey instruments included a combination of individual questions, validated questionnaires, and COVID-19-specific questionnaires, which were used to assess respondent attitudes, behaviors, and beliefs related to COVID-19 and its mitigation, as well as the social and behavioral health impacts of the COVID-19 pandemic.

§§ https://www.qualtrics.com/.

¶¶ Survey weighting was implemented according to the 2010 U.S. Census with respondents who reported gender, age, and race/ethnicity. Respondents who reported a gender of "Other," or who did not report race/ethnicity were assigned a weight of one.

*** Symptoms of anxiety disorder and depressive disorder were assessed via the four-item Patient Health Questionnaire (PHQ-4). Those who scored ≥3 out of 6 on the Generalized Anxiety Disorder (GAD-2) and Patient Health Questionnaire (PHQ-2) subscales were considered symptomatic for these respective disorders. This instrument was included in the April, May, and June surveys.

††† Symptoms of a TSRD attributed to the COVID-19 pandemic were assessed via the six-item Impact of Event Scale (IES-6) to screen for overlapping symptoms of PTSD, ASD, and ADs. For this survey, the COVID-19 pandemic was specified as the traumatic exposure to record peri- and posttraumatic symptoms associated with the range of stressors introduced by the COVID-19 pandemic. Those who scored ≥1.75 out of 4 were considered symptomatic. This instrument was included in the May and June surveys only.

The *MMWR* series of publications is published by the Center for Surveillance, Epidemiology, and Laboratory Services, Centers for Disease Control and Prevention (CDC), U.S. Department of Health and Human Services, Atlanta, GA 30329-4027.

**Suggested citation:** [Author names; first three, then et al., if more than six.] [Report title]. MMWR Morb Mortal Wkly Rep 2020;69:[inclusive page numbers].

whether they had started or increased substance use to cope with stress or emotions related to COVID-19 or seriously considered suicide in the 30 days preceding the survey.[§§§]

Analyses were stratified by gender, age, race/ethnicity, employment status, essential worker status, unpaid adult caregiver status, rural-urban residence classification,[¶¶¶] whether the respondent knew someone who had positive test results for SARS-CoV-2, the virus that causes COVID-19, or who had died from COVID-19, and whether the respondent was receiving treatment for diagnosed anxiety, depression, or posttraumatic stress disorder (PTSD) at the time of the survey. Comparisons within subgroups were evaluated using Poisson regressions with robust standard errors to calculate prevalence ratios, 95% confidence intervals (CIs), and p-values to evaluate statistical significance ($\alpha = 0.005$ to account for multiple comparisons). Among the 1,497 respondents who completed all three surveys, longitudinal analyses of the odds of incidence[****] of symptoms of adverse mental or behavioral health conditions by essential worker and unpaid adult caregiver status were conducted on unweighted responses using logistic regressions to calculate unadjusted and adjusted[††††] odds ratios (ORs), 95% CI, and p-values ($\alpha = 0.05$). The statsmodels package in Python (version 3.7.8; Python Software Foundation) was used to conduct all analyses.

Overall, 40.9% of 5,470 respondents who completed surveys during June reported an adverse mental or behavioral health condition, including those who reported symptoms of anxiety disorder or depressive disorder (30.9%), those with TSRD symptoms related to COVID-19 (26.3%), those who reported having started or increased substance use to cope with stress or emotions related to COVID-19 (13.3%), and those who reported having seriously considered suicide in the preceding 30 days (10.7%) (Table 1). At least one adverse mental or behavioral health symptom was reported by more than one half of respondents who were aged 18–24 years (74.9%) and 25–44 years (51.9%), of Hispanic ethnicity (52.1%), and who held less than a high school diploma (66.2%), as well as those who were essential workers (54.0%), unpaid caregivers for adults (66.6%), and who reported treatment for diagnosed anxiety (72.7%), depression (68.8%), or PTSD (88.0%) at the time of the survey.

Prevalences of symptoms of adverse mental or behavioral health conditions varied significantly among subgroups (Table 2). Suicidal ideation was more prevalent among males than among females. Symptoms of anxiety disorder or depressive disorder, COVID-19–related TSRD, initiation of or increase in substance use to cope with COVID-19–associated stress, and serious suicidal ideation in the previous 30 days were most commonly reported by persons aged 18–24 years; prevalence decreased progressively with age. Hispanic respondents reported higher prevalences of symptoms of anxiety disorder or depressive disorder, COVID-19–related TSRD, increased substance use, and suicidal ideation than did non-Hispanic whites (whites) or non-Hispanic Asian (Asian) respondents. Black respondents reported increased substance use and past 30-day serious consideration of suicide in the previous 30 days more commonly than did white and Asian respondents. Respondents who reported treatment for diagnosed anxiety, depression, or PTSD at the time of the survey reported higher prevalences of symptoms of adverse mental and behavioral health conditions compared with those who did not. Symptoms of a COVID-19–related TSRD, increased substance use, and suicidal ideation were more prevalent among employed than unemployed respondents, and among essential workers than nonessential workers. Adverse conditions also were more prevalent among unpaid caregivers for adults than among those who were not, with particularly large differences in increased substance use (32.9% versus 6.3%) and suicidal ideation (30.7% versus 3.6%) in this group.

Longitudinal analysis of responses of 1,497 persons who completed all three surveys revealed that unpaid caregivers for adults had a significantly higher odds of incidence of adverse mental health conditions compared with others (Table 3). Among those who did not report having started or increased substance use to cope with stress or emotions related to COVID-19 in May, unpaid caregivers for adults had 3.33 times the odds of reporting this behavior in June (adjusted OR 95% CI = 1.75–6.31; $p<0.001$). Similarly, among those who did not report having seriously considered suicide in the previous 30 days in May, unpaid caregivers for adults had 3.03 times the odds of reporting suicidal ideation in June (adjusted OR 95% CI = 1.20–7.63; $p = 0.019$).

[§§§] For this survey, substance use was defined as use of "alcohol, legal or illegal drugs, or prescriptions drugs that are taken in a way not recommended by your doctor." Questions regarding substance use and suicidal ideation were included in the May and June surveys only. Participants were informed that responses were deidentified and that direct support could not be provided to those who reported substance use behavior or suicidal ideation. Regarding substance use, respondents were provided the following: "This survey is anonymous so we cannot provide direct support. If you would like crisis support please contact the Substance Abuse and Mental Health Services Administration National Helpline, 1-800-662-HELP (4357), (also known as the Treatment Referral Routing Service) or TTY: 1-800-487-4889. This is a confidential, free, 24-hour-a-day, 365-day-a-year, information service, in English and Spanish, for persons and family members facing mental and/or substance use disorders." Regarding suicidal ideation, respondents were provided the following: "This survey is anonymous so we cannot provide direct support. If you would like crisis support please contact the National Suicide Prevention Lifeline, 1-800-273-TALK (8255, or chat line) for help for themselves or others."

[¶¶¶] Rural-urban classification was determined by using self-reported ZIP codes according to the Federal Office of Rural Health Policy definition of rurality. https://www.hrsa.gov/rural-health/about-us/definition/datafiles.html.

[****] Odds of incidence was defined as the odds of the presence of an adverse mental or behavioral health outcome reported during a later survey after previously having reported the absence of that outcome (e.g., having reported symptoms of anxiety disorder during June 24–30, 2020, after not having reported symptoms of anxiety disorder during April 2–8, 2020).

[††††] Adjusted for gender, employment status, and essential worker status or unpaid adult caregiver status.

TABLE 1. Respondent characteristics and prevalence of adverse mental health outcomes, increased substance use to cope with stress or emotions related to COVID-19 pandemic, and suicidal ideation — United States, June 24–30, 2020

| | | Weighted %* | | | | | | |
|---|---|---|---|---|---|---|---|---|
| | | Conditions | | | | | | |
| Characteristic | All respondents who completed surveys during June 24–30, 2020 weighted* no. (%) | Anxiety disorder[†] | Depressive disorder[†] | Anxiety or depressive disorder[†] | COVID-19–related TSRD[§] | Started or increased substance use to cope with pandemic-related stress or emotions[¶] | Seriously considered suicide in past 30 days | ≥1 adverse mental or behavioral health symptom |
| **All respondents** | **5,470 (100)** | **25.5** | **24.3** | **30.9** | **26.3** | **13.3** | **10.7** | **40.9** |
| **Gender** | | | | | | | | |
| Female | 2,784 (50.9) | 26.3 | 23.9 | 31.5 | 24.7 | 12.2 | 8.9 | 41.4 |
| Male | 2,676 (48.9) | 24.7 | 24.8 | 30.4 | 27.9 | 14.4 | 12.6 | 40.5 |
| Other | 10 (0.2) | 20.0 | 30.0 | 30.0 | 30.0 | 10.0 | 0.0 | 30.0 |
| **Age group (yrs)** | | | | | | | | |
| 18–24 | 731 (13.4) | 49.1 | 52.3 | 62.9 | 46.0 | 24.7 | 25.5 | 74.9 |
| 25–44 | 1,911 (34.9) | 35.3 | 32.5 | 40.4 | 36.0 | 19.5 | 16.0 | 51.9 |
| 45–64 | 1,895 (34.6) | 16.1 | 14.4 | 20.3 | 17.2 | 7.7 | 3.8 | 29.5 |
| ≥65 | 933 (17.1) | 6.2 | 5.8 | 8.1 | 9.2 | 3.0 | 2.0 | 15.1 |
| **Race/Ethnicity** | | | | | | | | |
| White, non-Hispanic | 3,453 (63.1) | 24.0 | 22.9 | 29.2 | 23.3 | 10.6 | 7.9 | 37.8 |
| Black, non-Hispanic | 663 (12.1) | 23.4 | 24.6 | 30.2 | 30.4 | 18.4 | 15.1 | 44.2 |
| Asian, non-Hispanic | 256 (4.7) | 14.1 | 14.2 | 18.0 | 22.1 | 6.7 | 6.6 | 31.9 |
| Other race or multiple races, non-Hispanic** | 164 (3.0) | 27.8 | 29.3 | 33.2 | 28.3 | 11.0 | 9.8 | 43.8 |
| Hispanic, any race(s) | 885 (16.2) | 35.5 | 31.3 | 40.8 | 35.1 | 21.9 | 18.6 | 52.1 |
| Unknown | 50 (0.9) | 38.0 | 34.0 | 44.0 | 34.0 | 18.0 | 26.0 | 48.0 |
| **2019 Household income (USD)** | | | | | | | | |
| <25,000 | 741 (13.6) | 30.6 | 30.8 | 36.6 | 29.9 | 12.5 | 9.9 | 45.4 |
| 25,000–49,999 | 1,123 (20.5) | 26.0 | 25.6 | 33.2 | 27.2 | 13.5 | 10.1 | 43.9 |
| 50,999–99,999 | 1,775 (32.5) | 27.1 | 24.8 | 31.6 | 26.4 | 12.6 | 11.4 | 40.3 |
| 100,999–199,999 | 1,301 (23.8) | 23.1 | 20.8 | 27.7 | 24.2 | 15.5 | 11.7 | 37.8 |
| ≥200,000 | 282 (5.2) | 17.4 | 17.0 | 20.6 | 23.1 | 14.8 | 11.6 | 35.1 |
| Unknown | 247 (4.5) | 19.6 | 23.1 | 27.2 | 24.9 | 6.2 | 3.9 | 41.5 |
| **Education** | | | | | | | | |
| Less than high school diploma | 78 (1.4) | 44.5 | 51.4 | 57.5 | 44.5 | 22.1 | 30.0 | 66.2 |
| High school diploma | 943 (17.2) | 31.5 | 32.8 | 38.4 | 32.1 | 15.3 | 13.1 | 48.0 |
| Some college | 1,455 (26.6) | 25.2 | 23.4 | 31.7 | 22.8 | 10.9 | 8.6 | 39.9 |
| Bachelor's degree | 1,888 (34.5) | 24.7 | 22.5 | 28.7 | 26.4 | 14.2 | 10.7 | 40.6 |
| Professional degree | 1,074 (19.6) | 20.9 | 19.5 | 25.4 | 24.5 | 12.6 | 10.0 | 35.2 |
| Unknown | 33 (0.6) | 25.2 | 23.2 | 28.2 | 23.2 | 10.5 | 5.5 | 28.2 |
| **Employment status[††]** | | | | | | | | |
| Employed | 3,431 (62.7) | 30.1 | 29.1 | 36.4 | 32.1 | 17.9 | 15.0 | 47.8 |
| Essential | 1,785 (32.6) | 35.5 | 33.6 | 42.4 | 38.5 | 24.7 | 21.7 | 54.0 |
| Nonessential | 1,646 (30.1) | 24.1 | 24.1 | 29.9 | 25.2 | 10.5 | 7.8 | 41.0 |
| Unemployed | 761 (13.9) | 32.0 | 29.4 | 37.8 | 25.0 | 7.7 | 4.7 | 45.9 |
| Retired | 1,278 (23.4) | 9.6 | 8.7 | 12.1 | 11.3 | 4.2 | 2.5 | 19.6 |
| **Unpaid adult caregiver status[§§]** | | | | | | | | |
| Yes | 1,435 (26.2) | 47.6 | 45.2 | 56.1 | 48.4 | 32.9 | 30.7 | 66.6 |
| No | 4,035 (73.8) | 17.7 | 16.9 | 22.0 | 18.4 | 6.3 | 3.6 | 31.8 |
| **Region[¶¶]** | | | | | | | | |
| Northeast | 1,193 (21.8) | 23.9 | 23.9 | 29.9 | 22.8 | 12.8 | 10.2 | 37.1 |
| Midwest | 1,015 (18.6) | 22.7 | 21.1 | 27.5 | 24.4 | 9.0 | 7.5 | 36.1 |
| South | 1,921 (35.1) | 27.9 | 26.5 | 33.4 | 29.1 | 15.4 | 12.5 | 44.4 |
| West | 1,340 (24.5) | 25.8 | 24.2 | 30.9 | 26.7 | 14.0 | 10.9 | 43 |
| **Rural-urban classification***** | | | | | | | | |
| Rural | 599 (10.9) | 26.0 | 22.5 | 29.3 | 25.4 | 11.5 | 10.2 | 38.3 |
| Urban | 4,871 (89.1) | 25.5 | 24.6 | 31.1 | 26.4 | 13.5 | 10.7 | 41.2 |

See table footnotes on the next page.

**TABLE 1.** (*Continued*) **Respondent characteristics and prevalence of adverse mental health outcomes, increased substance use to cope with stress or emotions related to COVID-19 pandemic, and suicidal ideation — United States, June 24–30, 2020**

| Characteristic | All respondents who completed surveys during June 24–30, 2020 weighted* no. (%) | Weighted %* | | | | | | |
|---|---|---|---|---|---|---|---|---|
| | | Conditions | | | | Started or increased substance use to cope with pandemic-related stress or emotions¶ | Seriously considered suicide in past 30 days | ≥1 adverse mental or behavioral health symptom |
| | | Anxiety disorder† | Depressive disorder† | Anxiety or depressive disorder† | COVID-19–related TSRD§ | | | |
| **Know someone who had positive test results for SARS-CoV-2** | | | | | | | | |
| Yes | 1,109 (20.3) | 23.8 | 21.9 | 29.6 | 21.5 | 12.9 | 7.5 | 39.2 |
| No | 4,361 (79.7) | 26.0 | 25.0 | 31.3 | 27.5 | 13.4 | 11.5 | 41.3 |
| **Knew someone who died from COVID-19** | | | | | | | | |
| Yes | 428 (7.8) | 25.8 | 20.6 | 30.6 | 28.1 | 11.3 | 7.6 | 40.1 |
| No | 5,042 (92.2) | 25.5 | 24.7 | 31.0. | 26.1 | 13.4 | 10.9 | 41 |
| **Receiving treatment for previously diagnosed condition** | | | | | | | | |
| **Anxiety** | | | | | | | | |
| Yes | 536 (9.8) | 59.6 | 52.0 | 66.0 | 51.9 | 26.6 | 23.6 | 72.7 |
| No | 4,934 (90.2) | 21.8 | 21.3 | 27.1 | 23.5 | 11.8 | 9.3 | 37.5 |
| **Depression** | | | | | | | | |
| Yes | 540 (9.9) | 52.5 | 50.6 | 60.8 | 45.5 | 25.2 | 22.1 | 68.8 |
| No | 4,930 (90.1) | 22.6 | 21.5 | 27.7 | 24.2 | 12.0 | 9.4 | 37.9 |
| **Posttraumatic stress disorder** | | | | | | | | |
| Yes | 251 (4.6) | 72.3 | 69.1 | 78.7 | 69.4 | 43.8 | 44.8 | 88 |
| No | 5,219 (95.4) | 23.3 | 22.2 | 28.6 | 24.2 | 11.8 | 9.0 | 38.7 |

**Abbreviations:** COVID-19 = coronavirus disease 2019; TSRD = trauma- or stress-related disorder.

* Survey weighting was employed to improve the cross-sectional June cohort representativeness of the U.S. population by gender, age, and race/ethnicity according to the 2010 U.S. Census with respondents in which gender, age, and race/ethnicity were reported. Respondents who reported a gender of "Other" or who did not report race/ethnicity were assigned a weight of one.

† Symptoms of anxiety disorder and depressive disorder were assessed via the four-item Patient Health Questionnaire (PHQ-4). Those who scored ≥3 out of 6 on the Generalized Anxiety Disorder (GAD-2) and Patient Health Questionnaire (PHQ-2) subscales were considered symptomatic for each disorder, respectively.

§ Disorders classified as TSRDs in the *Diagnostic and Statistical Manual of Mental Disorders* (DSM–5) include posttraumatic stress disorder (PTSD), acute stress disorder (ASD), and adjustment disorders (ADs), among others. Symptoms of a TSRD precipitated by the COVID-19 pandemic were assessed via the six-item Impact of Event Scale (IES-6) to screen for overlapping symptoms of PTSD, ASD, and ADs. For this survey, the COVID-19 pandemic was specified as the traumatic exposure to record peri- and posttraumatic symptoms associated with the range of stressors introduced by the COVID-19 pandemic. Those who scored ≥1.75 out of 4 were considered symptomatic.

¶ 104 respondents selected "Prefer not to answer."

** The Other race or multiple races, non-Hispanic category includes respondents who identified as not being Hispanic and as more than one race or as American Indian or Alaska Native, Native Hawaiian or Pacific Islander, or "Other."

†† Essential worker status was self-reported. The comparison was between employed respondents (n = 3,431) who identified as essential vs. nonessential. For this analysis, students who were not separately employed as essential workers were considered nonessential workers.

§§ Unpaid adult caregiver status was self-reported. The definition of an unpaid caregiver for adults was a person who had provided unpaid care to a relative or friend aged ≥18 years to help them take care of themselves at any time in the last three months. Examples provided included helping with personal needs, household chores, health care tasks, managing a person's finances, taking them to a doctor's appointment, arranging for outside services, and visiting regularly to see how they are doing.

¶¶ Region classification was determined by using the U.S. Census Bureau's Census Regions and Divisions of the United States. https://www2.census.gov/geo/pdfs/maps-data/maps/reference/us_regdiv.pdf.

*** Rural-urban classification was determined by using self-reported ZIP codes according to the Federal Office of Rural Health Policy definition of rurality. https://www.hrsa.gov/rural-health/about-us/definition/datafiles.html.

## Discussion

Elevated levels of adverse mental health conditions, substance use, and suicidal ideation were reported by adults in the United States in June 2020. The prevalence of symptoms of anxiety disorder was approximately three times those reported in the second quarter of 2019 (25.5% versus 8.1%), and prevalence of depressive disorder was approximately four times that reported in the second quarter of 2019 (24.3% versus 6.5%) (*2*). However, given the methodological differences and potential unknown biases in survey designs, this analysis might not be directly comparable with data reported on anxiety and depression disorders in 2019 (*2*). Approximately one quarter of respondents reported symptoms of a TSRD related to the pandemic, and approximately one in 10 reported that they started or increased substance use because of COVID-19. Suicidal ideation was also elevated; approximately twice as many respondents reported serious consideration of suicide in the previous 30 days than did adults in the United States in 2018, referring to the previous 12 months (10.7% versus 4.3%) (*6*).

Mental health conditions are disproportionately affecting specific populations, especially young adults, Hispanic persons, black persons, essential workers, unpaid caregivers for adults, and those receiving treatment for preexisting psychiatric conditions. Unpaid caregivers for adults, many of whom are currently providing critical aid to persons at increased risk

**TABLE 2. Comparison of symptoms of adverse mental health outcomes among all respondents who completed surveys (N = 5,470), by respondent characteristic* — United States, June 24–30, 2020**

| Characteristic | Prevalence ratio¶ (95% CI¶) | | | |
|---|---|---|---|---|
| | Symptoms of anxiety disorder or depressive disorder† | Symptoms of a TSRD related to COVID-19§ | Started or increased substance use to cope with stress or emotions related to COVID-19 | Serious consideration of suicide in past 30 days |
| **Gender** | | | | |
| Female vs. male | 1.04 (0.96–1.12) | 0.88 (0.81–0.97) | 0.85 (0.75–0.98) | 0.70 (0.60–0.82)** |
| **Age group (yrs)** | | | | |
| 18–24 vs. 25–44 | 1.56 (1.44–1.68)** | 1.28 (1.16–1.41)** | 1.31 (1.12–1.53)** | 1.59 (1.35–1.87)** |
| 18–24 vs. 45–64 | 3.10 (2.79–3.44)** | 2.67 (2.35–3.03)** | 3.35 (2.75–4.10)** | 6.66 (5.15–8.61)** |
| 18–24 vs. ≥65 | 7.73 (6.19–9.66)** | 5.01 (4.04–6.22)** | 8.77 (5.95–12.93)** | 12.51 (7.88–19.86)** |
| 25–44 vs. 45–64 | 1.99 (1.79–2.21)** | 2.09 (1.86–2.35)** | 2.56 (2.14–3.07)** | 4.18 (3.26–5.36)** |
| 25–44 vs. ≥65 | 4.96 (3.97–6.20)** | 3.93 (3.18–4.85)** | 6.70 (4.59–9.78)** | 7.86 (4.98–12.41)** |
| 45–64 vs. ≥65 | 2.49 (1.98–3.15)** | 1.88 (1.50–2.35)** | 2.62 (1.76–3.9)** | 1.88 (1.14–3.10) |
| **Race/Ethnicity††** | | | | |
| Hispanic vs. non-Hispanic black | 1.35 (1.18–1.56)** | 1.15 (1.00–1.33) | 1.19 (0.97–1.46) | 1.23 (0.98–1.55) |
| Hispanic vs. non-Hispanic Asian | 2.27 (1.73–2.98)** | 1.59 (1.24–2.04)** | 3.29 (2.05–5.28)** | 2.82 (1.74–4.57)** |
| Hispanic vs. non-Hispanic other race or multiple races | 1.23 (0.98–1.55) | 1.24 (0.96–1.61) | 1.99 (1.27–3.13)** | 1.89 (1.16–3.06) |
| Hispanic vs. non-Hispanic white | 1.40 (1.27–1.54)** | 1.50 (1.35–1.68)** | 2.09 (1.79–2.45)** | 2.35 (1.96–2.80)** |
| Non-Hispanic black vs. non-Hispanic Asian | 1.68 (1.26–2.23)** | 1.38 (1.07–1.78) | 2.75 (1.70–4.47)** | 2.29 (1.39–3.76)** |
| Non-Hispanic black vs. non-Hispanic other race or multiple races | 0.91 (0.71–1.16) | 1.08 (0.82–1.41) | 1.67 (1.05–2.65) | 1.53 (0.93–2.52) |
| Non-Hispanic black vs. non-Hispanic white | 1.03 (0.91–1.17) | 1.30 (1.14–1.48)** | 1.75 (1.45–2.11)** | 1.90 (1.54–2.36)** |
| Non-Hispanic Asian vs. non-Hispanic other race or multiple races | 0.54 (0.39–0.76)** | 0.78 (0.56–1.09) | 0.61 (0.32–1.14) | 0.67 (0.35–1.29) |
| Non-Hispanic Asian vs. non-Hispanic white | 0.62 (0.47–0.80)** | 0.95 (0.74–1.20) | 0.64 (0.40–1.02) | 0.83 (0.52–1.34) |
| Non-Hispanic other race or multiple races vs. non-Hispanic white | 1.14 (0.91–1.42) | 1.21 (0.94–1.56) | 1.05 (0.67–1.64) | 1.24 (0.77–2) |

See table footnotes on the next page.

for severe illness from COVID-19, had a higher incidence of adverse mental and behavioral health conditions compared with others. Although unpaid caregivers of children were not evaluated in this study, approximately 39% of unpaid caregivers for adults shared a household with children (compared with 27% of other respondents). Caregiver workload, especially in multigenerational caregivers, should be considered for future assessment of mental health, given the findings of this report and hardships potentially faced by caregivers.

The findings in this report are subject to at least four limitations. First, a diagnostic evaluation for anxiety disorder or depressive disorder was not conducted; however, clinically validated screening instruments were used to assess symptoms. Second, the trauma- and stressor-related symptoms assessed were common to multiple TSRDs, precluding distinction among them; however, the findings highlight the importance of including COVID-19–specific trauma measures to gain insights into peri- and posttraumatic impacts of the COVID-19 pandemic (*7*). Third, substance use behavior was self-reported; therefore, responses might be subject to recall, response, and social desirability biases. Finally, given that the web-based survey might not be fully representative of the United States population, findings might have limited generalizability. However, standardized quality and data inclusion screening procedures, including algorithmic analysis of click-through behavior, removal of duplicate responses and scrubbing methods for web-based panel quality were applied. Further the prevalence of symptoms of anxiety disorder and depressive disorder were largely consistent with findings from the Household Pulse Survey during June (*1*).

Markedly elevated prevalences of reported adverse mental and behavioral health conditions associated with the COVID-19 pandemic highlight the broad impact of the pandemic and the need to prevent and treat these conditions. Identification of populations at increased risk for psychological distress and unhealthy coping can inform policies to address health inequity, including increasing access to resources for clinical diagnoses and treatment options. Expanded use of telehealth, an effective means of delivering treatment for mental health conditions, including depression, substance use disorder, and suicidal ideation (*8*), might reduce COVID-19-related mental health consequences. Future studies should identify drivers of adverse mental and behavioral health during the COVID-19 pandemic and whether factors such as social isolation, absence of school structure, unemployment and other financial worries, and various forms of violence (e.g., physical,

**TABLE 2. (*Continued*) Comparison of symptoms of adverse mental health outcomes among all respondents who completed surveys (N = 5,470), by respondent characteristic* — United States, June 24–30, 2020**

| | Prevalence ratio¶ (95% CI¶) | | | |
|---|---|---|---|---|
| Characteristic | Symptoms of anxiety disorder or depressive disorder† | Symptoms of a TSRD related to COVID-19§ | Started or increased substance use to cope with stress or emotions related to COVID-19 | Serious consideration of suicide in past 30 days |
| **Employment status** | | | | |
| Employed vs. unemployed | 0.96 (0.87–1.07) | 1.28 (1.12–1.46)** | 2.30 (1.78–2.98)** | 3.21 (2.31–4.47)** |
| Employed vs. retired | 3.01 (2.58–3.51)** | 2.84 (2.42–3.34)** | 4.30 (3.28–5.63)** | 5.97 (4.20–8.47)** |
| Unemployed vs. retired | 3.12 (2.63–3.71)** | 2.21 (1.82–2.69)** | 1.87 (1.30–2.67)** | 1.86 (1.16–2.96) |
| **Essential vs. nonessential worker§§** | 1.42 (1.30–1.56)** | 1.52 (1.38–1.69)** | 2.36 (2.00–2.77)** | 2.76 (2.29–3.33)** |
| **Unpaid caregiver for adults vs. not¶¶** | 2.55 (2.37–2.75)** | 2.63 (2.42–2.86)** | 5.28 (4.59–6.07)** | 8.64 (7.23–10.33)** |
| **Rural vs. urban residence*** ** | 0.94 (0.82–1.07) | 0.96 (0.83–1.11) | 0.84 (0.67–1.06) | 0.95 (0.74–1.22) |
| **Knows someone with positive SARS-CoV-2 test result vs. not** | 0.95 (0.86–1.05) | 0.78 (0.69–0.88)** | 0.96 (0.81–1.14) | 0.65 (0.52–0.81)** |
| **Knew someone who died from COVID-19 vs. not** | 0.99 (0.85–1.15) | 1.08 (0.92–1.26) | 0.84 (0.64–1.11) | 0.69 (0.49–0.97) |
| **Receiving treatment for anxiety vs. not** | 2.43 (2.26–2.63)** | 2.21 (2.01–2.43)** | 2.27 (1.94–2.66)** | 2.54 (2.13–3.03)** |
| **Receiving treatment for depression vs. not** | 2.20 (2.03–2.39)** | 1.88 (1.70–2.09)** | 2.13 (1.81–2.51)** | 2.35 (1.96–2.82)** |
| **Receiving treatment for PTSD vs. not** | 2.75 (2.55–2.97)** | 2.87 (2.61–3.16)** | 3.78 (3.23–4.42)** | 4.95 (4.21–5.83)** |

**Abbreviations:** CI = confidence interval; COVID-19 = coronavirus disease 2019; PTSD = posttraumatic stress disorder; TSRD = trauma- or stress-related disorder.

* Number of respondents for characteristics: gender (female = 2,784, male = 2,676), age group in years (18–24 = 731; 25–44 = 1,911; 45–64 = 1,895; ≥65 = 933), race/ethnicity (non-Hispanic white = 3453, non-Hispanic black = 663, non-Hispanic Asian = 256, non-Hispanic other race or multiple races = 164, Hispanic = 885).

† Symptoms of anxiety disorder and depressive disorder were assessed via the four-item Patient Health Questionnaire (PHQ-4). Those who scored ≥3 out of 6 on the Generalized Anxiety Disorder (GAD-2) and Patient Health Questionnaire (PHQ-2) subscales were considered to have symptoms of these disorders.

§ Disorders classified as TSRDs in the *Diagnostic and Statistical Manual of Mental Disorders* (DSM–5) include PTSD, acute stress disorder (ASD), and adjustment disorders (ADs), among others. Symptoms of a TSRD precipitated by the COVID-19 pandemic were assessed via the six-item Impact of Event Scale (IES-6) to screen for overlapping symptoms of PTSD, ASD, and ADs. For this survey, the COVID-19 pandemic was specified as the traumatic exposure to record peri- and posttraumatic symptoms associated with the range of stressors introduced by the COVID-19 pandemic. Persons who scored ≥1.75 out of 4 were considered to be symptomatic.

¶ Comparisons within subgroups were evaluated on weighted responses via Poisson regressions used to calculate a prevalence ratio, 95% CI, and p-value (not shown). Statistical significance was evaluated at a threshold of a = 0.005 to account for multiple comparisons. In the calculation of prevalence ratios for started or increased substance use, respondents who selected "Prefer not to answer" (n = 104) were excluded.

** P-value is statistically significant (p<0.005).

†† Respondents identified as a single race unless otherwise specified. The non-Hispanic, other race or multiple races category includes respondents who identified as not Hispanic and as more than one race or as American Indian or Alaska Native, Native Hawaiian or Pacific Islander, or 'Other'.

§§ Essential worker status was self-reported. The comparison was between employed respondents (n = 3,431) who identified as essential vs. nonessential. For this analysis, students who were not separately employed as essential workers were considered nonessential workers.

¶¶ Unpaid adult caregiver status was self-reported. The definition of an unpaid caregiver for adults was having provided unpaid care to a relative or friend aged ≥18 years to help them take care of themselves at any time in the last three months. Examples provided included helping with personal needs, household chores, health care tasks, managing a person's finances, taking them to a doctor's appointment, arranging for outside services, and visiting regularly to see how they are doing.

*** Rural-urban classification was determined by using self-reported ZIP codes according to the Federal Office of Rural Health Policy definition of rurality. https://www.hrsa.gov/rural-health/about-us/definition/datafiles.html.

emotional, mental, or sexual abuse) serve as additional stressors. Community-level intervention and prevention efforts should include strengthening economic supports to reduce financial strain, addressing stress from experienced racial discrimination, promoting social connectedness, and supporting persons at risk for suicide (*9*). Communication strategies should focus on promotion of health services§§§§,¶¶¶¶,***** and culturally and linguistically tailored prevention messaging regarding practices to improve emotional well-being. Development and implementation of COVID-19–specific screening instruments for early identification of COVID-19–related TSRD symptoms would allow for early clinical interventions that might prevent progression from acute to chronic TSRDs. To reduce potential harms of increased substance use related to COVID-19, resources, including social support, comprehensive treatment options, and harm reduction services, are essential and should remain accessible. Periodic assessment of mental health, substance use, and suicidal ideation should evaluate the prevalence of psychological distress over time. Addressing mental health disparities and preparing support systems to mitigate mental health consequences as the pandemic evolves will continue to be needed urgently.

§§§§ Disaster Distress Helpline (https://www.samhsa.gov/disaster-preparedness): 1-800-985-5990 (press 2 for Spanish), or text TalkWithUs for English or Hablanos for Spanish to 66746. Spanish speakers from Puerto Rico can text Hablanos to 1-787-339-2663.

¶¶¶¶ Substance Abuse and Mental Health Services Administration National Helpline (also known as the Treatment Referral Routing Service) for persons and families facing mental disorders, substance use disorders, or both: https://www.samhsa.gov/find-help/national-helpline, 1-800-662-HELP, or TTY 1-800-487-4889.

***** National Suicide Prevention Lifeline (https://suicidepreventionlifeline.org/): 1-800-273-TALK for English, 1-888-628-9454 for Spanish, or Lifeline Crisis Chat (https://suicidepreventionlifeline.org/chat/).

**TABLE 3. Odds of incidence* of symptoms of adverse mental health, substance use to cope with stress or emotions related to COVID-19 pandemic, and suicidal ideation in the third survey wave, by essential worker status and unpaid adult caregiver status among respondents who completed monthly surveys from April through June (N = 1,497) — United States, April 2–8, May 5–12, and June 24–30, 2020**

| | Essential worker[†] vs. all other employment statuses (nonessential worker, unemployed, retired) | | | | Unpaid caregiver for adults[§] vs. not unpaid caregiver | | | |
|---|---|---|---|---|---|---|---|---|
| | Unadjusted | | Adjusted[¶] | | Unadjusted | | Adjusted** | |
| **Symptom or behavior** | **OR (95% CI)[††]** | **p-value[††]** | **OR (95% CI)[††]** | **p-value[††]** | **OR (95% CI)[††]** | **p-value[††]** | **OR (95% CI)[††]** | **p-value[††]** |
| Symptoms of anxiety disorder[§§] | 1.92 (1.29–2.87) | 0.001 | 1.63 (0.99–2.69) | 0.056 | 1.97 (1.25–3.11) | 0.004 | 1.81 (1.14–2.87) | 0.012 |
| Symptoms of depressive disorder[§§] | 1.49 (1.00–2.22) | 0.052 | 1.13 (0.70–1.82) | 0.606 | 2.29 (1.50–3.50) | <0.001 | 2.22 (1.45–3.41) | <0.001 |
| Symptoms of anxiety disorder or depressive disorder[§§] | 1.67 (1.14–2.46) | 0.008 | 1.26 (0.79–2.00) | 0.326 | 1.84 (1.19–2.85) | 0.006 | 1.73 (1.11–2.70) | 0.015 |
| Symptoms of a TSRD related to COVID-19[¶¶] | 1.55 (0.86–2.81) | 0.146 | 1.27 (0.63–2.56) | 0.512 | 1.88 (0.99–3.56) | 0.054 | 1.79 (0.94–3.42) | 0.076 |
| Started or increased substance use to cope with stress or emotions related to COVID-19 | 2.36 (1.26–4.42) | 0.007 | 2.04 (0.92–4.48) | 0.078 | 3.51 (1.86–6.61) | <0.001 | 3.33 (1.75–6.31) | <0.001 |
| Serious consideration of suicide in previous 30 days | 0.93 (0.31–2.78) | 0.895 | 0.53 (0.16–1.70) | 0.285 | 3.00 (1.20–7.52) | 0.019 | 3.03 (1.20–7.63) | 0.019 |

**Abbreviations:** CI = confidence interval, COVID-19 = coronavirus disease 2019, OR = odds ratio, TSRD = trauma- and stressor-related disorder.

* For outcomes assessed via the four-item Patient Health Questionnaire (PHQ-4), odds of incidence were marked by the presence of symptoms during May 5–12 or June 24–30, 2020, after the absence of symptoms during April 2–8, 2020. Respondent pools for prospective analysis of odds of incidence (did not screen positive for symptoms during April 2–8): anxiety disorder (n = 1,236), depressive disorder (n = 1,301) and anxiety disorder or depressive disorder (n = 1,190). For symptoms of a TSRD precipitated by COVID-19, started or increased substance use to cope with stress or emotions related to COVID-19, and serious suicidal ideation in the previous 30 days, odds of incidence were marked by the presence of an outcome during June 24–30, 2020, after the absence of that outcome during May 5–12, 2020. Respondent pools for prospective analysis of odds of incidence (did not report symptoms or behavior during May 5–12): symptoms of a TSRD (n = 1,206), started or increased substance use (n = 1,408), and suicidal ideation (n = 1,456).

† Essential worker status was self-reported. For Table 3, essential worker status was determined by identification as an essential worker during the June 24–30 survey. Essential workers were compared with all other respondents, not just employed respondents (i.e., essential workers vs. all other employment statuses [nonessential worker, unemployed, and retired], not essential vs. nonessential workers).

§ Unpaid adult caregiver status was self-reported. The definition of an unpaid caregiver for adults was having provided unpaid care to a relative or friend 18 years or older to help them take care of themselves at any time in the last three months. Examples provided included helping with personal needs, household chores, health care tasks, managing a person's finances, taking them to a doctor's appointment, arranging for outside services, and visiting regularly to see how they are doing.

¶ Adjusted for gender, employment status, and unpaid adult caregiver status.

** Adjusted for gender, employment status, and essential worker status.

†† Respondents who completed surveys from all three waves (April, May, June) were eligible to be included in an unweighted longitudinal analysis. Comparisons within subgroups were evaluated via logit-linked Binomial regressions used to calculate unadjusted and adjusted odds ratios, 95% confidence intervals, and p-values. Statistical significance was evaluated at a threshold of $\alpha = 0.05$. In the calculation of odds ratios for started or increased substance use, respondents who selected "Prefer not to answer" (n = 11) were excluded.

§§ Symptoms of anxiety disorder and depressive disorder were assessed via the PHQ-4. Those who scored ≥3 out of 6 on the two-item Generalized Anxiety Disorder (GAD-2) and two-item Patient Health Questionnaire (PHQ-2) subscales were considered symptomatic for each disorder, respectively.

¶¶ Disorders classified as TSRDs in the *Diagnostic and Statistical Manual of Mental Disorders* (DSM-5) include posttraumatic stress disorder (PTSD), acute stress disorder (ASD), and adjustment disorders (ADs), among others. Symptoms of a TSRD precipitated by the COVID-19 pandemic were assessed via the six-item Impact of Event Scale (IES-6) to screen for overlapping symptoms of PTSD, ASD, and ADs. For this survey, the COVID-19 pandemic was specified as the traumatic exposure to record peri- and posttraumatic symptoms associated with the range of potential stressors introduced by the COVID-19 pandemic. Those who scored ≥1.75 out of 4 were considered symptomatic.

## Acknowledgments

Survey respondents; Kristen Holland, Emily Kiernan, Meg Watson, CDC COVID-19 Response Team; Mallory Colys, Sneha Baste, Daniel Chong, Rebecca Toll, Qualtrics, LLC; Alexandra Drane, Sarah Stephens Winnay, Archangels; Emily Capodilupo, Whoop, Inc.; The Kinghorn Foundation; Australian-American Fulbright Commission.

Corresponding author: Rashon Lane for the CDC COVID-19 Response Team, Rlane@cdc.gov.

[1]Turner Institute for Brain and Mental Health, Monash University, Melbourne, Australia; [2]Austin Health, Melbourne, Australia; [3]CDC COVID-19 Response Team; [4]Brigham and Women's Hospital, Boston, Massachusetts; [5]Harvard Medical School, Boston, Massachusetts; [6]University of Melbourne, Melbourne, Australia.

All authors have completed and submitted the International Committee of Medical Journal Editors form for disclosure of potential conflicts of interest. Charles A. Czeisler reports an endowed professorship provided to Harvard Medical School by Cephalon, Inc. for educational and research support to Harvard Medical School and Brigham and Women's Hospital from Philips Respironics, Inc, which supported in part the contract with Qualtrics LLC to administer the survey. Elise R. Facer-Childs reports a grant from the Science and Industry Endowment Fund Ross Metcalf STEM+ Business Fellowship, administered by the Commonwealth Scientific and Industrial Research Organisation. Mark É. Czeisler reports a grant from the Australian-American Fulbright Commission for a research project that was cancelled because of COVID-19. Mark E. Howard reports a grant from the Institute for Breathing and Sleep, Austin Health (Australia). Shantha M.W. Rajaratnam reports a grant from the Turner Institute for Brain and Mental Health, Monash University (Australia). Charles A. Czeisler, Elise R. Facer-Childs, Laura K. Barger, Joshua F. Wiley, Matthew D. Weaver, Mark É. Czeisler, Mark E. Howard, Rebecca Robbins, and Shantha M.W. Rajaratnam report contributions by Archangels for the screener used to determine unpaid caregiver status in the survey; and a grant from Whoop, Inc, for

**Summary**

What is already known about this topic?

Communities have faced mental health challenges related to COVID-19–associated morbidity, mortality, and mitigation activities.

What is added by this report?

During June 24–30, 2020, U.S. adults reported considerably elevated adverse mental health conditions associated with COVID-19. Younger adults, racial/ethnic minorities, essential workers, and unpaid adult caregivers reported having experienced disproportionately worse mental health outcomes, increased substance use, and elevated suicidal ideation.

What are the implications for public health practice?

The public health response to the COVID-19 pandemic should increase intervention and prevention efforts to address associated mental health conditions. Community-level efforts, including health communication strategies, should prioritize young adults, racial/ethnic minorities, essential workers, and unpaid adult caregivers.

administration of the survey in June. No other potential conflicts of interest were disclosed.

## References

1. CDC, National Center for Health Statistics. Indicators of anxiety or depression based on reported frequency of symptoms during the last 7 days. Household Pulse Survey. Atlanta, GA: US Department of Health and Human Services, CDC, National Center for Health Statistics; 2020. https://www.cdc.gov/nchs/covid19/pulse/mental-health.htm
2. CDC, National Center for Health Statistics. Early release of selected mental health estimates based on data from the January–June 2019 National Health Interview Survey. Atlanta, GA: US Department of Health and Human Services, CDC, National Center for Health Statistics; 2020. https://www.cdc.gov/nchs/data/nhis/earlyrelease/ERmentalhealth-508.pdf
3. Czeisler MÉ, Tynan MA, Howard ME, et al. Public attitudes, behaviors, and beliefs related to COVID-19, stay-at-home orders, nonessential business closures, and public health guidance—United States, New York City, and Los Angeles, May 5 12, 2020. MMWR Morb Mortal Wkly Rep 2020;69:751–8. https://doi.org/10.15585/mmwr.mm6924e1
4. Löwe B, Wahl I, Rose M, et al. A 4-item measure of depression and anxiety: validation and standardization of the Patient Health Questionnaire-4 (PHQ-4) in the general population. J Affect Disord 2010;122:86–95. https://doi.org/10.1016/j.jad.2009.06.019
5. Hosey MM, Leoutsakos JS, Li X, et al. Screening for posttraumatic stress disorder in ARDS survivors: validation of the Impact of Event Scale-6 (IES-6). Crit Care 2019;23:276. https://doi.org/10.1186/s13054-019-2553-z
6. Substance Abuse and Mental Health Services Administration. Key substance use and mental health indicators in the United States: results from the 2018 National Survey on Drug Use and Health. Rockville, MD: US Department of Health and Human Services, Substance Abuse and Mental Health Services Administration; 2018. https://www.samhsa.gov/data/sites/default/files/cbhsq-reports/NSDUHNationalFindingsReport2018/NSDUHNationalFindingsReport2018.pdf
7. Horesh D, Brown AD. Traumatic stress in the age of COVID-19: call to close critical gaps and adapt to new realities. Psychol Trauma 2020;12:331–5. https://doi.org/10.1037/tra0000592
8. Hailey D, Roine R, Ohinmaa A. The effectiveness of telemental health applications: a review. Can J Psychiatry 2008;53:769–78. https://doi.org/10.1177/070674370805301109
9. Stone D, Holland K, Bartholow B, Crosby A, Davis S, Wilkins N. Preventing suicide: a technical package of policy, programs, and practices. Atlanta, GA: US Department of Health and Human Services, CDC, National Center for Injury Prevention and Control; 2017. https://www.cdc.gov/violenceprevention/pdf/suicideTechnicalPackage.pdf

# HIV SURVEILLANCE REPORT

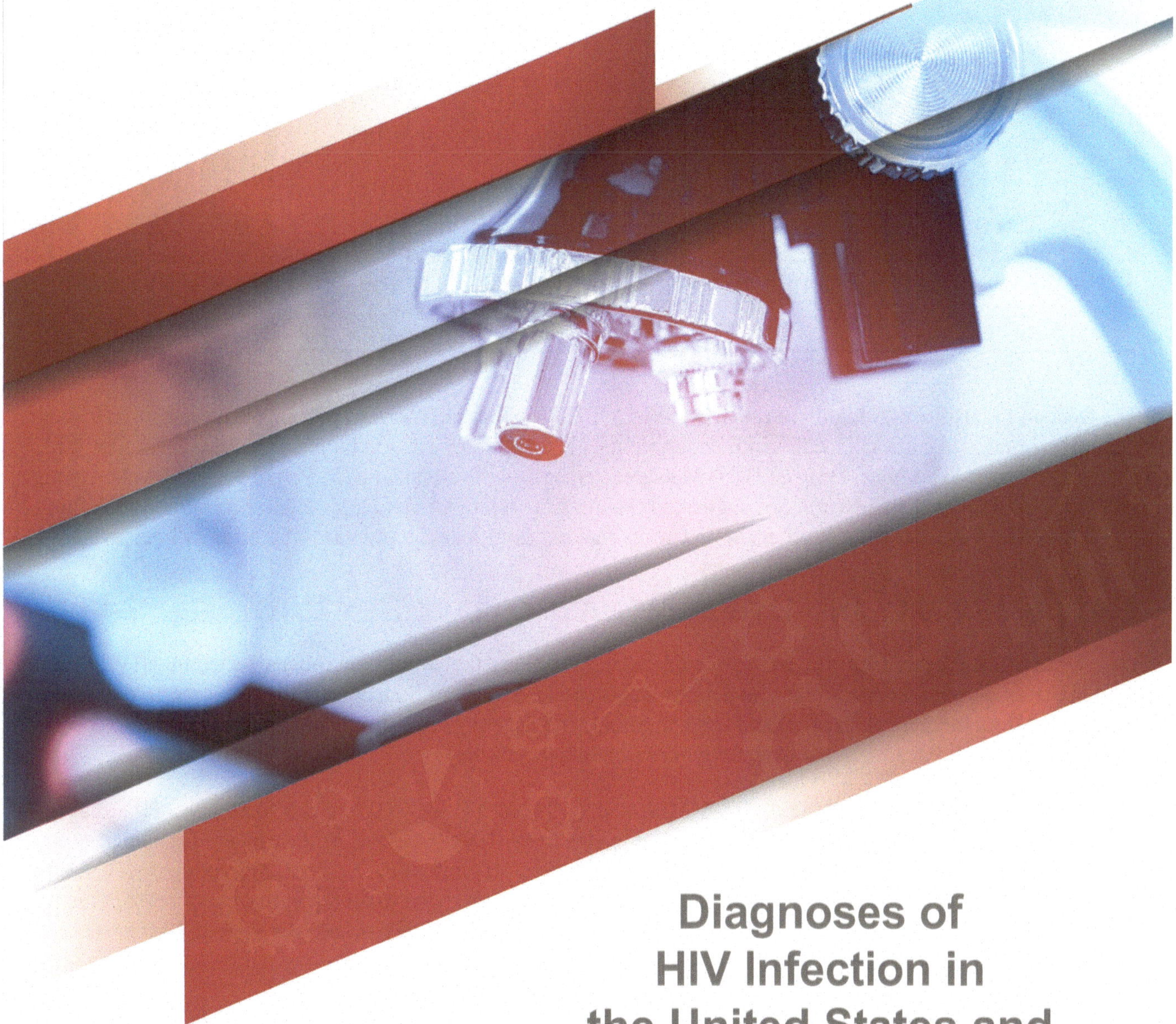

## Diagnoses of HIV Infection in the United States and Dependent Areas, 2020

Centers for Disease Control and Prevention
National Center for HIV, Viral Hepatitis, STD, and TB Prevention

# Special Focus Profiles

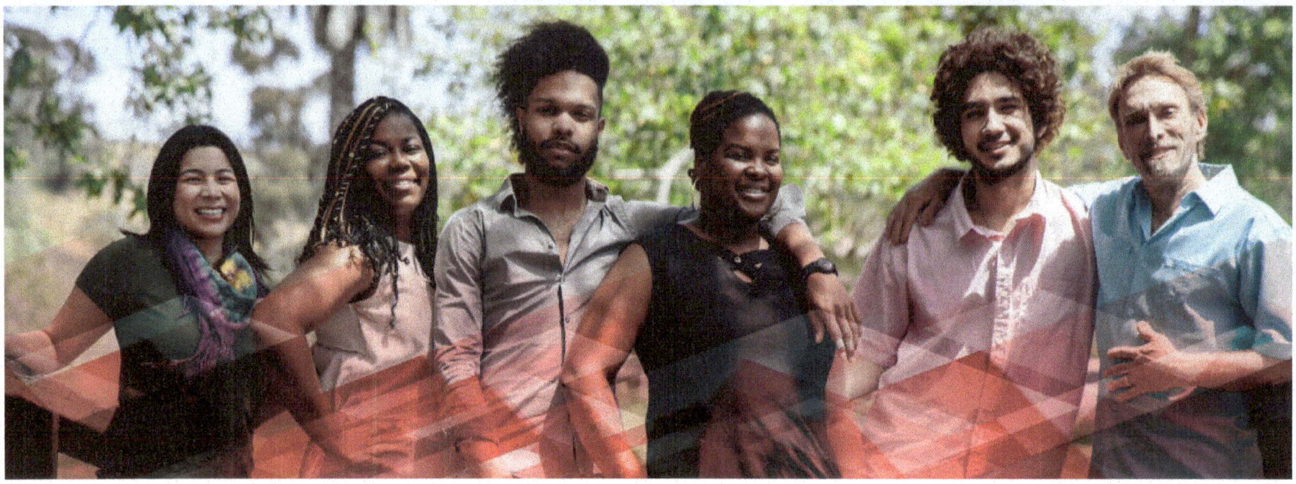

*Note.* This is not a stock image. The persons in this image are living with HIV or are advocates for those living with HIV.

---

The Special Focus Profiles highlight the distribution of HIV in 6 populations of particular interest to HIV prevention programs in state and local health departments: (1) Gay, Bisexual, and Other Men Who Have Sex With Men, (2) Persons Who Inject Drugs, (3) Transgender Persons, (4) Women, and (5) Persons Aged 13–24 Years, and (6) Children Aged <13 Years. See suggested readings for references and additional information including HIV risk behaviors, barriers to care, and prevention challenges for each population of particular interest.

## Gay, Bisexual, and Other Men Who Have Sex With Men

Gay, bisexual, and other men who have sex with men (MSM) are the population most affected by HIV in the United States. Stigma, homophobia, and discrimination make MSM of all races/ethnicities susceptible to multiple physical and mental health problems and can affect whether they seek and receive high-quality health services, including HIV testing, treatment, and other prevention services.

In 2020, MSM accounted for 71% (20,758 MMSC and 1,109 MMSC *and* IDU) of the 30,692 new HIV diagnoses in the United States and 6 dependent areas (Table 1b). Many Black/African American and Hispanic/Latino MSM with HIV, particularly young MSM, are unaware of their HIV infection. Lack of awareness of HIV status among young MSM may be due to recent infection, not getting tested due to underestimation of personal risk, or fewer opportunities to get tested. Persons who do not know they have HIV do not get medical care or receive treatment and can unknowingly infect others.

## Diagnoses of HIV infection among MSM

HIV diagnosis percentages for 2020 were as follows:

- **Age group** (Figure 12):
  - 13–24 years: 24%
  - 25–34 years: 40%
  - 35–44 years: 17%
  - 45–54 years: 11%
  - ≥55 years: 8%
- **Race/ethnicity** (Figure 12):
  - American Indian/Alaska Native: 1%
  - Asian: 2%
  - Black/African American: 39%
  - Hispanic/Latino: 31%
  - Native Hawaiian/other Pacific Islander: <1%
  - White: 25%
  - Multiracial: 3%
- **Region of residence** (Figure 12):
  - Northeast: 13%
  - Midwest: 14%
  - South: 50%
  - West: 23%
  - U.S. dependent areas: 1%

**Figure 12. Percentages of diagnoses of HIV infection among men who have sex with men, by selected characteristics, 2020 (COVID-19 pandemic)—United States and 6 dependent areas**

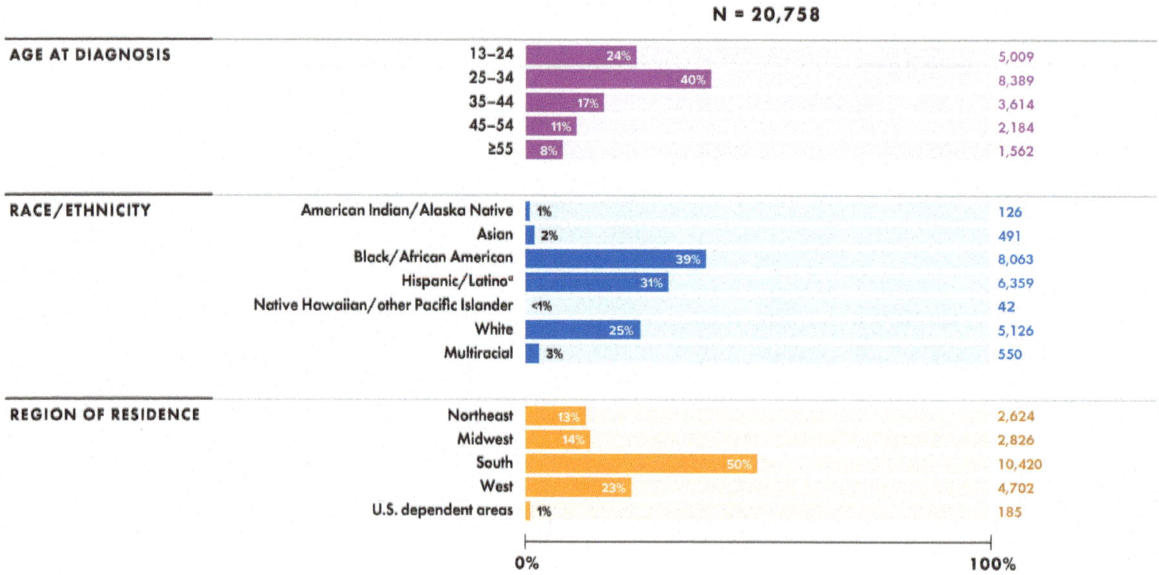


*Note.* Data have been statistically adjusted to account for missing transmission category. Data for 2020 should be interpreted with caution due to the impact of the COVID-19 pandemic on access to HIV testing, care-related services, and case surveillance activities in state/local jurisdictions.

[a] Hispanic/Latino persons can be of any race.

- **Age group and race/ethnicity—highest percentages by age group** (Figure 13):
  - ○ Aged 13–24 years: Black/African American (54%)
  - ○ Aged >24 years: Black/African American (34%)

**Figure 13. Percentages of diagnoses of HIV infection among men who have sex with men, by age group and race/ethnicity, 2020 (COVID-19 pandemic)—United States and 6 dependent areas**

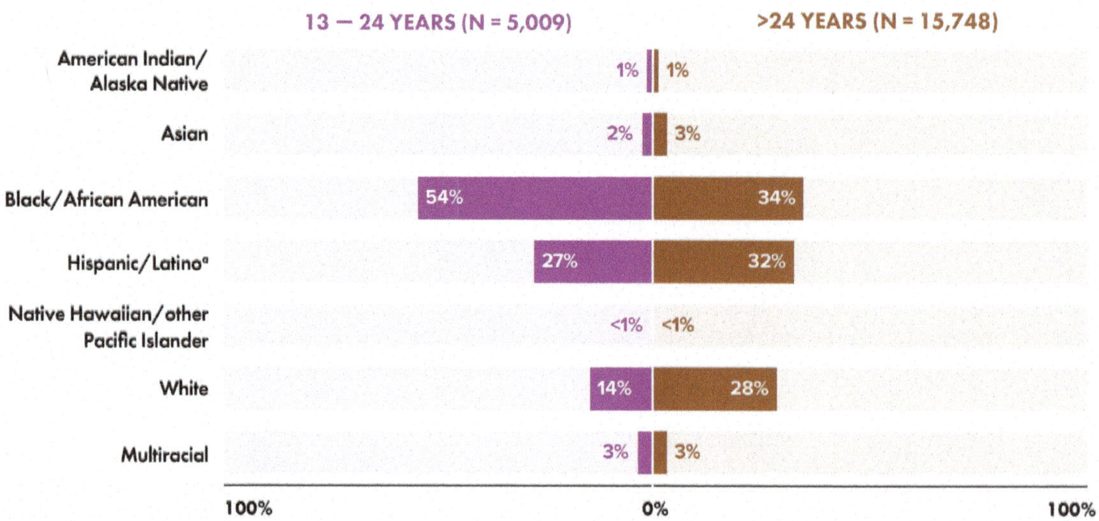


*Note.* Data have been statistically adjusted to account for missing transmission category. Data for 2020 should be interpreted with caution due to the impact of the COVID-19 pandemic on access to HIV testing, care-related services, and case surveillance activities in state/local jurisdictions.

[a] Hispanic/Latino persons can be of any race.

- **Region of residence and race/ethnicity—highest numbers and percentages by region** (Figure 14):
  - o Northeast: Black/African American (941; 36%)
  - o Midwest: Black/African American (1,323; 47%)
  - o South: Black/African American (5,079; 49%)
  - o West: Hispanic/Latino (2,199; 47%)
  - o U.S. dependent areas: Hispanic/Latino (183; 99%)

**Figure 14. Diagnoses of HIV infection among men who have sex with men, by region of residence and race/ethnicity, 2020 (COVID-19 pandemic)—United States and 6 dependent areas**

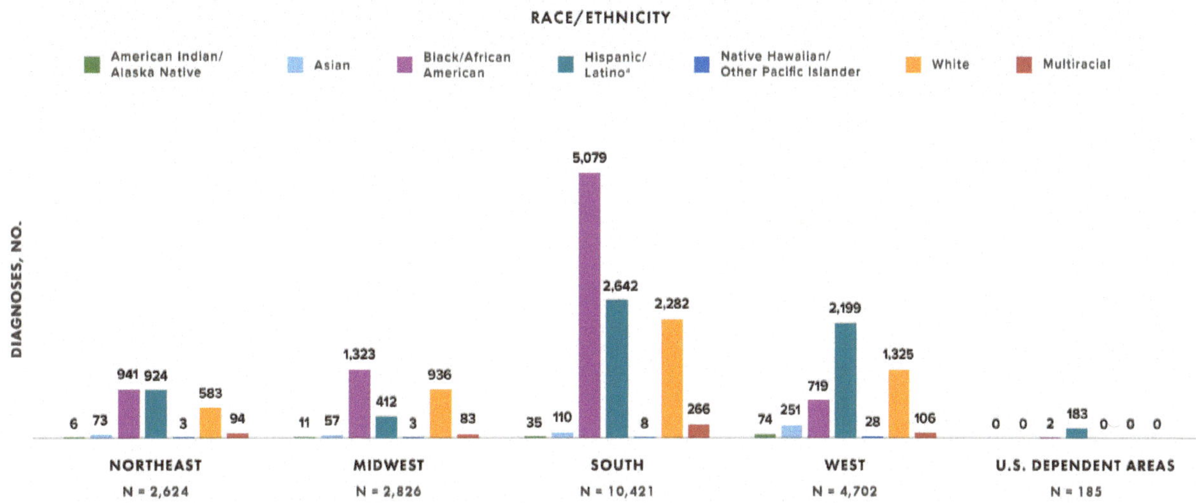


*Note*. Data have been statistically adjusted to account for missing transmission category. Data for 2020 should be interpreted with caution due to the impact of the COVID-19 pandemic on access to HIV testing, care-related services, and case surveillance activities in state/local jurisdictions.

[a] Hispanic/Latino persons can be of any race.

- **Prevalence and race/ethnicity** (Table 16b):

  At year-end 2020 in the United States and 6 dependent areas, 604,590 MSM were living with diagnosed HIV infection attributed to MMSC.

  Prevalence by race/ethnicity was as follows:

  - o American Indian/Alaska Native: <1%
  - o Asian: 2%
  - o Black/African American: 31%
  - o Hispanic/Latino: 26%
  - o Native Hawaiian/other Pacific Islander: <1%
  - o White: 36%
  - o Multiracial: 5%

## Persons Who Inject Drugs

Persons who inject drugs (PWID) can get HIV if they use and share needles, syringes, or other drug injection equipment (e.g., cookers) that someone with HIV has used. In 2020, persons who inject drugs account for about 1 in 15 HIV diagnoses in the United States. In recent years, the opioid (including prescription and synthetic opioids) and heroin crisis has led to increased numbers of PWID. HIV diagnoses among PWID have increased in the 50 states and District of Columbia. IDU in nonurban areas has created prevention challenges and brought attention to populations who would benefit from HIV prevention efforts.

## Diagnoses of HIV infection among PWID

In 2020, in the United States and 6 dependent areas, 2,055 diagnoses of HIV infection were attributed to IDU (1,198 among male and 857 among female PWID) (Table 6b).

HIV diagnosis percentages among PWID for 2020 were as follows:

- **Age group** (Figure 15):
  - 13–24 years: 6%
  - 25–34 years: 32%
  - 35–44 years: 27%
  - 45–54 years: 18%
  - ≥55 years: 17%

  For additional data by 5-year age groups, see Table 6b.
- **Race/ethnicity** (Figure 15):
  - American Indian/Alaska Native: 1%
  - Asian: 1%
  - Black/African American: 27%
  - Hispanic/Latino: 20%
  - Native Hawaiian/other Pacific Islander: <1%
  - White: 47%
  - Multiracial: 3%
- **Region of residence** (Figure 15):
  - Northeast: 21%
  - Midwest: 14%
  - South: 44%
  - West: 21%
  - U.S. dependent areas: 1%

**Figure 15. Percentages of diagnoses of HIV infection among persons who inject drugs, by selected characteristics, 2020 (COVID-19 pandemic)—United States and 6 dependent areas**

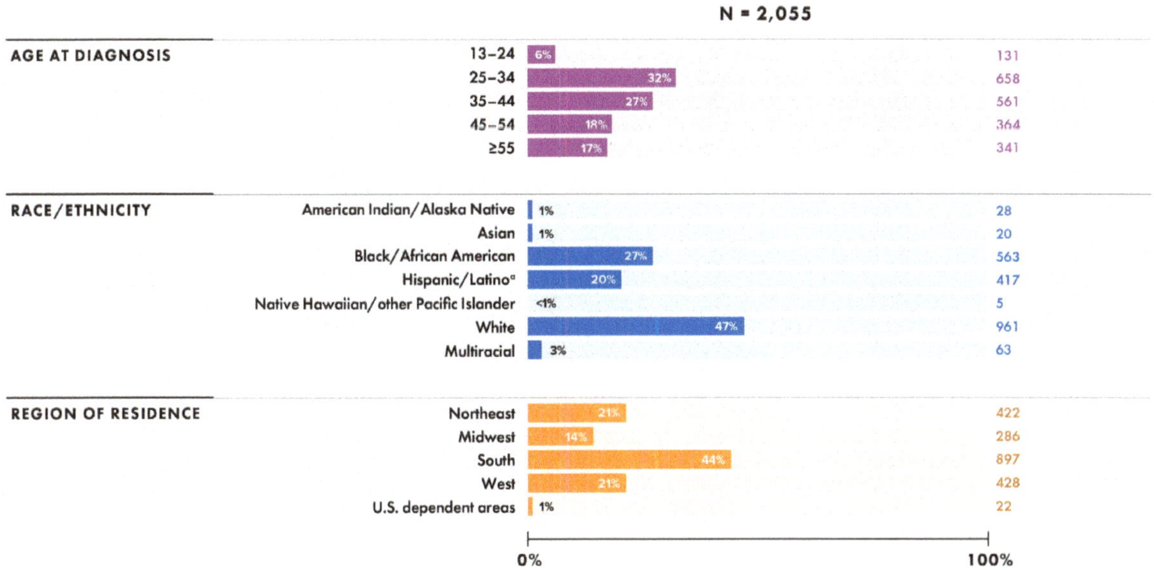


*Note.* Data have been statistically adjusted to account for missing transmission category. Data for 2020 should be interpreted with caution due to the impact of the COVID-19 pandemic on access to HIV testing, care-related services, and case surveillance activities in state/local jurisdictions.

[a] Hispanic/Latino persons can be of any race.

- **Sex assigned at birth and race/ethnicity—highest percentages** (Figure 16):
  - White female: 49%
  - White male: 45%
  - Black/African American female: 29%
  - Black/African American male: 26%

**Figure 16. Percentages of diagnoses of HIV infection among persons who inject drugs, by sex assigned at birth and race/ethnicity, 2020 (COVID-19 pandemic)—United States and 6 dependent areas**

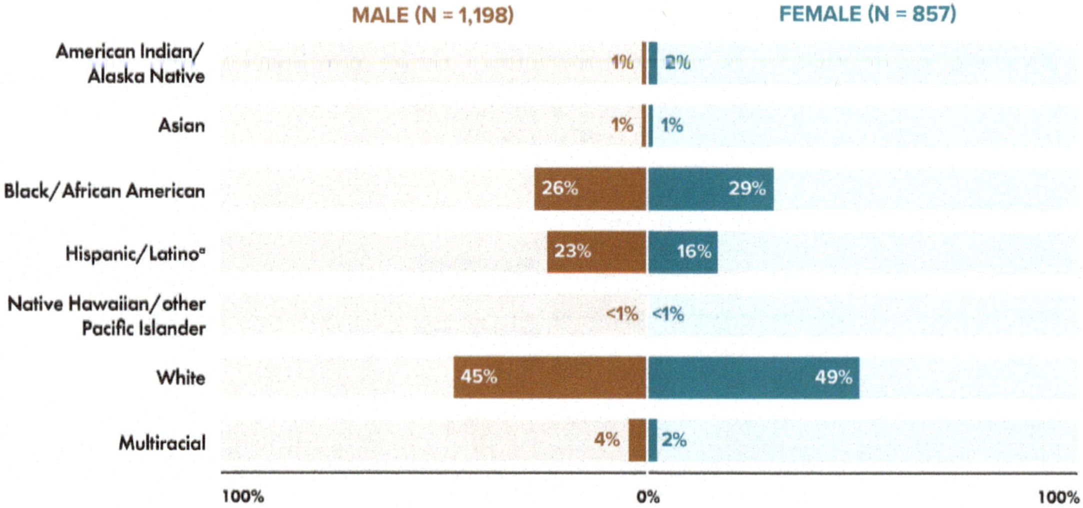


*Note.* Data have been statistically adjusted to account for missing transmission category. Data for 2020 should be interpreted with caution due to the impact of the COVID-19 pandemic on access to HIV testing, care-related services, and case surveillance activities in state/local jurisdictions.

[a] Hispanic/Latino persons can be of any race.

- **Region of residence and race/ethnicity—highest numbers and percentages by region** (Figure 17):
  - Northeast: White (157; 37%)
  - Midwest: White (152; 53%)
  - South: White (464; 52%)
  - West: White (188; 44%)
  - U.S. dependent areas: Hispanic/Latino (22; 100%)

**Figure 17. Diagnoses of HIV infection among persons who inject drugs, by region and race/ethnicity, 2020 (COVID-19 pandemic)—United States and 6 dependent areas**

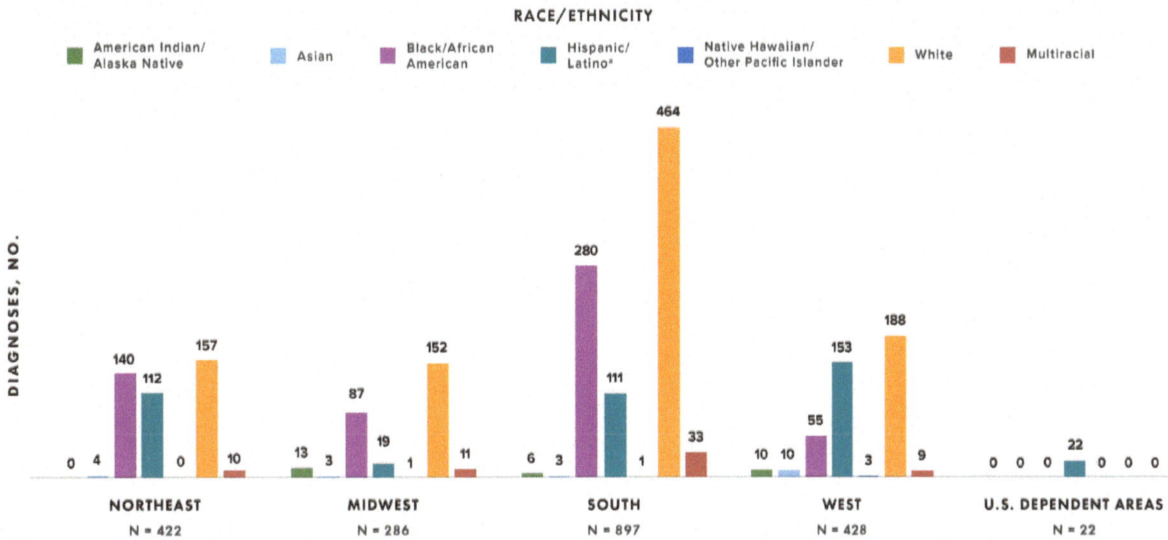


*Note.* Data have been statistically adjusted to account for missing transmission category. Data for 2020 should be interpreted with caution due to the impact of the COVID-19 pandemic on access to HIV testing, care-related services, and case surveillance activities in state/local jurisdictions.

[a] Hispanic/Latino persons can be of any race.

- **Prevalence and race/ethnicity** (Table 16b):
  - At year-end 2020 in the United States and 6 dependent areas, 118,213 PWID were living with diagnosed HIV infection. Prevalence by race/ethnicity was as follows:
  - American Indian/Alaska Native: <1%
  - Asian: 1%
  - Black/African American: 45%
  - Hispanic/Latino: 27%
  - Native Hawaiian/other Pacific Islander: <1%
  - White: 22%
  - Multiracial: 5%

## Transgender Persons

*Transgender* is an umbrella term that is used to identify persons whose sex assigned at birth does not match current gender identity or expression. *Gender identity* refers to one's internal understanding of one's own gender, or the gender with which a person identifies. *Gender expression* is a term used to describe people's outward presentation of their gender. Gender identity and sexual orientation are different facets of identity. Everyone has a gender identity and a sexual orientation, but a person's gender does not determine a person's sexual orientation. Transgender persons may identify as heterosexual, homosexual, bisexual, or none of the above. Transgender persons are understudied in HIV prevention (e.g., preexposure prophylaxis [PrEP]) and treatment interventions and face numerous prevention challenges, including social rejection and exclusion and lack of public/provider knowledge about transgender issues.

## Diagnoses of HIV infection

In 2020, in the United States and 6 dependent areas, 697 diagnoses of HIV infection were among transgender and AGI persons (Table 4b). Diagnoses of HIV infection among transgender persons accounted for approximately 2% of diagnoses. Transgender women accounted for the highest percentage of diagnoses of HIV infections (92%).

HIV diagnosis percentages among transgender and AGI persons for 2020 were as follows:

- **Age group** (Figure 18):
  - 13–24 years: 28%
  - 25–34 years: 49%
  - 35–44 years: 13%
  - 45–54 years: 7%
  - ≥55 years: 2%

  For additional data by 5-year age groups, see Table 4b.
- **Race/ethnicity** (Figure 18):
  - American Indian/Alaska Native: 1%
  - Asian: 2%
  - Black/African American: 47%
  - Hispanic/Latino: 31%
  - Native Hawaiian/other Pacific Islander: <1%
  - White: 13%
  - Multiracial: 5%
- **Exposure category** (Figure 18):
  - Sexual contact: 89%
  - IDU: <1%
  - Sexual contact and IDU: 6%
  - Other: 5%
- **Region of residence** (Figure 18):
  - Northeast: 16%
  - Midwest: 15%
  - South: 44%
  - West: 24%
  - U.S. dependent areas: <1%

**Figure 18. Percentages of diagnoses of HIV infection among transgender and additional gender identity persons aged ≥13 years, by selected characteristics, 2020 (COVID-19 pandemic)—United States and 6 dependent areas**

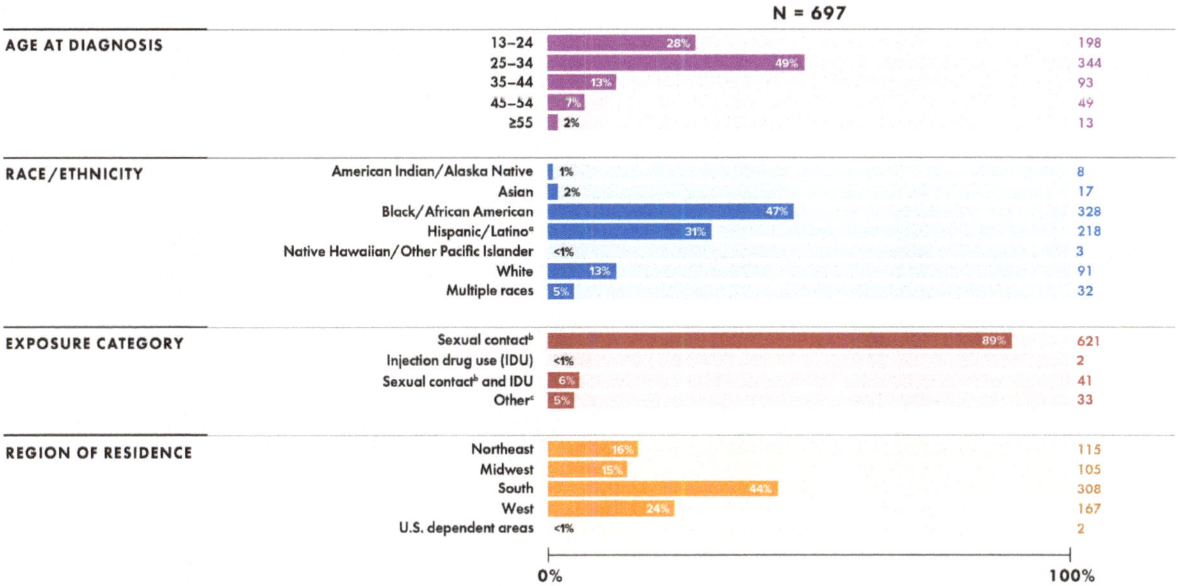


*Note.* Data for 2020 should be interpreted with caution due to the impact of the COVID-19 pandemic on access to HIV testing, care-related services, and case surveillance activities in state/local jurisdictions.

[a] Hispanic/Latino persons can be of any race.

[b] For persons assigned "male" sex at birth, sexual contact with any person. For persons assigned "female" sex at birth, sexual contact with a person assigned "male" sex at birth.

[c] Other risk factors, including perinatal, hemophilia, blood transfusion, and risk factor not reported or not identified. Data were not statistically adjusted to account for missing exposure category; therefore, case counts for "Other" might be high.

- **Gender and race/ethnicity—highest percentages** (Figure 19):
  - Transgender woman: Black/African American (48%)
  - Transgender man: White (38%)
  - AGI: Black/African American (47%)

**Figure 19. Percentages of diagnoses of HIV infection among transgender and additional gender identity persons aged ≥13 years, by gender and race/ethnicity, 2020 (COVID-19 pandemic)—United States and 6 dependent areas**

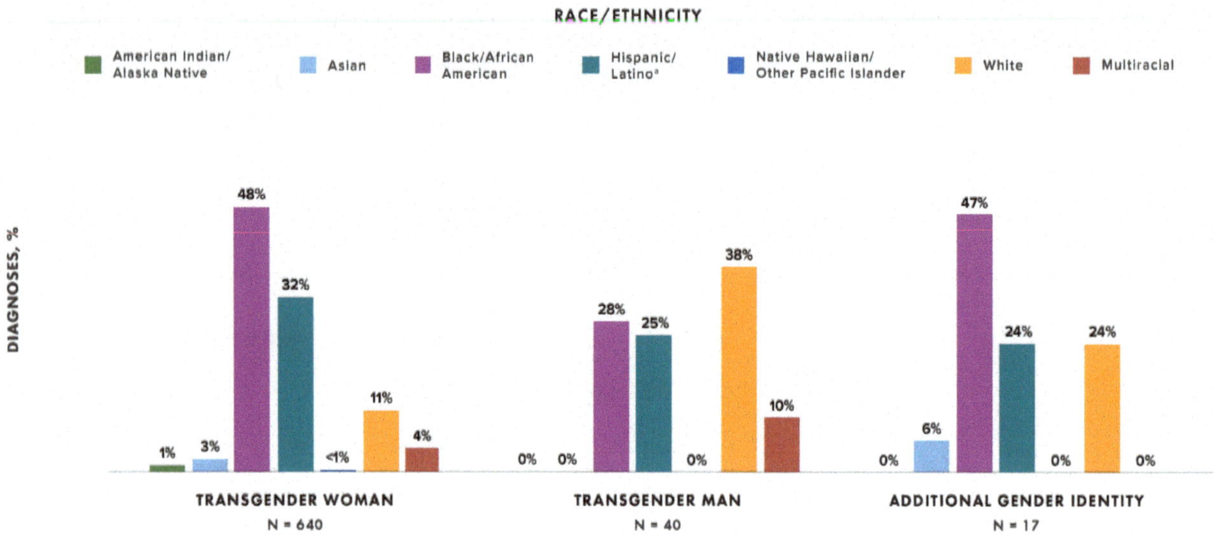


*Note.* Data for 2020 should be interpreted with caution due to the impact of the COVID-19 pandemic on access to HIV testing, care-related services, and case surveillance activities in state/local jurisdictions.

[a] Hispanic/Latino persons can be of any race.

- **Gender and exposure category—highest percentages** (Figure 20):
  - Transgender woman: sexual contact (90%)
  - Transgender man: sexual contact (73%)
  - AGI: sexual contact (82%)

**Figure 20. Percentages of diagnoses of HIV infection among transgender and additional gender identity persons aged ≥13 years, by gender and exposure category, 2020 (COVID-19 pandemic)—United States and 6 dependent areas**

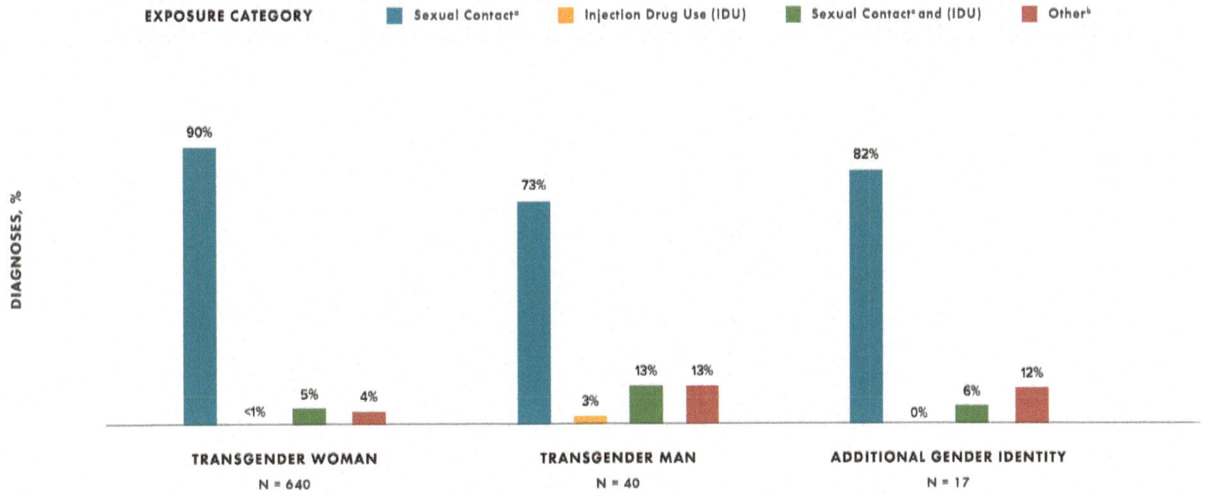


*Note.* Data for 2020 should be interpreted with caution due to the impact of the COVID-19 pandemic on access to HIV testing, care-related services, and case surveillance activities in state/local jurisdictions.

[a] For persons assigned "male" sex at birth, sexual contact with any person. For persons assigned "female" sex at birth, sexual contact with a person assigned "male" sex at birth.

[b] Other risk factors, including perinatal, hemophilia, blood transfusion, and risk factor not reported or not identified. Data were not statistically adjusted to account for missing exposure category; therefore, case counts for "Other" might be high.

## Women

More than 5,000 women received an HIV diagnosis in the United States and 6 dependent areas in 2020. One in nine women with HIV are unaware they have it. Because some women may be unaware of their male partner's risk factors for HIV (such as injection drug use or having sex with men), they may not use condoms or medicines to prevent HIV. Additionally, HIV testing rates within the past year were low among women with sexual behaviors that increase their risk of acquiring HIV and especially low among those who reported anal sex.

## Diagnoses of HIV infection

In 2020 in the United States and 6 dependent areas, the rate of diagnoses of HIV infection among females aged ≥13 years was 3.8 (Figure 21).

**Figure 21. Rates of diagnoses of HIV infection among females aged ≥13 years, 2020 (COVID-19 pandemic)—United States and 6 dependent areas**

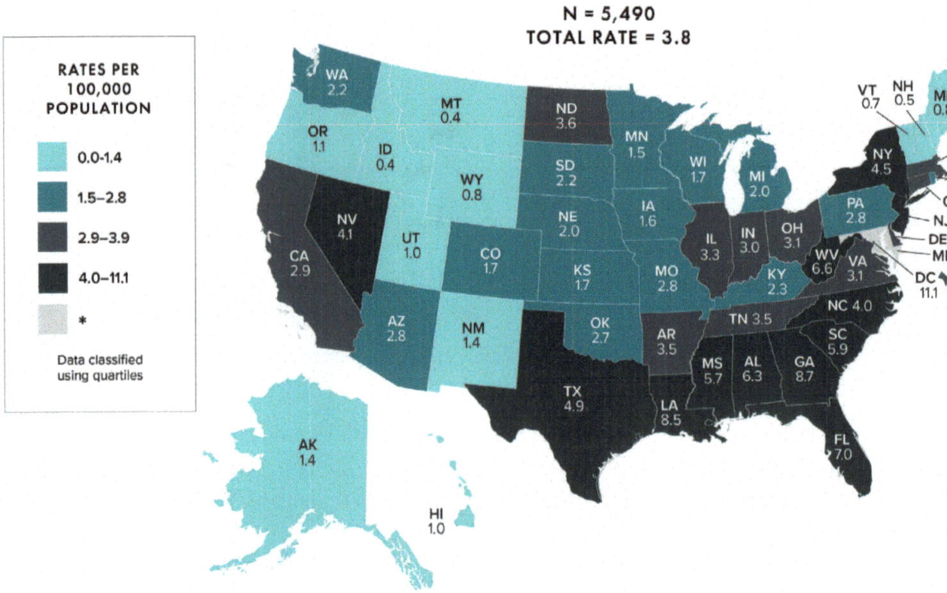


| | |
|---|---|
| American Samoa | 0.0 |
| Guam | 0.0 |
| Northern Mariana Islands | 0.0 |
| Puerto Rico | 2.8 |
| Republic of Palau | 0.0 |
| U.S. Virgin Islands | 0.0 |

*Note.* Data for 2020 should be interpreted with caution due to the impact of the COVID-19 pandemic on access to HIV testing, care-related services, and case surveillance activities in state/local jurisdictions. Asterisk (*) indicates incomplete reporting.

In 2020 in the United States (Figure 22):

- Black/African American females aged ≥13 years made up 13% of the female population but accounted for 54% of diagnoses of HIV infection among females.
- White females aged ≥13 years made up 62% of the female population and accounted for 24% of diagnoses of HIV infection.
- Hispanic/Latino females aged ≥13 years made up 17% of the female population and accounted for 17% of diagnoses of HIV infection.

**Figure 22. Percentages of diagnoses of HIV infection and population among females aged ≥13 years, by race/ethnicity, 2020 (COVID-19 pandemic)—United States**

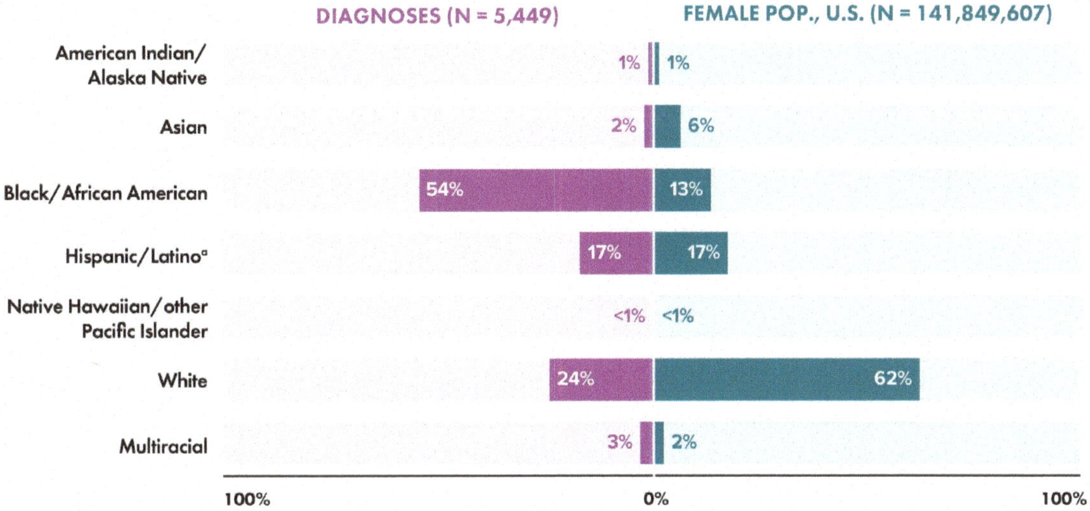


*Note.* Data for 2020 should be interpreted with caution due to the impact of the COVID-19 pandemic on access to HIV testing, care-related services, and case surveillance activities in state/local jurisdictions.

[a] Hispanic/Latino persons can be of any race.

HIV diagnosis rates among females aged ≥13 years were as follows:

- **Age group (U.S. only)** (Figure 23):
  - 13–24 years: 2.9
  - 25–34 years: 7.0
  - 35–44 years: 6.0
  - 45–54 years: 4.9
  - ≥55 years: 1.6

  For additional data by 5-year age groups, see Table 3a.

  - ***Disparities by age group***:
    - Absolute disparity (rate difference)—If persons aged 25–34 years had the same rate as persons aged ≥55 years, 5 cases per 100,000 population would have been prevented.
    - Relative disparity (rate ratio)—Persons aged 25–34 years had a rate that was 4.4 times as high as persons aged ≥55 years.
- **Race/ethnicity (U.S. only)** (Figure 23):
  - American Indian/Alaska Native: 4.2
  - Asian: 1.0
  - Black/African American: 16.4
  - Hispanic/Latino: 3.8
  - Native Hawaiian/other Pacific Islander: 6.0
  - White: 1.5
  - Multiracial: 5.3

- ***Disparities by race/ethnicity***:
  - Absolute disparity (rate difference)—If Black/African American persons aged ≥13 years had the same rate as White persons aged ≥13 years (1.5), 15 cases per 100,000 population would have been prevented.
  - Relative disparity (rate ratio)—Black/African American persons aged ≥13 years had a rate that was 10.9 times as high as White persons aged ≥13 years.

- **Region of residence (U.S. only)** (Figure 23):
  - Northeast: 3.6
  - Midwest: 2.5
  - South: 5.5
  - West: 2.4
    - ***Disparities by region***:
      - Absolute disparities (rate difference): if the South had the same rate as the West, 3 cases per 100,000 population would have been prevented.
      - Relative disparities (rate ratio): the South had a rate that was 2.3 times as high as the West.

**Figure 23. Rates and disparities of diagnoses of HIV infection among females aged ≥13 years, by selected characteristics, 2020 (COVID-19 pandemic)—United States and 6 dependent areas**

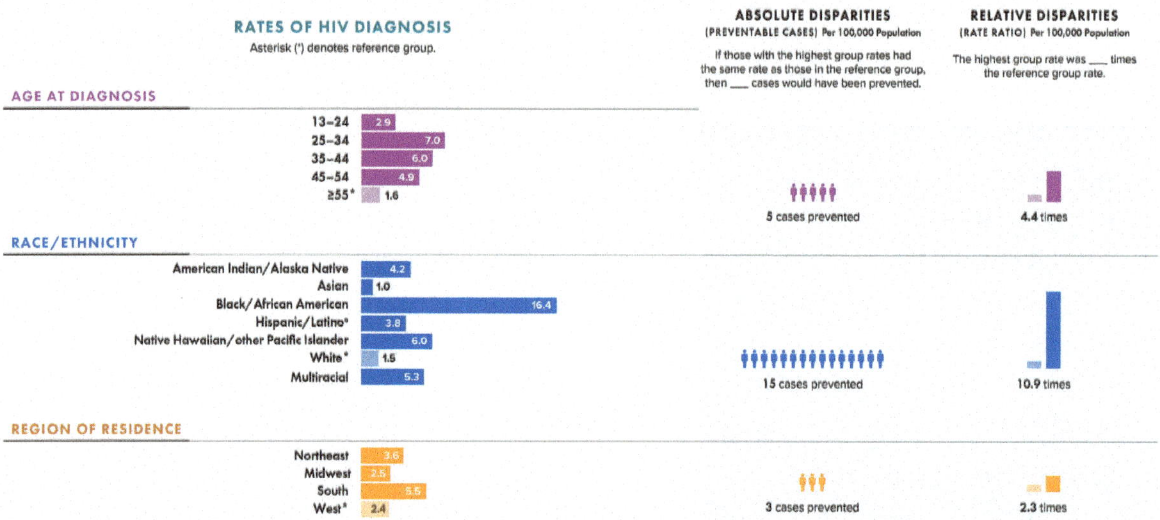


*Note.* Data for 2020 should be interpreted with caution due to the impact of the COVID-19 pandemic on access to HIV testing, care-related services, and case surveillance activities in state/local jurisdictions. Absolute disparity measures the difference between rates in groups with the highest rates and a reference group ($Rate_{highest\ group} - Rate_{reference\ group}$). Relative disparity (rate ratio) measures the rates in groups with the highest rates divided by a reference group ($Rate_{highest\ group} \div Rate_{reference\ group}$).

[a] Hispanic/Latino persons can be of any race.

- **Transmission category and race/ethnicity—highest percentages** (Figure 24):
  - PWID: American Indian/Alaska Native (47%)
  - Heterosexual contact: Asian (92%)

**Figure 24. Percentages of diagnoses of HIV infection among females aged ≥13 years, by transmission category and race/ethnicity, 2020 (COVID-19 pandemic)—United States and 6 dependent areas**

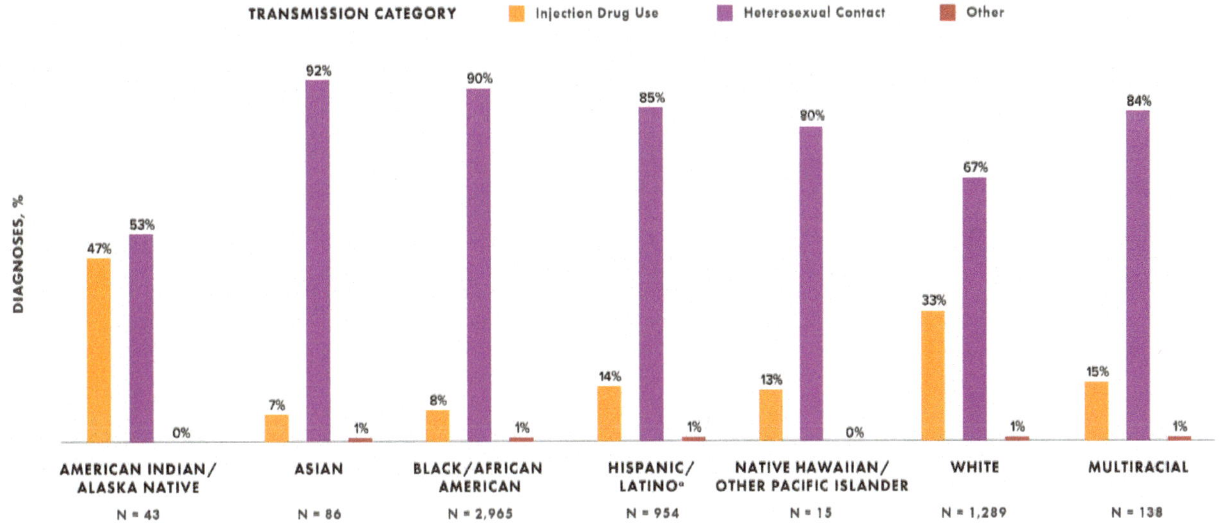


*Note.* Data have been statistically adjusted to account for missing transmission category. Data for 2020 should be interpreted with caution due to the impact of the COVID-19 pandemic on access to HIV testing, care-related services, and case surveillance activities in state/local jurisdictions.

[a] Hispanic/Latino persons can be of any race.

- **Region of residence and race/ethnicity—highest rates (U.S. only)** (Figure 25):
  - Northeast: Black/African American (16.3)
  - Midwest: Black/African American (13.8)
  - South: Black/African American (17.2)
  - West: Black/African American (15.9)

**Figure 25. Rates of diagnoses of HIV infection among females aged ≥13 years, by race/ethnicity and region, 2020 (COVID-19 pandemic)—United States**

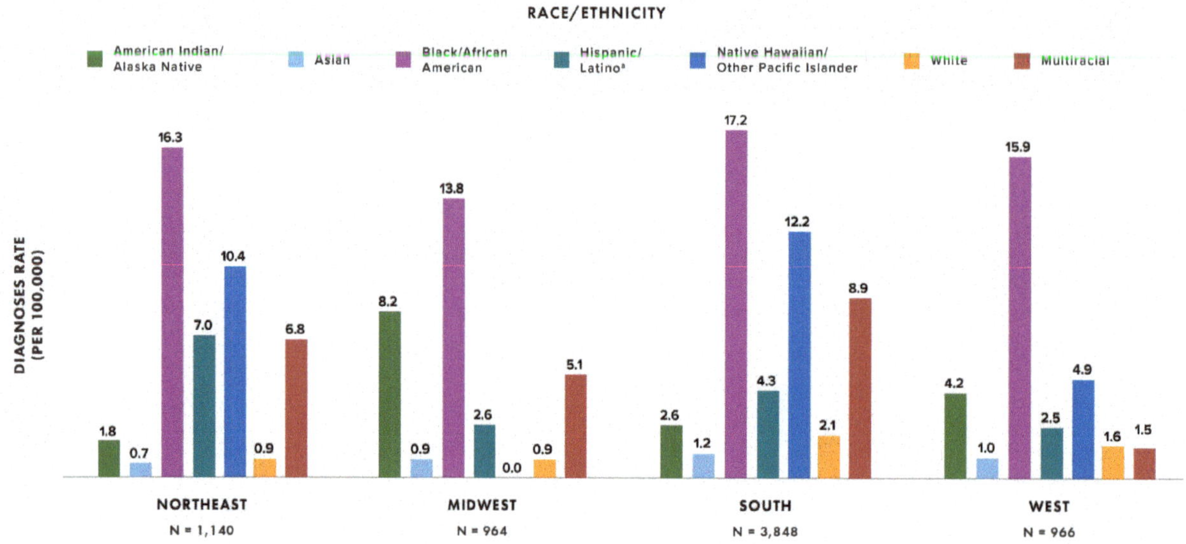


*Note.* Data for 2020 should be interpreted with caution due to the impact of the COVID-19 pandemic on access to HIV testing, care-related services, and case surveillance activities in state/local jurisdictions.

[a] Hispanic/Latino persons can be of any race.

- **Prevalence and race/ethnicity** (Table 16b):
  - At year-end 2020 in the United States and 6 dependent areas, 248,819 females aged ≥13 years were living with diagnosed HIV infection. Prevalence by race/ethnicity was as follows:
  - American Indian/Alaska Native: <1%
  - Asian: 1%
  - Black/African American: 57%
  - Hispanic/Latino: 20%
  - Native Hawaiian/other Pacific Islander: <1%
  - White: 16%
  - Multiracial: 5%

## Persons Aged 13–24 Years

Persons aged 13–24 years accounted for 20% of the 30,692 diagnoses of HIV infection in 2020 in the United States and 6 dependent areas. They are the least likely of any age group to be aware of their HIV infection, retained in care, or have a suppressed viral load. Lack of awareness of HIV status may be due to recent infection or low rates of HIV testing. Persons who do not know that they have HIV do not get medical care or receive treatment and can unknowingly infect others. In addition, persons aged 13–24 years have high rates of STDs and low rates of condom use, greatly increasing the chance of getting or transmitting HIV. Addressing HIV among persons aged 13–24 years requires that they have access to the information and tools they need to make healthy decisions, reduce their risk factors, get treatment, and stay in care.

## Diagnoses of HIV infection

In 2020 in the United States and 6 dependent areas, there were 6,135 diagnoses of HIV infection among persons aged 13–24 years (Figure 26, Table 8b).

The percentage and/or rates of diagnoses of HIV infection among persons aged 13–24 years were as follows:

- **Gender** (Figure 26):
  - Male: 85%
  - Female: 12%
  - Transgender woman: 3%
  - Transgender man: <1%
  - AGI: <1%
- **Age group** (Figure 26):
  - 13–14 years: <1%
  - 15–17 years: 5%
  - 18–19 years: 16%
  - 20–21 years: 45%
  - 23–24 years: 35%%
- **Race/ethnicity** (Figure 26):
  - American Indian/Alaska Native: 1%
  - Asian: 1%
  - Black/African American: 54%
  - Hispanic/Latino: 26%
  - Native Hawaiian/other Pacific Islander: <1%
  - White: 15%
  - Multiracial: 3%
- **Region of residence** (Figure 26):
  - Northeast: 12%
  - Midwest: 15%
  - South: 55%
  - West: 17%
  - U.S. dependent areas: 1%

**Figure 26. Percentages of diagnoses of HIV infection among persons aged 13–24 years, by selected characteristics, 2020 (COVID-19 pandemic)—United States and 6 dependent areas**

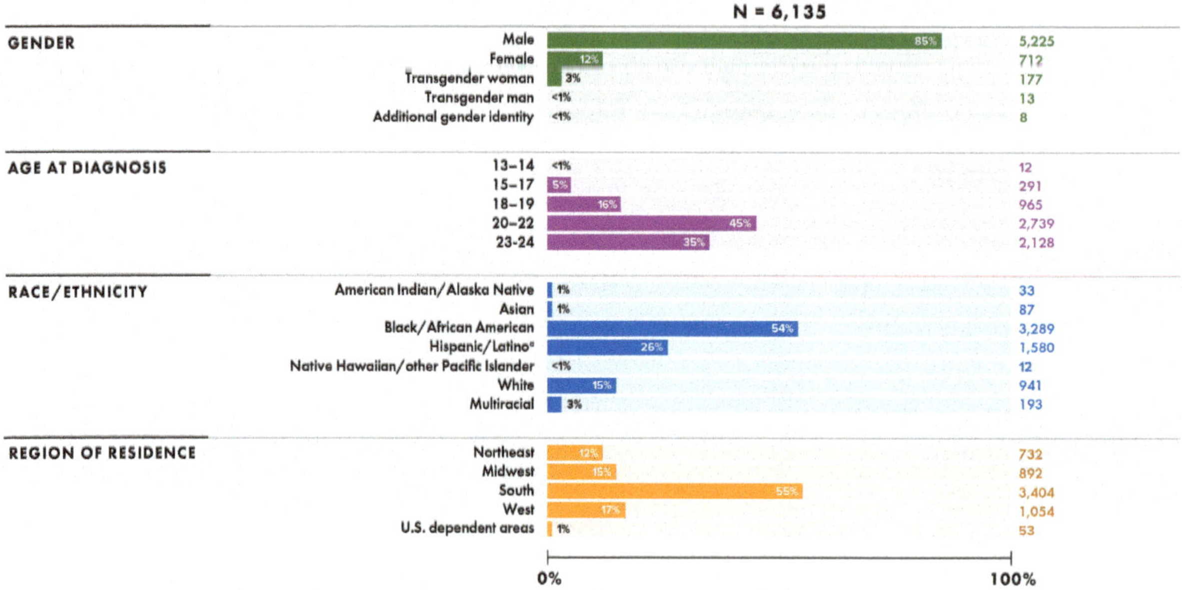


*Note*. Data for 2020 should be interpreted with caution due to the impact of the COVID-19 pandemic on access to HIV testing, care-related services, and case surveillance activities in state/local jurisdictions.

[a] Hispanic/Latino persons can be of any race.

- **Sex assigned at birth and transmission category—highest percentages** (Figure 27):
  - Male sex at birth: MMSC (82%)
  - Female sex at birth: heterosexual contact (10%)

**Figure 27. Percentages of diagnoses of HIV infection among persons aged 13–24 years, by sex assigned at birth and transmission category, 2020 (COVID-19 pandemic)—United States and 6 dependent areas**

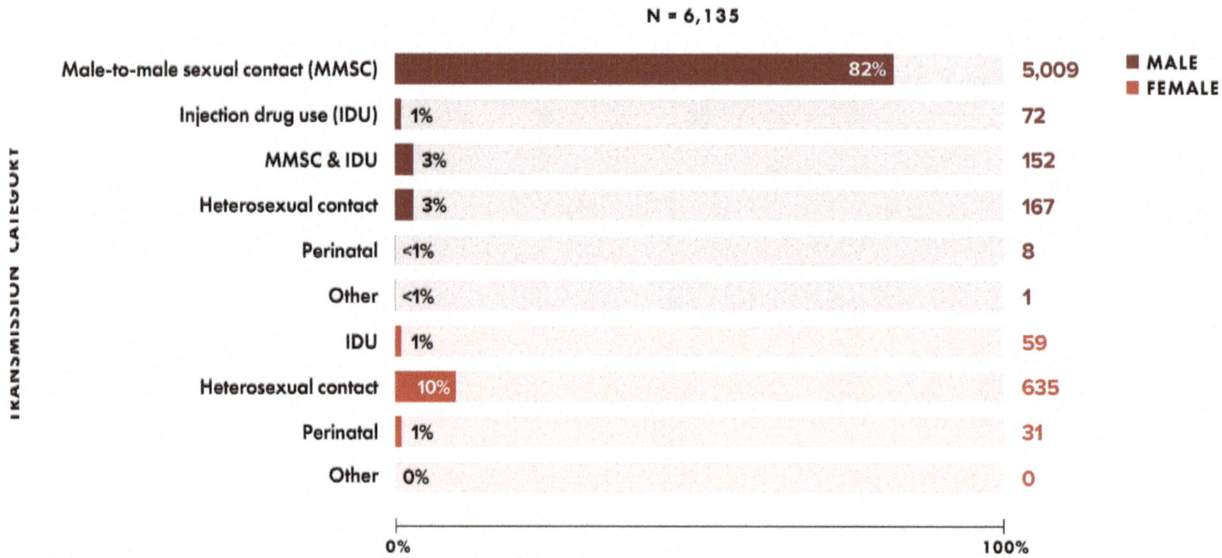


*Note*. Data for 2020 should be interpreted with caution due to the impact of the COVID-19 pandemic on access to HIV testing, care-related services, and case surveillance activities in state/local jurisdictions.

- **Rates (U.S. only)** (Figure 28):
  - o Highest: persons aged 23–24 years (24.2)
  - o Lowest: persons aged 13–14 years (0.1)
    - ▪ ***Disparities by age group***:
      - ▸ Absolute disparity (rate difference)—If persons aged 23–24 years had the same rate as persons aged 18–19 ycars (11.4), 13 cascs pcr 100,000 population would havc bccn prcvcntcd.
      - ▸ Relative disparity (rate ratio)—Persons aged 23–34 years had a rate that was 2.1 times as high as persons aged 18–19 years.
- **Rates (U.S. only)** (Figure 28):
  - o Highest: Black/African American (46.6)
  - o Lowest: Asian (3.1)
    - ▪ ***Disparities by race/ethnicity***:
      - ▸ Absolute disparity (rate difference)—If Black/African American persons aged 13–24 years had the same rate as White persons aged 13–24 years (3.5), 43 cases per 100,000 population would have been prevented.
      - ▸ Relative disparity (rate ratio)—Black/African American persons aged 13–24 years had a rate that was 13.3 times as high as White persons aged 13–24 years.
- **Rates (U.S. only)** (Figure 28):
  - o Highest: South (17.3)
  - o Lowest: Midwest (8.3)
    - ▪ ***Disparities by region***:
      - ▸ Absolute disparity (rate difference): if the South had the same rate as the Midwest, 9 cases per 100,000 population would have been prevented.
      - ▸ Relative disparity (rate ratio): the South had a rate that was 2.1 times as high as the Midwest.

**Figure 28. Rates and disparities of diagnoses of HIV infection among persons aged 13–24 years, by selected characteristics, 2020 (COVID-19 pandemic)—United States**

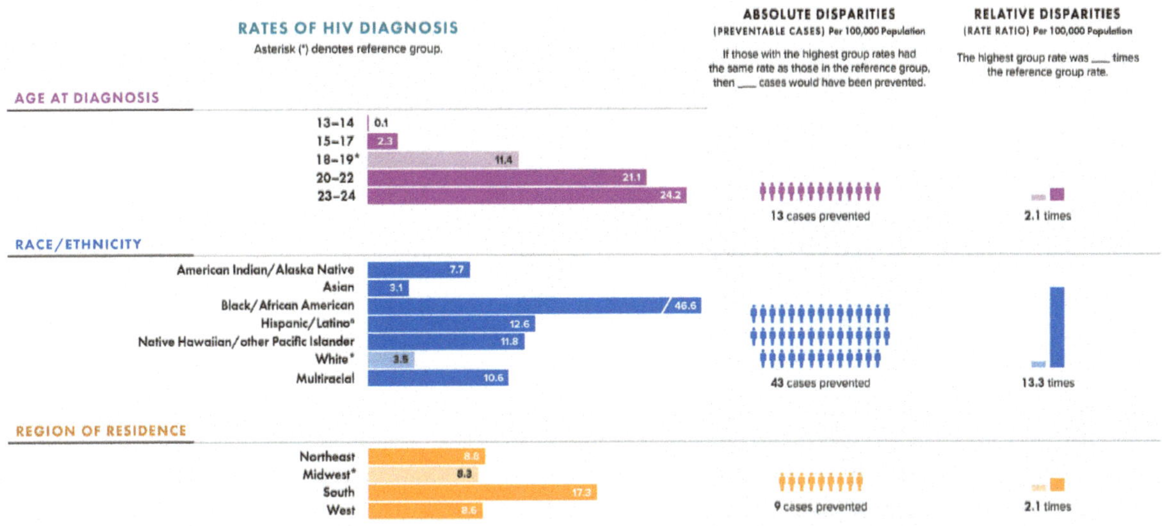


*Note*. Data for 2020 should be interpreted with caution due to the impact of the COVID-19 pandemic on access to HIV testing, care-related services, and case surveillance activities in state/local jurisdictions. Absolute disparity measures the difference between rates in groups with the highest rates and a reference group ($Rate_{highest\ group} - Rate_{reference\ group}$). Relative disparity (rate ratio) measures the rates in groups with the highest rates divided by a reference group ($Rate_{highest\ group} \div Rate_{reference\ group}$).

[a] Hispanic/Latino persons can be of any race.

## Children Aged <13 Years

To make informed decisions about antiretroviral therapy to reduce perinatal transmission of HIV to infants, pregnant women should know their HIV infection status. In 1995, the first recommendations for HIV counseling and voluntary testing for pregnant women were published. In 2006, CDC released revised recommendations for HIV testing which specified that opt-out HIV screening should be included in the routine panel of prenatal screening tests for all pregnant women.

In 2019, 37 areas reported no perinatally acquired infections among infants born. Because of delays in the reporting of births and diagnoses of HIV infection attributed to perinatal exposure, the exclusion of data for the most recent 2 years allowed at least 24 months for data from 2019 to be reported to CDC. Data reflect all infants with diagnosed, perinatally acquired HIV infection who were born in the United States and 6 dependent areas during 2019, regardless of year of diagnosis.

### Diagnoses of HIV infection

In the United States and 6 dependent areas, a total of 32 children born during 2019 received a diagnosis of HIV infection attributed to perinatal transmission (Figure 29).

**Figure 29. Diagnoses of perinatally acquired HIV infection among children born during 2019—United States and 6 dependent areas**

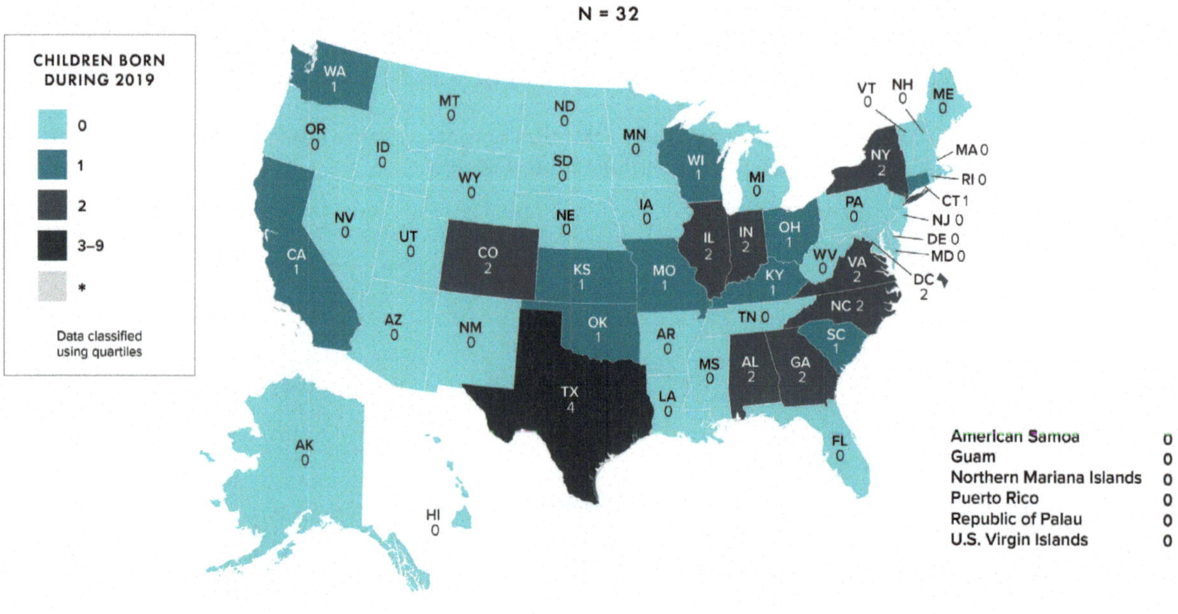


**Infected infants** (Figure 30): From 2016 through 2019 in the United States and Puerto Rico, among the 193 children born with diagnosed, perinatally acquired HIV infection, time of maternal HIV testing was as follows:

- 45% were born to mothers who were tested before pregnancy
- 19% were born to mothers who were tested during pregnancy

- 8% to mothers tested at the time of birth
- 21% of children with diagnosed, perinatally acquired HIV infection were born to mothers who were tested after the child's birth
- 7% were born to mothers whose time of maternal HIV testing was unknown

**Exposed but not infected** (Figure 30): From 2016 through 2019 in the United States and Puerto Rico, among the 11,757 children born who were exposed but not perinatally infected with HIV, time of maternal HIV testing was as follows:

- 82% were born to mothers who were tested before pregnancy
- 15% were born to mothers who were tested during pregnancy
- 1% to mothers tested at the time of birth
- 1% to mothers tested after birth
- 1% were born to mothers whose time of maternal HIV testing was unknown

*Note.* The number of areas contributing exposure data varied by year. Because not all jurisdictions have exposure reporting in place, the number presented is likely a minimum count of the number of exposed infants in the United States and Puerto Rico.

**Figure 30. Time of maternal HIV testing among children with diagnosed perinatally acquired HV infection and children exposed to HIV, birth years 2016–2019—United States and Puerto Rico**

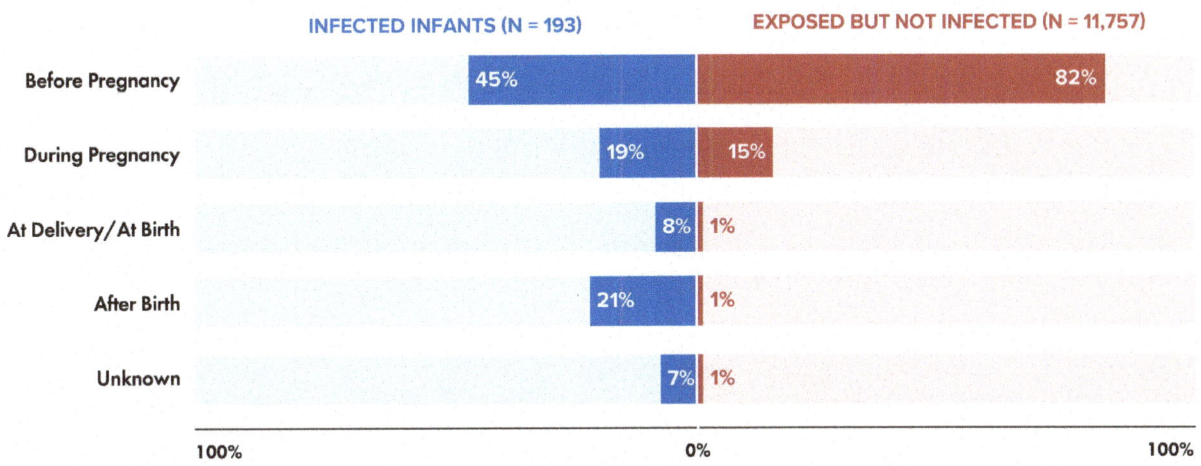


**Diagnoses** (Figure 31): In 2020, among children in the United States,

- Black/African American children made up approximately 14% of the population of children but accounted for 56% of diagnoses of HIV infection.
- Hispanic/Latino children made up 26% of the population of children but accounted for 16% of diagnoses.
- White children made up 49% of the population of children but accounted for 21% of diagnoses.

**Figure 31. Percentages of diagnoses of HIV infection among children, by race/ethnicity, 2020 (COVID-19 pandemic)—United States and 6 dependent areas**

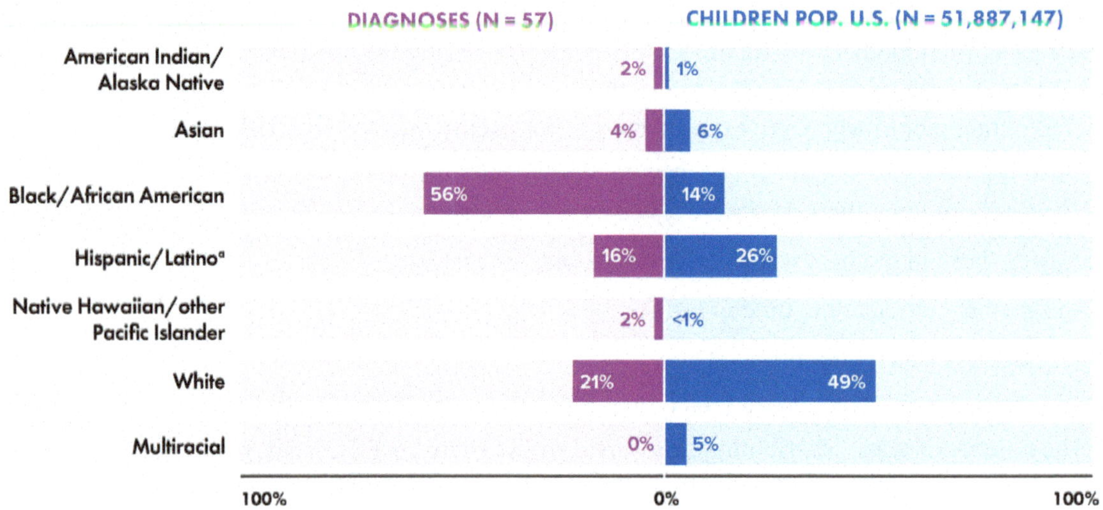


*Note.* Data for 2020 should be interpreted with caution due to the impact of the COVID-19 pandemic on access to HIV testing, care-related services, and case surveillance activities in state/local jurisdictions.

[a] Hispanic/Latino persons can be of any race.

- **Prevalence, children** (Figure 32):
  - At year-end 2020 in the United States and 6 dependent areas, approximately 1,447 children were living with diagnosed HIV infection.
  - The overall rate of persons living with diagnosed HIV infection was 2.8.

**Figure 32. Rates of children living with diagnosed HIV infection, year-end 2020 (COVID-19 pandemic)—United States and 6 dependent areas**

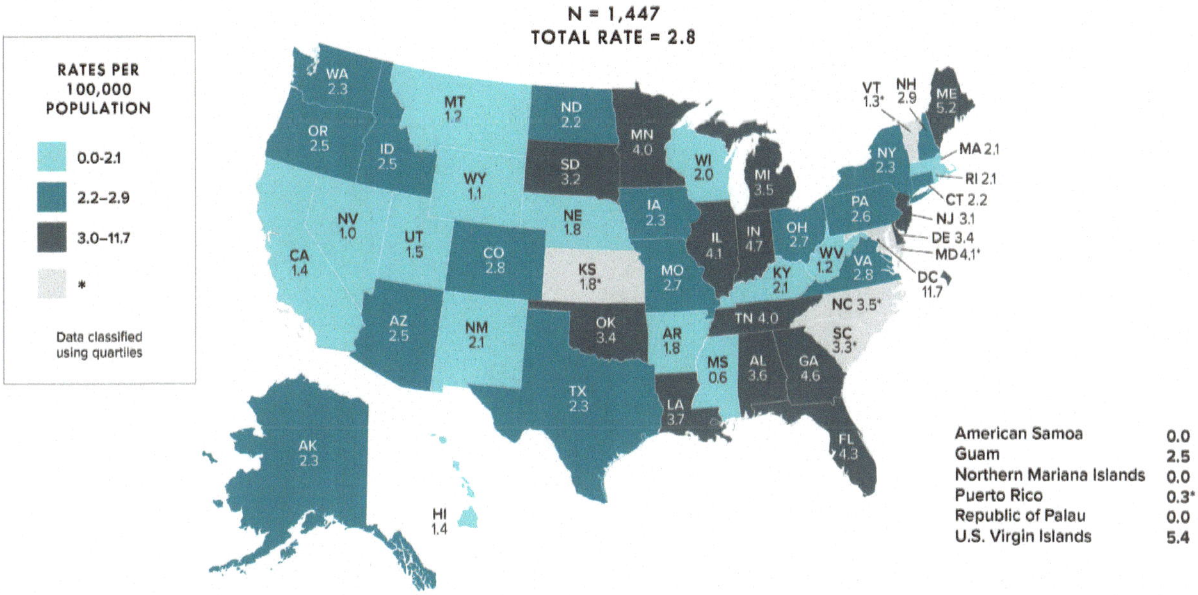


*Note.* Data for the year 2020 are preliminary and based on deaths reported to CDC as of December 2021. Data are based on address of residence as of December 31, 2020 (i.e., most recent known address). Data for 2020 should be interpreted with caution due to the impact of the COVID-19 pandemic on access to HIV testing, care-related services, and case surveillance activities in state/local jurisdictions. Asterisk (*) indicates incomplete reporting.

- **Prevalence and race/ethnicity, children** (Table 16b):
  - American Indian/Alaska Native: <1%
  - Asian: 7%
  - Black/African American: 58%
  - Hispanic/Latino: 13%
  - Native Hawaiian/other Pacific Islander: <1%
  - White: 13%
  - Multiracial: 8%
- **Prevalence, perinatally acquired HIV infection** (Figure 33):
  - At year-end 2020 in the United States and 6 dependent areas, there were 12,588 persons living with diagnosed, perinatally acquired HIV infection.
  - Data reflect all persons (i.e., children, adolescents, and adults) with diagnosed, perinatally acquired HIV infection who were alive at year-end 2020, regardless of their age at year-end 2020.

**Figure 33. Persons living with diagnosed, perinatally acquired HIV infection, year-end 2020 (COVID-19 pandemic)—United States and 6 dependent areas**

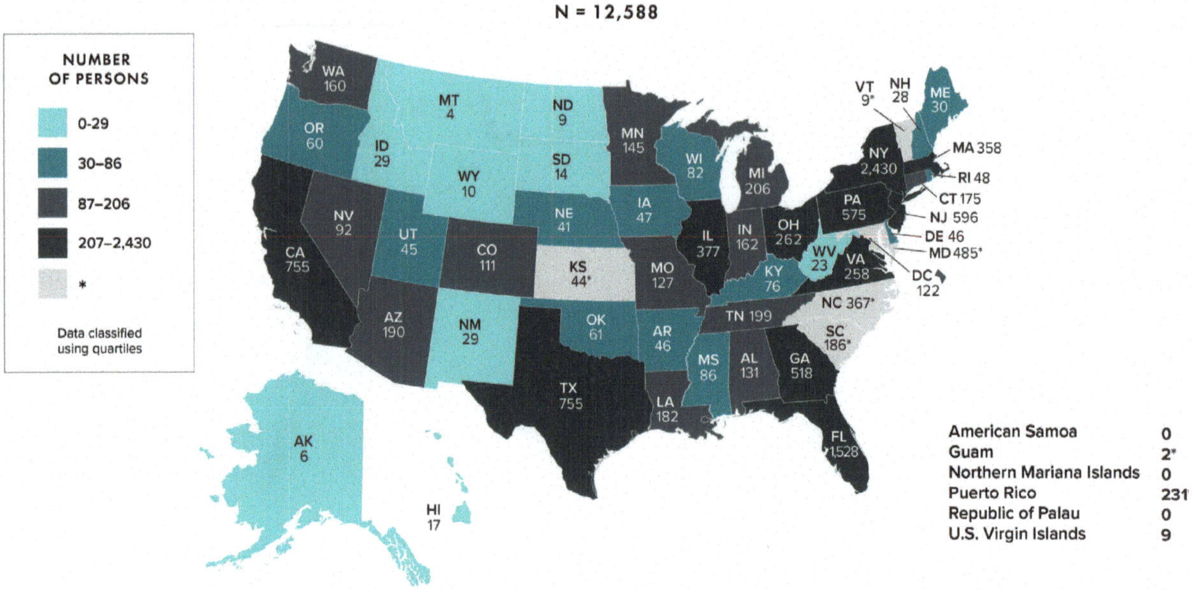


*Note.* Data for the year 2020 are preliminary and based on deaths reported to CDC as of December 2021. Data are based on address of residence as of December 31, 2020 (i.e., most recent known address). Data for 2020 should be interpreted with caution due to the impact of the COVID-19 pandemic on access to HIV testing, care-related services, and case surveillance activities in state/local jurisdictions. Asterisk (*) indicates incomplete reporting.

- **Prevalence and race/ethnicity, perinatally acquired HIV infection** (Table 16b):
  - American Indian/Alaska Native: <1%
  - Asian: 1%
  - Black/African American: 57%
  - Hispanic/Latino: 24%
  - Native Hawaiian/other Pacific Islander: <1%
  - White: 11%
  - Multiracial: 7%

# Living Well With Dementia in the Community

## Resources and Support

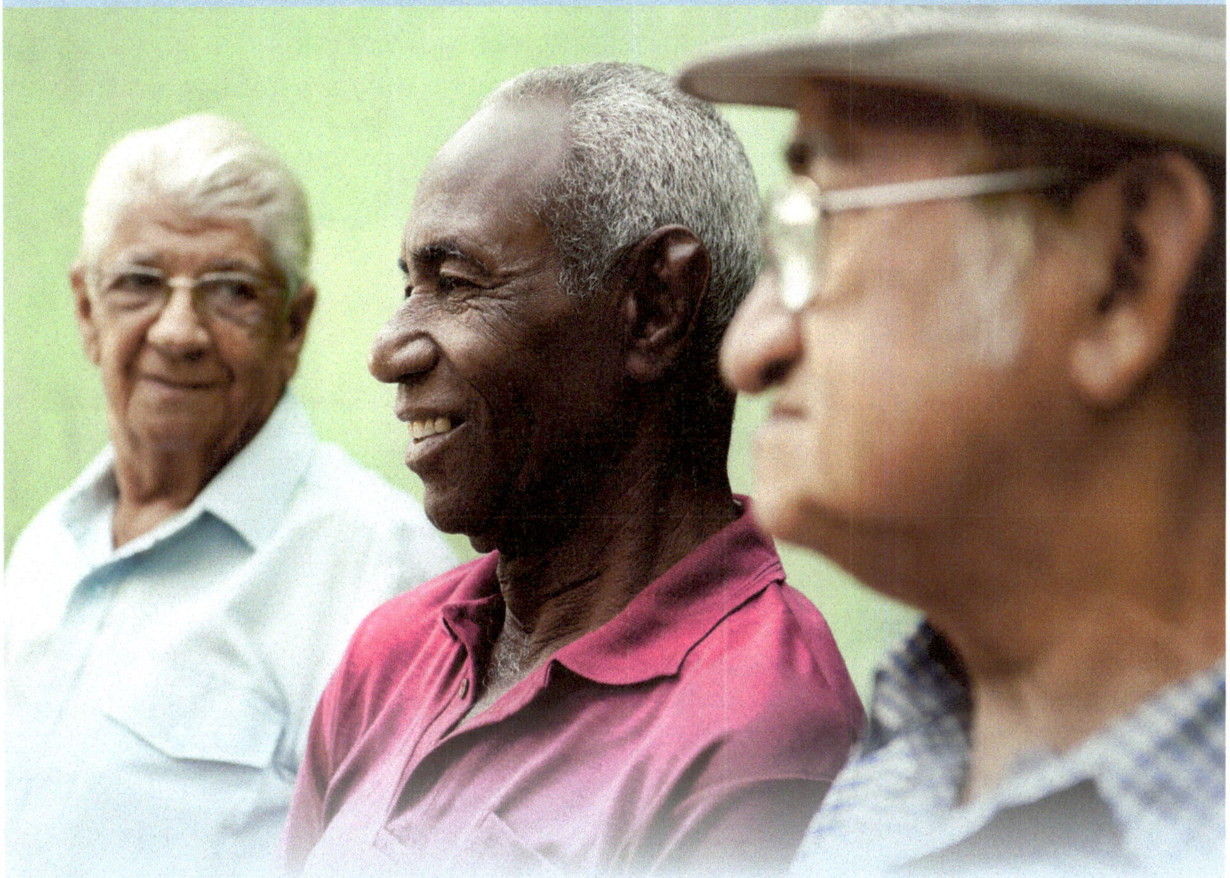

eldercare locator

Americans are living longer than ever before, and the rapidly growing older adult population is expected to reach 73 million people by the year 2030. While longer lifespans bring great opportunities, older adults face an increased risk of developing a chronic condition or cognitive disorder. If you or a loved one is experiencing changes in self-management abilities, judgement or behavior, it is important to recognize the differences between normal aging-related changes and something more serious like dementia.

One in 10 people age 65 and older lives with some form of dementia, the most common of which is Alzheimer's disease. Sixty percent of people with dementia live in their homes and in the community. **While living with the condition can be difficult, people with dementia and their caregivers can have independent, high-quality lives—especially when they are connected to local community services and supports.** Fortunately, there is more support for people with dementia and their caregivers than ever before.

## What is Dementia?

According to the Alzheimer's Association (www.alz.org), dementia is a general term that describes a range of symptoms an individual experiences that are associated with a decline in memory and mental ability that are severe enough to interfere with daily life. While each person with dementia is affected differently, symptoms include memory loss, language difficulty, a loss of motor function and difficulty problem solving. **Although there is currently no cure for dementia, early detection and treatment can greatly improve quality of life.**

### How Do Signs of Dementia Differ from the Typical Aging Process?

Many of dementia's symptoms can be confused with the normal aging process. But for people with dementia, these symptoms can change and accelerate over time, depending on the stage of dementia a person is in. The chart on the right differentiates signs of dementia from what many would classify to be characteristic of the aging process.

| TYPICAL AGE-RELATED CHANGES | SIGNS OF DEMENTIA |
|---|---|
| Making a bad decision once in a while | Poor judgment and decision-making |
| Missing a monthly payment | Inability to manage a budget |
| Forgetting which day it is and remembering it later | Losing track of the date or the season |
| Sometimes forgetting which word to use | Difficulty having a conversation |
| Losing things from time to time | Misplacing things and being unable to retrace steps to find them |

Source: Alzheimer's Association, 10 Early Signs and Symptoms of Alzheimer's

## If You Suspect That You or a Loved One Has Dementia…

### Seek Medical Advice

Reversible conditions—dehydration, thyroid issues and vitamin deficiencies, among others—can cause symptoms similar to dementia. If you suspect that you or a loved one is showing signs of dementia, the first step is to see a medical doctor who can make an assessment, possibly provide a diagnosis and make referrals to specialists such as a neurologist who can provide further information and care. **Early detection is vital.** Going to the doctor as soon as you or your loved one suspects dementia can speed access to essential treatments and other resources that may slow the progress of dementia and extend the period of time individuals living with dementia can stay in their homes and communities.

### Learn About Dementia

After receiving a dementia diagnosis, many people want to learn all they can about what living with dementia means. Because symptoms of dementia change over time, an individual's needs change depending on the stage of dementia they are in. Resources available from the Alzheimer's Association, Dementia Friendly America and others (see Resources section on the back panel) help people with dementia continue living independently in their homes and communities for years.

## Dementia by the Numbers

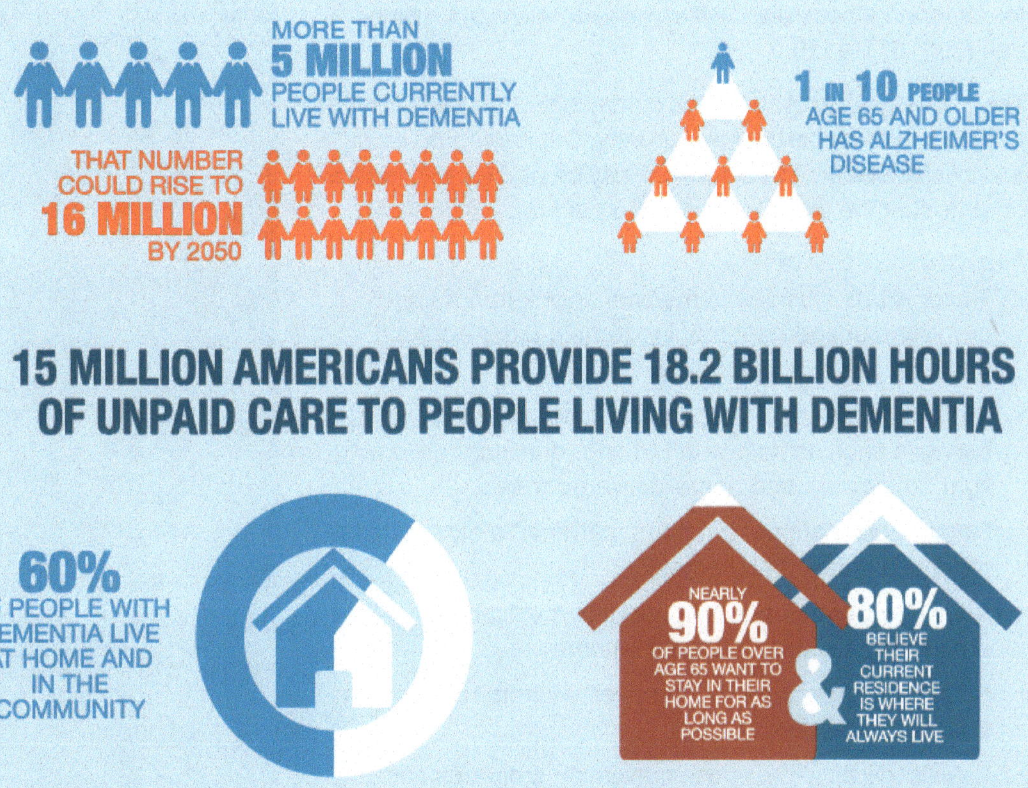


Source: Alzheimer's Association, Alzheimer's Disease Facts and Figures 2017

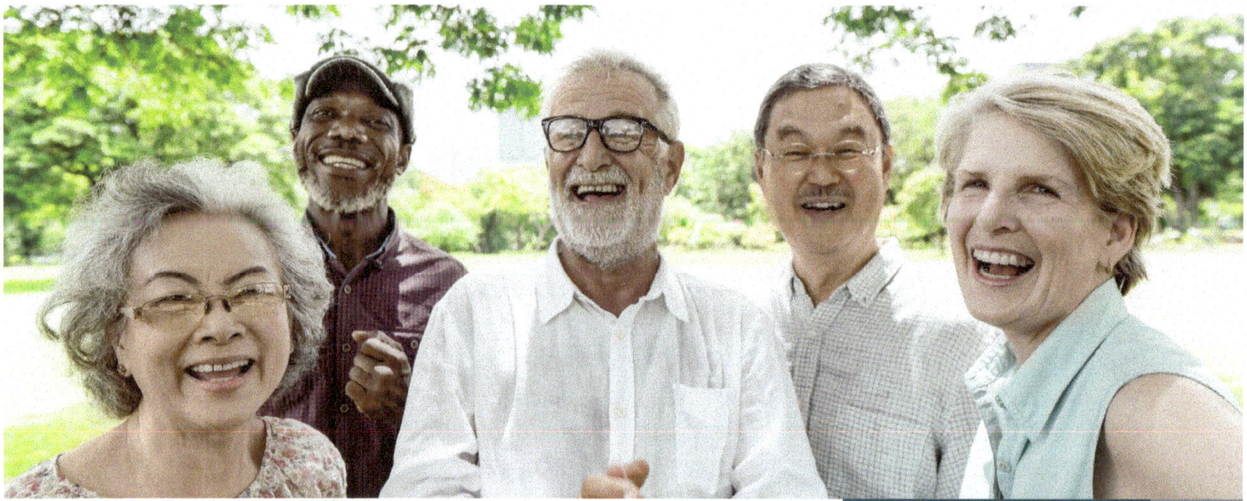

## Explore Local Community Services and Supports

For many, living at home and in the community will require supportive services to maintain independence and increase well-being, and this is especially important for people living with dementia. The Eldercare Locator connects people with dementia and their caregivers to a wide range of services. In doing so, people with dementia can live independently in their communities for as long as possible. Visit **www.eldercare.acl.gov or call (800) 677-1116.**

The following types of home and community-based services are available in most parts of the country. Depending on income and local availability, these services may be paid for with federal or state funding or may need to be paid out-of-pocket.

### Supportive Services

- Transportation: Rides to medical appointments and mobility management training to help older adults navigate public transportation
- In-Home Services: Personal care and other supportive services such as help with bathing, dressing, grooming, light housework and home-delivered meals
- Home modifications or repairs that enable older adults to remain safely their homes
- Adult Day Care: Supervised social or medical care provided in a setting outside the home
- Professional or "friendly volunteer" visitors to maintain social engagement
- Legal services, elder abuse prevention programs and Adult Protective Services

### Memory Cafés

Memory cafés are popping up across the country. Often located in central community locations—coffee houses, libraries and houses of faith, to name a few—memory cafés offer a welcoming, safe, supportive, engaging environment for people with dementia and caregivers alike. People attending memory cafés benefit from conversation and shared activities with individuals who are sharing their experience, in social and accepting settings.

## Health, Wellness and Social Activities

- Events and classes offered through senior centers and other community-based organizations that promote engagement and reduce social isolation such as memory cafés (see panel)
- Programs to prevent falls, manage chronic diseases and promote health and well-being
- Health insurance and Medicare counseling

## Programs for Caregivers

Those who provide support to individuals who have dementia face a unique set of challenges and often need support themselves. The Aging Network and dementia-specific organizations such as the Alzheimer's Association can connect caregivers to local resources, such as:

- Support groups with other family caregivers, either in person or online (e.g., the Alzheimer's Association's ALZConnected at www.alzconnected.org)
- Training for caregivers on health, nutrition and financial literacy
- Evidence-based trainings designed to help caregivers manage the behavioral symptoms that may accompany dementia (e.g., Powerful Tools for Caregivers, REACH, SAVVY Caregiver)
- Respite care to enable caregivers to be temporarily relieved of their caregiving responsibilities or allow them to attend caregiver trainings
- Supplemental services to better help caregivers manage their role (e.g., assistive technology, equipment)
- Technology solutions to support health and safety

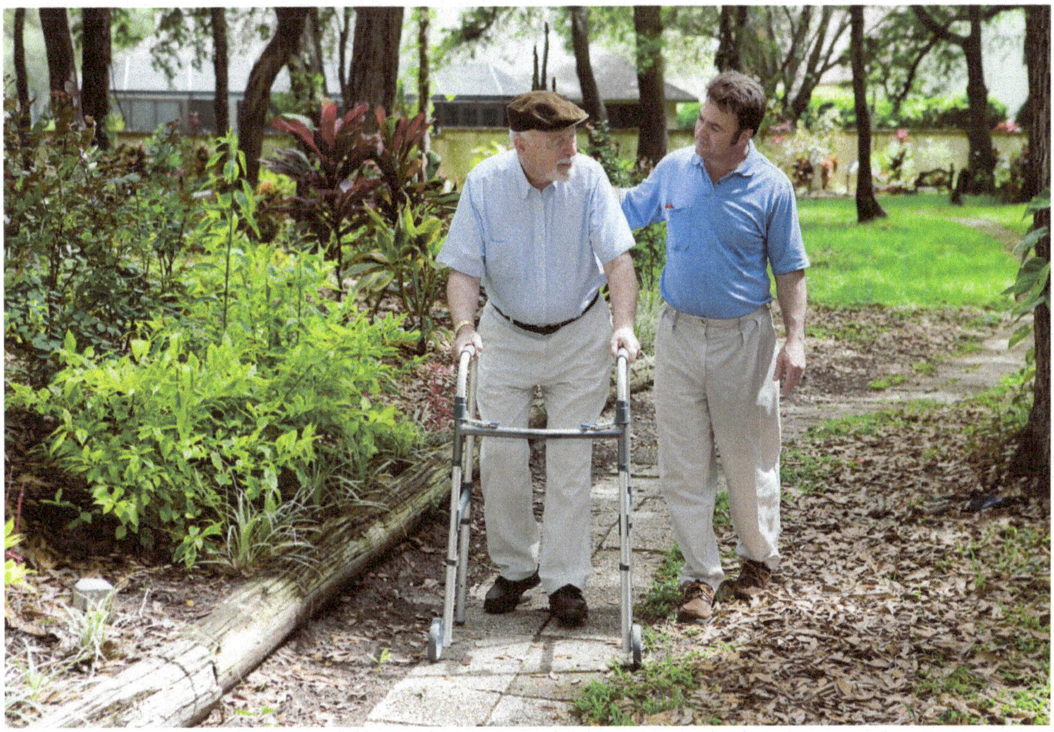

# Dementia Friendly America

Every part of the community can play a role in making life easier for people living with dementia and their caregivers. Already there are dozens of Dementia Friendly Communities in 28 states. And many sectors—banks, places of worship, law enforcement, local governments, businesses and first responders—can take steps to become "dementia friendly" by adopting practices to support people with dementia and their caregivers.

To find out how you can help make your community more dementia friendly, visit Dementia Friendly America (www.dfamerica.org). In addition, individuals can learn about dementia by becoming a Dementia Friend (www.dementiafriends.usa.org), which simply involves watching a few short videos that explain dementia and how to best interact with people living with dementia.

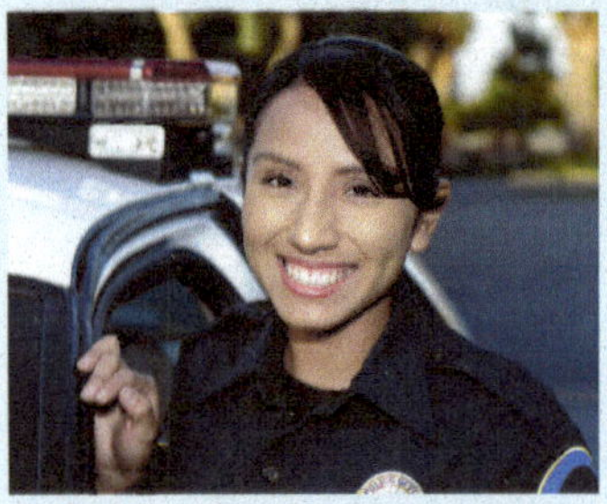

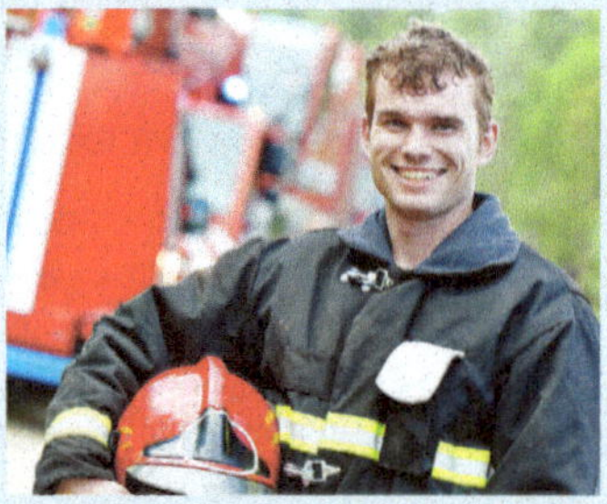

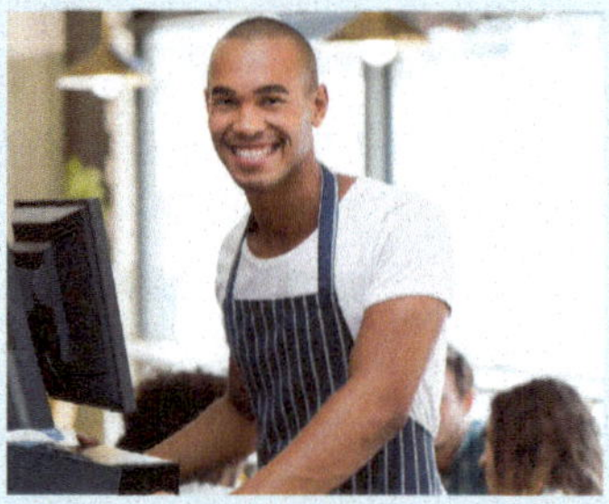

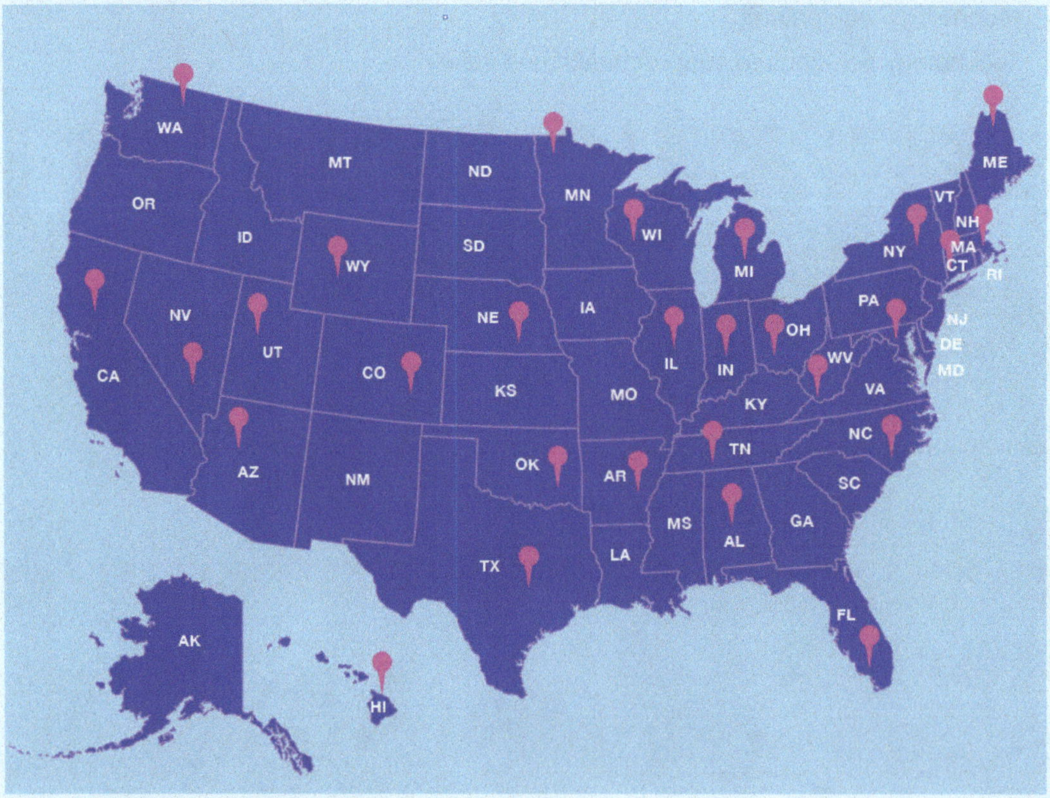

## Communicating Well With People With Dementia

- Greet people warmly even if you think they do not remember you. If they seem confused, remind them who you are.
- Slow the pace of conversation slightly and allow time for the person to process and respond.
- Speak clearly and calmly; be patient and understanding.
- Keep communication simple; ask one question at a time.
- Listen with empathy and seek to understand the person's reality or feelings.
- Connect on an emotional level even if conversation topics shift or do not make sense to you.
- Be aware of the person's and your body language: smile, make eye contact at eye level.
- Enjoy spending time with the person in the present moment.
- Offer hugs and hand-holding as appropriate.
- Avoid arguing with or embarrassing the person.
- Treat the person with dignity and respect.

## Projected Changes Between 2014 and 2025 in Alzheimer's Disease Prevalence by State

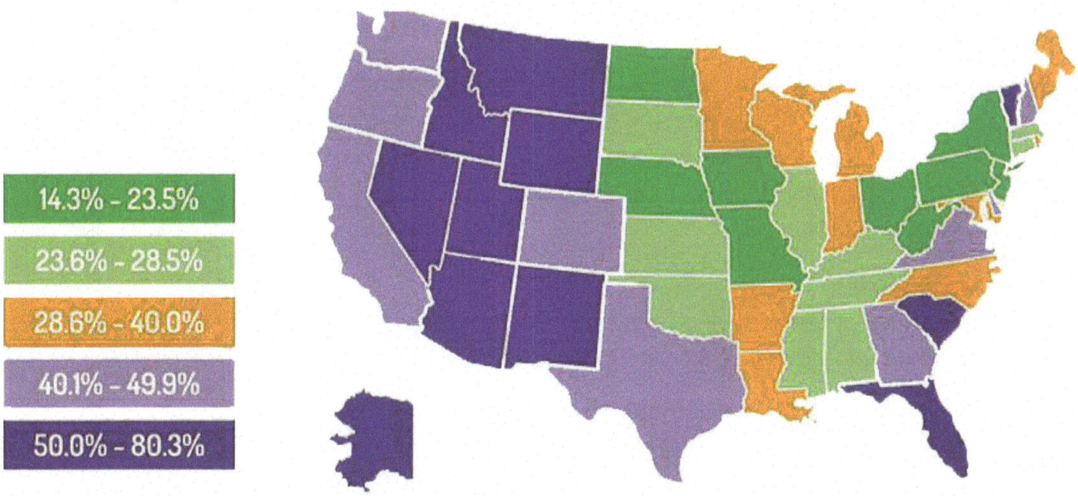


Source: Alzheimer's Association, Alzheimer's Disease Facts and Figures 2014

## Resources

**Eldercare Locator**
The only national information and referral resource to provide support to consumers across the spectrum of issues affecting older Americans.
www.eldercare.acl.gov and (800) 677-1116

**National Association of Area Agencies on Aging (n4a)**
The mission of n4a is to build the capacity of Area Agencies on Aging and Title VI Native American aging programs so they can better help older adults and people with disabilities live with dignity and choices in their homes and communities.
www.n4a.org

**Alzheimer's Association**
The leading voluntary health organization in Alzheimer's care, support and research.
www.alz.org

**Alzheimer's Association's Community Resource Finder**
This tool provides a comprehensive listing of Alzheimer's and dementia resources, community programs and services.
www.communityresourcefinder.org

**Dementia Friendly America**
Through the work of more than 35 national, leading organizations, the Dementia Friendly America initiative is catalyzing a movement to more effectively support and serve those across America who are living with dementia and their family and friend care partners.
www.dfamerica.org

**Dementia Friends USA**
A global movement that is changing the way people think, act and talk about dementia. Developed by the Alzheimer's Society in the U.K., the Dementia Friends initiative in the U.S. is administered by n4a.
www.dementiafriendsusa.org

### Acknowledgements
Thank you to the Alzheimer's Association and Dementia Friendly America for lending their expertise to the development of this brochure.

This brochure was published by the Eldercare Locator, a program established in 1991 and funded by the Administration for Community Living; it is administered by the National Association of Area Agencies on Aging (n4a).

This project was supported, in part, by grant number 901R0002, from the U.S. Administration for Community Living, Department of Health and Human Services, Washington, DC 20201. Grantees undertaking projects under government sponsorship are encouraged to express freely their findings and conclusions. Points of view or opinions do not, therefore, necessarily represent official Administration for Community Living policy.

# Autoimmune Diseases and Your Environment

A healthy immune system defends the body against disease and infection. But if the immune system malfunctions, it mistakenly attacks healthy cells, tissues, and organs. Called autoimmune disease, these attacks can affect any part of the body, weakening bodily function and even turning life-threatening.

Scientists know about more than 100 autoimmune diseases. Some are well known, such as Type 1 diabetes, multiple sclerosis, lupus, and rheumatoid arthritis, while others are rare and difficult to diagnose. With unusual autoimmune diseases, patients may suffer years before getting a proper diagnosis. Most of these diseases have no cure. Some require lifelong treatment to ease symptoms.

## Autoimmune diseases are on the rise

Collectively, these diseases affect 5-9% of the population and create considerable personal and public health burdens. Race, ethnicity, and sex are genetic characteristics linked to the chance of developing an autoimmune disease. These diseases afflict women more than men, and are among the leading causes of death for young and middle-aged women.[1]

Autoimmune diseases appear to be increasing throughout the world, yet the reasons are unexplained.[2] The prevalence of antinuclear antibodies, the most common indicator of autoimmunity in human cells, increased substantially over a recent 25-year span in the U.S.[3]

Research increasingly suggests that autoimmune diseases likely result from the interactions of environmental and genetic risk factors. Autoimmune diseases seem more common when people are in contact with certain environmental exposures, as described below.

## What is NIEHS Doing?

For decades, NIEHS has researched how the environment may affect development of autoimmune diseases.

In 2010, the institute gathered an interdisciplinary panel of 40 experts to evaluate the state of the science in this area. Among many conclusions, the panel stated:

- Solvent exposure, from working with products such as paint thinners and cleaners, is linked to systemic sclerosis.
- Crystalline silica exposure, from working with quartz or granite, for example, can contribute to the development of several autoimmune diseases.
- Smoking can contribute to the development of seropositive rheumatoid arthritis.

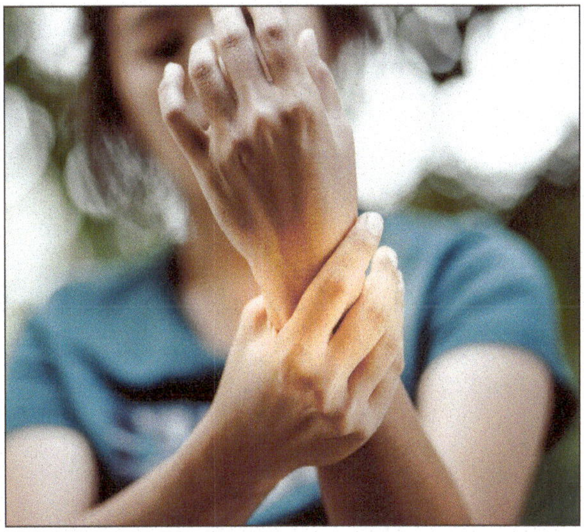

Unraveling the genetic and environmental underpinnings of autoimmune disease remains a focus at NIEHS and the National Toxicology Program (NTP). Research progress leads to discoveries such as:

- **Added risk from ultraviolet (UV) radiation –** Short-term ultraviolet radiation exposure, as from outdoor sunlight, may affect the onset of juvenile dermatomyositis, an illness with muscle weakness and skin rashes. The chance of illness increased as the UV index increased to its highest levels in the month before symptoms began.[4]
- **Links to childhood poverty –** Childhood in a household with lower socioeconomic status and education levels is linked to rheumatoid arthritis in adulthood.[5]
- **Agricultural chemical association –** Exposure to some pesticides may play a role in the development of rheumatoid arthritis in male farmers.[6]

  The same study shows that in farm wives, an increased chance of developing rheumatoid arthritis was associated with other types of farm-related exposures, such as painting and using solvents. More research is needed on these and other potential risk and protective factors.[7]
- **Genetic factors in autoimmune muscle disease –** Using DNA samples from myositis patients of European ancestry, NIEHS researchers identified primary genetic risk factors associated with this autoimmune muscle disease.[8]

- **Insight into genetic link to rheumatoid arthritis** – NIEHS-funded researchers are closer to explaining why a genetic risk that increases the chance of developing rheumatoid arthritis is amplified by environmental pollutants like cigarette smoke.[9]
- **Role of nutrition** – Vitamin D may help prevent immune dysfunction in older populations.[10] For lupus patients, NIEHS-funded researchers found that dietary micronutrients—choline, folate, and vitamin B12—may improve symptoms, but more research is needed.[11]

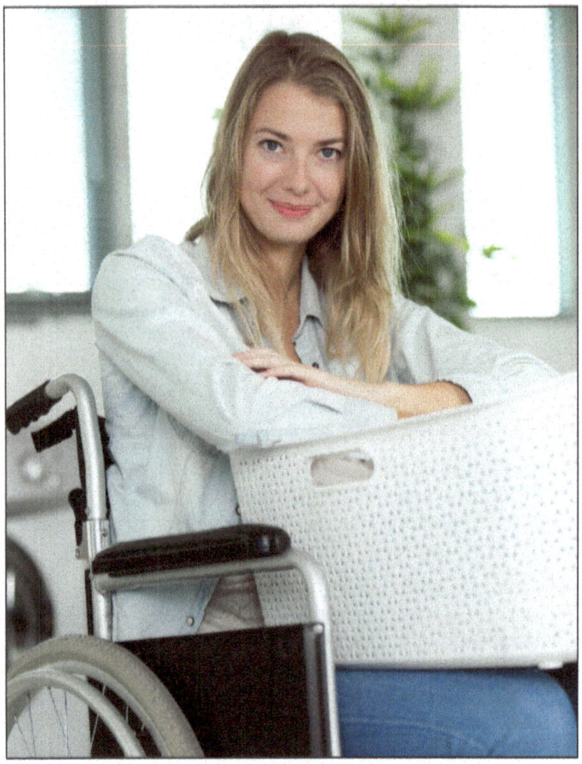

**NIEHS is conducting these clinical studies:**

- Immunity Cells in Blood studies how immune cells in the bloodstream may, under certain circumstances, contribute to inflammation.
- Adult and Juvenile Myositis investigates the causes, immune system changes, and medical problems associated with myositis, an inflammatory muscle disease that can damage muscles and other organs, resulting in significant disability.
- Myositis in Military Personnel compares people who developed myositis during active duty to military personnel without autoimmune diseases, to assess risk factors for myositis.
- Calcinosis Study examines the development of painful calcium deposits in people with dermatomyositis, a form of myositis associated with a skin rash, muscle weakness, and inflamed muscles.
- MYORISK Study seeks to understand the environmental factors that may result in dermatomyositis or polymyositis, a form of myositis that causes muscle weakness on both sides of the body.
- Rheumatic Disorders in Siblings identifies genetic and environmental factors by studying families with siblings or twins in which one of them has developed an autoimmune disease while the others have not.

To volunteer for a study on the causes of, and possible treatments for, autoimmune diseases, visit www.clinicaltrials.gov.

For more information on the National Institute of Environmental Health Sciences, go to **www.niehs.nih.gov.**


1 Ramos PS, et al. 2015. Genetics of autoimmune diseases: insights from population genetics. J Hum Genet. 60(11): 657–664.

2 Schiffenbauer A and FW Miller. Noninfectious environmental agents and autoimmunity [Book Chapter] *The Autoimmune Diseases* (2020) pp. 345-362.

3 Dinse GE, et al. Increasing Prevalence of Antinuclear Antibodies in the United States. April 8, 2020. Arthr & Rheumatol. doi: 10.1002/art.41214

4 Shah M, et al. Childhood Myositis Heterogeneity Collaborative Study Group. 2013. Ultraviolet radiation exposure is associated with clinical and autoantibody phenotypes in juvenile myositis. Arthritis Rheum. 65(7): 1934–1941.

5 Parks CG, et al. 2013. Childhood socioeconomic factors and perinatal characteristics influence development of rheumatoid arthritis in adulthood. Ann Rheum Dis. 72(3): 350–356.

6 Meyer A, et al. 2017. Pesticide exposure and risk of rheumatoid arthritis among licensed male pesticide applicators in the Agricultural Health Study. Environ Health Perspect 125(7): 077010.

7 Parks CG et al., 2016. Rheumatoid Arthritis in Agricultural Health Study Spouses: Associations with Pesticides and Other Farm Exposures. Environ Health Perspect. 124 (11): 1728-1734.

8 Miller FW, et al. 2015. Genome-wide association study identifies HLA 8.1 ancestral haplotype alleles as major genetic risk factors for myositis phenotypes. Genes Immun. 16(7):470–480.

9 Fu J, et al. 2018. Shared epitope-aryl hydrocarbon receptor crosstalk underlies the mechanism of gene-environment interaction in autoimmune arthritis. PNAS 115(18):4755-4760.

10 Meier HC, et al. 2016. Association between vitamin D deficiency and antinuclear antibodies in middle-aged and older U.S. adults. Cancer Epidemiol Biomarkers Prev 25(12):1559-1563.

11 Strickland FM, et al. 2013. Arthritis Rheum. 65(7):1872–1881. Diet influences expression of autoimmune associated genes and disease severity by epigenetic mechanisms in a transgenic lupus model.

GUT MICROBES
2021, VOL. 13, NO. 1, e1916278 (15 pages)
https://doi.org/10.1080/19490976.2021.1916278

Taylor & Francis
Taylor & Francis Group

REVIEW

OPEN ACCESS Check for updates

# Alcohol as friend or foe in autoimmune diseases: a role for gut microbiome?

Blaine Caslin, Kailey Mohler, Shreya Thiagarajan, and Esther Melamed

Department of Neurology, Dell Medical School, The University of Texas at Austin, Austin, United States

**ABSTRACT**

Alcohol is well known for promoting systemic inflammation and aggravating multiple chronic health conditions. Thus, alcohol may also be expected to serve as a risk factor in autoimmune diseases. However, emerging data from human and animal studies suggest that alcohol may in fact be protective in autoimmune diseases. These studies point toward alcohol's complex dose-dependent relationship in autoimmune diseases as well as potential modulation by duration and type of alcohol consumption, cultural background and sex. In this review, we will explore alcohol's pro- and anti-inflammatory properties in human and animal autoimmune diseases, including autoimmune diabetes, thyroid disease, systemic lupus erythematosus, rheumatoid arthritis, experimental autoimmune encephalomyelitis and multiple sclerosis. We will also discuss potential mechanisms of alcohol's anti-inflammatory effects mediated by the gut microbiome.

**ARTICLE HISTORY**
Received 28 August 2020
Revised 16 March 2021
Accepted 1 April 2021

**KEYWORDS**
Alcohol; autoimmunity; microbiome; inflammation; dysbiosis

## Introduction

Autoimmune diseases arise from aberrant immune system activation against self-antigens and affect approximately 24 million people in the United States, with rising incidence in recent years.[1] Women tend to be disproportionately affected, with female-to-male odds ratios of up to 9:1 in some autoimmune diseases.[2] While there are known genetic risk alleles,[3] environmental factors are increasingly seen as major contributors to triggering autoimmunity.[4] Among environmental factors, diet and the composition of the gut microbiome are being closely studied for their role in the initiation and progression of autoimmune disorders.[5,6]

Alcohol is a widely available dietary factor in our society and its pro-inflammatory effects and end-organ damage are well documented at high doses.[7] However, alcohol's role in inflammation and autoimmunity at moderate doses has been relatively less well understood. While it may be hypothesized that alcohol could serve as an environmental inflammatory risk factor, recent evidence actually points toward alcohol's protective effects in several autoimmune diseases, including autoimmune thyroid disease, autoimmune diabetes, systemic lupus erythematosus (SLE), rheumatoid arthritis (RA) and multiple sclerosis (MS), both in human and animal studies.[8–15] Although it is perplexing to explain alcohol's apparent protective role in autoimmune diseases given its pro-inflammatory properties, current evidence suggests that alcohol has pleiotropic tissue-specific and sex-specific anti-inflammatory actions in the body at different doses.

In this review, we will examine alcohol's dose-dependent effects and potential mechanisms in autoimmune diseases in human and animal studies with a focus on the role of alcohol in modulating the gut microbiome in autoimmunity.

## Alcohol metabolism and dosing in human and animal studies

Shortly after consumption, alcohol is absorbed into the bloodstream from the stomach and small intestine, and subsequently diffuses to different body organs. Alcohol is metabolized to acetaldehyde and acetate primarily within the gastrointestinal (GI) tract, but also in other organs, such as the brain.[16] Both alcohol and acetaldehyde can induce systemic inflammation via 1) activation of toll-like receptors (TLRs) 2, 3, 4 and NOD-like receptor family pyrin containing 3 (NLRP3) inflammasome complex on immune cells, 2) bacterial overgrowth in the GI tract and production of a bacterial

**CONTACT** Esther Melamed esther.melamed@austin.utexas.edu Department of Neurology, Dell Medical School, The University of Texas at Austin, Austin, United States

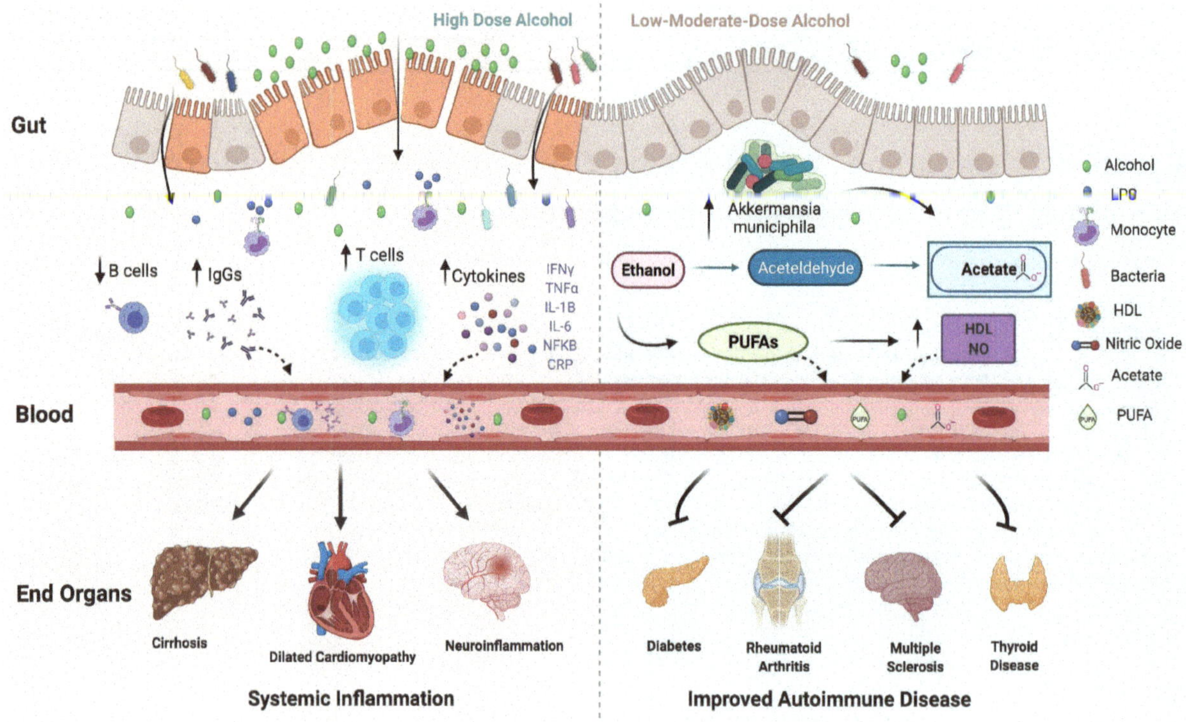


Figure 1. Alcohol has pleiotropic effects in the body. At high doses, alcohol destabilizes the gut barrier and can lead to dysbiosis, increase in bacterial wall product, liposaccharide (LPS), which can stimulate toll-like receptors (TLR) on immune cells and lead to an increase in monocytes, T cells, cytokines and immunoglobulin (IgG) levels as well as a decrease in B cells. In turn, circulating inflammatory cytokines, IgGs and immune cells contribute to end-organ damage. At low-moderate doses, alcohol has been demonstrated to improve autoimmune disease risk and progression. Although the precise mechanism is not well understood, low-moderate alcohol may have a positive impact on inflammation via increase in *Akkermansia muciniphila* and other protective gut microbes, as well as contribute to increases in acetate, polyunsaturated fatty acids (PUFAs), high-density lipoprotein (HDL) and nitric oxide (NO).

breakdown product, lipopolysaccharide (LPS) and 3) generation of free oxygen radical species and inducible nitric oxide synthase (iNOS), both of which directly affect the permeability of gut tight junctions leading to LPS leakage into the bloodstream[17–20]. LPS is a strong TLR agonist and leads to the activation and maturation of macrophages and other innate immune cells.[21] Thus, the combination of increased gut permeability, LPS translocation and alcohol-mediated immune activation can predispose to a pro-inflammatory state (Figure 1).

In interpreting human and animal alcohol studies, it is important to closely consider the administered quantity of alcohol. Patterns of human drinking are typically divided into light, moderate and heavy consumption. For humans, a standard alcoholic drink is defined as approximately 14 g of alcohol.[22] According to the CDC, light drinking is considered to be three or fewer alcoholic drinks per week. Moderate drinking is defined as one alcoholic drink per day for women and two drinks per day for men, though variations across studies exist for this definition. Heavy alcohol consumption is defined as having four or more drinks/day for females and five or more drinks/day for males.[22] Accurate human consumption can be challenging to quantify due to participant subjective memory and accurate reporting.

In animal studies, it is also important to account for variable physiological effects due to administered dose, route of administration (e.g. oral vs. gavage vs. intravenous), consumption pattern (e.g. voluntary vs. non-voluntary), as well as differences in body weight and metabolism between animal species. Rodents, for example, metabolize alcohol approximately five times faster than humans, which results in relatively lower voluntary consumption as rodents rapidly experience the deleterious effects of acetaldehyde accumulation.[23] In animal studies,

Table 1. Alcohol's therapeutic effects in autoimmune diseases.

| Disease | Study Design | No. cases/controls | Evaluated Alcohol Dose(s) | Study Duration/Region | Impact of Light-Moderate Alcohol on Disease Risk/ Morbidity | Reference |
|---|---|---|---|---|---|---|
| Systemic Lupus Erythematosus | Case Control | 150/300 | Light, Moderate, Binge (0–10 units of alcohol) | 1993–1995 Nottingham, UK | ↓ | Hardy CJ et al, 1998 |
| | Case Control | 85/205 | Moderate (1–150 g/month, >150 g/month) | 1981–1999 Sweden | ↓ | Bengtsson AA et al, 2002 |
| | Meta Analysis | 822/55,363 6 case control studies | Moderate | Japan, Sweden, US, UK | ↓ | Wang J et al 2008 |
| | Cohort | 127/64,500 | Moderate (wine >4 drinks/week) | 1995–2015 US Black Women's Health Study | ↓ | Cozier YC et al 2019 |
| | Cohort | 67/57,613 | Light, Moderate (<1; 1–6; >7 drinks/week) | 1997–1999 US Black Women's Health Study | No effect | Formica MK et al, 2003 |
| | Cross-sectional | 505 | Light drinkers (1–5; >6 glasses/week) | 2014–2016 Korean Lupus Network | No effect | Kim SK et al, 2017 |
| | Cross-sectional | 244/204,055 | Light to Moderate (0–5 g/d or >5 g/d) | 1988–1990 Nurse Health Study 1 and 1996–1999 Nurse Health Study 2 | ↓ | Hahn J et al, 2020, Barbhaiya M et al, 2017 |
| Rheumatoid Arthritis | Cross-sectional | 2800/2102 | Hazardous vs. non-hazardous (1–2 drinks, 3–4 drinks, 5–6 drinks, 7–9 drinks, >10 drinks) | 1992–2005 Sweden; Better Anti- Rheumatic FarmacOTherapy | ↓ | Bergman S et al, 2013 |
| | Cross-sectional | 3353/2836 | Low, Moderate (0–16 drinks/week) | 1996–2014 Sweden | ↓ | Hedstrom AK et al, 2019 |
| | Cohort | 11,839 | Mild (≤7 units per week); Moderate (8–14 unites/week); Moderate-High (15–21 units/week); High (>21 units/week) | 1987 and 2016 UK Clinical Practice Research Datalink | ↓ | Humphreys JH et al, 2017 |
| | Meta Analysis | 1878/195,029 8 prospective studies | Light to Moderate | Studies completed prior to 2013 | J shaped | Jin Z et al, 2014 |
| | Cross-sectional | 188 | Light to Moderate (nondrinkers, participants who consume 1–7 drinks/ week, 8–14 drinks/week and >14 drinks/week) | 2013–2014 Leiden Early Arthritis Clinic | J shaped | Mangnus L et al, 2018 |
| | Cohort | 596 | Moderate abstinent (0 g/d), moderate (≤20 g/d for women, ≤30 g/d for men), and abuse (>20 g/d for women, >30 g/d for men) | 2002–2005 France Étude et Suivi des Polyarthrites Indifférenciées Récentes | ↓ in males, ↑ in females | Sageloli F et al, 2018 |
| | Cohort | 166 | Moderate <15 or >15 beverages per month | 2002–2005 Consortium for the Longitudinal Evaluations of African Americans with Early Rheumatoid Arthritis (CLEAR) registry1 | J shaped | Davis ML et al, 2013 |
| | Cross-sectional | 174/204,055 | Moderate (0–25 g/d) | 1988–1990 Nurse Health Study 1 and 1996–1999 Nurse Health Study 2 | U shaped | Lu B et al, 2010 |
| | Cohort | 662/1100 | Moderate (5.1–10.0 g/d) | 2003–2010 Brigham and Women's Hospital Rheumatoid Arthritis Sequential Study | J shaped | Lu B et al, 2014 |
| | Animal Research | 5–10/group | Moderate Consumption (10% v/v ethanol) | 42 d | ↓ | Azizov V et al, 2020 |
| | Animal Research | 12/group | Moderate alcohol (10% ethanol in water) | 6 weeks | ↓ | Jonsson IM et al, 2007 |

*(Continued)*

Table 1. (Continued).

| Disease | Study Design | No. cases/controls | Evaluated Alcohol Dose(s) | Study Duration/Region | Impact of Light-Moderate Alcohol on Disease Risk/Morbidity | Reference |
|---|---|---|---|---|---|---|
| Thyroid Disease | Case Control | 140/560 | Low (1–10 units per week), moderate (11–20 units per week), high (>21 units/week) | 1997–2001 Denmark | ↓ | Carle A et al, 2012 |
| | Case Control | 272/1088 | Light, Moderate and hight (0, 3–10, 11–20 or ≥21 units/week) | 1997–2001 Denmark | ↓ | Carle A et al, 2013 |
| | Case Control | 803/1003 | <10 or >10 units/week | 5 year study Amsterdam Autoimmune thyroid disease | ↓ | Effraimidis G et al, 2012 |
| | Case Control | 140/5154 (hyperthyroidism) 206/5154 (hypothyroidism) | 35 g/d | 2007–2009 Chinese She population | ↓ | Huang Y et al 2019 |
| Diabetes | Cohort | 186/2781 | HUNT 1: abstainers, <1, 1–4, 5–10 and >10 times and HUNT 2: abstainers, very low (0.01–4.9 g/d), low (5–9.9 g/d), moderate (10–14.9 g/d) and high consumers (>15 g/d) | 1984–2008 Norway Nord-Trondelag Health Survey (HUNT) studies | ↓ | Rasouli B et al, 2013 |
| | Meta-analysis | 13 cohorts | Moderate (5–30 g alcohol/d) | Caucasians, Japanese, African Americans, Nauruans | ↓ | Carlsson S et al, 2005 |
| | Case Control | 1905/51,529 | Light (0–4.9 g/d) vs. Moderate (5.0–29.9 g/d) | 1986–2004 Health Professionals Follow-Up Study | ↓ | Joosten MM et al, 2011 |
| | Cohort | 8289 | 0, low (less than or equal to 14/7 (men/women) drinks/week), risky (more than 14/7 drinks and less than 28/14 drinks/week), and high (more than 28/14 drinks/week) | 1979–2012 US National Longitudinal Survey of Youth | ↓ | Kerr WC et al, 2018 |
| | Meta-analysis | 26 studies | Light (0–12 g/d), Moderate (12–24 g/d), or Heavy (>24 g/d) | | ↓ | Li XH et al, 2016 |
| | Case Control | 250/1012 | Nondrinkers, 0.01–4.9, 5–14.9, 15–24.9, and >25 g alcohol/d | 2010–2013 Sweden Epidemiological study of risk factors for LADA and type 2 diabetes | ↓ | Rasouli B et al, 2014 |
| Multiple Sclerosis | Animal Research | 19–20/group | Moderate (2.6% alcohol) | 65 d | ↓ | Caslin B, Maguire C et al, 2019 |
| | Case Control | 745/1761 | Low (<50 g/week for women and <100 g/week for men), moderate (50–112 g/week for women and 100–168 g/week for men), and high (>112 g/week for women and >168 g/week for men) | 2005–2011 Epidemiological Investigation of Multiple Sclerosis 2009–2011 Environment in Multiple Sclerosis studies Sweden | Dose-dependent inverse association | Hedstrom AK et al 2014 |
| | Case Control | 1717/4685 | No consumption, 0 units/week for women (men); low: 1–7 (1–14); moderate: 8–14 (15–21); and high > 14 | 2009–2014 Danish MS Biobank Denmark | Inverse association | Andersen C et al, 2019 |
| | Cohort | 923 | Non drinker, <1 drink/week, >1-4 drinks/week, >4 drinks/week | Comprehensive Longitudinal Investigation of Multiple Sclerosis at the Brigham and Women's Hospital United States | ↓ | Diaz-Cruz C et al, 2017 |
| | Cross-sectional | 429/547,288 | Alcohol abuse, alcohol dependence, and alcohol use | 1999–2011 English National Health Service hospitals | ↑ | Pakpoor J et al, 2014 |
| | Cross-sectional | 258/238,371 | 0 g/d, 0.1–4.9 g/d, 5.0–14.9 g/d, 15.0–29.9 g/d, and 30+ g/d | 1980–2004 Nurse Health Study 1 1991–2005 Nurse Health Study 2 | No effect | Mass J et al, 2013 |

alcohol consumption is usually measured in grams of pure ethanol per kilogram of body weight (g/kg), though some studies may report values as blood ethanol concentration (BEC) or as alcohol by volume (ABV).[24] For murine alcohol studies, light, moderate and heavy alcohol consumption are generally within 0–1.5 g/kg, 2.5 g/kg and 3–6 g/kg, respectively.[25–27]

## Protective role of light-moderate dose of alcohol in autoimmune diseases

Alcohol consumption may be expected to contribute toward an increased risk of or exacerbation of autoimmune diseases given its pro-inflammatory properties. Indeed, in some inflammatory diseases, such as irritable bowel syndrome (IBS) and perennial allergies, there is a direct correlation between consumption of high alcohol doses and disease onset.[28,29] However, impressively, in multiple studies across autoimmune diseases, light-moderate alcohol consumption appears to reduce the disease risk, severity and progression (Table 1). In the following section, we will delineate the known alcohol dose-dependent effects on autoimmune diseases.

### *Autoimmune diabetes*

The beneficial effects of moderate alcohol have been documented in both non-autoimmune type 2 diabetes and in autoimmune type 1 diabetes in adults (LADA)[30–34] (Table 1). In a study of LADA, there was a 60% risk reduction in patients who consumed 2–7 g/day compared with patients consuming 0.01–2 g/day. This study also noted higher anti-glutamic acid decarboxylase antibody (GAD Ab) levels and lower C-peptide in abstainers compared with alcohol consumers, with a more pronounced effect in men. In another LADA study, a 46% risk reduction was noted in men and women consuming greater than 25 g/day.[34] The effect appeared to be strongest in patients with low anti-GAD Ab levels and was restricted to wine drinkers compared to beer or liquor consumers.[34] The authors surmised that patients with low anti-GAD Ab levels may be most similar to patients with type 2 diabetes, and it may be polyphenols and hydroxystilbenes in wine that promote anti-oxidative or anti-inflammatory effects of alcohol in autoimmunity.[34]

### *Autoimmune thyroid diseases*

Similarly to diabetes, moderate alcohol has been demonstrated to be protective in both autoimmune hypothyroidism and hyperthyroidism (Table 1). For example, moderate alcohol was correlated with decreased risk of hypothyroidism and Grave's disease in a dose-dependent manner compared to controls, regardless of gender or type of alcohol consumed.[10,35] Several studies also found that moderate alcohol consumption of >10 units/week[36] or at least 35 g of alcohol per day[37] was associated with a lower probability of autoimmune thyroid disease and development of positive thyroid peroxidase antibodies.

### *Systemic lupus erythematosus*

A significant dose-dependent association between moderate alcohol and SLE risk has been identified in multiple case-control, cohort and cross-sectional studies[9,38–41] (Table 1). In a meta-analysis, protective effects of moderate alcohol were tied to the duration of SLE, with significance seen in patients treated for less than 10 years compared to patients treated for less than 5 years.[40] Another study concluded that moderate alcohol may lower the chance of ANA-positive patients to progress to SLE.[42] Smaller case-control SLE studies, which tend to be more prone to recall bias and reverse causation bias, have either not identified an association with alcohol consumption and SLE risk or have detected a slightly higher risk.[43,44]

### *Rheumatoid arthritis*

Similar to thyroid disease, diabetes and SLE, multiple epidemiological studies and several mechanistic studies support the protective role of light to moderate alcohol in RA in a J- or U-shaped dose-dependent manner[8,15,45–54] (Table 1). In a meta-analysis study, both men and women had a reduction in RA risk over 10 years, with women experiencing the highest risk reduction.[49] In other studies, women consuming moderate alcohol reported lower disease activity and higher quality of life compared to men.[48] However, it has also been documented that alcohol may prevent radiological progression in men and increase radiological progression in women.[53] A significantly lower Modified Health Assessment Questionnaire scores (suggestive of improved functional status) have also been found in RA patients consuming moderate alcohol compared to nondrinkers.[55] This effect was stronger in patients who were positive for *HLA-DRB1* shared epitope.[55] Thus, there is likely to be a beneficial but complex relationship between alcohol, gender and genetic make-up in RA.

### *Multiple sclerosis*

Likewise, in MS there is also evidence for protective effects of moderate alcohol in decreasing disease risk and/or disease progression (Table 1). Several large population studies have demonstrated a dose-dependent inverse association between alcohol and MS risk in both sexes.[12,56] Moderate consumption of red wine appears to correlate with a lower Expanded Disability Status Scale score, suggesting improved function, though patients drinking moderate alcohol exhibited an increase in T2 lesion volume on brain MRI.[57] Conversely, high doses of alcohol may contribute to increased risk of MS, particularly in men.[58,59]

Some studies have noted no association between different doses of alcohol and the risk of developing MS. In these studies, gender may be a variable that may explain alcohol's effects in MS. For example, in a female Nurses' Health Study (NHS) I and II, there was no association between different types of alcohol and the risk of MS.[60] Although this was a large study of >90,000 women between the two NHS studies, the cohort of MS patients of 258 cases was relatively smaller and it is also possible that females may not experience the degree of protective effects of alcohol compared to males. For example, in an animal model of MS, experimental autoimmune encephalomyelitis (EAE), it was recently shown that primarily male mice improved in disease scores on a moderate alcohol diet.[11]

## Alcohol's pro- and anti-inflammatory effects on the immune system

It is well known that chronic high-dose alcohol consumption can lead to a higher infectious disease burden in alcoholics and more difficulty in clearing pathogens such as *Listeria monocytogenes*, *Mycobacterium tuberculosis* and influenza.[61–63] However, while chronic high-level alcohol consumption is known to induce systemic inflammation, there is an increasing understanding that alcohol's effects on the innate and adaptive immune system are dose-dependent.

For example, alcohol has prominent dose-dependent effects on microglia, the innate immune cells of the central nervous system (CNS). In mouse models of acute alcohol abuse, cerebellar microglia display no inflammatory cytokine production following a single moderate-dose alcohol exposure of 3 g/kg and only a transient IL-1β/TNF-α increase following high-dose administration 5 g/kg.[64] At much higher alcohol doses of up to 10 g/kg/day, microglia display increased activation in association with the production of different inflammatory cytokines, including IL-1β, IL-18, IL-10, interferon-gamma (IFN-γ), transformative growth factor beta (TGF-β) and chemokines, CXCL2, CX3CL1. In turn, these cytokines and chemokines can lead to peripheral lymphocyte translocation across the blood–brain barrier (BBB) and further CNS inflammation.[65–68]

Alcohol also modulates the adaptive immune system in a dose-dependent manner. Chronic moderate alcohol consumption leads to T and B cell activation and proliferation,[69] while chronic heavy consumption is associated with T and B cell depletion and apoptosis as well as an increase in immunoglobulins.[70] Additionally, chronic binge alcohol consumption changes T cell phenotypes leading to a decreased percentage of naive T lymphocytes and higher percentages of memory T-cells.[71,72] Conversely, moderate alcohol consumption has been linked to modulation of T follicular helper ($T_{FH}$) cells.[8]

Cytokines and inflammatory markers are also affected by alcohol in a dose-dependent manner. For instance, C-reactive protein (CRP) and interleukin 6 (IL-6) are elevated in human heavy drinkers but relatively reduced in moderate drinkers compared to nondrinkers.[73] CRP effects may also be sexually dimorphic, with some studies indicating that alcohol-induced CRP reduction is specific to women,[74] though other studies suggest that moderate consumption reduces CRP in a U-shaped pattern regardless of sex.[75]

### *Pro- and anti-inflammatory dose-dependent alcohol effects on the immune system in rheumatoid arthritis*

In RA, a J-shaped association has been noted with CRP levels, with patients consuming 1–7 drinks/week had the lowest CRP levels.[51] RA patients consuming moderate alcohol display a U-shaped association with IL-6 levels prior to symptom development and an inverse relationship between alcohol consumption and soluble tumor necrosis factor receptor 2 (TNFR2) levels.[76] As alcohol can contribute to liver damage, a study evaluating the relationship between alcohol consumption and liver inflammation reported that >21 units per week correlated with transaminitis, while <14 units per week did not.[48] Moderate alcohol consumption has also been associated with 50% reduction in RA risk in patients positive for anticitrullinated protein antibodies (ACPA), and a 30% disease risk reduction in ACPA-negative RA in an inverse dose–response relationship.[47]

Dose-dependent effects of alcohol on the immune system are also noted in RA mouse models. In a model of collagen-induced arthritis (CIA), mice on a moderate alcohol diet experienced a 40% lower incidence of CIA and >50% decrease in radiological disease severity compared to non-alcohol controls.[8] Alcohol-consuming mice also had lower levels of IL-21 and IL-17A, neutrophils, monocytes, plasma B cells and IgG levels.[8] The authors also found that both alcohol and acetate affected the functional state of T follicular helper ($T_{FH}$) cells in vitro and in vivo, leading to suppression of IL-21 secretion.[8] These findings are intriguing as $T_{FH}$ cells are often found in synovial joints in RA patients and are also important mediators of gut immunity, suggesting a possible link between immune processes in the gut and RA. In another CIA study, moderate alcohol (10% ethanol in water) delayed the onset and ameliorated the progression of CIA via an increase in endogenous testosterone, inhibition of nuclear factor B activation and down-regulation of leukocyte migration.[77]

## Alcohol's pro- and anti-inflammatory effects on the gut

The gut microbiome, composed of trillions of microorganisms, is increasingly considered to be one of the critical environmental factors in modulating the immune system and risk of autoimmune diseases. For example, fecal transplantation of gut bacteria from patients with SLE and MS to animal models can reproduce disease symptoms in animals.[78,79] Conversely, supplementation of a dysbiotic microbiome with diverse commensal species through fecal transplant has therapeutic benefits in IBS and MS.[80–82] Similarly, in animal studies, antibiotic ablation of the gut flora is sufficient to prevent EAE onset entirely, while the introduction of strains of Erysipelotrichaceae and *Lactobacillus reuteri* exacerbates EAE symptoms and increases autoreactive T-cells.[83] In an RA model in germ-free mice, the introduction of segmented filamentous bacteria (SFB) was sufficient for the development of arthritis via Th17 response.[84] Likewise, in non-germ-free RA mice, oral gavage of SFB drove the differentiation and migration of $T_{FH}$ cells systemically, leading to autoantibody generation and arthritis exacerbation.[85]

As alcohol is largely metabolized within the GI tract, it is a prime factor to impact gut microbiome composition, gut immune system and downstream systemic immune communications with other organs. In the following section, we will focus on alcohol's effects on the gut, gut immune system and gut metabolism of fatty acids and how these effects may translate into pro-inflammatory vs protective effects in autoimmune diseases.

### *Pro-inflammatory effects of high-dose alcohol on the gastrointestinal tract, gut microbiome, gut metabolites and nutrients*

Microbiome transfer from high-dose alcohol-fed mice to alcohol-naïve germ-free mice has been shown to induce intestinal inflammation in the recipient mice.[86] Potential explanations for how high-dose alcohol may induce gut inflammation include alteration of the gut microbiome (dysbiosis) in alcohol-metabolizing species, bacterial cytotoxicity, changes to enteric peristalsis and hepatotoxicity (liver steatosis and cirrhosis).[87–90] Microbiome dysbiosis can lead to impaired intestinal permeability and promote inflammation via systemic translocation of gut bacterial endotoxin, LPS, activation of TLR and nuclear factor-κB (NF-kB) on immune cells and induction of inflammatory iNOS[17,19,20.] In turn, hepatotoxicity interferes with the liver's ability to detoxify substances, which results in systemic accumulation of alcohol's toxic metabolite, acetaldehyde.[91] In addition, LPS-mediated activation of liver-resident macrophages, Kupffer cells, further contributes to pro-inflammatory cytokine release and propagation of systemic inflammation.[92]

There are also specific microbiota changes that have been described in animal and human high-dose alcohol studies (Table 2). In human alcohol use disorder (AUD) studies, dysbiosis has been characterized by lower Bacteroidetes,[89,93] lower *Akkermansia muciniphila*,[9412195] and higher Proteobacteria.[89] In animal models of high-dose alcohol consumption, alcohol-consuming animals have reduced bacterial diversity along with lower Bacteroidetes, elevated Proteobacter, elevated Actinobacter,[94] reduction in Firmicutes and elevation in Bacteroidetes.[96] However, not all studies have noted a reduction in Firmicutes in response to high-dose alcohol. For example, voluntary self-administration of chronic high-dose alcohol in macaques resulted in reduced Bacteroidetes, elevated Firmicutes and a complete absence of *Akkermansia muciniphila* during the drinking period, while abstinence from drinking restored baseline bacterial species.[90]

In addition to changes in microbiota, high-dose alcohol can also decrease immunomodulatory gut metabolites such as aryl hydrocarbon receptor (AhR).[97] AhR is a transcriptional factor expressed in immune cells and is known to impact T cell differentiation, effector and regulatory T cell functions. AhR aberrant expression has also been linked to autoimmune dysregulation.[98,99] As AhR ligand administration is beneficial in autoimmune diseases, lower levels of AhR due to chronic high-dose alcohol may potentially contribute to autoimmune disease exacerbation.

Lastly, chronic high-dose alcohol intake can cause malabsorption and nutrient deficiencies.[100] In turn, nutrient deficiencies for vitamins such as thiamine, cyanocobalamin and vitamin D can exacerbate different autoimmune conditions.[101]

### *Anti-inflammatory effects of low-to-moderate alcohol on the gut microbiome, gut metabolites and fatty acids*

An important way in which alcohol may beneficially impact autoimmune inflammation is via its effects on fatty acid metabolism in the gut. While at high doses alcohol is known to lead to fatty acid dysregulation and development of fatty liver disease,[102–104] at lower doses, alcohol may contribute to the generation of gut-derived anti-inflammatory fatty acids, such as short-chain fatty acids (SCFAs) and polyunsaturated fatty acids (PUFAs)[103,104] (Figure 1).

SCFAs, including formate, acetate, propionate and butyrate, are a class of carboxylic acids produced primarily through microbial fermentation of dietary fiber.[106] Importantly, SCFAs are known to have important anti-microbial and anti-inflammatory properties and to reduce inflammation in autoimmune diseases.[107,108] Oral supplementation of SCFA cocktail has been shown to be sufficient to reduce autoreactive Th1 and Th17 cell activity and to dampen disease severity in animal models of autoimmune colitis and EAE.[109,110]

There are potentially two ways in which low-to-moderate alcohol consumption can modulate SCFA production. First, low-to-moderate alcohol can alter SCFA-producing microbial communities in the gut, such as *Akkermansia muciniphila*.[111] Caslin, Maguire et al. showed that moderate alcohol consumption (2.6% ABV Lieber-DeCarli diet) increased levels of *Akkermansia muciniphila* in the gut in association with reducing disease severity in EAE.[11] Similarly, Lee et al. found that short-term alcohol consumption (5 days of 0.8 g/kg intragastric) elevated *Akkermansia muciniphila* levels in mice, an elevation not observed in groups consuming fermented rice liquor (FRL) of equivalent alcoholic strength.[112] In addition, alcohol itself is metabolized into the SCFA, acetate,[113] and animals fed a Lieber-DeCarli diet for 8 weeks show

Table 2. Alcohol induced gut microbiota alterations by dose and alcohol diet duration.

| Alcohol Model | Alcohol Model Details | Diet Duration | Subject Model | Microbiota | Reference |
|---|---|---|---|---|---|
| Chronic (Alcohol Liver Disease) | National Institute on Alcohol Abuse and Alcoholism, criteria for alcoholism (Men: >14 drinks/wk or >4 drinks/occasion Women: >7 drinks/wk or >3 drinks/occasion) | Alcohol consumption ≥10 yrs | Human | ↑ Proteobacteria<br>↑ Gammaproteobacteria<br>↑ Bacilli<br>↓ Clostridia<br>↓ Bacteriodetes<br>↓ Verrucomicrobiae | Mutlu et al., 2012 |
| Chronic (Alcohol Dependence (AD)) | Diagnostic and Statistical Manual of Mental Disorders IV criteria for AD | 19 days of rehab/alcohol abstinence in patients with AD | Human | ↑ Ruminococcaceae<br>↑ Bifidobacterium<br>↑ Lactobacillus<br>↓ Erysipelotrichaceae<br>↓ Holdemania | Leclercq et al., 2014 |
| Chronic (Alcohol Use Disorder (AUD)) | Less heavy drinkers (<10 drinks/d) vs high heavy drinkers (≥10 drinks/d) | 4 weeks of abstinence in patients with AUD | Human | Less Heavy Drinkers<br>↑ Erysipelotrichaceae<br>↑ Lachnospiraceae | Ames et al., 2020 |
| Chronic (Alcohol Dependence Syndrome (ADS)) | ICD-10 definition of alcohol dependence syndrome +/- liver cirrhosis | ADS: ≥8 years | Human | ↑ *Klebsiella*<br>↑ *Lactobacillus*<br>↑ *Bifidobacterium*<br>↓ *Prevotella,*<br>↓ *Faecalibacterium prausnitzii*<br>↓ *Acidaminococcus*<br>↓ *Clostridiales* | Dubinkina et al., 2017 |
| Chronic | 0.8-2.2 g/kg | 5 years | Macaque | ↑ Firmicutes: Streptococcaceae<br>↑ Firmicutes : Bacteriodes ratio | Zhang et al., 2019 |
| Chronic | 2.6% Lieber-DeCarli diet | 65 days | Mouse | ↑ *Turicibacter*<br>↑ *Akkermansia*<br>↑ *Prevotella*<br>↑ *Clostridium*<br>↑ *Verrucomirobia : Firmicute* | Caslin, Maguire et al., 2019 |
| Chronic | Vapor chamber 175 ± 25 mg/dL | 4 weeks | Mouse | ↑ Rikenellaceae<br>↑ Alistipes<br>↓ Clostridium IV<br>↓ Clostridium XiVb<br>↓ Dorea<br>↓ Coprococcus<br>↓ Propionibacterium | Peterson et al., 2017 |

elevated levels of acetic acid compared to controls.[114] Thus, low-to-moderate alcohol could impact SCFA balance both by influencing SCFA producing bacteria and via acetate production (Figure 1).

Another potential mechanism of low-to-moderate alcohol's protection in autoimmune diseases may rely on alcohol's important role in the metabolism of essential PUFAs, such as docosahexaenoic acid (DHA) and eicosapentaenoic acid (EPA).[103,105] These PUFAs can reduce reactive oxygen species formation and act as anti-inflammatory molecules. Low-to-moderate dose alcohol has been shown to increase PUFA production,[115] while at high alcohol doses, PUFA concentration decreases due to increased fatty acid catabolism.[103] Of note, PUFAs and PUFA derivatives, such as resolvins, lipoxins and protection, have been linked to the mitigation of autoimmune diseases.[116,117] In addition, an increase in PUFAs has also been shown to be cardioprotective in multiple studies.[118–120] As cardiovascular health is becoming an important factor in autoimmune disease outcomes, it is possible that this may be another protective mechanism mediated by low-to-moderate alcohol (Figure 1).

### *Protective effects of low-moderate alcohol on the gut microbiome in models of multiple sclerosis*

In an animal model of MS, EAE, Caslin, Maguire et al. administered a 2.6% moderate alcohol or isocaloric diet to both male and female C57BL/6 J mice and observed that males on the diet exhibited a greater long-term disease remission while females initially experienced remission and a subsequent disease exacerbation.[11] In this study, a moderate alcohol diet resulted in sex-specific gut microbiota alterations in individual immunoregulatory taxa, such as *Turicibacter, Akkermansia* and *Prevotella*, and also led to significant enrichment in beneficial Clostridial and Firmicute networks of bacteria.[11] Another study evaluating a moderate alcohol model of 10% (vol/vol) in EAE also documented EAE amelioration in alcohol-consuming C57BL/6 J mice and implicated gut-related $T_{FH}$ cells mechanistically.[8]

## Conclusions and future directions

Overall, current evidence points to a dose-dependent association between alcohol and disease severity in multiple autoimmune diseases, including autoimmune thyroid disease, diabetes, SLE, RA and MS. At low-to-moderate doses, alcohol appears to have protective effects, while at higher consumption patterns, alcohol can be addictive and can contribute to detrimental symptomatic effects on the host and worse autoimmune disease outcomes.

Though the exact mechanism by which low-to-moderate alcohol mediates autoimmune disease amelioration remains to be fully understood, emerging mechanistic studies suggest that low-to-moderate alcohol likely has both a systemic immunomodulatory role, such as shifting the balance of anti-inflammatory innate and adaptive immune cells and cytokines/chemokines, as well as a role in sculpting the composition of the gut microbiome and their fatty acid metabolites, such as SCFAs and PUFAs.

Future prospective patient studies that account for sex, age, cultural and socioeconomic background, alcohol type, timing of administration and mechanistic animal model studies on the gut microbiome and the immune system will be critical to better understand alcohol's role in autoimmune diseases. In turn, this knowledge will help guide the creation of specific clinical recommendations on alcohol consumption in patients with autoimmune diseases as well as help identify protective immune and gut-derived biomarkers that could be used in the treatment of autoimmune diseases independently of alcohol.

## Acknowledgments

We are grateful to Dr R. Adron Harris, Dr William Schwartz and Cole Maguire for their advice and support in preparing this review. Figure 1 was created with Biorender.com.

## Disclosure statement

The authors report no conflict of interest.

## Funding

This work was supported by Dell Medical School start-up funding to EM, and NIAAA funding under grants T32AA007471 to BC and K08 1K08AA027837-01A1 to EM.

## ORCID

Blaine Caslin http://orcid.org/0000-0002-4658-2945
Esther Melamed http://orcid.org/0000-0001-5571-3591

## Contributions

BC, KM, ST and EM wrote the first draft of the paper. ST and KM made the first draft of the tables. EM edited the manuscript, created the figure and final tables.

## References


1. Roberts MH, Erdei E. Comparative United States autoimmune disease rates for 2010-2016 by sex, geographic region, and race. Autoimmun Rev. 2020;19(1):102423. doi:10.1016/j.autrev.2019.102423.
2. Ngo ST, Steyn FJ, McCombe PA. Gender differences in autoimmune disease. Front Neuroendocrinol. 2014;35:347–369.
3. Ceccarelli F, Agmon-Levin N, Perricone C. Genetic factors of autoimmune diseases 2017. J Immunol Res. 2017;2017:2789242. doi:10.1155/2017/2789242.
4. Costenbader KH, Gay S, Alarcon-Riquelme ME, Iaccarino L, Doria A. Genes, epigenetic regulation and environmental factors: which is the most relevant in developing autoimmune diseases? Autoimmun Rev. 2012;11:604–609. doi:10.1016/j.autrev.2011.10.022.
5. Yamamoto EA, Jørgensen TN. Relationships between vitamin D, gut microbiome, and systemic autoimmunity. Front Immunol. 2020;10:3141. doi:10.3389/fimmu.2019.03141.
6. Hills RD, Pontefract BA, Mishcon HR, Black CA, Sutton SC, Theberge CR. Gut microbiome: profound implications for diet and disease. Nutrients. 2019;11:1613. doi:10.3390/nu11071613.
7. Bishehsari F, Magno E, Swanson G, Desai V, Voigt RM, Forsyth CB, Keshavarzian A. Alcohol and gut-derived inflammation. Alcohol Res. 2017;38:163–171.
8. Azizov V, Dietel K, Steffen F, Dürholz K, Meidenbauer J, Lucas S, Frech M, Omata Y, Tajik N, Knipfer L, et al. Ethanol consumption inhibits TFH cell responses and the development of autoimmune

arthritis. Nat Commun. 2020;11:1998. doi:10.1038/s41467-020-15855-z.
9. Barbhaiya M, Lu B, Sparks JA, Malspeis S, Chang S-C, Karlson EW, Costenbader KH. Influence of alcohol consumption on the risk of systemic lupus erythematosus among women in the nurses' health study cohorts. Arthritis Care Res (Hoboken). 2017;69:384–392. doi:10.1002/acr.22945.
10. Carle A, Pedersen IB, Knudsen N, Perrild H, Ovesen L, Rasmussen LB, Jørgensen T, Laurberg P. Moderate alcohol consumption may protect against overt autoimmune hypothyroidism: a population-based case-control study. Eur J Endocrinol. 2012;167(4):483–490. doi:10.1530/EJE-12-0356.
11. Caslin B, Maguire C, Karmakar A, Mohler K, Wylie D, Melamed E. Alcohol shifts gut microbial networks and ameliorates a murine model of neuroinflammation in a sex-specific pattern. Proc Natl Acad Sci U S A. 2019;116:25808–25815. doi:10.1073/pnas.1912359116.
12. HedströmAK,HillertJ,OlssonT,AlfredssonL. Alcoholasamodifiablelifestylefactoraffectingmultiplesclerosisrisk.JAMANeurol.2014;71:300–305. doi:10.1001/jamaneurol.2013.5858.
13. Kiyohara C, Washio M, Horiuchi T, Asami T, Ide S, Atsumi T, Kobashi G, Tada Y, Takahashi H. Cigarette smoking, alcohol consumption, and risk of systemic lupus erythematosus: a case-control study in a Japanese population. J Rheumatol. 2012;39:1363–1370. doi:10.3899/jrheum.111609.
14. Lu B, Solomon DH, Costenbader KH, Karlson EW. Alcohol consumption and risk of incident rheumatoid arthritis in women: a prospective study. Arthritis Rheumatol. 2014;66:1998–2005. doi:10.1002/art.38634.
15. Rasouli B, Ahlbom A, Andersson T, Grill V, Midthjell K, Olsson L, Carlsson S. Alcohol consumption is associated with reduced risk of type 2 diabetes and autoimmune diabetes in adults: results from the Nord-Trondelag health study. Diabet Med. 2013;30:56–64. doi:10.1111/j.1464-5491.2012.03713.x.
16. Cederbaum AI. Alcohol metabolism. Clin Liver Dis. 2012;16:667–685. doi:10.1016/j.cld.2012.08.002.
17. Lawrimore CJ, Crews FT. Ethanol, TLR3, and TLR4 agonists have unique innate immune responses in neuron-like SH-SY5Y and microglia-like BV2. Alcohol Clin Exp Res. 2017;41:939–954. doi:10.1111/acer.13368.
18. Iracheta-Vellve A, Petrasek J, Gyogyosi B, Bala S, Csak T, Kodys K, Szabo G. Interleukin-1 inhibition facilitates recovery from liver injury and promotes regeneration of hepatocytes in alcoholic hepatitis in mice. Liver Int. 2017;37:968–973. doi:10.1111/liv.13430.
19. Wang H, Khor TO, Saw CL, Lin W, Wu T, Huang Y, Kong ANT. Role of Nrf2 in suppressing LPS-induced inflammation in mouse peritoneal macrophages by polyunsaturated fatty acids docosahexaenoic acid and eicosapentaenoic acid. Mol Pharm. 2010;7:2185–2193. doi:10.1021/mp100199m.
20. Keshavarzian A, Farhadi A, Forsyth CB, Rangan J, Jakate S, Shaikh M, Banan A, Fields JZ. Evidence that chronic alcohol exposure promotes intestinal oxidative stress, intestinal hyperpermeability and endotoxemia prior to development of alcoholic steatohepatitis in rats. J Hepatol. 2009;50:538–547. doi:10.1016/j.jhep.2008.10.028.
21. Lien E, Means TK, Heine H, Yoshimura A, Kusumoto S, Fukase K, Fenton MJ, Oikawa M, Qureshi N, Monks B, et al. Toll-like receptor 4 imparts ligand-specific recognition of bacterial lipopolysaccharide. J Clin Invest. 2000;105:497–504. doi:10.1172/JCI8541.
22. Rolland B, Chazeron I, Carpentier F, Moustafa F, Viallon A, Jacob X, Lesage P, Ragonnet D, Genty A, Geneste J, et al. Comparison between the WHO and NIAAA criteria for binge drinking on drinking features and alcohol-related aftermaths: results from a cross-sectional study among eight emergency wards in France. Drug Alcohol Depend. 2017;175:92–98. doi:10.1016/j.drugalcdep.2017.01.034.
23. Holmes RS, Duley JA, Algar EM, Mather PB, Rout UK. Biochemical and genetic studies on enzymes of alcohol metabolism: the mouse as a model organism for human studies. Alcohol Alcohol. 1986;21:41–56.
24. Leeman RF, Heilig M, Cunningham CL, Stephens DN, Duka T, O'Malley SS. Ethanol consumption: how should we measure it? Achieving consilience between human and animal phenotypes. Addict Biol. 2010;15:109–124. doi:10.1111/j.1369-1600.2009.00192.x.
25. Bjork JM, Gilman JM. The effects of acute alcohol administration on the human brain: insights from neuroimaging. Neuropharmacology. 2014;84:101–110. doi:10.1016/j.neuropharm.2013.07.039.
26. Kanuri G, Wagnerberger S, Landmann M, Prigl E, Hellerbrand C, Bischoff SC, Bergheim I. Effect of acute beer ingestion on the liver: studies in female mice. Eur J Nutr. 2015;54:465–474. doi:10.1007/s00394-014-0730-z.
27. Pruett S, Tan W, Howell GE 3rd, Nanduri B. Dosage scaling of alcohol in binge exposure models in mice: an empirical assessment of the relationship between dose, alcohol exposure, and peak blood concentrations in humans and mice. Alcohol. 2020;89:9–17. doi:10.1016/j.alcohol.2020.03.011.
28. Bendtsen P, Gronbaek M, Kjaer SK, Munk C, Linneberg A, Tolstrup JS. Alcohol consumption and the risk of self-reported perennial and seasonal allergic rhinitis in young adult women in a population-based cohort study. Clin Exp Allergy. 2008;38:1179–1185. doi:10.1111/j.1365-2222.2008.02945.x.
29. Hsu TY, He GY, Wang YC, Chen C-Y, Wang S-H, Chen W-K, Kao C-H. Alcohol use disorder increases the risk of irritable bowel disease: a nationwide retrospective cohort study. Medicine (Baltimore). 2015;94:e2334. doi:10.1097/MD.0000000000002334.

30. Carlsson S, Hammar N, Grill V. Alcohol consumption and type 2 diabetes meta-analysis of epidemiological studies indicates a U-shaped relationship. Diabetologia. 2005;48:1051–1054. doi:10.1007/s00125-005-1768-5.
31. Joosten MM, Chiuve SE, Mukamal KJ, Hu FB, Hendriks HF, Rimm EB. Changes in alcohol consumption and subsequent risk of type 2 diabetes in men. Diabetes. 2011;60:74–79. doi:10.2337/db10-1052.
32. Kerr WC, Williams E, Li L, Lui CK, Ye Y, Greenfield TK, Lown EA. Alcohol use patterns and risk of diabetes onset in the 1979 National Longitudinal Survey of Youth Cohort. Prev Med. 2018;109:22–27. doi:10.1016/j.ypmed.2018.01.010.
33. Li XH, Yu FF, Zhou YH, He J. Association between alcohol consumption and the risk of incident type 2 diabetes: a systematic review and dose-response meta-analysis. Am J Clin Nutr. 2016;103:818–829. doi:10.3945/ajcn.115.114389.
34. Rasouli B, Andersson T, Carlsson PO, Dorkhan M, Grill V, Groop L, Martinell M, Tuomi T, Carlsson S. Alcohol and the risk for latent autoimmune diabetes in adults: results based on Swedish ESTRID study. Eur J Endocrinol. 2014;171:535–543. doi:10.1530/EJE-14-0403.
35. Carle A, Bulow Pedersen I, Knudsen N, Perrild H, Ovesen L, Rasmussen LB, Jørgensen T, Laurberg P. Graves' hyperthyroidism and moderate alcohol consumption: evidence for disease prevention. Clin Endocrinol (Oxf). 2013;79:111–119. doi:10.1111/cen.12106.
36. Effraimidis G, Tijssen JG, Wiersinga WM. Alcohol consumption as a risk factor for autoimmune thyroid disease: a prospective study. Eur Thyroid J. 2012;1:99–104. doi:10.1159/000338920.
37. Huang Y, Cai L, Zheng Y, Pan J, Li L, Zong L, Lin W, Liang J, Huang H, Wen J, et al. Association between lifestyle and thyroid dysfunction: a cross-sectional epidemiologic study in the She ethnic minority group of Fujian Province in China. BMC Endocr Disord. 2019;19:83. doi:10.1186/s12902-019-0414-z.
38. Hardy CJ, Palmer BP, Muir KR, Sutton AJ, Powell RJ. Smoking history, alcohol consumption, and systemic lupus erythematosus: a case-control study. Ann Rheum Dis. 1998;57:451–455. doi:10.1136/ard.57.8.451.
39. Bengtsson AA, Rylander L, Hagmar L, Nived O, Sturfelt G. Risk factors for developing systemic lupus erythematosus: a case-control study in southern Sweden. Rheumatology (Oxford). 2002;41:563–571. doi:10.1093/rheumatology/41.5.563.
40. Wang J, Pan HF, Ye DQ, Su H, Li XP. Moderate alcohol drinking might be protective for systemic lupus erythematosus: a systematic review and meta-analysis. Clin Rheumatol. 2008;27:1557–1563. doi:10.1007/s10067-008-1004-z.
41. Cozier YC, Barbhaiya M, Castro-Webb N, Conte C, Tedeschi S, Leatherwood C, Costenbader KH, Rosenberg L. A prospective study of obesity and risk of systemic lupus erythematosus (SLE) among Black women. Semin Arthritis Rheum. 2019;48(6):1030–1034. doi:10.1016/j.semarthrit.2018.10.004.
42. Hahn J, Leatherwood C, Malspeis S, Liu X, Lu B, Roberts AL, Sparks JA, Karlson EW, Feldman CH, Munroe ME, et al. Associations between daily alcohol consumption and systemic lupus erythematosus-related cytokines and chemokines among US female nurses without SLE. Lupus. 2020;29:976–982. doi:10.1177/0961203320929427.
43. Formica MK, Palmer JR, Rosenberg L, McAlindon TE. Smoking, alcohol consumption, and risk of systemic lupus erythematosus in the Black women's health study. J Rheumatol. 2003;30:1222–1226.
44. Kim SK, Lee SS, Choe JY, Park SH, Lee H. Effect of alcohol consumption and smoking on disease damage in systemic lupus erythematosus: data from the Korean Lupus Network (KORNET) registry. Lupus. 2017;26:1540–1549. doi:10.1177/0961203317709346.
45. Baker JF, England BR, Mikuls TR, Hsu JY, George MD, Pedro S, Sayles H, Michaud K. Changes in alcohol use and associations with disease activity, health status, and mortality in rheumatoid arthritis. Arthritis Care Res (Hoboken). 2020;72:301–308. doi:10.1002/acr.23847.
46. Bergman S, Symeonidou S, Andersson ML, Soderlin MK, Group B. Alcohol consumption is associated with lower self-reported disease activity and better health-related quality of life in female rheumatoid arthritis patients in Sweden: data from BARFOT, a multicenter study on early RA. BMC Musculoskelet Disord. 2013;14:218. doi:10.1186/1471-2474-14-218.
47. Hedstrom AK, Hossjer O, Klareskog L, Alfredsson L. Interplay between alcohol, smoking and HLA genes in RA aetiology. RMD Open. 2019;5:e000893. doi:10.1136/rmdopen-2019-000893.
48. Humphreys JH, Warner A, Costello R, Lunt M, Verstappen SMM, Dixon WG. Quantifying the hepatotoxic risk of alcohol consumption in patients with rheumatoid arthritis taking methotrexate. Ann Rheum Dis. 2017;76:1509–1514. doi:10.1136/annrheumdis-2016-210629.
49. Jin Z, Xiang C, Cai Q, Wei X, He J. Alcohol consumption as a preventive factor for developing rheumatoid arthritis: a dose-response meta-analysis of prospective studies. Ann Rheum Dis. 2014;73:1962–1967. doi:10.1136/annrheumdis-2013-203323.
50. Kallberg H, Jacobsen S, Bengtsson C, Pedersen M, Padyukov L, Garred P, Frisch M, Karlson EW, Klareskog L, Alfredsson L, et al. Alcohol consumption is associated with decreased risk of rheumatoid arthritis: results from two Scandinavian case-control studies. Ann Rheum Dis. 2009;68:222–227. doi:10.1136/ard.2007.086314.

51. Mangnus L, Van Steenbergen HW, Nieuwenhuis WP, Reijnierse M, Van Der Helm-van Mil AHM. Moderate use of alcohol is associated with lower levels of C reactive protein but not with less severe joint inflammation: a cross-sectional study in early RA and healthy volunteers. RMD Open. 2018;4:e000577. doi:10.1136/rmdopen-2017-000577.
52. Maxwell JR, Gowers IR, Moore DJ, Wilson AG. Alcohol consumption is inversely associated with risk and severity of rheumatoid arthritis. Rheumatology (Oxford). 2010;49:2140–2146. doi:10.1093/rheumatology/keq202.
53. Sageloli F, Quesada JL, Fautrel B, Salliot C, Gaudin P, Baillet A. Moderate alcohol consumption is associated with increased radiological progression in women, but not in men, with early rheumatoid arthritis: results from the ESPOIR cohort (Etude et Suivi des Polyarthrites Indifferenciees Recentes). Scand J Rheumatol. 2018;47:440–446. doi:10.1080/03009742.2018.1437216.
54. Scott IC, Tan R, Stahl D, Steer S, Lewis CM, Cope AP. The protective effect of alcohol on developing rheumatoid arthritis: a systematic review and meta-analysis. Rheumatology (Oxford). 2013;52:856–867. doi:10.1093/rheumatology/kes376.
55. Lu B, Rho YH, Cui J, Iannaccone CK, Frits ML, Karlson EW, Shadick NA. Associations of smoking and alcohol consumption with disease activity and functional status in rheumatoid arthritis. J Rheumatol. 2014;41:24–30. doi:10.3899/jrheum.130074.
56. Andersen C, Sondergaard HB, Bang Oturai D, Laursen JH, Gustavsen S, Larsen NK, Magyari M, Just-Østergaard E, Thørner LW, Sellebjerg F, et al. Alcohol consumption in adolescence is associated with a lower risk of multiple sclerosis in a Danish cohort. Mult Scler. 2019;25:1572–1579. doi:10.1177/1352458518795418.
57. Diaz-Cruz C, Chua AS, Malik MT, Kaplan T, Glanz BI, Egorova S, Guttmann CRG, Bakshi R, Weiner HL, Healy BC, et al. The effect of alcohol and red wine consumption on clinical and MRI outcomes in multiple sclerosis. Mult Scler Relat Disord. 2017;17:47–53. doi:10.1016/j.msard.2017.06.011.
58. Gili-Miner M, Lopez-Mendez J, Vilches-Arenas A, Ramírez-Ramírez G, Franco-Fernández D, Sala-Turrens J, Béjar-Prado L. Multiple sclerosis and alcohol use disorders: in-hospital mortality, extended hospital stays, and overexpenditures. Neurologia. 2016. doi:10.1016/j.nrl.2016.07.008.
59. Pakpoor J, Goldacre R, Disanto G, Giovannoni G, Goldacre MJ. Alcohol misuse disorders and multiple sclerosis risk. JAMA Neurol. 2014;71:1188–1189. doi:10.1001/jamaneurol.2014.1795.
60. Massa J, O'Reilly EJ, Munger KL, Ascherio A. Caffeine and alcohol intakes have no association with risk of multiple sclerosis. Multiple Sclerosis. 2013;19:53–58. doi:10.1177/1352458512448108.
61. Gurung P, Young BM, Coleman RA, Wiechert S, Turner LE, Ray NB, Waldschmidt TJ, Legge KL, Cook RT. Chronic ethanol induces inhibition of antigen specific CD8+ but not CD4+ immunodominant T cell responses following *Listeria monocytogenes* inoculation. J Leukoc Biol. 2009;85:34–43. doi:10.1189/jlb.0208101.
62. Meyerholz DK, Edsen-Moore M, McGill J, Coleman RA, Cook RT, Legge KL. Chronic alcohol consumption increases the severity of murine influenza virus infections. J Immunol. 2008;181:641–648. doi:10.4049/jimmunol.181.1.641.
63. Mason CM, Dobard E, Zhang P, Nelson S. Alcohol exacerbates murine pulmonary tuberculosis. Infect Immun. 2004;72:2556–2563. doi:10.1128/IAI.72.5.2556-2563.2004.
64. Ahlers KE, Karacay B, Fuller L, Bonthius DJ, Dailey ME. Transient activation of microglia following acute alcohol exposure in developing mouse neocortex is primarily driven by BAX-dependent neurodegeneration. Glia. 2015;63:1694–1713. doi:10.1002/glia.22835.
65. Alfonso-Loeches S, Urena-Peralta J, Morillo-Bargues MJ, Gomez-Pinedo U, Guerri C. Ethanol-induced TLR4/NLRP3 neuroinflammatory response in microglial cells promotes leukocyte infiltration across the BBB. Neurochem Res. 2016;41:193–209. doi:10.1007/s11064-015-1760-5.
66. Warden AS, Azzam M, DaCosta A, Mason S, Blednov YA, Messing RO, Mayfield RD, Harris RA. Toll-like receptor 3 activation increases voluntary alcohol intake in C57BL/6J male mice. Brain Behav Immun. 2019;77:55–65. doi:10.1016/j.bbi.2018.12.004.
67. Warden AS, Wolfe SA, Khom S, Varodayan FP, Patel RR, Steinman MQ, Bajo M, Montgomery SE, Vlkolinsky R, Nadav T, et al. Microglia control escalation of drinking in alcohol-dependent mice: genomic and synaptic drivers. Biol Psychiatry. 2020;88:910–921. doi:10.1016/j.biopsych.2020.05.011.
68. Marshall SA, Geil CR, Nixon K. Prior binge ethanol exposure potentiates the microglial response in a model of alcohol-induced neurodegeneration. Brain Sci. 2016;6:6. doi:10.3390/brainsci6020016.
69. Romeo J, Warnberg J, Nova E, Diaz LE, Gomez-Martinez S, Marcos A. Moderate alcohol consumption and the immune system: a review. Br J Nutr. 2007;98 (Suppl 1):S111–115. doi:10.1017/S0007114507838049.
70. Slukvin II, Jerrells TR. Different pathways of in vitro ethanol-induced apoptosis in thymocytes and splenic T and B lymphocytes. Immunopharmacology. 1995;31:43–57. doi:10.1016/0162-3109(95)00032-4.
71. Appay V, Sauce D. Naive T cells: the crux of cellular immune aging?Exp Gerontol. 2014;54:90–93. doi:10.1016/j.exger.2014.01.003.
72. Zhang H, Meadows GG. Chronic alcohol consumption in mice increases the proportion of peripheral memory T cells by homeostatic proliferation. J Leukoc Biol. 2005;78:1070–1080. doi:10.1189/jlb.0605317.
73. Volpato S, Pahor M, Ferrucci L, Simonsick EM, Guralnik JM, Kritchevsky SB, Fellin R, Harris TB. Relationship of alcohol intake with inflammatory markers and plasminogen activator inhibitor-1 in

well-functioning older adults: the health, aging, and body composition study. Circulation. 2004;109:607–612. doi:10.1161/01.CIR.0000109503.13955.00.

74. Oliveira A, Rodriguez-Artalejo F, Lopes C. Alcohol intake and systemic markers of inflammation–shape of the association according to sex and body mass index. Alcohol Alcohol. 2010;45:119–125. doi:10.1093/alcalc/agp092.
75. Imhof A, Froehlich M, Brenner H, Boeing H, Pepys MB, Koenig W. Effect of alcohol consumption on systemic markers of inflammation. Lancet. 2001;357:763–767. doi:10.1016/S0140-6736(00)04170-2.
76. Lu B, Solomon DH, Costenbader KH, Keenan BT, Chibnik LB, Karlson EW. Alcohol consumption and markers of inflammation in women with preclinical rheumatoid arthritis. Arthritis Rheum. 2010;62:3554–3559. doi:10.1002/art.27739.
77. Jonsson IM, Verdrengh M, Brisslert M, Lindblad S, Bokarewa M, Islander U, Carlsten H, Ohlsson C, Nandakumar KS, Holmdahl R, et al. Ethanol prevents development of destructive arthritis. Proc Natl Acad Sci U S A. 2007;104:258–263. doi:10.1073/pnas.0608620104.
78. Ma Y, Xu X, Li M, Cai J, Wei Q, Niu H. Gut microbiota promote the inflammatory response in the pathogenesis of systemic lupus erythematosus. Mol Med. 2019;25:35. doi:10.1186/s10020-019-0102-5.
79. Berer K, Gerdes LA, Cekanaviciute E, Jia X, Xiao L, Xia Z, Liu C, Klotz L, Stauffer U, Baranzini SE, et al. Gut microbiota from multiple sclerosis patients enables spontaneous autoimmune encephalomyelitis in mice. Proc Natl Acad Sci U S A. 2017;114:10719–10724. doi:10.1073/pnas.1711233114.
80. Meighani A, Hart BR, Bourgi K, Miller N, John A, Ramesh M. Outcomes of fecal microbiota transplantation for *Clostridium difficile* infection in patients with inflammatory bowel disease. Dig Dis Sci. 2017;62:2870–2875. doi:10.1007/s10620-017-4580-4.
81. Li K, Wei S, Hu L, Yin X, Mai Y, Jiang C, Peng X, Cao X, Huang Z, Zhou H, et al. Protection of fecal microbiota transplantation in a mouse model of multiple sclerosis. Mediators Inflamm. 2020;2020:2058272. doi:10.1155/2020/2058272.
82. Makkawi S, Camara-Lemarroy C, Metz L. Fecal microbiota transplantation associated with 10 years of stability in a patient with SPMS. Neurol Neuroimmunol Neuroinflamm. 2018;5:e459. doi:10.1212/NXI.0000000000000459.
83. Miyauchi E, Kim SW, Suda W, Kawasumi M, Onawa S, Taguchi-Atarashi N, Morita H, Taylor TD, Hattori M, Ohno H, et al. Gut microorganisms act together to exacerbate inflammation in spinal cords. Nature. 2020;585:102–106. doi:10.1038/s41586-020-2634-9.
84. Wu YY, Hsu JL, Wang HC, Wu SJ, Hong CJ, Cheng IH. Alterations of the neuroinflammatory markers IL-6 and TRAIL in Alzheimer's disease. Dement Geriatr Cogn Dis Extra. 2015;5:424–434. doi:10.1159/000439214.
85. Teng F, Klinger CN, Felix KM, Bradley C, Wu E, Tran N, Umesaki Y, Wu H-J. Gut microbiota drive autoimmune arthritis by promoting differentiation and migration of Peyer's patch T follicular helper cells. Immunity. 2016;44:875–888. doi:10.1016/j.immuni.2016.03.013.
86. Canesso MCC, Lacerda NL, Ferreira CM, Jl G, D A, C G, G C, Sh P, C M, Fs M, et al. Comparing the effects of acute alcohol consumption in germ-free and conventional mice: the role of the gut microbiota. BMC Microbiol. 2014;14:240. doi:10.1186/s12866-014-0240-4.
87. Bode JC, Bode C, Heidelbach R, Durr HK, Martini GA. Jejunal microflora in patients with chronic alcohol abuse. Hepatogastroenterology. 1984;31:30–34.
88. Chang CS, Chen GH, Lien HC, Yeh HZ. Small intestine dysmotility and bacterial overgrowth in cirrhotic patients with spontaneous bacterial peritonitis. Hepatology. 1998;28:1187–1190. doi:10.1002/hep.510280504.
89. Mutlu EA, Gillevet PM, Rangwala H, Sikaroodi M, Naqvi A, Engen PA, Kwasny M, Lau CK, Keshavarzian A. Colonic microbiome is altered in alcoholism. Am J Physiol Gastrointest Liver Physiol. 2012;302:G966–978. doi:10.1152/ajpgi.00380.2011.
90. Zhang X, Yasuda K, Gilmore RA, Westmoreland SV, Platt DM, Miller GM, Vallender EJ. Alcohol-induced changes in the gut microbiome and metabolome of rhesus macaques. Psychopharmacology (Berl). 2019;236:1531–1544. doi:10.1007/s00213-019-05217-z.
91. Tuma DJ. Role of malondialdehyde-acetaldehyde adducts in liver injury. Free Radic Biol Med. 2002;32:303–308. doi:10.1016/S0891-5849(01)00742-0.
92. Zeng T, Zhang CL, Xiao M, Yang R, Xie KQ. Critical roles of Kupffer cells in the pathogenesis of alcoholic liver disease: from basic science to clinical trials. Front Immunol. 2016;7:538. doi:10.3389/fimmu.2016.00538.
93. Puri P, Liangpunsakul S, Christensen JE, Shah VH, Kamath PS, Gores GJ, Walker S, Comerford M, Katz B, Borst A, et al. The circulating microbiome signature and inferred functional metagenomics in alcoholic hepatitis. Hepatology. 2018;67:1284–1302. doi:10.1002/hep.29623.
94. Dubinkina VB, Tyakht AV, Odintsova VY, Yarygin KS, Kovarsky BA, Pavlenko AV, Ischenko DS, Popenko AS, Alexeev DG, Taraskina AY, et al. Links of gut microbiota composition with alcohol dependence syndrome and alcoholic liver disease. Microbiome. 2017;5:141. doi:10.1186/s40168-017-0359-2.
95. Bull-Otterson L, Feng W, Kirpich I, Wang Y, Qin X, Liu Y, Gobejishvili L, Joshi-Barve S, Ayvaz T, Petrosino J, et al. Metagenomic analyses of alcohol induced pathogenic alterations in the intestinal microbiome and the effect of *Lactobacillus rhamnosus* GG treatment. PLoS One. 2013;8:e53028. doi:10.1371/journal.pone.0053028.
96. Yan AW, Schnabl B. Bacterial translocation and changes in the intestinal microbiome associated with alcoholic liver disease. World J Hepatol. 2012;4:110–118. doi:10.4254/wjh.v4.i4.110.

97. Zhang HF, Lin XH, Yang H, Zhou LC, Guo YL, Barnett JV, Guo ZM. Regulation of the activity and expression of aryl hydrocarbon receptor by ethanol in mouse hepatic stellate cells. Alcohol Clin Exp Res. 2012;36:1873–1881. doi:10.1111/j.1530-0277.2012.01787.x.
98. Quintana FJ, Basso AS, Iglesias AH, Korn T, Farez MF, Bettelli E, Caccamo M, Oukka M, Weiner HL. Control of T reg and TH 17 cell differentiation by the aryl hydrocarbon receptor. Nature. 2008;453:65–71. doi:10.1038/nature06880.
99. Veldhoen M, Hirota K, Westendorf AM, Buer J, Dumoutier L, Renauld J-C, Stockinger B. The aryl hydrocarbon receptor links TH 17-cell-mediated autoimmunity to environmental toxins. Nature. 2008;453:106–109. doi:10.1038/nature06881.
100. Barr TM. Impact of alcohol on intestinal homeostasis: UC Riverside, 2018.
101. Ogunsakin O, Hottor T, Mehta A, Lichtveld M, McCaskill M. Chronic ethanol exposure effects on vitamin D levels among subjects with alcohol use disorder. Environ Health Insights. 2016;10(EHI):S40335. doi:10.4137/EHI.S40335.
102. Mann RE, Smart RG, Govoni R. The epidemiology of alcoholic liver disease. Alcohol Res Health. 2003;27:209.
103. Pawlosky RJ, Salem N Jr. Perspectives on alcohol consumption: liver polyunsaturated fatty acids and essential fatty acid metabolism. Alcohol. 2004;34:27–33. doi:10.1016/j.alcohol.2004.07.009.
104. Bjørkhaug ST, Aanes H, Neupane SP, Bramness JG, Malvik S, Henriksen C, Skar V, Medhus AW, Valeur J. Characterization of gut microbiota composition and functions in patients with chronic alcohol overconsumption. Gut Microbes. 2019;10:663–675. doi:10.1080/19490976.2019.1580097.
105. De Lorgeril M, Salen P, Martin J-L, Boucher F, De Leiris J. Interactions of wine drinking with omega-3 fatty acids in patients with coronary heart disease: a fish-like effect of moderate wine drinking. Am Heart J. 2008;155:175–181. doi:10.1016/j.ahj.2007.08.009.
106. Flint HJ, Duncan SH, Scott KP, Louis P. Links between diet, gut microbiota composition and gut metabolism. Proc Nutr Soc. 2015;74:13–22. doi:10.1017/S0029665114001463.
107. Correa-Oliveira R, Fachi JL, Vieira A, Sato FT, Vinolo MA. Regulation of immune cell function by short-chain fatty acids. Clin Transl Immunol. 2016;5:e73. doi:10.1038/cti.2016.17.
108. Parada Venegas D, De La Fuente MK, Landskron G, González MJ, Quera R, Dijkstra G, Harmsen HJM, Faber KN, Hermoso MA. Short chain fatty acids (SCFAs)-mediated gut epithelial and immune regulation and its relevance for inflammatory bowel diseases. Front Immunol. 2019;10:277. doi:10.3389/fimmu.2019.00277.
109. Luu M, Visekruna A. Short-chain fatty acids: bacterial messengers modulating the immunometabolism of T cells. Eur J Immunol. 2019;49:842–848. doi:10.1002/eji.201848009.
110. Mizuno M, Noto D, Kaga N, Chiba A, Miyake S, Ashour HM. The dual role of short fatty acid chains in the pathogenesis of autoimmune disease models. PLoS One. 2017;12:e0173032. doi:10.1371/journal.pone.0173032.
111. Morrison DJ, Preston T. Formation of short chain fatty acids by the gut microbiota and their impact on human metabolism. Gut Microbes. 2016;7:189–200. doi:10.1080/19490976.2015.1134082.
112. Lee JE, Ha JS, Park HY, Lee E. Alteration of gut microbiota composition by short-term low-dose alcohol intake is restored by fermented rice liquor in mice. Food Res Int. 2020;128:108800. doi:10.1016/j.foodres.2019.108800.
113. Edenberg HJ. The genetics of alcohol metabolism: role of alcohol dehydrogenase and aldehyde dehydrogenase variants. Alcohol Res Health. 2007;30:5–13.
114. Xie G, Zhong W, Li H, Li Q, Qiu Y, Zheng X, Chen H, Zhao X, Zhang S, Zhou Z, et al. Alteration of bile acid metabolism in the rat induced by chronic ethanol consumption. FASEB J. 2013;27:3583–3593. doi:10.1096/fj.13-231860.
115. Denkins Y, Woods J, Whitty J, Hannigan JH, Martier SS, Sokol RJ, Salem N. Highly unsaturated fatty acids in nutrition and disease prevention-maternal nutrition-effects of gestational alcohol exposure on the fatty acid composition of umbilical cord serum in humans. Am J Clin Nutr. 2000;71:300S. doi:10.1093/ajcn/71.1.300s.
116. Cas MD, Roda G, Li F, Secundo F. Functional lipids in autoimmune inflammatory diseases. Int J Mol Sci. 2020;21:3074. doi:10.3390/ijms21093074.
117. Abdolmaleki F, Kovanen PT, Mardani R, Gheibi-hayat SM, Bo S, Sahebkar A. Resolvins: emerging players in autoimmune and inflammatory diseases. Clin Rev Allergy Immunol. 2020;58:82–91. doi:10.1007/s12016-019-08754-9.
118. Massaro M, Scoditti E, Carluccio MA, De Caterina R. Nutraceuticals and prevention of atherosclerosis: focus on ω3 polyunsaturated fatty acids and Mediterranean diet polyphenols. Cardiovasc Ther. 2010;28:e13–e19. doi:10.1111/j.1755-5922.2010.00211.x.
119. Skulas-Ray AC, Wilson PW, Harris WS, Brinton EA, Kris-Etherton PM, Richter CK, Jacobson TA, Engler MB, Miller M, Robinson JG, et al. Omega-3 fatty acids for the management of hypertriglyceridemia: a science advisory from the American Heart Association. Circulation. 2019;140:e673–e691. doi:10.1161/CIR.0000000000000709.
120. Chaddha A, Eagle KA. Omega-3 fatty acids and heart health. Circulation. 2015;132:e350–e352. doi:10.1161/CIRCULATIONAHA.114.015176.
121. Yagi S, Fukuda D, Aihara K-I, Akaike M, Shimabukuro M, Sata M. N-3 polyunsaturated fatty acids: promising nutrients for preventing cardiovascular disease. J Atheroscler Thromb. 2017;24(10):999–1010. doi:10.5551/jat.RV17013.

# Substance abuse and cancer

**G.I. Moussas,[1] A.G. Papadopoulou[2]**

[1]*Department of Psychiatry, "Sotiria" General Hospital for Chest Diseases, Athens,*
[2]*2nd Department of Psychiatry, "Attikon" General Hospital, Athens University Medical School, Athens, Greece*

Psychiatriki 2017, 28:234–241

Substance abuse is a health problem with serious psychological and psychiatric dimensions and multiple social and economic consequences. Cancer is a disease that threatens not only life and physical integrity but mental health as well. Oncology patients suffer from mental disorders in high rates, especially from depression and anxiety. The role of substance abuse in the pathogenesis of cancer is studied systematically, since there are research data supporting the mutagenic effects of certain substances. It has been supported that a possible dysregulation of the immune system is linked to the oncogenic processes induced by substances of abuse. Specifically, opioids are the first addictive substances that have been identified as oncogenic factors. However, conflicting results have been offered by experimental animal studies, which showed that opioids, such as morphine, depending on the dosage administered, may not only enhance the process of tumor growth, but also inhibit it. Additionally, research data indicate that the use of cannabis may be associated with cancer, either as an independent factor or in relation to other mutagenics, although it is not yet clear to which extent these effects may be connected to the disease, especially once the consumption of tobacco and alcohol by these patients are taken into account. However, it has been argued that certain cannabinoids may have biological –anticancer– activities which could be used therapeutically without being accompanied by the corresponding 9-tetrahydrocannabinol psychoactive effects. It is well known that alcohol is a risk factor for developing head and neck cancer, and epidemiological studies indicate that the higher the consumption of alcohol, the more mortality due to cancer increases. In addition, it is suggested that there is no safety level for alcohol consumption regarding the risk of developing cancer; that is even a minimum daily consumption is associated with the occurrence of certain types of cancer. Specific components have been identified in tobacco, which are considered to be carcinogenic and responsible for tumor development in various sites. Moreover, complicated psychiatric problems arise due to substance abuse in cancer patients, either in the context of pain treatment, or under pre-existing dependence. The rational use of opioid analgesics, when it is medically required as suggested by the health professionals specialized in the treatment of acute pain in cancer patients, could be a therapeutic option. Substance abuse reduces treatment compliance, worsens cancer prognosis and seems to be a negative factor for the quality of life of these patients. Current literature highlights the importance of appropriate psychiatric interventions to address substance abuse in cancer patients.

**Key words**: Substances abuse, alcohol, smoking, cancer, immune system, pain.

## Introduction

The use and the abuse of addictive substances –legal and illegal– are among the greatest public health problems of the developed world and may lead to serious social complications. The use of alcohol and other substances has been associated with reduced productivity, absence from work and accidents which may lead to financial hardship.[1] Furthermore, the significant health problems that accompany substances abuse lead to a serious burden on the health system, especially in countries such as Greece, where the health system is still in development and maturation process. The comorbidity of mental disorders with other medical conditions in patients with substance abuse disorders constitutes a major health problem that requires targeted medical interventions and the securing of financial resources.

Cancer is the most common cause of death after heart disease. These patients experience high levels of stress and –depending on each person's vulnerability– they suffer from mental disorders at high rates such as depression and anxiety disorders.[2] Cancer is not only a life-threatening disease, but it also constitutes a psychotraumatic factor that may trigger negative feelings and affect functionality.

Many environmental factors have been studied and implicated for their mutagenic action.[3,4] Current research offers some scientific evidence supporting the link of addictive substances with cancer.[5] Moreover, both these serious health problems are investigated in the light of psychosocial issues which result from the substance abuse by cancer patients, either in the context of pain management, or under a preexisting psychiatric history of dependency.

## The role of addictive substances in pathogenesis of cancer

### *Opioids*

Opioids are the first substances which were identified as oncogenetics. Research studies support that opioid receptors, mainly the μ-receptors, are associated with the increase and growth of cancer cells and the enhancement of angiogenesis and metastasis. These data refer to the endogenous opioids but also to the exogenous opioids which are administered to cancer patients for pain management.[6,7] It is under question if drugs which act as antagonists of opioid receptors could inhibit, in some degree, the carcinogenesis process.[8]

### *Heroin*

Early cytogenetic studies show that the use of heroin affects and leads to significant changes in the chromosomes. The withdrawal from heroin use and the admission into a drug treatment program are associated with a significant reduction of chromosomal damage within a year.[9] Indeed, studies with newborns of mothers addicted to heroin showed that the chromosome alterations were six to seven times more compared to the control group with newborns of normal mothers. Previous studies showed a high prevalence of approximately 10% of these alterations in cells that were studied prenatally and postpartum in mothers who had used heroin or were in methadone treatment program.[10] Similar findings were reported in primates that received heroin. Chromosome damage of these newborns was ten times more than newborns of healthy animals.[11] A study showed the association of heroin with carcinogenesis. Specifically, it showed an unexpected increase in the CNS of M2 protein in patients with acute myeloid leukemia which is associated with heroin addiction in the past.[12] In a recent study, 44,000 patients attended a program for heroin over 10 years. In this program, high death rates from cancer were reported, which according to the authors may be related to the increased frequency of infections due to immunosuppression and with the significant consumption of tobacco and alcohol.[13] However, it should be considered that the earliness of deaths among heroin users might not permit a full research regarding its influence in the development of neoplasms.

### *Morphine*

Morphine is a derivative of heroin and is mainly used for the treatment of pain. In *in vivo* studies (animal studies), its impact on the chromosome was confirmed, while it wasn't possible to confirm these findings by in vitro studies. Morphine is classified as a co-mutagenic and it is supported that it could act in a long term through inhibition of copying or in relation to procedures of the repair of mutations leading to the conversion of temporary changes in permanent mutations.[14] In animal studies, it was shown that morphine does not cause the development of new tumors but increases the growth of existing neoplasms, thus reducing the life of the animal.[15] However, research data are conflicting, since there are both *in vivo* and *in vitro* studies which support not only the enhancement but also the reduction of tumors. It seems that the difference in the results is associated with the administered dose of this opioid. Specifically, larger doses for significant periods of time may limit the tumor's growth, while lower doses may be associated with adverse effects.[16] Moreover, the immunosuppressive activity and the effect of morphine in cell apoptosis may be involved in the biological pathways that lead to carcinogenesis.[17,18]

### Codeine

Due to its widespread and systematic use as an analgesic, codeine has been included in the substances for evaluation by the National Cancer Institute and the FDA in the United States' national research program for the effects of toxic substances on public health. No evidence was found regarding carcinogenesis, however it is considered to belong to the substances that may potentially cause cancer in laboratory animals.[19,20]

### Cocaine

Cocaine is known for its teratogenic properties, the disruption of the neurotransmitters function, and its concomitant alterations in brain structures such as cortical areas.[21] Furthermore, cocaine is associated with severe perinatal lesions and with abortions.[22] In laboratory animals it causes severe liver damage accompanied by significant changes in DNA.[23] Although the carcinogenetic properties of cocaine have not been established, the automated electronic evaluation [Computer Automated Structure Evaluation (CASE)] classifies cocaine among carcinogenic agents. This is an advanced artificial intelligence program that identifies molecular infrastructure which is responsible for different biological activities.[24] Furthermore, the adulteration of cocaine with levamisole, a powerful and toxic anti-inflammatory and anti-cancer agent, causes many side effects such as agranulocytosis, while studies estimating the danger of mixing the two substances are in progress.[25] Additionally, the cocaine use has been found to reduce the response to the administration of chemotherapeutic agents, such as imatinib in patients with chronic myeloid leukemia, probably because of cocaine's effect on cytochrome P450.[26]

### Cannabis

Cannabis, also known as marijuana, originates from the plant Cannabis Sativa and is used as a psychoactive substance, as well as a pharmaceutical agent. The component with the principal psychoactive activity is 9-tetrahydrocannabinol which is one of the 483 known components. Eighty three are cannabinoids.[27] Research data indicate that cannabis smoking may be involved in carcinogenesis, either as an independent factor, or in connection with other mutagens, especially in studies concerning the respiratory and gastrointestinal system of young adults.[28] Indeed, important histopathologic and molecular changes have been observed in the bronchial epithelium of systematic hashish smokers. In particular, in systematic smokers, more histopathologic lesions were identified compared to the control group which included nonsmokers.[29] However, from a recent meta-analysis of 6 case-control studies which included 2,150 patients who suffered from lung cancer, only some indications were found as concerns the association of lung cancer with chronic cannabis, taking into consideration the tobacco smoking and the severity of cannabis abuse,[30] Although research data support the adverse effects of cannabis in the respiratory system, it is not clear yet to what extent these effects are associated with cancer.[31] Additionally, the findings of epidemiological studies regarding the risk of head and neck cancer are contradicting, especially after controlling for tobacco and alcohol use in these patients.[32] Similar studies have also been conducted as regards other cancer types, such as the testicular cancer. A study indicated that among the oncological patients, those who had a history of cannabis use were twice as like to develop certain histological types of cancer with worse prognosis, compared to patients who had no relevant history.[33] However, some preclinical animal studies showed that certain cannabinoids such is cannabidiol (CBD), may have biological effects, which can be used therapeutically as anti-cancer, anti-inflammatory and analgesic substances, without 9-tetrahydrocannabinol psychoactive effect. The anticancer effects of cannabinoids are related to a variety of mechanisms such as the reduction of apoptosis in healthy cells, the inhibition of proliferation in cancer cells, and the minimization of tumor angiogenesis and metastasis process. In particular, *in vitro* studies of breast and lung cancer cells, it has been argued that CBD through its action in receptors, such as the receptor cannabinoid type 1(CB1) and the intercellular adhesion molecule-1 (ICAM-1 is associated with the immune system) may restrict the survival of cancer cells, with small effect on health cells, while it reduces the migration of malignant cells. Moreover, there is strong evidence from *in vitro* studies that this specific cannabinoid increases the chemopreventive action of certain drugs, and helps the uptake of chemotherapeutic agents into tumor cells.[34]

### Alcohol

It is known that the abuse and alcohol dependence is one of the greatest and most intractable public health problems with high costs and serious social effects. The degree of consumption and the frequency of abuse are related to a variety of physical and psychological problems. Furthermore, according to the World Health Organization it is one of the five major risk factors internationally associated with disease, disability and death. Additionally, it constitutes a causative agent for more than 200 diseases, with cancer among them.[35] Indeed, there is evidence that the prenatal fetal exposure to alcohol increases in adulthood the probability of dependence behaviors through mechanisms that cause changes in neurotransmitters' function and eventually neurophysiological changes with adverse effects on learning processes.[36] In this context it appears that early brain exposure to alcohol during its primary development stages increases indirectly carcinogenesis, since it is a risk factor for alcoholism.

A review of genetic epidemiology studies of head and neck cancer showed that these types of cancer are associated with polymorphisms in the alcohol metabolism genes. Specifically, they are associated with three variants of ADH (Alcohol dehydrogenase) gene, which controls the metabolism of ethanol. This risk can be modified by the genes that control ADH, especially polymorphisms ADH1B and ADH1C, which oxidizes ethanol to its carcinogenic metabolite, acetaldehyde.[37]

Epidemiological studies indicate that the higher the consumption of alcohol, the greater the mortality from cancer, and furthermore that there is no security level in alcohol use in relation to the risk of cancer development. Even a minimum daily consumption is associated with the occurrence of certain types of cancer.[38]

It is well known that alcohol is a risk factor for head and neck cancer, especially in the oral cavity, pharynx, larynx and esophagus.[39] The results of various studies show that stopping alcohol consumption is associated with a reduced risk of cancer development in the larynx and pharynx. A study concludes that for the heavy drinkers 35 years of discontinuing consumption are required, so that the relative risk would become equal to that of individuals' who do not consume alcohol. However, it is noteworthy that significant reduction of risk is recorded in a short time, which demonstrates the major importance of discontinuing alcohol in order to prevent cancer.[40] Also, alcohol consumption is a risk factor for various other cancer types; such are in upper digestive tract, liver, bowel and in breast.[41–43] Indeed, an even small dose of ethanol increases the risk for breast cancer. Specifically, moderate alcohol consumption is found to increase the risk for breast cancer by 4%, while heavy consumption increases it by 40–50%. It has been suggested that alcohol increases the levels of estrogen and thus enhances carcinogenic effect of hormones in mammary gland. Also, the role of acetaldehyde and some epigenetic changes that involve methyl-1-transferase which affect the life cycle cell are studied.[44] Prevention strategies should be designed to include early detection of alcohol abuse in women in order to reduce the risk for breast cancer. A significant proportion of depressive women abuse alcohol and that may not be recognized by mental health professionals.[45] Furthermore, the results of a recent meta-analysis support the existence of a casual relationship between heavy alcohol consumption and an increased risk for colon cancer, and also provide further evidence for the association between moderate alcohol intake and a relative risk for colon cancer. Nevertheless, many issues remain unsolved, including the quantification of consumption, since there are indications of risk even for mild consumption (a drink per day). However, moderate (2–3 drinks/day) alcohol consumption was found to increase by 21% the development of cancer and heavy one (>4 drinks/day, which is equivalent to >50 gr/day of ethanol) is associated with 52% increased risk for colorectal cancer.[46] The aforementioned findings along with the fact that a great number of women and especially men consume alcohol in a regular basis as well as with the high global incidence of colorectal cancer (particularly in developed countries) are of great significance due to their impact on public health. Abstinence from alcohol should be included in prevention strategies for colon cancer.

### Smoking

In tobacco, specific components are identified which are considered to be carcinogenic and responsible for the development of disease in various locations on the head, neck, lung, prostate and kidney.[47] Indeed, a total of 30% of cancers are thought to be related to smoking and tobacco consumption.[48] Smoking has been implicated in the development of lung cancer and studies have explored the correlation of specific histological types such as adenocarcinoma which is related to lower diversification in smokers.[49] In fact, lung cancer patients who smoke report higher levels of stress in comparison with cancer patients suffering from any other type of cancer, which is associated with strong feelings of guilt and shame about their behavior and the casual relationship of this behavior with lung cancer.[50]

### Abuse of addictive substances in cancer

The use of addictive substances has been studied in adult patients who have survived from cancer that appeared in childhood. One study suggested that cancer survivors, who were diagnosed in older age, were at greater risk for substance abuse and the appropriate psychiatric interventions could reduce this risk.[51]

#### *The use of opioids analgesics to control pain in cancer*

Cancer is accompanied by serious and persistent physical complaints including chronic pain which is an important negative prognostic factor for survival in cancer patients.[52] The use of opioids as analgesics to treat cancer is a common treatment option. However, various clinical issues arise related to their administration, particularly in terminally ill patients. Frequently, due to their concern that their patients may develop dependence, doctors avoid to administer analgesics to such an extent that the patients cannot experience the therapeutic benefits of analgesia. Moreover, the patient's relatives, based on the same rationale, may also feel concerned and thus may reject the idea of their family member using opioids. Therefore, the fear of stigma may influence and hinder medical care.[53]

Additionally, the use of opioids for pain treatment and specifically acute pain or pain at terminally ill patients is associated with lower risk for developing abuse behaviors. In contrast, the use of these drugs in chronic pain and especially in patients with substance abuse history, increase the relative risk, which generally is identified in 8 to 17% of cancer patients who receive opioids for treating chronic pain.[54] When medically necessary, the careful use of opioids analgesics for acute pain management in cancer patients is suggested.[55] The appropriate education and training of healthcare professionals is necessary in order to ensure an integrative medical approach, free from prejudiced beliefs.[56]

#### *Alcohol abuse in cancer patients*

Alcohol abuse is a risk factor for certain cancers types; such are head and neck cancer. Some of the patients continue to abuse alcohol even after their cancer's diagnosis and that is a frequent practice with bad consequences both in the quality of life and in the survival of these patients.[57] Indeed, a study which assessed the habits of cancer patients with head–cervical cancer according to alcohol, found that half of these patients continued to consume alcohol.[58] Psychiatric interventions in these patients aiming at psycho-educating them regarding the possible consequences of alcohol use, as well as treating depressive symptoms, that often appear in cancer patients who abuse alcohol, could lead to the reduction of alcohol intake, with beneficial results in the prognosis of cancer.[59]

#### *Tobacco use in cancer patients*

Many patients despite being diagnosed with cancer continue to smoke or relapse quickly in case they had quit smoking. Specifically, a study which recorded the behavior of smoker patients with non-small cell lung cancer during a four-year period found that only almost 40% of them had permanently quit smoking in the first two years.[60] It has been observed that critically ill patient quit smoking more frequently and more constantly than those with less serious disease. Indeed, in a study for smoking cessation of patients with head and neck cancer, patients who were treated with a surgery as laryngectomy, had significantly higher rates of abstinence from smoking compared with those who received radiotherapy.[61] Therefore, several factors may influence smoking cessation and the duration of abstinence in cancer patients, such as the stage of the disease and the treatment selected. Moreover, it has been suggested that the time period during the diagnosis of cancer could be used in order to implement the appropriate interventions, since the high motive and the therapeutic relationship may facilitate smoking cessation. Also, it is required to address possible problems that follow smoke cessation, such as depression and weight gain. The use of drug therapies, such as nicotine replacement therapy (e.g., skin patches or nicotine gum) and problem solving training may be used in combination to achieve the best possible therapeutic result.[62]

## Conclusions

The abuse of legal and illegal substances through direct and indirect mechanisms increases inflammatory activity at a molecular level.[63] Meanwhile, evidence from epidemiological, preclinical and clinical studies, suggest that dysregulated inflammatory activity plays a central role in a variety of chronic diseases, including cancer. These inflammatory processes may be triggered by a number of environmental factors as well as by unhealthy lifestyle that includes tobacco use, stress, bad diet, obesity and alcohol use. The aforementioned factors are believed to be involved in the development of 90% of all cancer types.[64] Therefore, it seems that the odds of developing cancer are significantly affected by our lifestyle choices. Several uncontrollable risk factors are involved in the majority of cancer types; however we can change our daily habits in order to reduce this threat.

The use of opioids analgesics for pain management in cancer patients constitutes an appropriate therapeutic option when medical reasons dictate it, such as in acute pain. Providing information to the patients and their relatives regarding the treatment plan contributes to a higher level of compliance and reduces the risk of abusing these drugs.

Tobacco and alcohol abuse in cancer patients aggravates the prognosis of cancer and acts as a negative factor for the quality of life of these patients. These data highlight the need for the development and implementation of appropriate interventions regarding these patients.

## References

1. van Boekel LC, Brouwers EP, van Weeghel J, Garretsen HF. Stigma among health professionals towards patients with substance use disorders and its consequences for health care delivery: systematic review. *Drug Alcohol Depend* 2013, 131:23–35, doi: 10.1016/j.drugalcdep.2013.02.018
2. Razavi D, Stiefel F. Common psychiatric disorders in cancer patients. I. Adjustment disorders and depressive disorders. *Support Care Cancer* 1994, 2:223–232, PMID: 8087440
3. Dhaini HR, Kobeissi L. Toxicogenetic profile and cancer risk in Lebanese. *J Toxicol Environ Health B Crit Rev* 2014, 17:95–125, doi: 10.1080/10937404.2013.878679
4. Adams BD, Kasinski AL, Slack FJ. Aberrant regulation and function of microRNAs in cancer. *Curr Biol* 2014, 24:R762–76, doi: 10.1016/j.cub.2014.06.043
5. Varela-Rey M, Woodhoo A, Martinez-Chantar ML, Mato JM, Lu SC. Alcohol, DNA methylation, and cancer. *Alcohol Res* 2013, 35:25–35, PMID: 24313162
6. Lennon FE, Mirzapoiazova T, Mambetsariev B, Poroyko VA, Salgia R, Moss J et al. The Mu opioid receptor promotes opioid and growth factor-induced proliferation, migration and Epithelial Mesenchymal Transition (EMT) in human lung cancer. *PLoS One* 2014, 9:e91577, doi: 10.1371/journal.pone.0091577
7. Leo S, Nuydens R, Meert TF. Opioid-induced proliferation of vascular endothelial cells. *J Pain Res* 2009, 2:59–66, PMID: 21197294
8. Lennon FE, Moss J, Singleton PA. The μ-opioid receptor in cancer progression: is there a direct effect? *Anesthesiology* 2012, 116:940–945, doi: 10.1097/ALN.0b013e31824b9512
9. Falek A, Hollingsworth F. Heroin and chromosome damage. *Arch Gen Psychiatry* 1980, 37:227–228, doi:10.1001/archpsyc.1980.01780150117012
10. Amarose AP, Norusis MJ. Cytogenetics of methadone-managed and heroin-addicted pregnant women and their newborn infants. *Am J Obstet Gynecol* 1976, 124:635–640, PMID: 1258915
11. Fischman HK, Roizin L, Moralishvili E, Albu P, Ross D, Rainer JD. Clastogenic effects of heroin in pregnant monkeys and their offspring. *Mutat Res* 1983, 118:77–89, PMID: 6866001
12. Romani C, Pettinau M, Dessalvi P, Murru R, Angelucci E. Unexpected CNS localization in M2 acute myeloid leukemia: a link with past heroin addiction? *Am J Hematol* 2008, 83:682–683, doi: 10.1002/ajh.21190.
13. Degenhardt L, Larney S, Randall D, Burns L, Hall W. Causes of death in a cohort treated for opioid dependence between 1985 and 2005. *Addiction* 2014, 109:90–99, doi: 10.1111/add.12337
14. Li JH, Lin LF. Genetic toxicology of abused drugs: a brief review. *Mutagenesis* 1998, 13:557–565, PMID: 9862186
15. Nguyen J, Luk K, Vang D, Soto W, Vincent L, Robiner S et al. Morphine stimulates cancer progression and mast cell activation and impairs survival in transgenic mice with breast cancer. *Br J Anaesth* 2014, 113(Suppl 1):i4–13, doi: 10.1093/bja/aeu090
16. Gach K, Wyrebska A, Fichna J, Janecka A. The role of morphine in regulation of cancer cell growth. *Naunyn Schmiedebergs Arch Pharmacol* 2011, 384:221–230, doi: 10.1007/s00210-011-0672-4
17. Odunayo A, Dodam JR, Kerl ME, DeClue AE. Immunomodulatory effects of opioids. *J Vet Emerg Crit Care* (San Antonio) 2010, 20:376–385, doi: 10.1111/j.1476-4431.2010.00561.x
18. Kaufmann SH, Hengartner MO. Programmed cell death: alive and well in the new millennium. *Trends Cell Biol* 2001, 11:526–534, PMID: 11719060
19. Program NT. NTP Toxicology and Carcinogenesis Studies of Codeine (CAS No. 76-57-3) in F344 Rats and B6C3F1 Mice (Feed Studies). *National Toxicology Program Technical Report Series* 1996, 455:1
20. Zhang YP, Sussman N, Macina OT, Rosenkranz HS, Klopman G. Prediction of the carcinogenicity of a second group of organic chemicals undergoing carcinogenicity testing. *Environ Health Perspect* 1996, 104(Suppl 5):1045–1050, PMID: 8933053
21. Behnke M, Smith VC. Prenatal substance abuse:short- and long-term effects on the exposed fetus. *Pediatrics* 2013, 131:e1009–1024, doi: 10.1542/peds.2012-3931
22. Cain MA, Bornick P, Whiteman V. The maternal, fetal, and neonatal effects of cocaine exposure in pregnancy. *Clin Obstet Gynecol* 2013, 56:124–132, doi: 10.1097/GRF.0b013e31827ae167
23. Cascales M, Alvarez A, Gasco P, Fernandez-Simon L, Sanz N, Bosca L. Cocaine-induced liver injury in mice elicits specific changes in DNA ploidy and induces programmed death of hepatocytes. *Hepatology* 1994, 20:992–1001, PMID: 7927241
24. Rosenkranz HS, Klopman G. The carcinogenic potential of cocaine. *Cancer Lett* 1990, 52:243–246, PMID: 2379147
25. Wolford A, McDonald TS, Eng H, Hansel S, Chen Y, Bauman J et al. Immune-mediated agranulocytosis caused by the cocaine adulterant levamisole: a case for reactive metabolite(s) involvement. *Drug Metab Dispos* 2012, 40:1067–1075, doi: 10.1124/dmd.112.045021
26. Breccia M, Gentilini F, Alimena G. Cocaine abuse may influence the response to imatinib in CML patients. *Haematologica* 2007, 92:e41–42, doi: 10.3324/haematol.10976
27. Grotenhermen F. Cannabinoids. *Curr Drug Targets CNS Neurol Disord* 2005, 4:507–530, PMID: 16266285
28. Mao L, Oh Y. Does marijuana or crack cocaine cause cancer? *J Natl Cancer Inst* 1998, 90:1182–1184, PMID: 9719073

29. Fligiel SE, Roth MD, Kleerup EC, Barsky SH, Simmons MS, Tashkin DP. Tracheobronchial histopathology in habitual smokers of cocaine, marijuana, and/or tobacco. *Chest* 1997, 112:319–326, PMID: 9266864
30. Zhang LR, Morgenstern H, Greenland S, Chang SC, Lazarus P, Teare MD et al. Cannabis smoking and lung cancer risk: Pooled analysis in the International Lung Cancer Consortium. *Int J Cancer* 2015, 136:894–903, doi: 10.1002/ijc.29036
31. Gates P, Jaffe A, Copeland J. Cannabis smoking and respiratory health: consideration of the literature. *Respirology* 2014, 19:655–662, doi: 10.1111/resp.12298
32. Hashibe M, Straif K, Tashkin DP, Morgenstern H, Greenland S, Zhang ZF. Epidemiologic review of marijuana use and cancer risk. *Alcohol* 2005, 35:265–275, doi: 10.1016/j.alcohol.2005.04.008
33. Lacson JC, Carroll JD, Tuazon E, Castelao EJ, Bernstein L, Cortessis VK. Population-based case-control study of recreational drug use and testis cancer risk confirms an association between marijuana use and nonseminoma risk. *Cancer* 2012, 118:5374–5383, doi: 10.1002/cncr.27554
34. National Cancer Institute HPV, Laboratory/Animal/Preclinical Studies Cannabis and Cannabinoids, http://www.cancer.gov/cancertopics/pdq/cam/cannabis/healthprofessional
35. WHO. *Global status report on alcohol and health*. WHO Press, Geneva, 2014
36. Parker MO, Evans AM, Brock AJ, Combe FJ, Teh MT, Brennan CH. Moderate alcohol exposure during early brain development increases stimulus-response habits in adulthood. *Addict Biol* 2016, 21:49–60, doi: 10.1111/adb.12176
37. Chang JS, Straif K, Guha N. The role of alcohol dehydrogenase genes in head and neck cancers: a systematic review and meta-analysis of ADH1B and ADH1C. *Mutagenesis* 2012, 27:275–286, doi: 10.1093/mutage/ger073
38. Nelson DE, Jarman DW, Rehm J, Greenfield TK, Rey G, Kerr WC et al. Alcohol-attributable cancer deaths and years of potential life lost in the United States. *Am J Public Health* 2013, 103:641–648, doi: 10.2105/AJPH.2012.301199
39. Boyle P, Macfarlane GJ, Zheng T, Maisonneuve P, Evstifeeva T, Scully C. Recent advances in epidemiology of head and neck cancer. *Curr Opin Oncol* 1992, 4:471–477, PMID: 1498155
40. Ahmad Kiadaliri A, Jarl J, Gavriilidis G, Gerdtham UG. Alcohol drinking cessation and the risk of laryngeal and pharyngeal cancers: a systematic review and meta-analysis. *PLoS One* 2013, 8:e58158, doi: 10.1371/journal.pone.0058158
41. Heckley GA, Jarl J, Asamoah BO, U GG. How the risk of liver cancer changes after alcohol cessation: a review and meta-analysis of the current literature. *BMC Cancer* 2011, 11:446, doi: 10.1186/1471-2407-11-446
42. Moskal A, Norat T, Ferrari P, Riboli E. Alcohol intake and colorectal cancer risk: a dose-response meta-analysis of published cohort studies. *Int J Cancer* 2007, 120:664–671, doi: 10.1002/ijc.22299
43. IARC Working Group on the Evaluation of Carcinogenic Risk to Humans. Alcohol consumption and ethyl carbamate. *IARC Monogr Eval Carcinog Risks Hum* 2010, 96:3–1383, PMID: 21735939
44. Seitz HK, Pelucchi C, Bagnardi V, La Vecchia C. Epidemiology and pathophysiology of alcohol and breast cancer: Update 2012. *Alcohol Alcohol* 2012, 47:204–212, doi: 10.1093/alcalc/ags011
45. Advani P, Moreno-Aspitia A. Current strategies for the prevention of breast cancer. *Breast Cancer* (Dove Med Press) 2014, 6:59–71, doi: 10.2147/BCTT.S39114
46. Cai S, Li Y, Ding Y, Chen K, Jin M. Alcohol drinking and the risk of colorectal cancer death: a meta-analysis. *Eur J Cancer Prev* 2014, 23:532–539, doi: 10.1097/CEJ.0000000000000076
47. Scully C. Oral cancer aetiopathogenesis, past, present and future aspects. *Med Oral Patol Oral Cir Bucal* 2011, 16:e306–311, PMID: 21441876
48. Toll BA, Rojewski AM, Duncan LR, Latimer-Cheung AE, Fucito LM, Boyer JL et al. "Quitting smoking will benefit your health": the evolution of clinician messaging to encourage tobacco cessation. *Clin Cancer Res* 2014, 20:301–309, doi: 10.1158/1078-0432.CCR-13-2261
49. Khan N, Afaq F, Mukhtar H. Lifestyle as risk factor for cancer: Evidence from human studies. *Cancer Lett* 2010, 293:133–143, doi: 10.1016/j.canlet.2009.12.013
50. Dirkse D, Lamont L, Li Y, Simonic A, Bebb G, Giese-Davis J. Shame, guilt, and communication in lung cancer patients and their partners. *Curr Oncol* 2014, 21:e718–722, doi: 10.3747/co.21.2034
51. Thompson AL, Gerhardt CA, Miller KS, Vannatta K, Noll RB. Survivors of childhood cancer and comparison peers: the influence of peer factors on later externalizing behavior in emerging adulthood. *J Pediatr Psychol* 2009, 34:1119–1128, doi: 10.1093/jpepsy/jsp019
52. Montazeri A. Quality of life data as prognostic indicators of survival in cancer patients: an overview of the literature from 1982 to 2008. *Health Qual Life Outcomes* 2009, 7:102, doi: 10.1186/1477-7525-7-102
53. Shah S, Diwan S. Methadone: does stigma play a role as a barrier to treatment of chronic pain? *Pain Physician* 2010, 13:289–293, PMID: 20495594
54. Ballantyne JC. Chronic pain following treatment for cancer: the role of opioids. *Oncologist* 2003, 8:567–575, doi: 10.1634/theoncologist.8-6-567
55. Ballantyne JC. Treating pain in patients with drug-dependence problems. *BMJ* 2013, 347:f3213, doi: 10.1136/bmj.f3213
56. Welshman A. Palliative care. Some organisational considerations. *Minerva Anestesiol* 2005, 71:439–443, PMID: 16012417
57. Mehanna HM, De Boer MF, Morton RP. The association of psycho-social factors and survival in head and neck cancer. *Clin Otolaryngol* 2008, 33:83–89, doi: 10.1111/j.1749-4486.2008.01666.x
58. Duffy SA, Terrell JE, Valenstein M, Ronis DL, Copeland LA, Connors M. Effect of smoking, alcohol, and depression on the quality of life of head and neck cancer patients. *Gen Hosp Psychiatry* 2002, 24:140–147, PMID: 12062138
59. Potash AE, Karnell LH, Christensen AJ, Vander Weg MW, Funk GF. Continued alcohol use in patients with head and neck cancer. *Head Neck* 2010, 32:905–912, doi: 10.1002/hed.21281
60. Gritz ER, Nisenbaum R, Elashoff RE, Holmes EC. Smoking behavior following diagnosis in patients with stage I non-small cell lung cancer. *Cancer Causes Control* 1991, 2:105–112, PMID: 1651777
61. Gritz ER, Carr CR, Rapkin D, Abemayor E, Chang LJ, Wong WK et al. Predictors of long-term smoking cessation in head and neck cancer patients. *Cancer Epidemiol Biomarkers Prev* 1993, 2:261–270, PMID: 8318879
62. Cox LS, Africano NL, Tercyak KP, Taylor KL. Nicotine dependence treatment for patients with cancer. *Cancer* 2003, 98:632–644, doi: 10.1002/cncr.11538
63. Ray LA, Roche DJ, Heinzerling K, Shoptaw S. Opportunities for the development of neuroimmune therapies in addiction. *Int Rev Neurobiol* 2014, 118:381–401, doi: 10.1016/B978-0-12-801284-0.00012-9
64. Sethi G, Shanmugam MK, Ramachandran L, Kumar AP, Tergaonkar V. Multifaceted link between cancer and inflammation. *Biosci Rep* 2012, 32:1–15, doi: 10.1042/BSR20100136

*Corresponding author:* G.I. Moussas, Psychiatric Department, "Sotiria" General Hospital, Athens
Tel: (+30) 210-77 78 611
e-mail: gmpsuoa@gmail.com

## Rate of New Alcohol-associated Cancers by Cancer Type All Alcohol-associated Cancers, Male and Female, United States, 2019

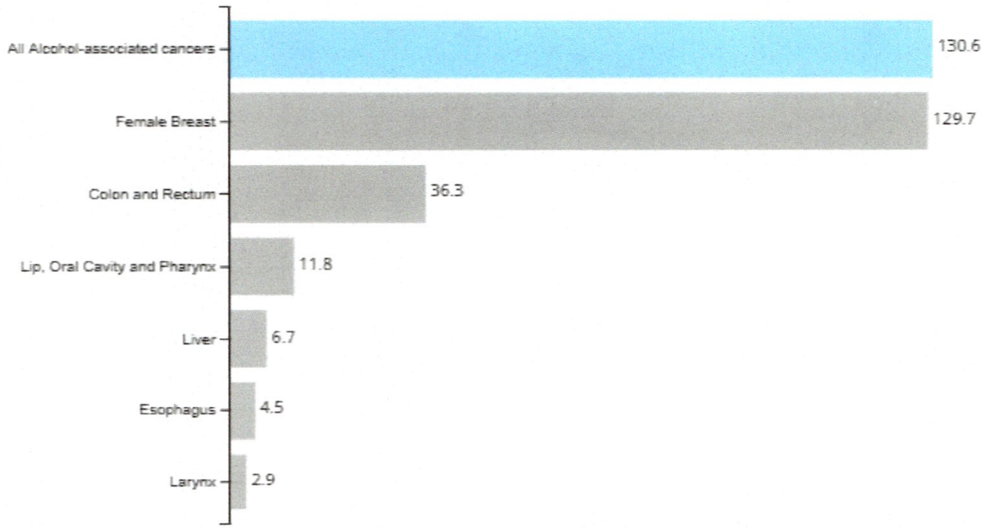


Rate per 100,000 people

Source - U.S. Cancer Statistics Working Group. U.S. Cancer Statistics Data Visualizations Tool, based on 2021 submission data (1999-2019): U.S. Department of Health and Human Services, Centers for Disease Control and Prevention and National Cancer Institute; https://www.cdc.gov/cancer/dataviz, released in November 2022.

Rate of New Alcohol-associated Cancers By State
All Alcohol-associated Cancers,
Male and Female, United States, 2019

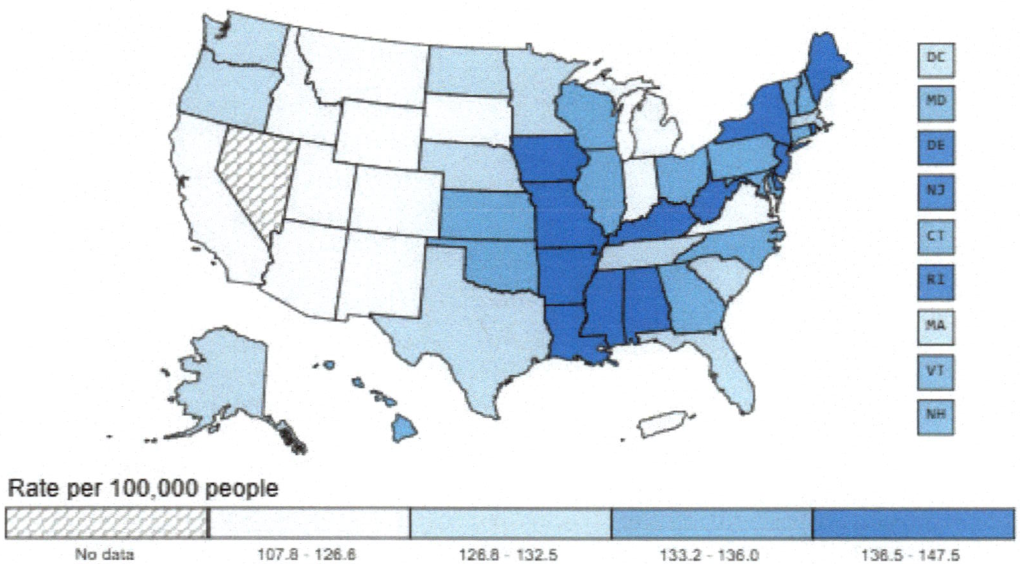


Source - U.S. Cancer Statistics Working Group. U.S. Cancer Statistics Data Visualizations Tool, based on 2021 submission data (1999-2019): U.S. Department of Health and Human Services, Centers for Disease Control and Prevention and National Cancer Institute; https://www.cdc.gov/cancer/dataviz, released in November 2022.

## Rate of New Alcohol-associated Cancers By Race and Ethnicity
## All Alcohol-associated Cancers,
## Male and Female, United States, 2019

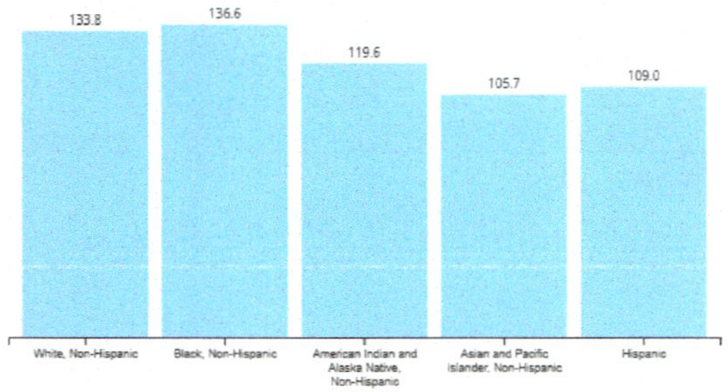


Rate per 100,000 people

Source - U.S. Cancer Statistics Working Group. U.S. Cancer Statistics Data Visualizations Tool, based on 2021 submission data (1999-2019): U.S. Department of Health and Human Services, Centers for Disease Control and Prevention and National Cancer Institute; https://www.cdc.gov/cancer/dataviz, released in November 2022.

Rate of New Alcohol-associated Cancers By Age Group (years)
All Alcohol-associated Cancers,
Male and Female, United States, 2019

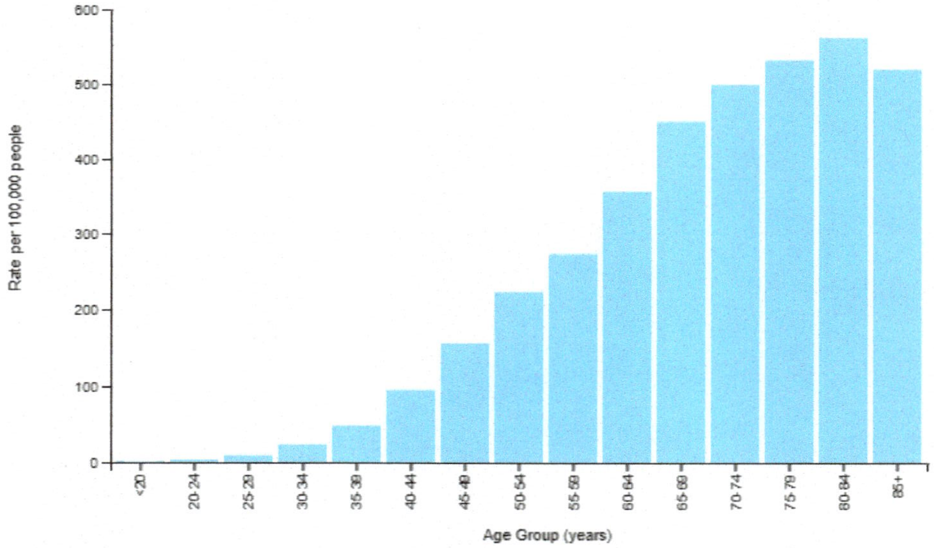


Source - U.S. Cancer Statistics Working Group. U.S. Cancer Statistics Data Visualizations Tool, based on 2021 submission data (1999-2019): U.S. Department of Health and Human Services, Centers for Disease Control and Prevention and National Cancer Institute; https://www.cdc.gov/cancer/dataviz, released in November 2022.

## Rate of New Tobacco-associated Cancers by Cancer Type
## All Tobacco-associated Cancers, Male and Female, United States, 2019

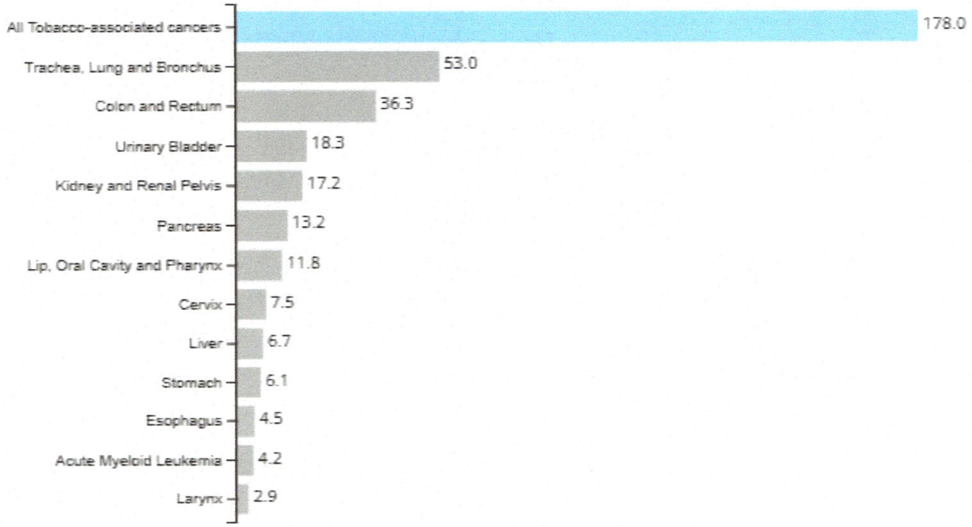


Rate per 100,000 people

Source - U.S. Cancer Statistics Working Group. U.S. Cancer Statistics Data Visualizations Tool, based on 2021 submission data (1999-2019): U.S. Department of Health and Human Services, Centers for Disease Control and Prevention and National Cancer Institute; https://www.cdc.gov/cancer/dataviz, released in November 2022.

## Rate of New Tobacco-associated Cancers By State
## All Tobacco-associated Cancers, Male and Female, United States, 2019

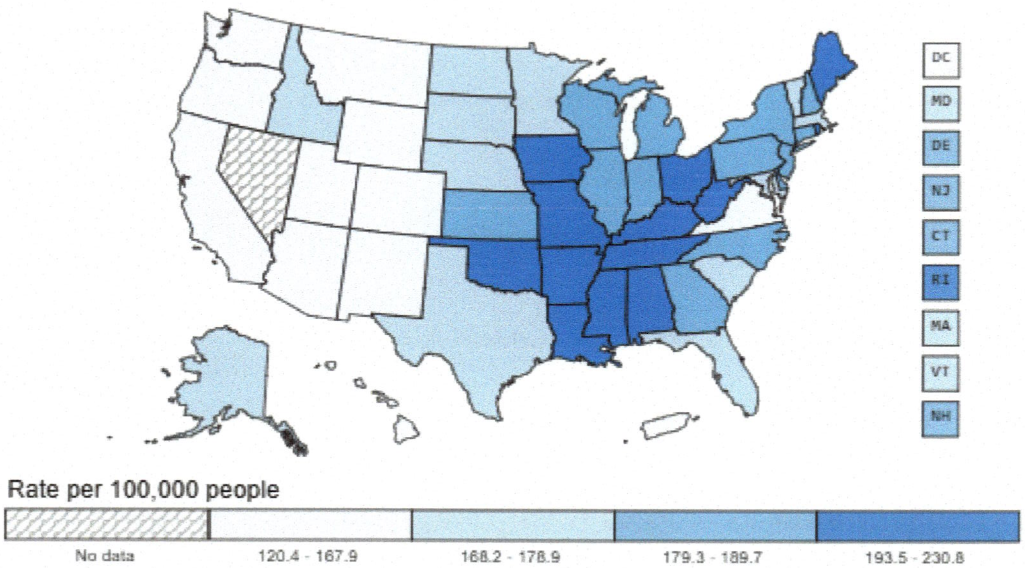


Source - U.S. Cancer Statistics Working Group. U.S. Cancer Statistics Data Visualizations Tool, based on 2021 submission data (1999-2019): U.S. Department of Health and Human Services, Centers for Disease Control and Prevention and National Cancer Institute; https://www.cdc.gov/cancer/dataviz, released in November 2022.

## Rate of New Tobacco-associated Cancers By Race and Ethnicity
## All Tobacco-associated Cancers,
## Male and Female, United States, 2019

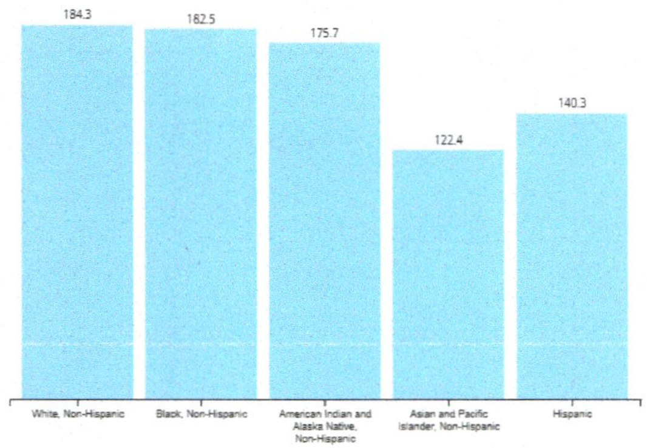


Rate per 100,000 people

Source - U.S. Cancer Statistics Working Group. U.S. Cancer Statistics Data Visualizations Tool, based on 2021 submission data (1999-2019): U.S. Department of Health and Human Services, Centers for Disease Control and Prevention and National Cancer Institute; https://www.cdc.gov/cancer/dataviz, released in November 2022.

## Rate of New Tobacco-associated Cancers By Age Group (years)
## All Tobacco-associated Cancers,
## Male and Female, United States, 2019

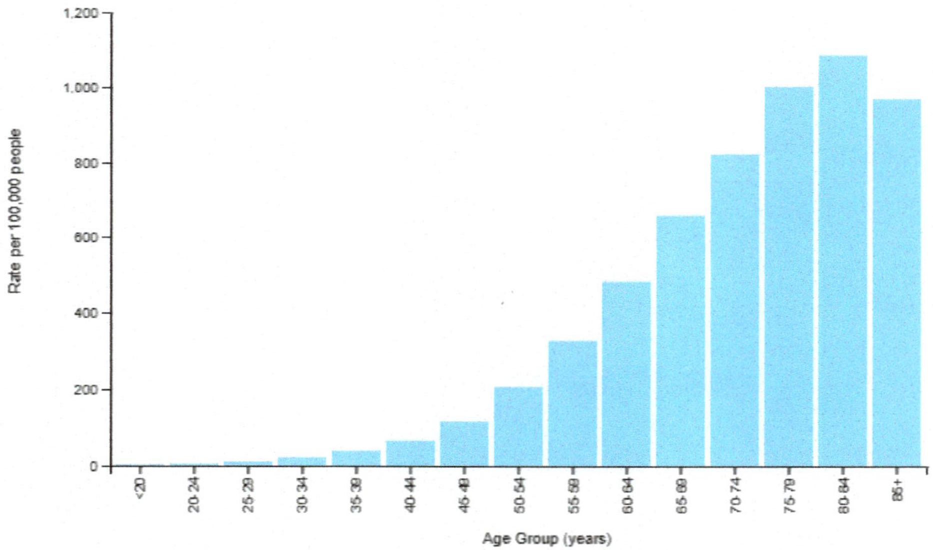


Source - U.S. Cancer Statistics Working Group. U.S. Cancer Statistics Data Visualizations Tool, based on 2021 submission data (1999-2019): U.S. Department of Health and Human Services, Centers for Disease Control and Prevention and National Cancer Institute; https://www.cdc.gov/cancer/dataviz, released in November 2022.

YOUR GUIDE TO

# Living Well With Heart Disease

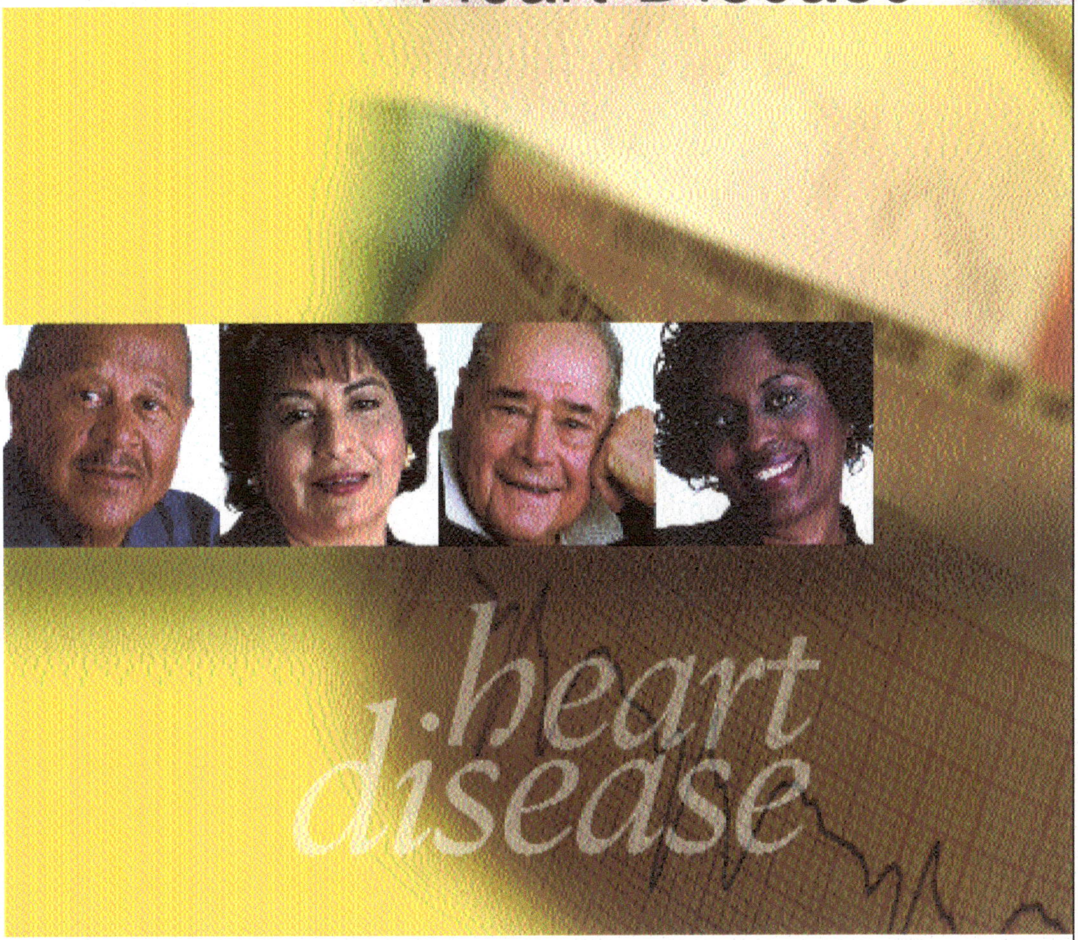


U.S. DEPARTMENT OF HEALTH AND HUMAN SERVICES
National Institutes of Health
National Heart, Lung, and Blood Institute

NIH Publication No. 06-5270
November 2005

# What Is Heart Disease?

Coronary heart disease is the main form of heart disease. It occurs when the coronary arteries, which supply blood to the heart muscle, become hardened and narrowed due to a buildup of plaque on the arteries' inner walls. Plaque is the accumulation of cholesterol, fat, and other substances. As plaque continues to build up in the arteries, blood flow to the heart is reduced.

Coronary heart disease—often simply called heart disease—can lead to a heart attack. A heart attack happens when a cholesterol-rich plaque bursts and releases its contents into the bloodstream. This causes a blood clot to form over the plaque, totally blocking blood flow through the artery and preventing vital oxygen and nutrients from getting to the heart. A heart attack can cause permanent damage to the heart muscle.

Heart disease includes a number of other serious conditions, including:

**Angina.** More than 6 million Americans live with angina, which is chest pain or discomfort that occurs when the heart muscle is not getting enough blood. The inadequate blood flow is caused by narrowed coronary arteries, due to an accumulation of plaque. A bout of angina is not a heart attack, but it means that you're more likely to have a heart attack than someone who doesn't have angina. There are two kinds of angina:

**Stable angina** has a recognizable pattern. It may feel like pressure or a squeezing pain in your chest. The pain may also occur in your shoulders, arms, neck, jaw, or back. It may also feel like indigestion. Stable angina pain is generally brought on by some kind of exertion or strain (such as climbing stairs or experiencing emotional stress), and it is usually relieved by rest or medicine.

**Unstable angina** is more serious than stable angina. Occurring at any time, unstable angina often reflects a change in a previously stable pattern of angina. Episodes of unstable angina are usually more frequent, painful, and longer lasting than bouts of stable angina, and a re less often relieved by rest or medicine. Unstable angina is a sign that you may have a heart attack very soon. The symptoms are the same as if you are having a heart attack. (See page 46 for heart attack warning signs.) If you have any of these symptoms, you should call 9–1–1 right away so that you can get immediate treatment.

**Congestive heart failure.** Congestive heart failure is a life-threatening condition in which the heart cannot pump enough blood to supply the body's needs. Affecting nearly 5 million Americans, heart failure occurs when excess fluid collects in the body as a result of heart weakness or injury. This condition leads to a buildup of fluid in the lungs, causing swelling of the feet, tiredness, weakness, and breathing difficulties.

High blood pressure is the leading cause of congestive heart failure in the United States. Heart disease and diabetes are also major underlying causes of heart failure. People who have had a heart attack are at high risk of developing this condition.

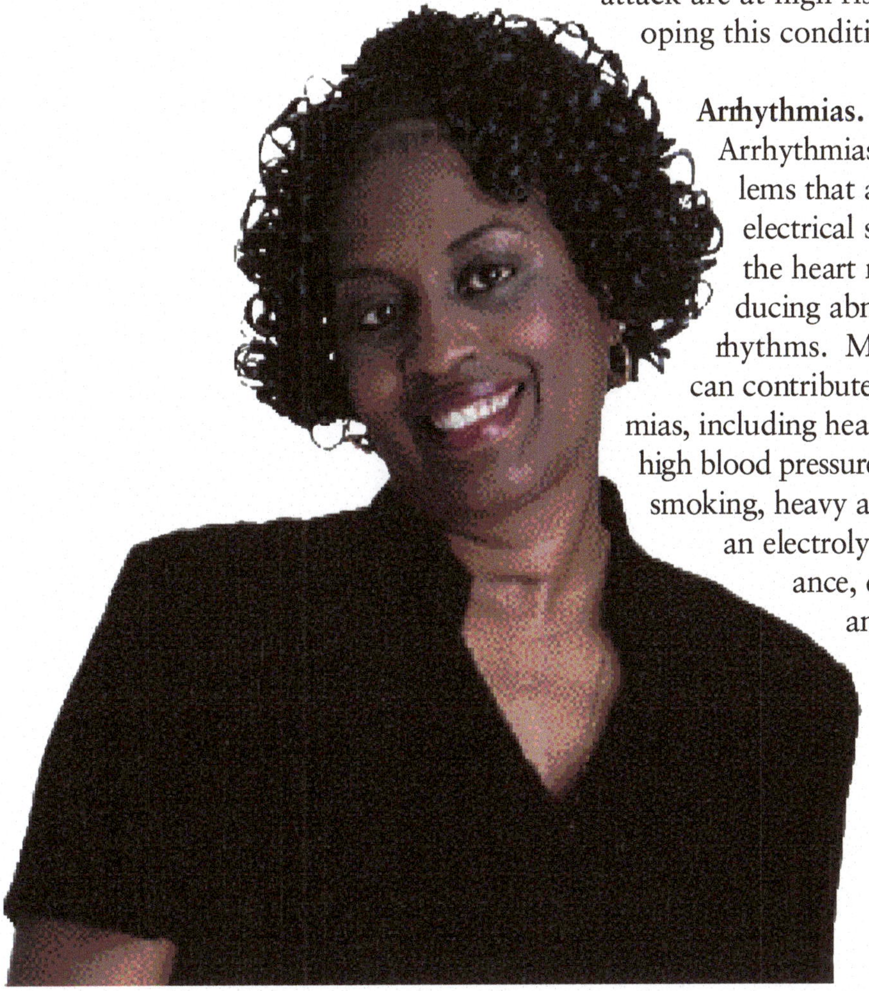

**Arrhythmias.** Arrhythmias are problems that affect the electrical system of the heart muscle, producing abnormal heart rhythms. Many factors can contribute to arrhythmias, including heart disease, high blood pressure, diabetes, smoking, heavy alcohol use, an electrolyte imbalance, drug abuse, and stress. Certain medicines, dietary supplements, and herbal remedies also cause arrhythmias in some people.

A common type of arrhythmia is called **atrial fibrillation,** a disorder affecting 2.2 million Americans. It is more common in older people and those with certain inborn heart problems. Atrial fibrillation occurs when the heart's two upper chambers (the atria) quiver instead of beating normally. Blood isn't pumped completely out of these chambers, making it more likely to pool and clot. If a clot leaves the heart and becomes lodged in an artery in the brain, a stroke results. About 15 percent of strokes occur in people with atrial fibrillation.

Another type of arrhythmia called **ventricular fibrillation** occurs when the lower heart chambers (the ventricles) quiver, preventing the heart from effectively pumping blood. This is the most dangerous type of heart rhythm disturbance. To prevent collapse and sudden cardiac death, it is vital to get immediate emergency medical help for ventricular fibrillation.

# Controlling Your Risk Factors

If you have heart disease, you may wonder *why* you have it. The answer is that many personal characteristics, health conditions, and lifestyle habits can contribute to heart disease. These are called risk factors.

But risk factors do more than simply contribute to heart problems. They also increase the chances that existing heart disease will worsen. Since you already have heart disease, it is very important to find out about all of your risk factors and take active steps to control them.

Certain risk factors, such as getting older, can't be changed. Starting at age 45, a man's risk of heart disease begins to rise, while a woman's risk begins to increase at age 55. Family history of early heart disease is another risk factor that can't be changed. If your father or brother had a heart attack before age 55, or if your mother or sister had one before age 65, you are more likely to develop heart disease yourself.

While certain risk factors can't be changed, it's important to realize that you do have control over many others. Regardless of your age or family history, or how serious your heart disease is, you can take steps to reduce your risk of a first or repeat heart attack. You can also manage other problems associated with heart disease, such as angina, heart failure, and arrhythmias.

It may be tempting to believe that doing just one healthy thing will be enough to control heart disease. For example, you may hope that if you walk or swim regularly, you can still eat a lot of fatty foods and stay safe. Not so. To reduce your risk of a heart attack and other complications, it is vital to make changes that address each risk factor you have. You can make the changes gradually, one at a time. But making them is very important.

While each risk factor may contribute to worsened heart disease, the more risk factors you have, the higher your risk. That's because risk factors tend to "gang up" and worsen each other's effects. For example, if you have high blood cholesterol and diabetes, your heart attack risk increases enormously. The message is clear: If you have heart disease, you must take immediate steps to reduce your risk of life-threatening medical problems. It's your heart and you have everything to gain from taking good care of it.

### You and Your Doctor: A Healthy Partnership

Your doctor can be an important partner in helping you manage heart disease. He or she may already have spoken with you about your heart disease risk factors, but if not, be sure to ask about how to control all of them to help prevent future problems. Here are some tips for establishing good, clear communication with your doctor.

**Speak up.** Tell your doctor that you want to keep your heart disease from getting worse and would like help in achieving that goal. Ask questions about your chances of having a first heart attack or a repeat heart attack, your risk of other heart complications, and ways to lower those risks. If you haven't done so already, ask for tests that will determine your personal risk factors.

**Be open.** When your doctor asks you questions, answer them as honestly and fully as you can. While certain topics may seem quite personal, discussing them openly can help your doctor work with you more effectively to manage your heart condition.

**Keep it simple.** If you don't understand something your doctor says, ask for an explanation in plain language. Be especially sure you understand how to make the lifestyle changes your doctor recommends, as well as why and how to take each medication you're given. If you're worried about understanding what the

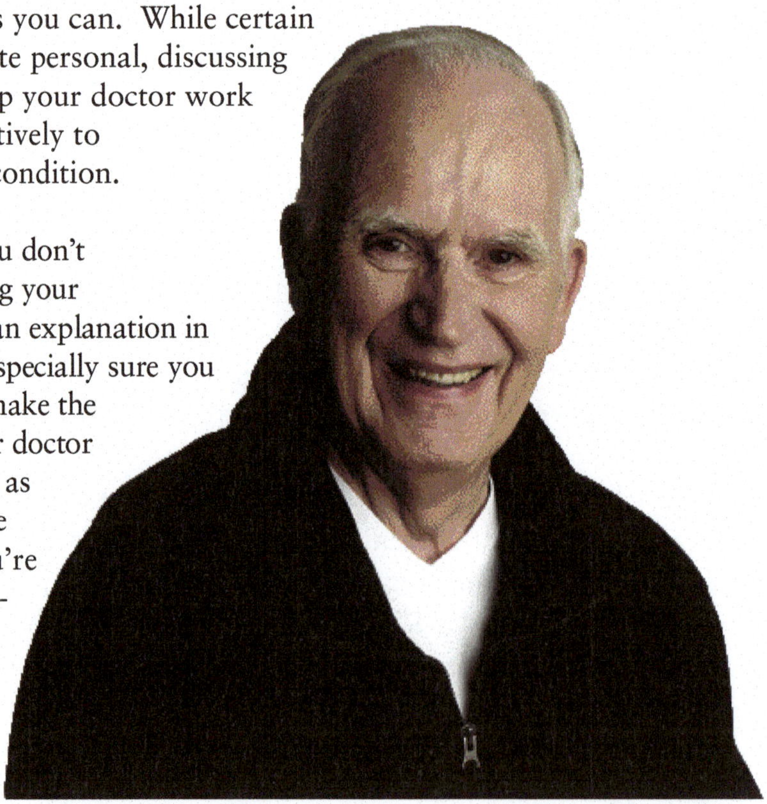

doctor says, or if you have trouble hearing, bring a friend or relative with you to your appointment. You may want to ask that person to write down the doctor's instructions for you.

## Major Risk Factors

A strong partnership with your doctor is an important first step in managing heart disease. But to make a lasting difference, you'll also need to learn more about the kinds of habits and conditions that can worsen heart disease and what you can do about them. What follows is a guide to major risk factors for heart disease, heart attack, and other heart problems, and steps you can take to control or eliminate them.

## Smoking

Smoking is the "leading cause of preventable death and disease in the United States," according to the Centers for Disease Control and Prevention. If you have heart disease and continue to smoke, your risk of having a heart attack is very high. If you live or work with others, your "secondhand" smoke can cause them numerous health problems, including a higher risk of heart attack—even if they don't smoke themselves. By the same token, if you have heart disease and live or work with someone who smokes, your own risk of heart attack goes up considerably.

Smoking puts stress on the heart in many ways. The nicotine in cigarettes constricts the coronary arteries, which raises blood pressure and forces the heart to work harder. Smoking also raises carbon monoxide levels and reduces oxygen levels in the blood. It's a double whammy: Smoking both increases the heart's need for oxygen and restricts the amount of oxygen it receives.

There is simply no safe way to smoke. Low-tar and low-nicotine cigarettes do not lessen the risks of a heart attack. The only safe and healthful course is not to smoke at all.

The good news is that quitting smoking will immediately and significantly reduce your risk of further heart disease complications. After a few days, once nicotine and carbon monoxide are cleared from your body, your blood pressure will go down and the levels of oxygen and carbon monoxide in your blood can return to normal. Within 1 year after quitting, your blood flow and breathing will be improved and your coughing and shortness of breath will be reduced.

Some people prefer to quit on their own, while others find group support helpful. A number of free or low-cost programs are available to help people stop smoking. They include classes offered by local chapters of the American Lung Association and the American Cancer Society. Other low-cost programs can be found through hospitals, health maintenance organizations (HMOs), workplaces, and community groups.

Also consider using a medicine that can help you stay off cigarettes. Some medications contain very small amounts of nicotine, which can help to lessen the urge to smoke. They include nicotine gum (available over the counter), a nicotine patch (available over the counter and by prescription), a nicotine inhaler (by prescription only), and a nicotine nasal spray (by prescription only). Another quitting aid is Bupropion SR, a medicine that contains no nicotine but reduces the craving for cigarettes. It is available only by prescription. While all of these medications can help people quit smoking, they are not safe for everyone. Talk with your doctor about whether you should try any of these medicines.

### High Blood Pressure

High blood pressure, also known as hypertension, is another major risk factor for heart disease and heart attack. For those who already have heart disease, high blood pressure raises heart attack risk even higher. Hypertension also raises the risks of stroke, congestive heart failure, and kidney disease.

Blood pressure is the amount of force exerted by the blood against the walls of the arteries. Everyone has to have some blood pressure, so that blood can get to all of the body's organs. Blood pressure is usually expressed as two numbers, such as 120/80, and is measured in millimeters of mercury (mmHg).

The first number is the systolic blood pressure, the amount of force produced when the heart beats. The second number, or diastolic blood pressure, is the pressure that exists in the arteries between heartbeats. The higher your blood pressure, the harder your heart has to work, and the more "wear and tear" on your blood vessels.

High blood pressure is often called the silent killer because it usually doesn't cause symptoms. According to a national survey, two-thirds of people with high blood pressure do not have it under control.

# Blood Pressure: How High Is High?

Your blood pressure category is determined by the higher number of either your systolic or your diastolic measurement. For example, if your systolic number is 115 but your diastolic number is 85, your category is prehypertension.

| | Systolic | | Diastolic |
|---|---|---|---|
| **Normal blood pressure** | Less than 120 | and | Less than 80 |
| **Prehypertension** | 120–139 | or | 80–89 |
| **High blood pressure** | 140 or higher | or | 90 or higher |

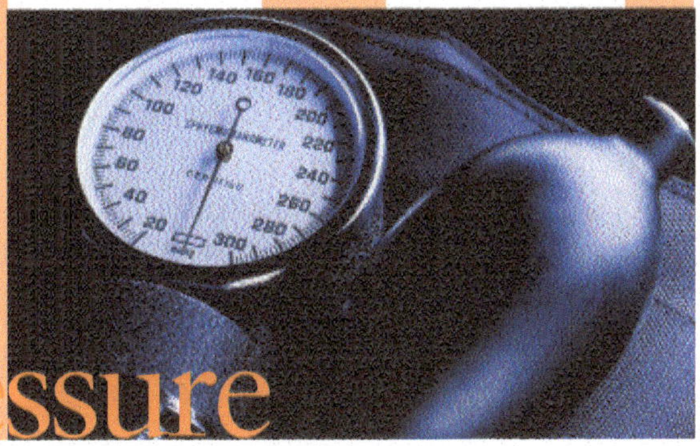


But you can take action to control high blood pressure, and thereby avoid many life-threatening disorders.

Your health care provider should check your blood pressure on several different days before deciding whether it is too high. Blood pressure is considered high when it stays at or above 140/90 over a period of time. However, if you have diabetes, it is important to keep your blood pressure below 130/80.

For those with heart disease, it is especially important to control blood pressure to reduce the risks of stroke and heart attack. Even if you don't have high blood pressure, it is important to avoid developing prehypertension, a condition that increases your risk for high blood pressure.

Be aware, too, that a high systolic blood pressure level (first number) is dangerous. If your systolic blood pressure is 140 or higher (or 130 or higher if you have diabetes), you are more likely to develop heart disease complications and other problems even if your diastolic blood pressure (second number) is in the normal range. High systolic blood pressure is high blood pressure. If you have this condition, you will need to take steps to control it. High blood pressure can be controlled in two ways: by changing your lifestyle and by taking medication.

**Changing your lifestyle.** If your blood pressure is not too high, you may be able to control it entirely by losing weight if you are overweight, getting regular physical activity, limiting the salt in your food, cutting down on alcohol, and changing your eating habits. A special eating plan called DASH can help to lower blood pressure. DASH stands for Dietary Approaches to Stop Hypertension. The DASH eating plan emphasizes fruits, vegetables, whole-grain foods, and low-fat dairy products. It is rich in magnesium, potassium, calcium, protein, and fiber, but low in saturated fat, *trans* fat, total fat, and cholesterol. (*Trans* fat is a harmful type of dietary fat that forms when vegetable oil is hardened.) The diet also limits red meat, sweets, and sugar-containing beverages.

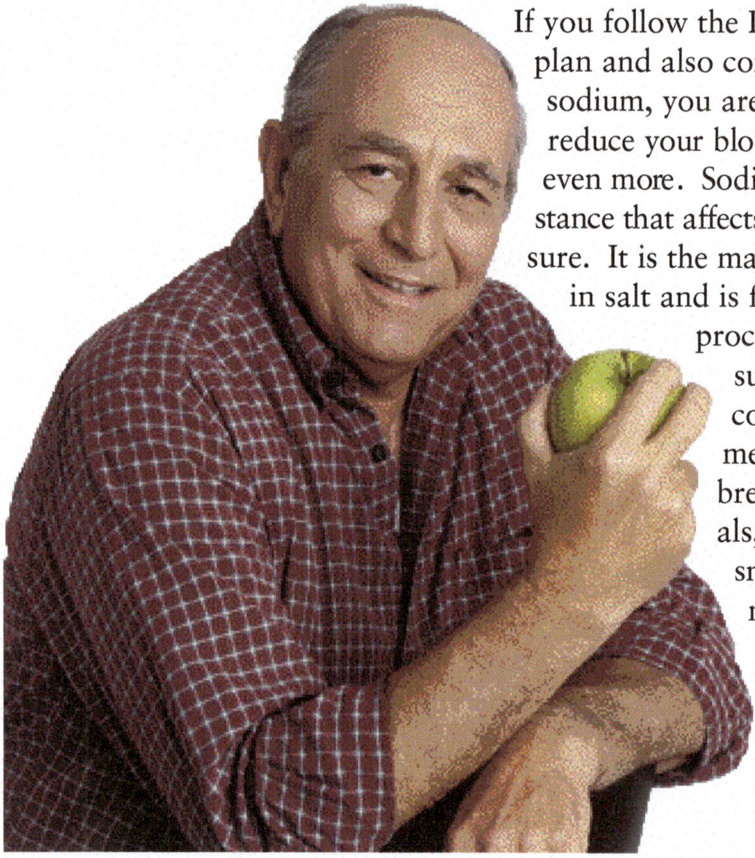

If you follow the DASH eating plan and also consume less sodium, you are likely to reduce your blood pressure even more. Sodium is a substance that affects blood pressure. It is the main ingredient in salt and is found in many processed foods, such as soups, convenience meals, some breads and cereals, and salted snacks. For more on the DASH eating plan and other changes you can make to lower and prevent high blood pressure, see the National Heart, Lung, and Blood Institute's (NHLBI's) Web page, Your Guide to Lowering High Blood Pressure, which is listed in the "To Learn More" section of this guidebook.

**Taking medication.** If your blood pressure remains high even after you make lifestyle changes, your doctor will probably prescribe medicine. Depending on your health needs, your doctor may prescribe medication from the start, along with changes in your living habits. One recent study found that diuretics (water pills) work better than newer drugs to treat high blood pressure in many people. Other research shows that using a diuretic can reduce the risk of death from heart and blood vessel diseases, especially among people with diabetes. Talk with your doctor about making one of your high blood pressure medications a diuretic.

Keep in mind that lifestyle changes will help the medicine work more effectively. In fact, if you are successful with the changes you make in your daily habits, you may be able to gradually reduce the amount of medication you take.

Taking medicine to lower blood pressure can reduce your risk of heart attack, stroke, congestive heart failure, and kidney disease. Be sure to take your blood pressure medicine exactly as your doctor has prescribed it. Before you leave your physician's office, make sure you understand the amount of medicine you are supposed to take each day, and the specific times of day you should be taking it. If you take a drug and notice any uncomfortable side effects, ask your doctor about changing the dosage or switching to another type of medicine.

### High Blood Cholesterol

The higher your blood cholesterol level, the greater your risk of having a heart attack. Because you have heart disease, your heart attack risk is already high, which means it is especially important to lower your cholesterol level. If you have diabetes as well as heart disease, your heart attack risk rises still higher. If you have both diseases, it is extremely important to take steps to keep both your cholesterol and your diabetes under control. Studies have proven that lowering cholesterol in people with heart disease reduces the risks for heart attack and death from heart disease and can actually prolong life.

*How Cholesterol Causes Heart Problems*

The body needs cholesterol to function normally. However, your body makes all the cholesterol it needs. Over time, extra cholesterol and fat circulating in the blood build up in the walls of the arteries that supply blood to the heart. This buildup, called plaque, makes the arteries narrower and narrower. If enough oxygen-rich blood cannot reach your heart, you may suffer chest pain, or angina. If the blood supply to a portion of the heart is completely cut off, the result is a heart attack. This usually happens when a cholesterol-rich plaque bursts, releasing the cholesterol into the bloodstream and causing a blood clot to form over the plaque.

*Types of Cholesterol*

Cholesterol travels in the blood in packages of fat (lipid) and protein called lipoproteins. Cholesterol packaged in low-density lipoprotein (LDL) is often called "bad" cholesterol, because too high a level of LDL in your blood can lead to blockages in your arteries. Another type of cholesterol is high-density lipoprotein (HDL) known as "good" cholesterol. That's because HDL helps to remove cholesterol from the body, preventing it from building up in your arteries.

*Getting Tested*

High blood cholesterol itself does not cause symptoms, so if your cholesterol level is too high, you may not be aware of it. So it is important to get your cholesterol levels checked regularly, especially if you have heart disease. A blood test called a "lipoprotein profile" measures the levels of all types of lipids, or fats, in your blood.

Total cholesterol is a measure of the cholesterol in all of your lipoproteins, including the bad cholesterol in LDL and the good cholesterol in HDL. Let's start with LDL levels. The higher your LDL number, the higher your risk of heart disease and heart attack. Knowing your LDL number is very important because it will determine the kind of treatment you may need. *The bottom line: If you have heart disease, reducing LDL cholesterol will reduce your risk of heart attack and can actually lengthen your life.*

Your HDL number tells a different story. The lower your HDL number, the higher your risk of heart disease and heart attack. Your lipoprotein profile test will also measure levels of triglycerides, which are another fatty substance in the blood.

*HDL Cholesterol Level*

An HDL cholesterol level of less than 40 mg/dL is a major risk factor for heart disease and heart attack. An HDL level of 60 mg/dL or higher is somewhat protective.

*Your LDL Goal*

The main goal of cholesterol-lowering treatment is to lower your LDL level enough to reduce your risk of heart attack. Reaching this goal is critically important if you have heart disease. The higher your risk category, the lower your LDL goal will be. For most people with heart disease or diabetes who are at high risk for heart attack, the goal of cholesterol-lowering treatment is an LDL level below 100 mg/dL.

| If You Are in This Risk Category | Your LDL Goal |
|---|---|
| High risk | Is less than 100 mg/dL* |
| Very high risk | May be less than 70 mg/dL* |

* *Cholesterol levels are measured in milligrams (mg) of cholesterol per deciliter (dL) of blood.*

*Even Lower May Be Better*

Because recent studies show a direct relationship between lower LDL cholesterol and reduced risk for heart attack, doctors now may prescribe more intensive cholesterol-lowering treatment for people at very high risk for a heart attack. For example, those with heart disease as well as diabetes, or those who have just had a heart attack, may have their LDL goal level lowered by their doctors to less than 70 mg/dL.

*A Special Type of Risk*

Nearly one-quarter of Americans have a group of risk factors known as metabolic syndrome. This condition is usually caused by overweight or obesity, and by not getting enough physical activity. If you have heart disease, this cluster of risk factors greatly increases your risk of heart attack regardless of your LDL cholesterol level. You have metabolic syndrome if you have three or more of the following conditions:

- A waist measurement of 35 inches or more for a woman, and 40 inches or more for a man

What's Your Number?

# Blood Cholesterol Levels for Preventing Heart Disease

| Total Cholesterol Level | Category |
|---|---|
| Less than 200* | Desirable |
| 200–239 | Borderline high |
| 240 and above | High |

| LDL Cholesterol Level | Category |
|---|---|
| Less than 100[†] | Optimal |
| 100–129 | Near optimal |
| 130–159 | Borderline high |
| 160–189 | High |
| 190 and above | Very high |

**All numbers refer to milligrams of cholesterol per deciliter (mg/dL) of blood.*

*† These cholesterol numbers and levels and goals are for the prevention of heart disease. If you already have heart disease, your LDL goal is less than 100 mg/dL. (See "Your LDL Goal" and "Even Lower May Be Better," page 20.)*

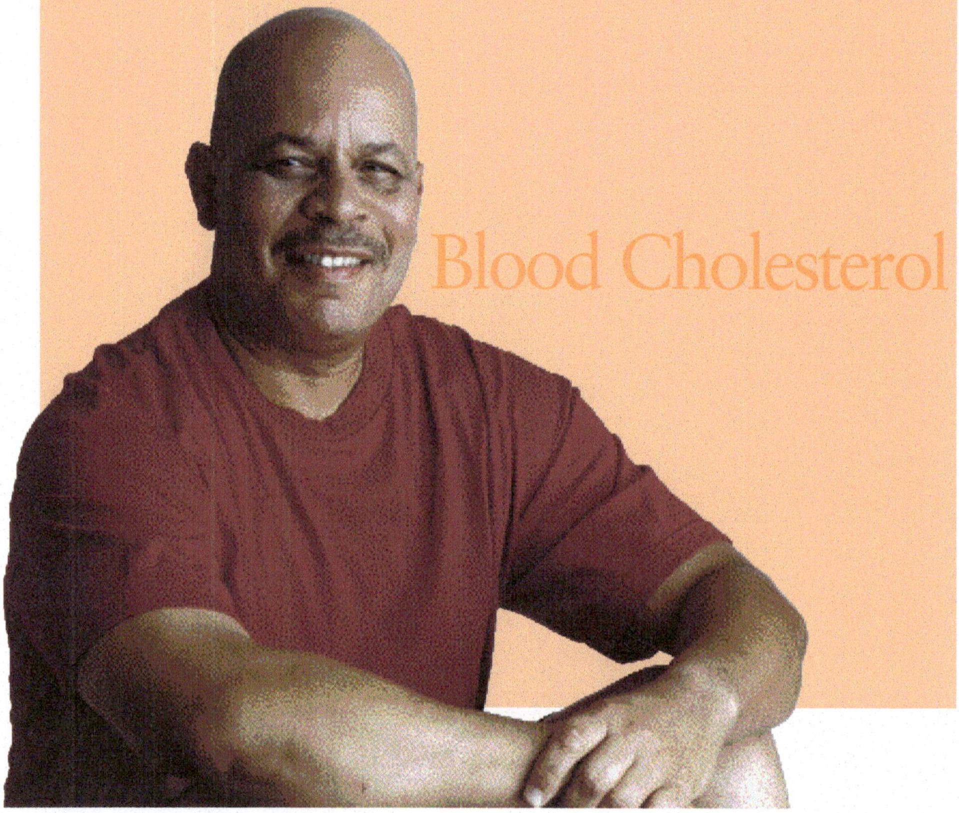

- Triglycerides of 150 mg/dL or more
- An HDL level of less than 50 mg/dL for a woman, and less than 40 mg/dL for a man
- Blood pressure of 130/85 mmHg or more (either number counts)
- Blood sugar of 100 mg/dL or more

If you have metabolic syndrome in addition to heart disease, your doctor will assess your risk factors and decide whether an LDL goal of less than 70 is right for you (especially if your triglycerides are 200 or higher, and your HDL is less than 40). You should make a particularly strong effort to reach and maintain your LDL goal. If you are overweight or obese, you will also need to take steps to lose weight by cutting back on high-calorie foods and increasing physical activity. Becoming physically active will help you correct the risk factors of the metabolic syndrome even if you don't need to lose weight.

*How To Lower Your LDL*

There are two main ways to lower your LDL cholesterol—through lifestyle changes alone, or through lifestyle changes combined with medication.

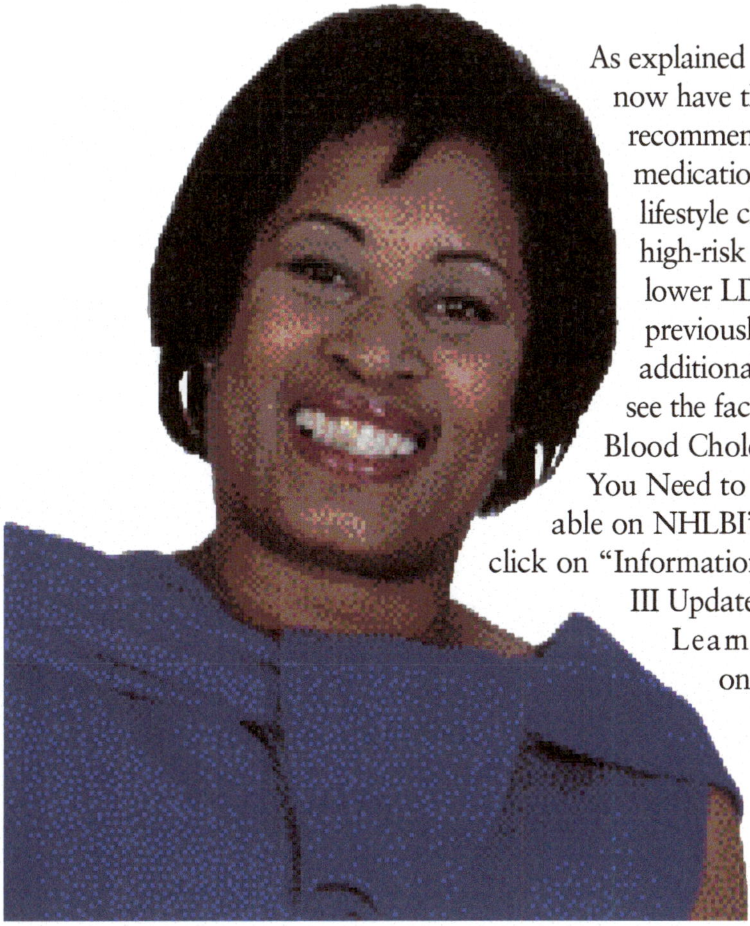

As explained before, doctors now have the option to recommend cholesterol medication, as well as lifestyle changes, to high-risk patients at lower LDL levels than previously advised. For additional information, see the fact sheet, "High Blood Cholesterol: What You Need to Know," available on NHLBI's Web site and click on "Information on the ATP III Update." (See "To Learn More" on page 64.)

**Lifestyle changes.** One important treatment approach is called TLC, which stands for Therapeutic Lifestyle Changes. This treatment helps to reduce LDL cholesterol through a diet that is low in saturated fat (the main dietary culprit that raises blood cholesterol), *trans* fat, and dietary cholesterol, as well as through regular physical activity and weight management.

Everyone who needs to lower LDL cholesterol should use this TLC program. Maintaining a healthy weight and getting regular physical activity are especially important for people who have metabolic syndrome. Adopt the TLC approach and you'll lower your chances of having a heart attack and other heart disease complications. Both the TLC eating plan and DASH eating plan recommend foods that are lower in saturated fats, *trans* fats, and cholesterol, such as vegetables and fruits, whole grains, low-fat milk products; and lean meats, fish, or poultry. The TLC plan simply puts more emphasis on decreasing saturated fat, *trans* fat, and cholesterol to lower blood cholesterol levels.

For a complete description of the TLC program, see the section on "Therapeutic Lifestyle Changes," available on NHLBI's Web site at www.nhlbi.nih.gov/chd/. This Web page also includes tips on shopping, cooking, and eating out for those who need to lower their cholesterol.

**Medication.** If your LDL level is above your goal, your doctor will prescribe medications at the same time you are making lifestyle changes. If you do need medication, be sure to use it along with the TLC approach. This will keep the dose of medicine as low as possible, and will lower your risk in other ways as well. You will also need to control all of your other heart disease risk factors, including high blood pressure, diabetes, and smoking.

## Overweight and Obesity

If you have heart disease and are overweight or obese (extremely overweight), your risks of heart attack and other heart complications rise sharply. This is true even if you have no other risk factors. Being overweight or obese also increases your chances of developing other major risk factors for heart disease and heart attack, such as diabetes, high blood pressure, and high blood cholesterol. Overall, obese people are more likely to die of heart disease than normal-

# Are You at a Healthy Weight?

Here is a chart for men and women that gives the BMI for various heights and weights*

**BODY MASS INDEX**

| | 21 | 22 | 23 | 24 | 25 | 26 | 27 | 28 | 29 | 30 | 31 |
|---|---|---|---|---|---|---|---|---|---|---|---|
| 4'10" | 100 | 105 | 110 | 115 | 119 | 124 | 129 | 134 | 138 | 143 | 148 |
| 5'0" | 107 | 112 | 118 | 123 | 128 | 133 | 138 | 143 | 148 | 153 | 158 |
| 5'1" | 111 | 116 | 122 | 127 | 132 | 137 | 143 | 148 | 153 | 158 | 164 |
| 5'3" | 118 | 124 | 130 | 135 | 141 | 146 | 152 | 158 | 163 | 169 | 175 |
| 5'5" | 126 | 132 | 138 | 144 | 150 | 156 | 162 | 168 | 174 | 180 | 186 |
| 5'7" | 134 | 140 | 146 | 153 | 159 | 166 | 172 | 178 | 185 | 191 | 198 |
| 5'9" | 142 | 149 | 155 | 162 | 169 | 176 | 182 | 189 | 196 | 203 | 209 |
| 5'11" | 150 | 157 | 165 | 172 | 179 | 186 | 193 | 200 | 208 | 215 | 222 |
| 6'1" | 159 | 166 | 174 | 182 | 189 | 197 | 204 | 212 | 219 | 227 | 235 |
| 6'3" | 168 | 176 | 184 | 192 | 200 | 208 | 216 | 224 | 232 | 240 | 248 |

** Weight is measured with underwear but not shoes.*

### What Does Your BMI Mean?

**Categories:**

**Normal weight: BMI =18.5–24.9.** Good for you! Try not to gain weight.

**Overweight: BMI = 25–29.9.** Do not gain any weight, especially if your waist measurement is high. You need to lose weight if you have two or more risk factors for heart disease and are overweight, or have a high waist measurement.

**Obese: BMI = 30 or greater.** You need to lose weight. Lose weight slowly—about 1/2 to 2 pounds a week. See your doctor or nutritionist if you need help.

*Source: Clinical Guidelines on the Identification, Evaluation and Treatment of Overweight and Obesity in Adults: The Evidence Report; National Heart, Lung, and Blood Institute, in cooperation with the National Institute of Diabetes and Digestive and Kidney Diseases, National Institutes of Health; NIH Publication 98-4083; June 1998.*

weight individuals. The bottom line: Maintaining a healthy weight is a necessary part of controlling heart disease.

*Should You Choose To Lose?*

Do you need to lose weight to help protect your heart? You can find out by taking these simple steps.

**Step 1: Get your number.** Take a look at the chart on page 24. You'll see that your weight in relation to your height gives you a number called a body mass index (BMI). A BMI from 18.5 to 24.9 indicates a normal weight. A person with a BMI from 25 to 29.9 is overweight, while someone with a BMI of 30 or higher is obese. Those in the overweight and obese categories have a higher risk of heart attack and other heart disease complications. The higher your BMI, the greater your risk.

**Step 2: Take out a tape measure.** The second step is to take your waist measurement. For women, a waist measurement of over 35 inches increases the risk of heart attack, as well as the risks of high blood pressure, diabetes, and other serious health conditions. For men, a waist measurement of more than 40 inches raises these risks. To measure your waist correctly, stand and place a tape measure around your middle, just above your hipbones. Measure your waist just after you breathe out.

Once you've taken these steps—found out your BMI and taken your waist measurement—you can use the information to decide whether you need to take off pounds. While you should talk with your doctor about whether you should lose weight, keep these guidelines in mind:

- If you have heart disease and are overweight or obese, you should lose weight.
- If you have heart disease and a high waist measurement (over 35 inches for a woman; over 40 inches for a man), you should lose weight.
- If you have two or more risk factors for heart disease and are overweight or obese, you should lose weight.
- If your weight and waist measurement are in the normal range, keep them that way! Avoid becoming overweight or adding extra inches around your middle.

*Lose a Little, Win a Lot*

If you need to lose weight, here's some good news: A small weight loss—just 5 to 10 percent of your current weight—can help to lower the risks of heart attack and other serious medical disorders. The best way to take off pounds is to do so gradually, by getting more physical activity and eating a balanced diet that is lower in calories and fat. For some people at very high risk, medication also may be necessary. To develop a weight-loss or weight-maintenance program that works well for you, consult with your doctor, registered dietitian, or qualified nutritionist. For ideas on how to lose weight safely and keep it off, see the section on "Aim for a Healthy Weight," available on NHLBI's Web site. (See "To Learn More" on page 64.)

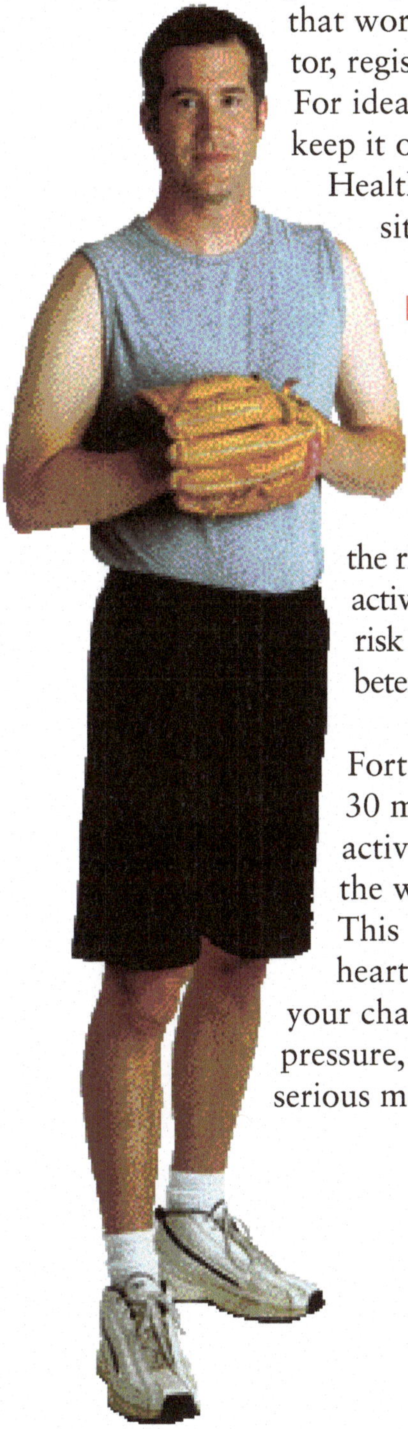

## Physical Inactivity

Many of us put off getting regular physical activity—and then put it off some more. But to protect our hearts, we must keep moving. For people with heart disease, physical inactivity greatly increases the risk of worsened disease. Lack of physical activity also contributes to other heart disease risk factors, such as high blood pressure, diabetes, and overweight.

Fortunately, research shows that as little as 30 minutes of moderate-intensity physical activity on most and preferably all days of the week helps to protect heart health. This level of activity can reduce your risk of heart disease complications, as well as lessen your chances of having a stroke, high blood pressure, diabetes, colon cancer, and other serious medical disorders.

Examples of moderate activity are taking a brisk walk, light weight-lifting, dancing, raking leaves, washing a car, housecleaning, or gardening. If you prefer, you can divide your 30-minute activity into shorter periods of at least 10 minutes each. If you have heart disease or another type of heart problem, be sure to see your doctor before starting a program of regular physical activity. To find out about easy, enjoyable ways to boost your activity level, see the "Guide to Physical Activity" page on NHLBI's Web site at: www.nhlbi.nih.gov/health/public/heart/obesity/lose_wt/phy_act.htm.

### Diabetes

If you have diabetes, you have about the same high risk for heart attack as someone who has heart disease itself. Those who have heart disease and diabetes have an even higher risk for heart attack than those who have either heart disease or diabetes alone. Up to three-quarters of those who have diabetes die of some type of heart or blood vessel disease. However, if you have diabetes, there is much you can do to prevent the complications of this condition.

The type of diabetes that most commonly develops in adulthood is called type 2 diabetes. In this type of diabetes, the pancreas makes insulin but the body cannot use it properly and gradually loses the ability to produce it. Type 2 diabetes is a serious disease. In addition to increasing the risks for heart disease and heart attack, diabetes is the #1 cause of kidney failure, blindness, and lower limb amputation in adults. Diabetes can also lead to nerve damage, difficulties in fighting infection, and delayed wound healing.

A major risk factor for type 2 diabetes is overweight, especially having extra weight around the waist. Other risk factors include physical inactivity and a family history of diabetes. Type 2 diabetes is more common among American Indians, Hispanic Americans, Asian Americans, and Pacific Islanders. Women who have had diabetes during pregnancy (gestational diabetes), or who gave birth to a baby weighing more than 9 pounds, are also more likely to develop type 2 diabetes in later life.

Symptoms of diabetes may include fatigue, nausea, frequent urination, unusual thirst, weight loss, blurred vision, frequent infections, and slow healing of sores. But type 2 diabetes develops gradually and sometimes has no symptoms. In fact, nearly 6 million Americans who have this serious disease are not aware of it. Even if you have no symptoms, if you are overweight or have any other risk factors for type 2 diabetes, ask your doctor about getting tested for it. You have diabetes if your fasting blood glucose level is 126 mg/dL or higher.

If you have diabetes, controlling your blood glucose (blood sugar) levels will help to prevent complications. Because diabetes is so strongly linked with heart disease and heart attack, you must manage your diabetes very carefully. It is also especially important to control your blood pressure and cholesterol levels. (See "The ABCs of Diabetes Control" on the next page.) Recommended levels of blood pressure and blood cholesterol are lower for people with diabetes than for most others. Not smoking, getting regular physical activity, and taking aspirin daily (if your doctor recommends it) also are important ways to prevent heart disease complications if you have diabetes.

Some people do not yet have diabetes, but are at high risk for developing the disease. About 40 percent of Americans aged 40–74 have a condition known as prediabetes, where blood glucose levels are higher than normal but not yet in the diabetic range. Prediabetes is defined as a fasting blood glucose level of 100–125 mg/dL.

If you have heart disease and also have prediabetes, it is extremely important to improve your blood glucose levels in order to prevent the development of diabetes. The good news: A recent study shows that many people with prediabetes can prevent or delay diabetes by eating a lower fat, lower calorie diet and getting 30 minutes of moderate physical activity at least 5 days per week.

# What Else Affects Heart Disease?

A number of other factors also contribute to heart disease, including certain health conditions, medicines, and other substances. Here is what you need to know:

## Stress

Stress is linked to heart disease in a number of ways. Research shows that the most commonly reported "trigger" for a heart attack is an emotionally upsetting event, particularly one involving anger. In addition, some common ways of coping with stress, such as overeating, heavy drinking, and smoking are clearly bad for your heart.

The good news is that sensible health habits can have a protective effect. For people with heart disease, regular physical activity not only relieves stress but also can directly lower the risk of heart disease complications. Participating in a stress management program can help to prevent recurrent heart attacks and repeat heart procedures. Good relationships count, too. Developing strong personal ties can help to improve recovery after a heart attack.

Much remains to be learned about the connections between stress and heart disease, but a few things are clear. Staying physically active, developing a wide circle of supportive people in your life, and sharing your feelings and concerns with them can help you to be happier and live longer.

## Alcohol

Recent research suggests that moderate drinkers are less likely to develop heart disease than people who don't drink any alcohol or who drink too much. Small amounts of alcohol may help protect against heart disease by raising levels of "good" HDL cholesterol.

If you are a nondrinker, this is not a recommendation to start drinking. Moreover, if you already have heart disease, you should be especially careful about using alcohol. Talk with your doctor about the impact of alcohol use on heart disease and other health conditions you may have. If you do decide to drink, moderation is the key. Moderate drinking is defined as no more than one drink per day for women, and no more than two drinks per day for men.

Heavy drinking is hazardous to your heart. More than three drinks per day can raise blood pressure. Meanwhile, binge drinking can contribute to stroke and doubles the risk of dying after a heart attack. Too much alcohol also can damage the heart muscle, leading to heart failure. Heavy drinking also raises the risk of developing metabolic syndrome, a cluster of heart disease risk factors that is particularly dangerous for people who already have heart disease.

### Sleep Apnea

Sleep apnea is a serious disorder in which a person briefly and repeatedly stops breathing for short periods of time during sleep. People with untreated sleep apnea are more likely to have a heart attack, stroke, high blood pressure, and congestive heart failure.

Sleep apnea tends to develop in middle age, and men are twice as likely as women to have the condition. Other factors that increase risk are overweight and obesity, smoking, use of alcohol or sleeping pills, and a family history of sleep apnea. Symptoms include heavy snoring and gasping or choking during sleep, along with extreme daytime sleepiness.

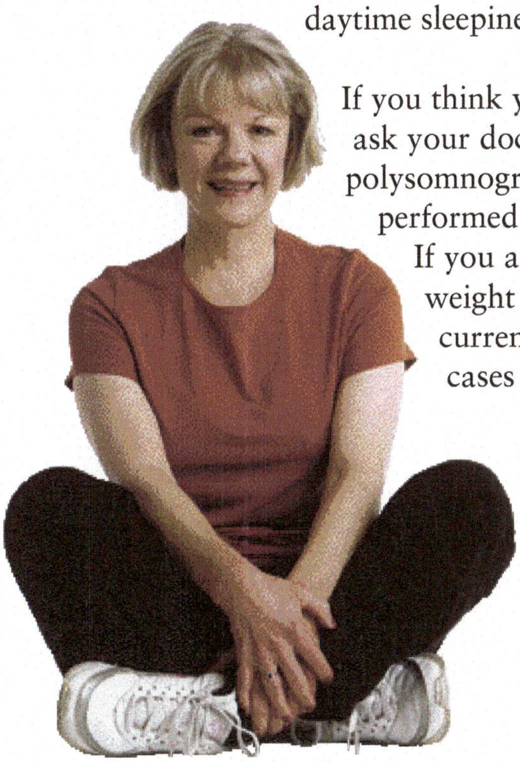

If you think you might have sleep apnea, ask your doctor for a test called polysomnography, which is usually performed overnight in a sleep center. If you are overweight, even a small weight loss—10 percent of your current weight—can relieve mild cases of sleep apnea.

Other self-help treatments include quitting smoking and avoiding alcohol and sleeping pills. Sleeping on your side rather than on your back also may help. Some people benefit from a mechanical device that helps to maintain a regular breathing pattern by increasing air pressure through the nasal passages. For very serious cases, surgery may be needed.

### Menopausal Hormone Therapy

Until recently, it was thought that menopausal hormone therapy could lower the risks of heart attack and stroke for women with heart disease. But research now shows that **women with heart disease should *not* take this medication.** Menopausal hormone therapy can involve the use of an estrogen-plus-progestin medicine or an estrogen-alone medicine. Studies on each type of medicine show that:

- Estrogen-plus-progestin medication increases the risk of heart attack during the first few years of use, and also increases the risks of stroke, blood clots, and breast cancer.
- Estrogen-only medication increases the risks of stroke and venous thrombosis (a blood clot that usually occurs in one of the deep veins of the legs). Estrogen-only medicine will not prevent heart attacks.

If you have heart disease and are currently taking or considering taking menopausal hormone therapy, talk with your doctor about safer medicines for controlling heart disease, for preventing osteoporosis, and/or for relieving menopausal symptoms.

### C-Reactive Protein (CRP)

An elevated level of this blood protein is a sign of inflammation. Studies indicate that people with low CRP levels tend to have a slower progression of heart disease as well as fewer heart attacks and deaths from heart disease, than those with higher levels of the protein. Whether CRP plays a role in causing heart disease is not known.

A high-sensitivity CRP blood test can measure the level of this protein in your blood. Elevated levels can be lowered with the same statin medications that lower LDL cholesterol. Getting more physical activity, losing weight if you are overweight, eating a healthy diet, and quitting smoking will also reduce CRP levels.

# Getting Help for a Heart Attack

For many people, the first symptom of heart disease is a heart attack. That means everyone should know how to identify the symptoms of a heart attack and how to get immediate medical help. Ideally, treatment should start within 1 hour of the first symptoms. Recognizing the warning signs and getting help quickly can save your life.

## Know the Warning Signs

Not all heart attacks begin with sudden, crushing pain, as is often shown on TV or in the movies. Many heart attacks start slowly with mild pain or discomfort. The most common warning signs are:

- **Chest discomfort.** Most heart attacks involve discomfort in the center of the chest that lasts for more than a few minutes. It may feel like uncomfortable pressure, squeezing, fullness, or pain. The discomfort can be mild or severe, and it may come and go.
- **Discomfort in other areas of the upper body,** including one or both arms, the back, neck, jaw, or stomach.
- **Shortness of breath.** This symptom may occur with or without chest discomfort.
- **Other signs include nausea,** light-headedness, or breaking out in a cold sweat.

## Get Help Quickly

If you think that you or someone else may be having a heart attack, you must act quickly to prevent disability or death, and to get the most benefit from current treatments. Wait no more than a few minutes—5 at most—before calling 9–1–1.

It is important to call 9–1–1 because emergency medical personnel can begin treatment even before you get to the hospital. They also have the equipment and training to start your heart beating again if it stops. Calling 9–1–1 quickly can save your life.

Even if you're not sure you're having a heart attack, call 9–1–1 if your symptoms last up to 5 minutes. If your symptoms stop completely in less than 5 minutes, you should still call your doctor right away.

You must also act at once because hospitals have clot-dissolving medicines and other artery-opening treatments that can stop a heart attack if given quickly. These treatments work best when given within the first hour after a heart attack starts.

When you get to the hospital, don't be afraid to speak up for what you need—or bring someone who can speak up for you. Ask for tests that can determine if you are having a heart attack. Commonly given initial tests include an electrocardiogram (EKG or ECG) and a cardiac blood test (to check for heart damage). You have the right to be thoroughly examined for a possible heart attack. If you are having a heart attack, you have the right to immediate treatment to help stop the attack.

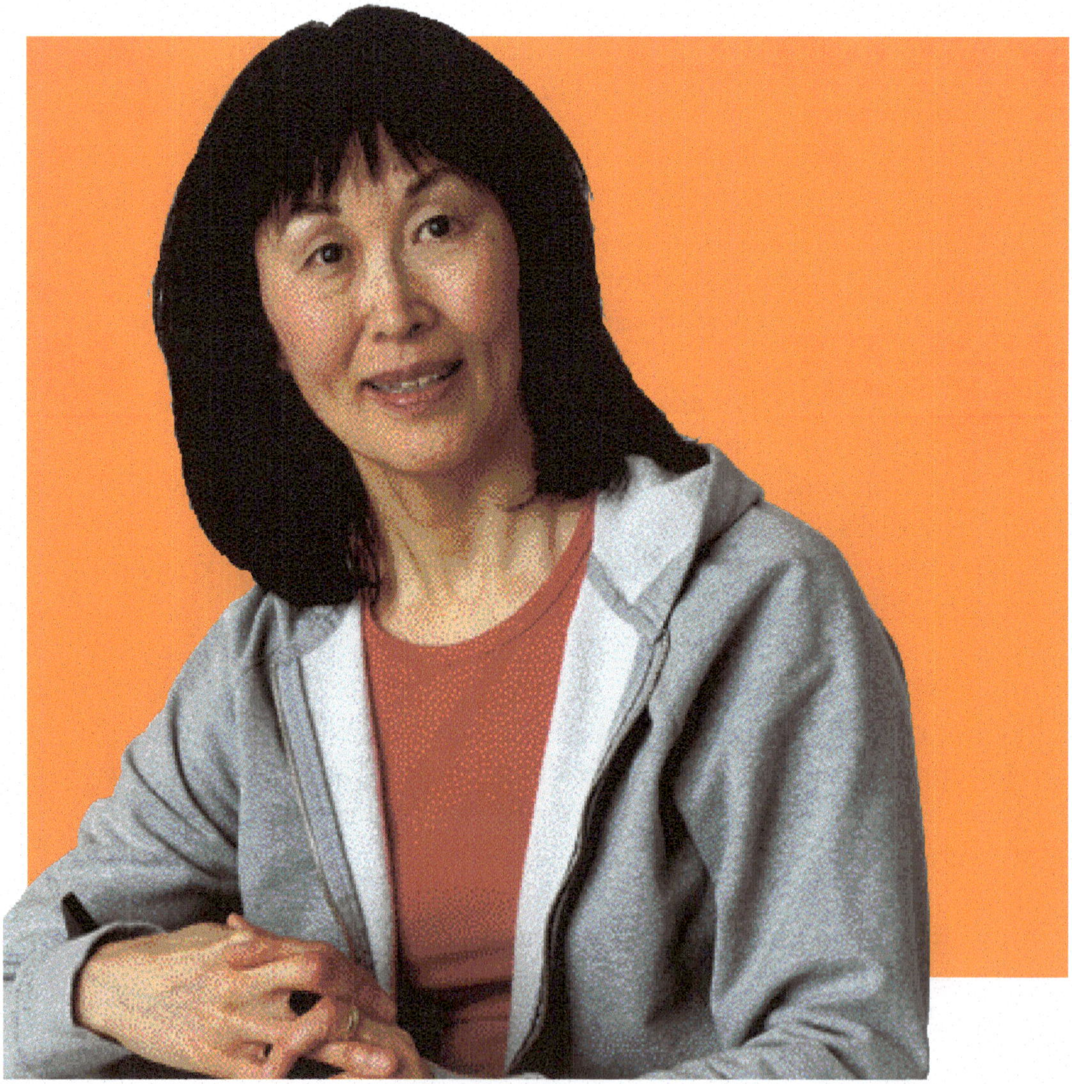

### Plan Ahead

Nobody plans on having a heart attack. But just as many people have a plan in case of fire, it is important to make a plan to deal with a possible heart attack. Taking the following steps can preserve your health—and your life.

- Learn the heart attack warning signs "by heart."
- Talk with family and friends about the warning signs and the need to call 9–1–1 quickly.
- Talk with your doctor about your risk factors for heart attack and how to reduce them.
- Write out a "heart attack survival plan" that includes important medical information and keep it handy. (Use the accompanying box on page 50 as a guide.)
- Arrange in advance to have someone else care for your children or other dependents in an emergency.

## Delay Can Be Deadly

Most people who have a heart attack wait too long to seek medical help—and that can be a fatal mistake. Some delay because they don't understand the symptoms of a heart attack and think that what they're feeling is due to something else. Others put off getting help because they don't want to worry others or "cause a scene," especially if their symptoms turn out to be a false alarm. Women are especially likely to delay. A large study of heart attack patients found that, on average, women waited 22 minutes longer than men did before going to the hospital.

Don't wait. When you're facing something as serious as a possible heart attack, it's much better to be safe than sorry. Waiting too long can cause permanent disability or death. If you have any symptoms of a possible heart attack that last up to 5 minutes, call 9–1–1 right away.

Don't Delay

# Heart Attack Survival Plan

Fill out the form below and make several copies. Keep one copy near your home phone, where you can easily see it. Keep another copy at work, and a third copy in your wallet or purse.

**Information To Share With Emergency Medical Personnel and Hospital Staff**

Medicines you are taking:

________________________________________

________________________________________

________________________________________

________________________________________

________________________________________

Medicines you are allergic to:

________________________________________

________________________________________

________________________________________

________________________________________

________________________________________

**How To Contact Your Doctor**

If symptoms stop completely in less than 5 minutes, you should still call your doctor right away.

Phone number during office hours:____________________

Phone number after office hours:____________________

**Person To Contact If You Go to the Hospital**

Name:____________________________________

Home phone number:____________________________

Work phone number:____________________________

Survival Plan

# 7 Strategies to Live a **Heart-Healthy** Lifestyle

When you choose healthy behaviors, you can lower your heart disease risk while also preventing other **serious chronic conditions** like **type 2 diabetes** and some kinds of **cancer**.

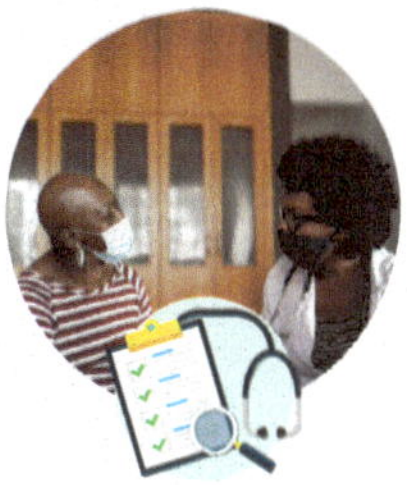

**1**

### Learn Your Health History

Know your risks and talk to your family and doctor about your health history.

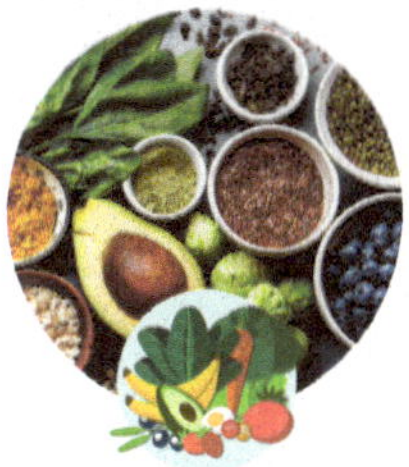

**2**

### Eat a Healthy Diet

Make healthy food choices like more fruits, vegetables, whole grains, lean meats, and low-fat dairy products. Eat less salt, saturated fat, and added sugar.

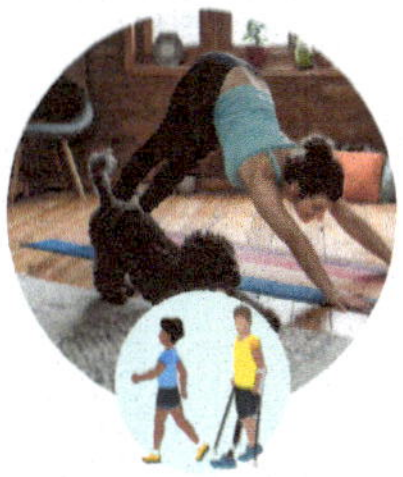

**3**

### Move More, Sit Less

Get at least 150 minutes of moderate-intensity aerobic activity every week, plus muscle-strengthening activities at least 2 days a week.

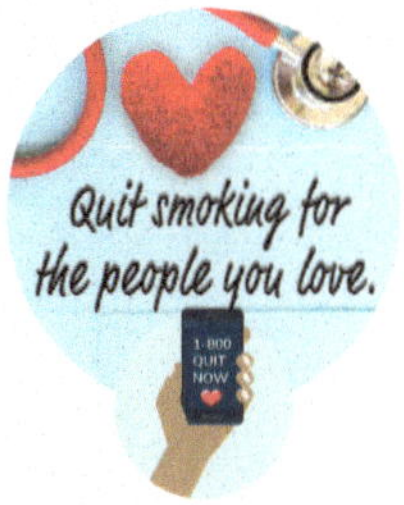
Quit smoking for the people you love.
1-800 QUIT NOW

**4**

### Quit Smoking!

Call 1-800-QUIT-NOW for free help and take the first step on your journey to quit.

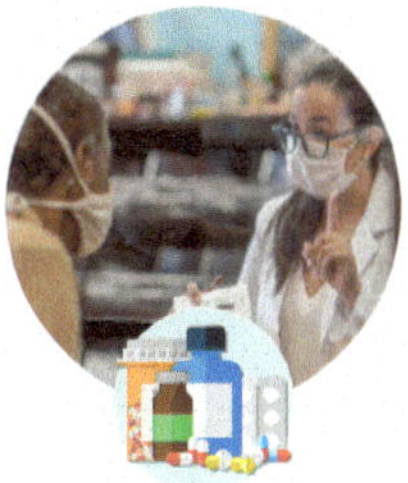

**5**

### Take Medicines as Directed

If you take medicine to treat high cholesterol, high blood pressure, or diabetes, follow your doctor's instructions carefully. Always ask questions if you don't understand something. Never stop taking your medicine without talking to your doctor, nurse, or pharmacist.

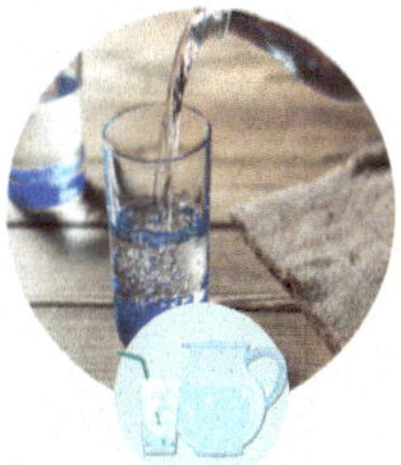

**6**

### Choose Your Drinks Wisely

Substitute water for sugary drinks to reduce calories. If you drink alcohol, do so in moderation by limiting consumption to no more than 1 drink a day for women (2 for men) on days that alcohol is consumed.

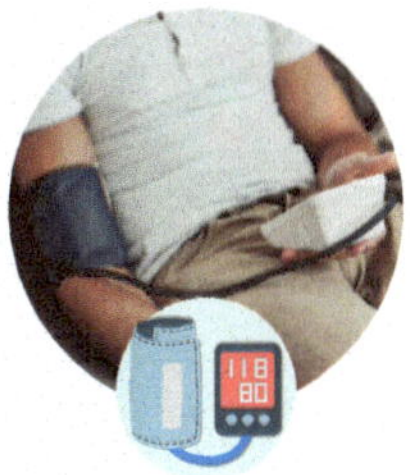

**7**

### Monitor Your Blood Pressure at Home

Self-measured blood pressure monitors are easy and safe to use, and your doctor can show you how to use one if you need help.

---

Learn more about keeping your heart healthy by visiting www.cdc.gov/heartdisease/prevention.htm.

Centers for Disease Control and Prevention
National Center for Chronic Disease Prevention and Health Promotion
@CDCChronic | www.cdc.gov/chronicdisease

# Infective Endocarditis

**Infective endocarditis** is a life-threatening inflammation of the heart's chambers and valves that can be difficult and expensive to treat.

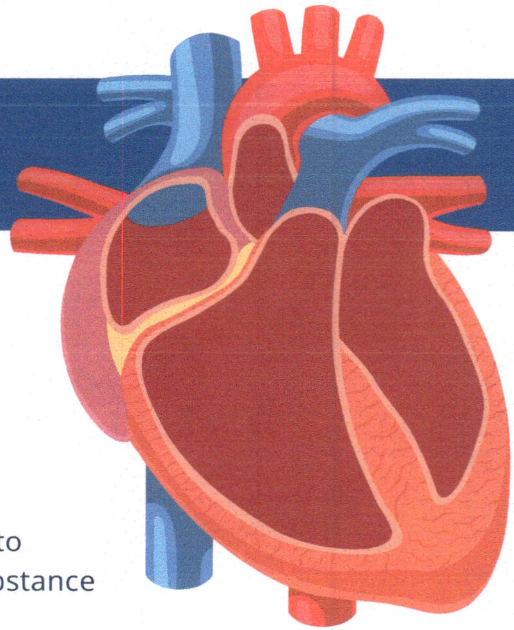

Like hepatitis and HIV, **infective endocarditis** can be caused by using needles that are not sterile.

**Infective endocarditis** associated with injection drug use can be **prevented** by:

- Providing **harm reduction services,** including access to sterile injection equipment and promoting safer injection practices
- Increasing access to **treatment** for substance use disorders

*Source: CDC, NHLBI*

NIH National Institute on Drug Abuse

nida.nih.gov

A TREATMENT IMPROVEMENT PROTOCOL

# Managing Chronic Pain in Adults With or in Recovery From Substance Use Disorders

# TIP 54

DEPARTMENT OF HEALTH & HUMAN SERVICES · USA

Substance Abuse and Mental Health Services Administration

SAMHSA

www.samhsa.gov • 1-877-SAMHSA-7 (1-877-726-4727)

# 1 Introduction

**IN THIS CHAPTER**



## Chronic Pain Impact

Chronic noncancer pain (CNCP) is common in the general population as well as in people who have a substance use disorder (SUD) (Exhibit 1-1). Chronic pain is not harmless; it has physiological, social, and psychological dimensions that can seriously harm health, functioning, and well-being. As a multidimensional condition with both objective and subjective aspects, CNCP is difficult to assess and treat. Although CNCP can be managed, it usually cannot be completely eliminated. When patients with CNCP have comorbid SUD or are recovering from SUD, a complex condition becomes even more difficult to manage.

**Exhibit 1-1 Statistics on Substance Use and Chronic Pain in the United States**

| Category | Statistic |
|---|---|
| Chronic pain patients who may have addictive disorders | 32% (Chelminski et al., 2005) |
| People ages 20 and older who report pain that lasted more than 3 months | 56% (National Center for Health Statistics, 2006) |
| People experiencing disabling pain in the previous year | 36% (Portenoy, Ugarte, Fuller, & Haas, 2004) |
| People ages 65 and older who experience pain that has lasted more than 12 months | 57% (National Center for Health Statistics, 2006) |
| Civilian, noninstitutionalized U.S. residents ages 12 and older who report nonmedical use* of pain relievers in past year | 5% (Substance Abuse and Mental Health Services Administration [SAMHSA], 2007) |
| People ages 12 and older who report that they initiated illegal drug use with pain relievers | 19% (SAMHSA, 2008) |
| People with opioid addiction who report chronic pain | 29–60% (Peles, Schreiber, Gordon, & Adelson, 2005; Potter, Shiffman, & Weiss, 2008; Rosenblum et al., 2003; Sheu et al., 2008) |

**Nonmedical use* is use for purposes other than that for which the medication was prescribed.

## Audience

This Treatment Improvement Protocol (TIP) is for primary care providers who treat or are likely to treat adult patients with or in recovery from SUDs who present with CNCP. Given the prevalence of CNCP in the population, this audience includes virtually all primary care providers. Addiction specialists, psychiatrists, nurses, and other clinicians may find information here that will help them ensure that their patients with CNCP receive adequate pain treatment. By providing a shared basic understanding of and a common language for these two chronic conditions, this TIP facilitates cooperation and communication between healthcare professionals treating pain and those treating addiction.

## Purpose

This TIP equips clinicians with practical guidance and tools for treating CNCP in adults with histories of SUDs. It does not describe how to treat SUDs or other behavioral health disorders in patients with CNCP; however, it provides readers with information about SUD assessments and referrals for further evaluation. For patients with histories of SUDs, the most controversial and possibly hazardous pain treatment in widespread use is opioid treatment. For this reason, this topic receives significant attention in Chapters 3 and 4.

## Definitions

Many terms important to the treatment of CNCP in people with SUDs are used inconsistently. Clinicians should not assume that their definitions of *addiction*, *CNCP*, *physical dependence*, *recovery*, *tolerance*, or other terms are shared by others, especially by patients and their families.

It is especially important that clinicians clarify with their patients terms related to substance use. For example, patients with histories of SUDs who are no longer using substances may or may not consider themselves to be in recovery. Likewise, some mutual-help groups may not regard patients as abstinent if they are treated for SUDs with medications such as naltrexone, buprenorphine, or methadone. Many people equate physical dependence or tolerance with addiction. However, if clinicians prescribing opioids for CNCP equate these terms, they may misdiagnose their patients on opioids as having an addiction, when in fact they do not.

In 2001, the American Academy of Pain Medicine, the American Pain Society, and the American Society of Addiction Medicine formed a Liaison Committee on Pain and Addiction to standardize the use of the terms *addiction*, *physical dependence*, and *tolerance* among pain professionals. Shared understandings of these and other terms facilitate research, advance dialog among professionals in the fields of addiction and pain, and help patients make informed decisions about their treatment.

Definitions used in this TIP are presented below.

- **addiction.** A primary, chronic, neurobiologic disease, with genetic, psychosocial, and environmental factors influencing its development and manifestations. It is characterized by behaviors that include one or more of the following: impaired *control* over drug use or compulsive use, *continued use* despite harm, and *craving* (Savage et al., 2003); clinicians commonly refer to these behaviors as the "3Cs."
- **addictive substance.** The phrase *addictive substance* is controversial. The phrase draws attention to the properties of the substance; however, some experts prefer to

emphasize the importance of individual variability, environment, and situational factors in addiction. Evidence suggests that animals will self-administer all drugs commonly sought by humans (with the exception of hallucinogens). Evidence also suggests that, if animals are exposed to a sufficient dose for a sufficient time, a substantial percentage will develop behaviors remarkably similar to those that suggest addiction in humans (e.g., "drug seeking" despite electrical shocks). Nonrewarding drugs (see Neurobiology of Addiction, below) do not elicit these behaviors in animals or humans. In this TIP, drugs or medications that elicit "drug seeking" behaviors are referred to as *addictive.*

- **behavioral health.** The term comprises substance use issues, mental health issues, and the prevention of both.
- **chronic noncancer pain (CNCP).** Pain that is (1) unassociated with an imminently terminal condition, and (2) unlikely to abate as a result of tissue healing, thus requiring long-term management. The term often refers to pain not caused by ongoing tissue pathology (e.g., backache, fibromyalgia). The term is problematic because it includes pain associated with sickle cell disease or recurrent pancreatitis, in which both neurological sensitization and tissue damage, at least in part, are likely. Inflammatory arthritis, connective tissue diseases, ischemia, and other conditions cause pain that persists for years yet are not, at least initially, life threatening.
- **chronic pain syndrome.** Intractable pain of 6 months or longer, with marked alteration of behavior; depression or anxiety; marked restriction in daily activities; frequent use of medication and medical services; no clear relationship to organic disorder; and a history of multiple, nonproductive tests, treatment, and surgeries (U.S. Commission on the Evaluation of Pain, 1987). This term is used casually and imprecisely to refer to pain, distress, and dysfunction that are not fully attributable to an identifiable medical condition.
- **hyperalgesia.** An abnormally intense response to a normally noxious stimulus.
- **narcotic.** Substance used to induce narcosis or stupor. *Narcotic* is not a synonym for the opioid class of medications.
- **opioid-induced hyperalgesia.** Hyperalgesia that results from the effects of opioids on the central nervous system (CNS).
- **pain.** An unpleasant sensory or emotional experience associated with actual or potential tissue damage or described in terms of such damage (International Association for the Study of Pain, 1986). Pain is subjective and may not always be corroborated by objective data.
- **physical dependence.** A state of adaptation that is manifested by a drug-class-specific withdrawal syndrome that can be produced by abrupt cessation, rapid dose reduction, decreasing the level of the drug in the blood, or administration of an antagonist (a substance that opposes the action of the drug) (Savage et al., 2003).
- **pseudoaddiction.** A controversial term coined to describe aberrant drug-related behaviors (e.g., clock watching, drug seeking), that resemble those of patients with addiction but that actually result from inadequate treatment of pain (Weissman & Haddox, 1989).
- **recovery.** A process of change through which an individual with an SUD achieves abstinence, wellness, and improved health and quality of life (Center for Substance Abuse Treatment [CSAT], 2007).

- **relapse.** A return to substance abuse after a period of abstinence.
- **substance use disorder** (SUD). A condition that includes alcohol and drug problems. SAMHSA recognizes that several terminologies (e.g., substance abuse and addiction) can be applied and respects that some individuals and communities may choose to use different terminologies (CSAT, 2007).
- **tolerance**. A state of adaptation in which exposure to a substance induces changes that result in a diminution of one or more of the substance's effects over time (Savage et al., 2003).

## Pain and Addiction Basics

Studies indicate that CNCP and addiction frequently co-occur (Chelminski et al., 2005; Rosenblum et al., 2003; Savage, Kirsh, & Passik, 2008). Chronic pain and addiction have many shared neurophysiological patterns. Most chronic pain involves abnormal neural processing, which can occur at various levels of the peripheral and CNS. Similarly, the disease of addiction results when normal neural processes, primarily in the brain's memory, reward, and stress systems, are altered into dysfunctional patterns. A full understanding of each condition is still emerging, and there is much to be learned regarding neurobiologic interactions between the conditions when they co-exist.

Chronic pain and addiction are not static conditions. Both fluctuate in intensity over time and under different circumstances and require ongoing management. Treatment for one condition can support or conflict with treatment for the other; a medication that may be appropriately prescribed for a particular chronic pain condition may be inappropriate given the patient's substance use history. Other commonalities include the following:

- Both are neurobiological conditions with evidence of disordered CNS function.
- Both are mediated by genetics and environment.
- Both may have significant behavioral components.
- Both may have serious harmful consequences if untreated.
- Both often require multifaceted treatment.

Chronic pain and SUDs have similar physical, social, emotional, and economic effects on health and well-being (Green, Baker, Smith, & Sato, 2003). Patients with one or both of these conditions may report insomnia, depression, impaired functioning, and other symptoms. Effective CNCP management in patients with or in recovery from SUDs must address both conditions simultaneously (Trafton, Oliva, Horst, Minkel, & Humphreys, 2004).

## Neurobiology of Pain

Both pain and responses to pain are shaped by culture, temperament, psychological state, memory, cognition, beliefs and expectations, co-occurring health conditions, gender, age, and other biopsychosocial factors. Because pain is both a sensory and an emotional experience, it is by nature subjective.

When nociceptors are excited, the stimulus is converted through transduction into action potentials that travel to the dorsal horn of the spinal cord. Signals then continue from the dorsal horn to the brain along multiple pathways in the cord: to the somatosensory cortex, where pain is evaluated; to the limbic system, where emotional reactions are mediated; to the autonomic centers that control such automatic functions as breathing, perspiration, and heart rate; and to other parts of the brain, where a behavioral response to the stimuli is determined. Nociceptive impulses are also transmitted to nearby terminals of the same nerve, where they may lead to diffuse pain and release of inflammatory substances that produce the flare and swelling that is a protective response to tissue injury (Exhibit 1-2).

Nociceptive input triggers a pain-inhibiting response. Signals traveling the ascending pathways are met by descending signals that emerge at various points along the spinal cord and brain. This antinociceptive response involves a panoply of chemicals, including endorphins, enkephalins, gamma-aminobutyric acid, norepinephrine, serotonin, oxytocin, and relaxin. Inhibitory signaling serves to attenuate nociceptive input, dampening the formation of pain sensation and providing pain relief (Brookoff, 2005).

Pain may be acute (e.g., postoperative pain), acute intermittent (e.g., migraine headache, pain caused by sickle cell disease), or chronic (persistent pain that may or may not have a known etiology). These categories are not mutually exclusive; for example, acute pain may be superimposed on chronic pain. Acute nociceptive or neuropathic pain can transform into chronic neuropathic pain in which the original sensations are extended and amplified.

**Exhibit 1-2 The Pain Pathways**

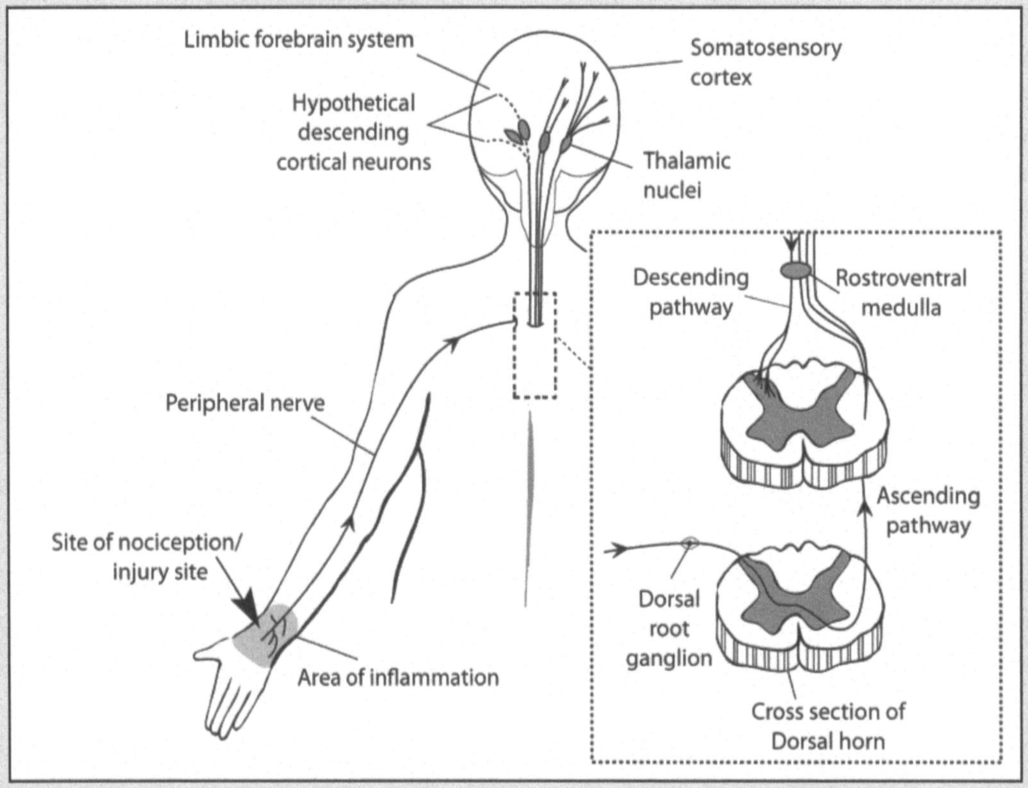

## Chronic Pain

Chronic pain can be nociceptive, neuropathic, or a mixture of both (Exhibit 1-3). Pains such as migraine and fibromyalgia, in which there is no noxious stimulus and no apparent neurological lesion, are attributed to dysfunction of a structurally intact CNS.

Chronic pain often results from a process of neural sensitization following injury or illness in which thresholds are lowered, responses are amplified (hyperalgesia), normally non-noxious stimulation becomes painful (allodynia), and spontaneous neural discharges occur. Increased signaling disconnected from nociceptive input can become autonomous, self-sustaining, and progressive, leading to the continuous perception of pain even in the absence of ongoing tissue damage. Thus, chronic pain is not equivalent to prolonged acute pain and for clinical purposes is best considered a distinct disorder (Brookoff, 2005).

The etiology of the abnormal processing in chronic pain is not fully understood. However, there are two main, nonexclusive causes. First, tissue damage can trigger the release of chemicals that sensitize the nerve fibers and alter gene expression, causing changes in signaling through many different mechanisms. Some of these changes enable non-pain-conducting fibers to trigger pain in the CNS. Second, pain can result from injured nerve fibers that regenerate in a neuroma, which generates pain signals with little or no stimulation.

When injury occurs to key pain-processing sectors of the CNS (e.g., the dorsal horn, thalamus), neural signals that pass through them may be interpreted as pain. Injury may also lead to degeneration of pain inhibitory cells. Modulation of nociceptive stimuli and inhibitory responses can occur at one or more locations in the CNS: the peripheral nerves, spinal cord neurons and tracts, thalamus, and cortex (Compton & Gebhart, 2003). Accurate identification of the source of the chronic pain, and of the neurological processes that modulate it, can lead to rational therapeutic approaches that target the source of aberrant signaling on the CNS pathway.

### Exhibit 1-3 Pain Types

| Type | Description |
|---|---|
| Nociceptive Pain | Pain that results from suprathreshold stimulation of nociceptors, which are neural receptors specialized for the detection of potentially harmful situations. This is an adaptive function of the nervous system. Nociceptors can be excited by mechanical, thermal, or chemical stimulation. The immediate physical response is reflexive and protective, causing a person to pull a hand away from a hot surface, for example. Nociceptive pain persists while the injurious agent remains or until healing occurs. Prolonged nociceptive input can cause central hypersensitization and the experience of spontaneous or amplified pain. |
| Neuropathic Pain | Pain that results from lesion or dysfunction of the sensory nervous system. A compressed, injured, or severed nerve can trigger neuropathic pain, as can disorders that affect the neural axis (e.g., metabolic diseases, infections, autoimmune disorders, vascular diseases, neoplasia [Campbell & Meyer, 2006]). |
| Mixed Nociceptive/ Neuropathic Pain | A combination of the two types of pain. For example, patients with degenerative disc disease may suffer from mechanical (nociceptive) back pain and radicular (neuropathic) pain. |

## Pain's Effect on Health

Persistent pain can have significant adverse effects on health. When pain stimuli continuously trigger the stress response, the acute signs of sympathetic activation (e.g., rapid heart rate, sweating) may cease or appear intermittently, yet the body continues to be stressed. This situation contributes to a sense of exhaustion.

Continued pain can trigger emotional responses, including sleeplessness, anxiety, and depressive symptoms, which in turn produce more pain. Such feedback cycles may continue to cause pain after the physiological causes have been addressed. Several studies show that the outcome of pain treatment is worse in the presence of depression, or when depression does not respond to treatment, and that the future course of pain syndromes can be, in part, predicted by emotional status. The physiological and psychological sequelae of CNCP can be exacerbated by such factors as inactivity and overuse of sedating drugs. Physical inactivity and a lack of engagement with life may also lead to increased levels of anxiety, depression, and an increased risk for suicidal ideation; these increases may lead a person to use substances in an attempt to treat these sequelae of CNCP and the losses that occur due to its presence.

## Neurobiology of Addiction

A person may use substances initially for several reasons, such as to experience the euphoric effects, to relieve stress, to overcome anxiety or depression (or both), or to blunt the pain (National Institute on Drug Abuse [NIDA], 2007). With repeated exposure, however, substance use in some people can become uncontrollable. The defining characteristics of the disease of addiction have been summarized as the "3Cs" (see the definition of *addiction*). Changes to the brain occur in a process that is mediated by both genetic and environmental factors, which result in an overvaluation of the substance, a devaluation of other things, and impaired control of substance-related behavior. Evidence indicates that addiction is a chronic disease.

The primary rewarding effects of addictive substances occur in the cortico-mesolimbic dopamine systems, where several structures link to control the basic emotions and connect them to memories, which drive behavior. These systems produce sensations of pleasure in response to actions that support survival (e.g., eating, sex) and sensations of fear in response to potential dangers. In a cascading effect, these sensations trigger the endocrine and autonomic nervous systems, stimulating bodily responses. The prefrontal cortex also plays a role in the formation of addictions, modifying pleasure and pain signals based on other considerations. Thus, the brain's reward and stress systems reinforce life-sustaining behaviors.

### *Reward Response*

Feelings of reward emerge from the core of the limbic system after neurons in the ventral tegmental area (VTA) release the neurotransmitter dopamine into the nucleus accumbens (NAc). Neural activity within this VTA–NAc circuit is necessary to experience reward, but other areas within the broader brain reward circuit also exert a strong influence. For example, the hippocampus contributes information from the past that may be relevant to the current experience. The amygdala adds critical information about the emotional valence of the stimulus that activated the reward circuit, thus contributing to the overall motivational power of the experience. In addition, parts of the prefrontal cortex (i.e., anterior cingulate and orbitofrontal cortices) help integrate all the information, a vital function that allows the individual to decide whether to initiate or suppress a particular behavior in response to the stimulus.

Most addictive substances increase the levels of dopamine in limbic targets well beyond what occurs in naturally rewarding situations (e.g., sex, food). Some drugs (e.g., marijuana, heroin) produce dopaminergic effects indirectly. Amphetamines cause the release of dopamine, and cocaine prevents its reuptake; both effects result in amplified messaging that eventually disrupts normal neuronal signaling.

It appears that the brain adjusts to excess dopamine levels by producing less dopamine and by reducing the number of receptors that respond to it in the receiving (postsynaptic) neuron. As a result, the pleasurable effects of a drug become diminished with continued use. The pleasurable effects of normal activities also are blunted, creating a state called *anhedonia* (an inability to experience pleasure).

It is commonly believed that continued substance use is driven by the need to prevent symptoms of withdrawal; however, this idea is misleading. Withdrawal, as commonly conceptualized, involves rebound symptoms resulting from the drug's absence. In the case of opioids, these symptoms include, but are not limited to, anxiety, sweating, tachycardia, diarrhea, piloerection, and chills. Although unpleasant, these symptoms are typically absent after a relatively brief period of detoxification or weaning and do not explain phenomena such as addiction relapse and prolonged craving. Even though detoxification is quick and technically easy, the prevention of relapse is extremely difficult and, in fact, the majority of those who attain abstinence experience at least one relapse (Dennis, Foss, & Scott, 2007). These more difficult problems are thought to result from the prolonged impairment of hedonic tone and conditioned responses that lead to intense craving.

### *Stress Response*

The dysregulation of the brain's reward system that occurs through substance use is paralleled by similar dysregulating effects in the stress system. Use of an addictive substance increases the flow of neurochemicals (e.g., corticotropin-releasing factor, norepinephrine, dynorphin). These chemicals can produce a negative emotional state that manifests as chronic irritability, emotional pain, lethargy, disinterest in natural rewards, and other dysphoric conditions. The stress response becomes more sensitive with repeated withdrawal and can persist into abstinence (Koob, 2009).

An individual may seek to avert the stress response by again using the substance. This negative reinforcement combines with the positive reinforcement of the substance's euphoric effects in an operant process that creates a compulsion for substance use. Thus, addiction is reflected in compulsive use combined with loss of control mediated by memory (cue-induced triggers for reuse), substance-induced reductions in executive functioning that hamper rational decisionmaking, and habit formation (Koob, 2009).

## Risk Factors for Addiction

People who use substances with addictive potential may develop tolerance to some of their effects and develop some degree of physical dependence. However, only a minority develops the disease of addiction. Important risk factors for addiction include genetics, psychological factors, and environmental factors.

Genetics plays a substantial role in risk factors for addiction: NIDA (2007) estimates that between 40 and 60 percent of a person's vulnerability to addiction may be genetic. The disease of addiction may be more heritable than type 2 diabetes, hypertension, and breast cancer (Nestler, 2005). Genes also underlie human variability in drug metabolism, susceptibility to psychiatric disorders that commonly co-occur with addiction, and response to environmental risk factors (e.g., drug availability, peer group pressure [Vaillant, 2003]).

Mental illness is another major risk factor for addiction (Volkow & Li, 2009), and the two conditions have high comorbidity (NIDA, 2009). One condition can follow the other (NIDA, 2007). For example, a person may attempt to relieve depression or anxiety with substances, and this behavior may lead to addiction. Conversely, chronic substance use may lead to mental disorders, such as psychosis, or make existing mental illness worse (NIDA, 2007). Environmental influences on addiction include, but are not limited to, poverty, poor parental support, living in a community with high drug availability, and using substances at an early age (NIDA, 2007, 2009; Volkow & Li, 2009).

## Cross-Addiction

Addiction to one substance can be linked with addiction to other substances in a pattern termed *cross-addiction*. An individual who voluntarily or involuntarily decreases use of one substance may increase use of another substance with similar effects on the brain (e.g., the person with an alcohol use disorder may use barbiturates for the sedative effects). The term cross-addiction is also used to describe simultaneous addiction (e.g., co-occurring addictions to nicotine, alcohol, and marijuana).

Cross-addiction is not official diagnostic nomenclature; rather, it refers to the observation that a person with an addiction to one substance may develop addiction to a subsequent substance, especially if the original drug of choice becomes inaccessible or is relinquished for other reasons. For example, a study of patients hospitalized for controlled-release oxycodone addiction found that the majority (77 percent) had previously had a non-opioid SUD (Potter, Hennessey, Borrow, Greenfield, & Weiss, 2004).

Individuals with chronic pain and histories of SUDs may be at increased risk of cross-addiction to any medication that acts on the brain as a reinforcing agent (Edlund, Sullivan, Steffick, Harris, & Wells, 2007). Because of cross-addiction, persons who abuse marijuana may be at increased risk for opioid addiction. People with alcohol use disorders have been found to be more than 18 times as likely to report nonmedical use of prescription medications as people who do not drink (McCabe, Cranford, & Boyd, 2006).

## The Cycle of Chronic Pain and Addiction

Although multiple factors influence the course of addiction, CNCP provides both positive and negative reinforcement of substance use. Positive reinforcement occurs when a behavior is followed by a consequence that is desirable—a donkey's walking may be rewarded by a carrot. Negative reinforcement occurs when a behavior is followed by the elimination of a negative consequence—a donkey's walking may eliminate the blows from a stick. For example, euphoria is a positive reinforcer for taking heroin, and pain reduction is a negative reinforcer for taking heroin. Prescribed opioids, benzodiazepines, or other medications may dramatically relieve pain or distress (e.g., depression, anxiety). Unprescribed substances may be used for similar reasons; for example, alcohol may promote relaxation or sleep. Such relief is a strong reinforcement for repeated consumption of the substance.

Unfortunately, analgesic and anxiolytic efficacy may diminish over the course of weeks, months, or years as tolerance develops. This loss of efficacy often elicits dose escalation to recapture efficacy. This escalation is rewarded, as the increased dose is initially more effective than the lower dose.

If the drug produces physical dependence, the person may have not only increased pain when the substance is absent, but also withdrawal symptoms (e.g., anxiety, nausea, cramps, insomnia). Withdrawal symptoms may lead to an increase in symptoms of depression and an increase in the potential risk for suicide. All these symptoms are relieved by ingesting more of the drug that caused the dependence. A similar situation may occur if the drug is one that elicits rebound symptoms. For example, ergot relieves migraine, but excessive use leads to rebound headaches that are more persistent and treatment resistant than were the original headaches.

An illusion of benefit produced by reinforcing drugs can create a paradoxical situation in which long-term use of the substance creates the very symptoms the person hopes to alleviate. People commonly drink to relax or "cheer up," yet chronic alcohol abuse leads to depression and anxiety.

In some people, a cycle develops in which pain or distress elicits severe preoccupation with the substance that previously provided relief. This cycle—seeking pain relief, experiencing relief, and then having pain recur—can be very difficult to break, even in the person without an addiction, and the development of addiction markedly exacerbates the difficulty. The propensity to develop this cycle is influenced by genetic and environmental factors; some people will experience greater degrees of analgesia than others, and some will have more severe or prolonged abstinence symptoms. Genetic variability in susceptibility to these experiences may explain some cases of iatrogenic addiction.

NCHS Data Brief ■ No. 379 ■ September 2020

# Symptoms of Depression Among Adults: United States, 2019

Maria A. Villarroel, Ph.D., and Emily P. Terlizzi, M.P.H.

## Key findings

### Data from the National Health Interview Survey

- In 2019, 2.8% of adults experienced severe symptoms of depression, 4.2% experienced moderate symptoms, and 11.5% experienced mild symptoms in the past 2 weeks.
- The percentage of adults who experienced any symptoms of depression was highest among those aged 18–29 (21.0%), followed by those aged 45–64 (18.4%) and 65 and over (18.4%), and lastly, by those aged 30–44 (16.8%).
- Women were more likely than men to experience mild, moderate, or severe symptoms of depression.
- Non-Hispanic Asian adults were least likely to experience mild, moderate, or severe symptoms of depression compared with Hispanic, non-Hispanic white, and non-Hispanic black adults.

Depression is characterized by the presence of feelings of sadness, emptiness, or irritability, accompanied by bodily and cognitive changes lasting at least 2 weeks that significantly affect the individual's capacity to function (1). The eight-item Patient Health Questionnaire (PHQ–8) is a validated diagnostic and severity measure of symptoms of depressive disorders (2,3). Adults with scores of 0–4 are considered to have no or minimal symptoms of depression, while those with scores of 5–9, 10–14, or 15–24 are considered to have mild, moderate, or severe symptoms, respectively (2,3). This report examines the percentage of adults aged 18 and over with symptoms of depression in the past 2 weeks in 2019, by symptom severity and select demographic characteristics, using the PHQ–8 scale.

## In 2019, 18.5% of adults had symptoms of depression that were either mild, moderate, or severe in the past 2 weeks.

Figure 1. Percent distribution of severity of depression symptoms in the past 2 weeks among adults aged 18 and over: United States, 2019

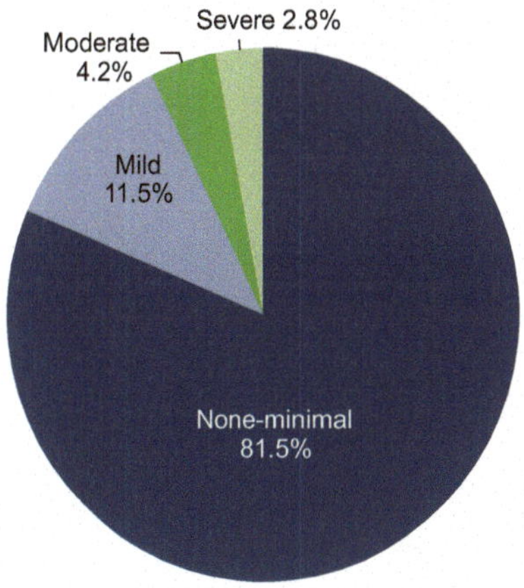


NOTES: Severity of depression symptoms was based on the eight-item Patient Health Questionnaire depression scale (PHQ–8), and summarized into none-minimal (values 0–4), mild (values 5–9), moderate (values 10–14), and severe (values 15–24). Estimates are based on household interviews of a sample of the civilian noninstitutionalized U.S. population. Access data table for Figure 1 at: https://www.cdc.gov/nchs/data/databriefs/db379-tables-508.pdf#1.
SOURCE: National Center for Health Statistics, National Health Interview Survey, 2019.

U.S. DEPARTMENT OF HEALTH AND HUMAN SERVICES
Centers for Disease Control and Prevention
National Center for Health Statistics

*NCHS reports can be downloaded from: https://www.cdc.gov/nchs/products/index.htm.*

- During 2019, 81.5% of adults aged 18 and over experienced no or minimal symptoms of depression in the past 2 weeks (Figure 1).
- Among adults, 11.5% experienced mild symptoms of depression, 4.2% experienced moderate symptoms, and 2.8% experienced severe symptoms.

## Severity of depression symptoms in the past 2 weeks varied by age.

- The total percentage of adults who experienced symptoms of depression that were either mild, moderate, or severe in the past 2 weeks was highest among those aged 18–29 (21.0%) and lowest among those aged 30–44 (16.8%) (Figure 2).
- The percentage of adults who experienced mild depression symptoms was highest among those aged 18–29 (13.9%), followed by those aged 65 and over (12.0%), and lowest among those aged 45–64 (10.7%) and 30–44 (10.3%).
- The percentage of adults who experienced moderate depression symptoms was higher among those aged 45–64 (4.5%) compared with those aged 30–44 (3.8%) and those aged 65 and over (3.8%). The observed difference between adults aged 18–29 (4.4%) and the older age groups was not significant.
- The percentage of adults who experienced severe depression symptoms did not vary significantly by age and was 2.7% among those aged 18–29, 2.7% among those aged 30–44, 3.1% among those aged 45–65, and 2.6% among those aged 65 and over.

Figure 2. Percentage of adults aged 18 and over with symptoms of depression in the past 2 weeks, by symptom severity and age group: United States, 2019

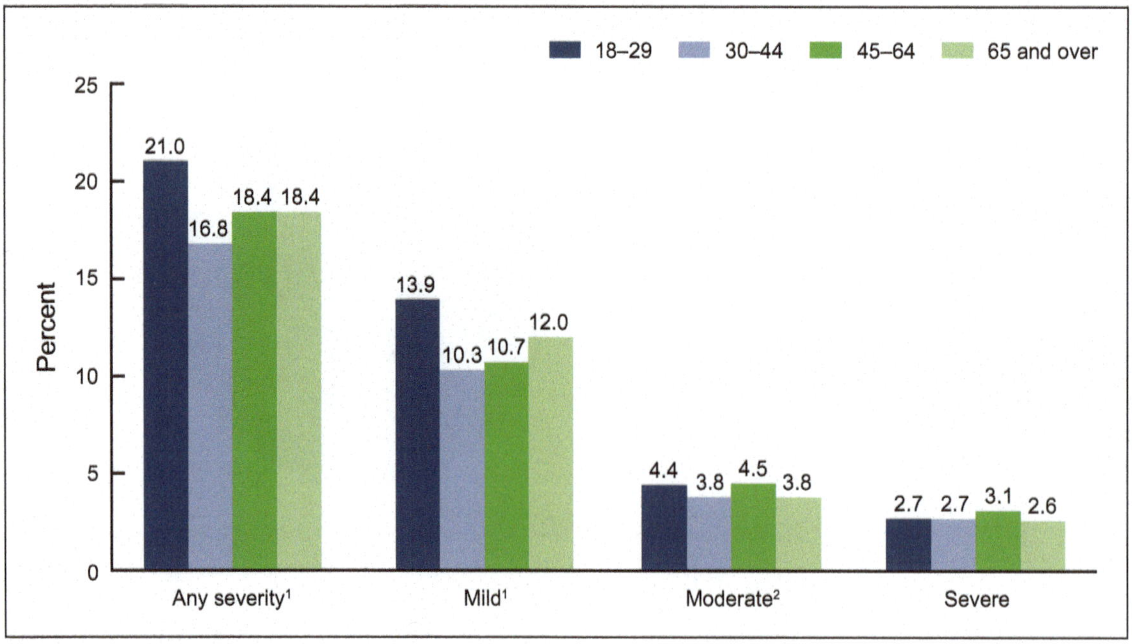


[1]Significant quadratic trend ($p < 0.05$).
[2]Significant cubic trend ($p < 0.05$).
NOTES: Severity of depression symptoms was based on the eight-item Patient Health Questionnaire depression scale (PHQ–8), and summarized into none-minimal (values 0–4), mild (values 5–9), moderate (values 10–14), and severe (values 15–24). Those categorized as having no or minimal symptoms of depression are not shown in this figure. Any severity includes those categorized as having either mild, moderate, or severe symptoms of depression in the past 2 weeks. Estimates are based on household interviews of a sample of the civilian noninstitutionalized U.S. population. Access data table for Figure 2 at: https://www.cdc.gov/nchs/data/databriefs/db379-tables-508.pdf#2.
SOURCE: National Center for Health Statistics, National Health Interview Survey, 2019.

## Women were more likely than men to experience mild, moderate, and severe depression symptoms in the past 2 weeks.

- In 2019, 21.8% of women experienced depression symptoms in the past 2 weeks that were either mild, moderate, or severe, which was higher than men (15.0%) (Figure 3).
- Women were more likely than men to have experienced depression symptoms that were mild (13.4% and 9.6%, respectively), moderate (4.9% and 3.4%, respectively), and severe (3.5% and 2.1%, respectively).

Figure 3. Percentage of adults aged 18 and over with symptoms of depression in the past 2 weeks, by symptom severity and sex: United States, 2019

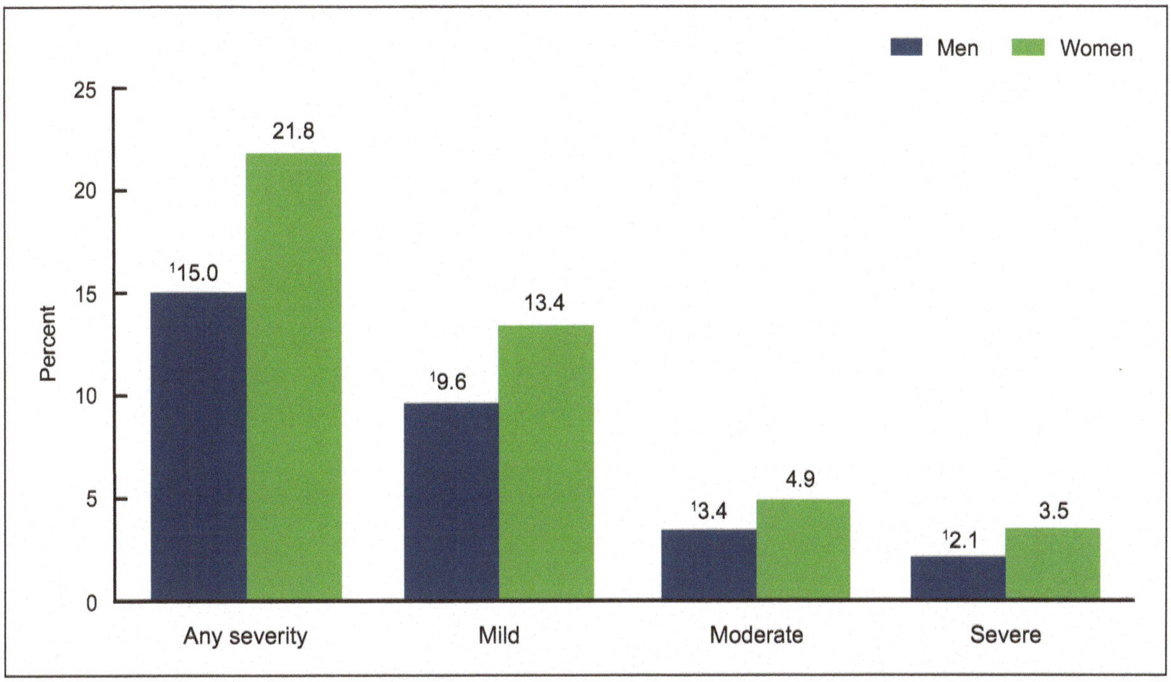


[1]Significantly different from women ($p < 0.05$).

NOTES: Severity of depression symptoms was based on the eight-item Patient Health Questionnaire depression scale (PHQ–8), and summarized into none-minimal (values 0–4), mild (values 5–9), moderate (values 10–14), and severe (values 15–24). Those categorized as having no or minimal symptoms of depression are not shown in this figure. Any severity includes those categorized as having either mild, moderate, or severe symptoms of depression in the past 2 weeks. Estimates are based on household interviews of a sample of the civilian noninstitutionalized U.S. population. Access data table for Figure 3 at: https://www.cdc.gov/nchs/data/databriefs/db379-tables-508.pdf#3.

SOURCE: National Center for Health Statistics, National Health Interview Survey, 2019.

## The percentage of adults who experienced depression symptoms in the past 2 weeks varied by Hispanic origin and race.

- Non-Hispanic white (19.3%) and non-Hispanic black (19.3%) adults were the most likely to have experienced any severity of depression symptoms in the past 2 weeks, followed by Hispanic (16.9%) adults, while non-Hispanic Asian (10.2%) adults were least likely (Figure 4).
- Non-Hispanic white (12.0%) and non-Hispanic black (12.2%) adults were the most likely to have experienced mild depression symptoms in the past 2 weeks, followed by Hispanic (10.2%) adults, while non-Hispanic Asian (7.9%) adults were least likely.
- Non-Hispanic Asian (1.2%) adults were least likely to have experienced moderate depression symptoms, compared with non-Hispanic black (4.6%), non-Hispanic white (4.4%), and Hispanic (4.0%) adults.
- Non-Hispanic Asian (1.2%) adults were least likely to have experienced severe depression symptoms, compared with non-Hispanic white (2.9%), Hispanic (2.7%), and non-Hispanic black (2.5%) adults.

Figure 4. Percentage of adults aged 18 and over with symptoms of depression in the past 2 weeks, by symptom severity and race and Hispanic origin: United States, 2019

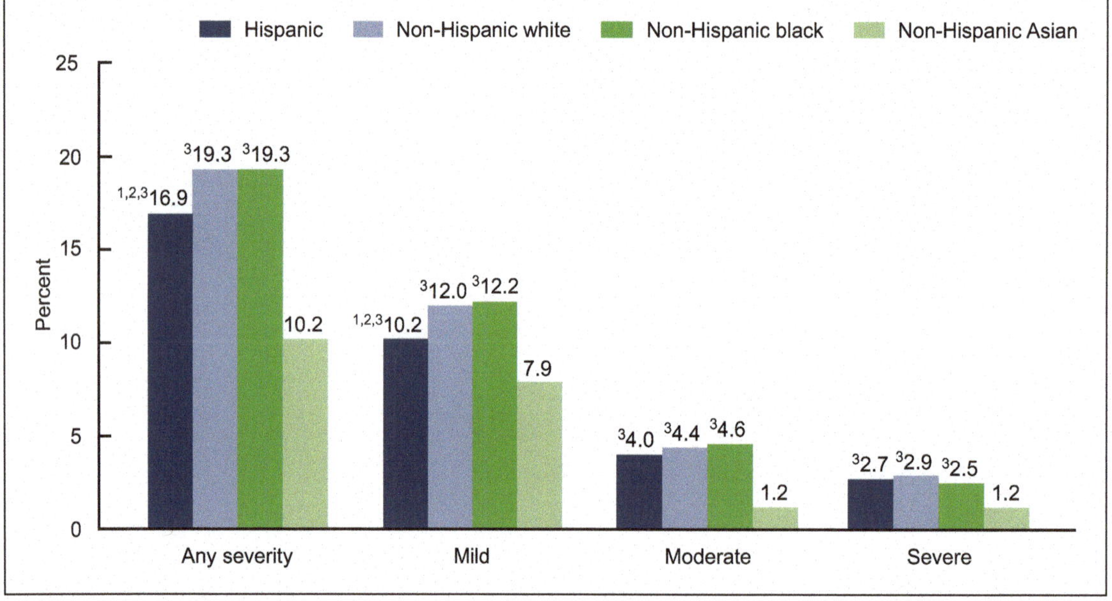


[1]Significantly different from non-Hispanic white ($p < 0.05$).
[2]Significantly different from non-Hispanic black ($p < 0.05$).
[3]Significantly different from non-Hispanic Asian ($p < 0.05$).
NOTES: Severity of depression symptoms was based on the eight-item Patient Health Questionnaire depression scale (PHQ–8), and summarized into none-minimal (values 0–4), mild (values 5–9), moderate (values 10–14), and severe (values 15–24). Those categorized as having no or minimal symptoms of depression are not shown in this figure. Any severity includes those categorized as having either mild, moderate, or severe symptoms of depression in the past 2 weeks. Estimates are based on household interviews of a sample of the civilian noninstitutionalized U.S. population. Access data table for Figure 4 at: https://www.cdc.gov/nchs/data/databriefs/db379-tables-508.pdf#4.
SOURCE: National Center for Health Statistics, National Health Interview Survey, 2019.

# The Voice of the Patient

A series of reports from the U.S. Food and Drug Administration's (FDA's) Patient-Focused Drug Development Initiative

**Functional Gastrointestinal Disorders**

**Public Meeting: May 11, 2015**
**Report Date: January 2016**

Center for Drug Evaluation and Research (CDER)
U.S. Food and Drug Administration (FDA)

## Introduction

On May 11, 2015, FDA held a public meeting to hear perspectives from patients living with functional gastrointestinal (GI) disorders, their caregivers, and other patient representatives on the most significant effects of these disorders and currently available therapies. FDA conducted the meeting as part of the agency's Patient-Focused Drug Development initiative, an FDA commitment under the fifth authorization of the Prescription Drug User Fee Act (PDUFA V) to more systematically gather patients' perspectives on their condition and available therapies to treat their condition. As part of this commitment, FDA is holding at least 20 public meetings between Fiscal Years 2013 - 2017, each focused on a specific disease area. More information on this initiative can be found at http://www.fda.gov/ForIndustry/UserFees/PrescriptionDrugUserFee/ucm326192.htm.

### Overview of functional gastrointestinal disorders

Functional gastrointestinal (GI) disorders describes a group of common, chronic GI conditions that affect a part of the GI tract and are often characterized by chronic time course and unpredictable symptom exacerbations. Generally, there are no anatomical, structural, or biochemical abnormalities. Diagnosis of these disorders is based on signs and symptoms using Rome Criteria. There are 28 adult and 17 pediatric functional GI disorders based on the Rome III diagnostic criteria.[1] These disorders include irritable bowel syndrome, chronic idiopathic constipation, functional dyspepsia, gastroparesis, and functional abdominal pain. Functional GI disorders are highly prevalent and impact across all demographics; approximately two out of every five people are affected by a functional GI disorder. There is much overlap between these disorders, and many patients suffer from two or more functional GI disorders.

The effects of functional GI disorders vary depending on the underlying disorder; however, common signs and symptoms of functional GI disorders relate to abnormal intestinal motility, abnormal intestinal perception, and/or abnormal brain-gut communication. Common symptoms include abdominal pain, heartburn, abdominal distention, nausea, vomiting, bloating, constipation, and/or diarrhea.

Current therapies are limited for functional GI disorders. Prescription therapies such as lubiprostone, linaclotide, metoclopramide, and alosetron are available to manage some of the symptoms. Over-the-counter treatments, including antidiarrheals, pro-motility agents, proton pump inhibitors, and H2 blockers, are also often incorporated into treatment regimens. Other therapies include dietary management, off-label, and investigational therapies. In severe cases, gastric electrical stimulation, feeding tubes, or surgical intervention may be required.

## Meeting overview

This meeting gave FDA the opportunity to hear directly from patients, caretakers, and other patient representatives about their experiences with functional GI disorders and their treatments. Discussion focused on two key topics: (1) the effects of functional GI disorders that matter most to patients and (2) patients' perspectives on treatments for functional GI disorders. The discussion questions (*Appendix 1*) were published in a Federal Register notice that announced the meeting.

---

[1] The Rome criteria is a system developed to classify functional gastrointestinal (GI) disorders, disorders of the digestive system in which symptoms cannot be explained by the presence of structural or tissue abnormality, based on clinical symptoms. For more information: http://www.romecriteria.org/

For each topic, a panel of patients and patient representatives (*Appendix 2*) shared comments to begin the dialogue. Panel comments were followed by a facilitated discussion inviting comments from other patients and patient representatives in the audience. An FDA facilitator led the discussion, and a panel of FDA staff *(Appendix 2)* asked follow-up questions. Participants who joined the meeting via live webcast (referred to in this report as web participants) were also able to contribute comments. In addition, in-person and web participants were periodically invited to respond to polling questions (*Appendix 3*), which provided a sense of the demographic makeup of participants as well as how many participants shared a particular perspective on a given topic.

Approximately 25 functional GI disorder patients or patient representatives attended the meeting in-person, and approximately 40 patients or patient representatives provided input through the live webcast. According to their responses to the polling questions, the majority of meeting participants were women, ranging from 18 years to 60 years old. In-person and web participants represented a number of functional GI disorders, including (but not limited to): irritable bowel syndrome, gastroparesis, chronic persistent symptomatic gastroesophageal reflux, and chronic idiopathic constipation. Although participants at this meeting may not fully represent the population living with functional GI disorders, FDA believes that the input received during the meeting reflects a range of experiences of those conditions described above.

To supplement the input gathered at the meeting, patients and others were encouraged to submit comments on the topic to a public docket,[2] which was open until July 13, 2015. Forty comments were submitted to the public docket by patients and other stakeholders. The comments received via the public docket have been incorporated into this summary.

More information, including the archived webcast and meeting transcript, is available on the meeting website: http://www.fda.gov/ForIndustry/UserFees/PrescriptionDrugUserFee/ucm430885.htm.

**Report overview and key themes**

This report summarizes the input provided by patients and patient representatives at the meeting or through the webcast. It also includes a summary of comments submitted to the public docket. To the extent possible, the terms used in this summary to describe specific signs, symptoms, impacts, and treatment experiences of functional GI disorders reflect the words used by in-person attendees, web participants, or docket commenters. The report is not meant to be representative in any way of the views and experiences of any specific group of individuals or entities. There may be signs, symptoms, impacts, treatments, or other aspects of the disease that are not included in the report.

The input from the meeting and docket comments emphasized the challenge of living with a functional GI disorder, its impact on daily life, and the difficulties involved in diagnosing and treating the disorder. Several key themes emerged from this meeting:

- Functional GI disorders are a group of chronic diseases that place a significant burden on daily life and have a severe impact on how patients feel and function. Most meeting participants were diagnosed with a primary underlying functional GI disorder, in addition to a range of other

[2] A *docket* is a repository through which the public can submit electronic and written comments on specific topics to U.S. federal agencies such as FDA. More information can be found at www.regulations.gov.

GI-related disorders. Participants frequently discussed the overlap of conditions and the cyclic and recurrent tendency of symptoms. Most participants focused their comments on abdominal pain and discomfort, vomiting and nausea, fatigue, and gas and flatulence as the most burdensome signs and symptoms of their disease.

- Daily life for many patients living with a functional GI disorder revolves around managing their condition and their treatments. Participants described their inability to eat, difficulty with basic tasks requiring exertion, difficulty interacting with friends and family, limitations on their ability to work, and the emotional impact on patients and caregivers.

- Although the specific treatments vary widely across the spectrum of functional GI disorders, participants shared common experiences while using a combination of drug and non-drug treatments. Participants commented on their experiences with pharmaceutical treatments addressing specific symptoms (such as nausea), strict dietary control, and non-drug therapies. Participants largely focused on the downsides of these treatments and the significant burden of a trial and error therapy regimen.

The patient input generated through this Patient-Focused Drug Development meeting and public docket comments strengthens FDA's understanding of the burden of functional GI disorders on patients and the treatments currently used to treat functional GI disorders and their symptoms. FDA staff will carefully consider this input as it fulfills its role in the drug development process, including when advising sponsors on their drug development programs and when assessing products under review for marketing approval. For example, *Appendix 4* shows how this input may directly support our benefit-risk assessments for products under review. This input may also be of value to the drug development process more broadly. For example, the report may be useful to drug developers as they explore potential areas of unmet need for patients with a functional GI disorder. It could also point to the potential need for a better understanding of particular effects of disease, such as the manifestation of fatigue or for the development and qualification of a more appropriate pain scale in clinical trials.

## Topic 1: Disease Symptoms and Daily Impacts That Matter Most to Patients

The first discussion topic focused on patients' experiences with symptoms of their functional GI disorder(s) and the impact these symptoms have on their daily lives. FDA was particularly interested in hearing patients describe how their condition and symptoms have changed over time, as well as specific activities patients could no longer do at all, or as fully as they would like to, due to their condition.

Four panelists provided comments to start the open dialogue. They included:

- Panelist 1: a woman diagnosed with gastroparesis, esophageal dysmotility, small intestinal dysmotility, and colonic inertia (which led to the removal of her colon)

- Panelist 2: a woman diagnosed with irritable bowel syndrome (IBS) a year and a half ago, although she experienced symptoms for many years before her diagnosis

- Panelist 3: a 35-year old woman diagnosed with severe gastroparesis

- Panelist 4: a woman diagnosed with a mitochondrial disorder, autonomic dysfunction, gastroparesis, overall gut dysmotility of her entire GI tract, esophageal spasms, intestinal spasms, biliary dyskinesia with a smooth muscle disorder, pancreatitis, chronic constipation, and hypoglycemia myoclonus.

The panelists detailed the difficulty of living with their respective conditions and the physical, emotional, and social impacts of their disease symptoms on their daily lives and on the lives of their loved ones. Their comments highlighted the wide variability in functional GI disorders and their manifestations. Patients and patient representatives in the audience indicated by a show of hands that the panelist comments resonated with their own experiences. The large-group discussion that followed the panel comments provided further insight into how symptoms manifest and how they change over time. The range of symptoms discussed in-person and web participants are described in more detail below.

## Perspectives on most significant symptoms

*Discomfort and abdominal pain*

In a polling question (*Appendix 3, Q7*), participants were asked to identify up to three upper-GI related symptoms that have the most significant impact on daily life. Abdominal pain or discomfort was identified by over three-fourths of in-person and web participants as being one of their most significant symptoms. Throughout the discussion, many participants echoed that these symptoms are among the most impactful on the daily life and well-being of patients with a functional GI disorder.

Participants distinguished abdominal discomfort and abdominal pain as separate symptoms. They described abdominal discomfort as a pervasive issue that lasts "hours and hours" or is present on a "daily basis," while abdominal pain was described as often temporary and triggered by specific foods and drinks. Discomfort was described as a "duller pain," and a participant elaborated, "I can do things to... ignore [the discomfort], but it's still there." Abdominal pain was described as "crippling," and one participant shared that during a "flare-up...it gets so bad it hurts to breathe, because [the stomach] pushed up on your lungs and it hurts."

Participants also commented on the need for an appropriate pain scale that helps patients and their medical providers differentiate between discomfort and pain. One participant shared, "our pain is not on that scale." Other participants added that there needs to be an increased awareness in the medical community that there are varying types of abdominal pain (e.g., constipation pain, intestinal spasms), and such distinctions would in turn help with proper diagnosis and treatment.

Participants identified eating and drinking as frequent triggers of "flare ups" or abdominal pain. A participant commented, "vegetables, even if they're juiced, will turn my stomach and make it into such pain that I'm on the floor... or in my bed in a ball." Other participants shared similar experiences; some commented that their pain was triggered by dairy, high fiber or fatty food consumptions.

*Nausea and Vomiting*

In a polling question (*Appendix 3, Q7*), two-thirds of in-person and web participants identified nausea and vomiting as significant signs and symptoms that impacted their daily life. Many participants described living with chronic nausea, which as one participant explained is like "being seasick all the time." Some participants described persistent and debilitating vomiting; in one example, one participant described vomiting 20 to 30 times per day in the early stage of her disease. A few participants acknowledged that as their disease progressed, they "managed to get a handle" or decrease the number of times they vomited daily, but that the nausea remained constant. Participants also shared the resulting impacts of persistent nausea and vomiting; these included pain, inability to eat a full meal, and inability to concentrate.

*Fatigue*

Many participants identified fatigue as one of the most significant symptoms of functional GI disorders impacting their daily life. As one participant summarized, "I have fatigue a large part of the day...any amount of physical activity will fatigue me." Other participants shared that their fatigue resulted in difficulty focusing and eating.

Participants commented on the lack of energy that affects their daily life. One participant shared, "On my best days, it takes an hour to get washed up and that includes the rest time." Another participant commented, "I was so tired, I'd start to fall asleep at work and go straight to bed when I got home." One web participant commented that her fatigue worsened as the day progressed, and shared that by the end of the day "I end up dragging myself on the floor." Several participants also discussed muscle fatigue, with one participant saying "my muscles hurt so bad, it hurts to walk."

*Abdominal distention or bloating*

Nearly half of the participants indicated abdominal distention or bloating as a significant symptom. A panelist diagnosed with IBS shared that bloating is a daily occurrence for her, and often leads to other symptoms including pain and unpredictable bowel movements. She explained further, "I have bloating so bad, I can't even fit into my work clothes. I just have a range of clothes that I...pick on a daily basis." A webcast participant added that her bloating is "so intense that it makes it difficult to breathe."

*Lower-GI related symptoms*

In a polling question (*Appendix 3, Q8*), participants were asked to identify the lower-GI related symptoms that have the most significant impact on daily life. Nearly all of the meeting participants indicated gas or flatulence as a significant symptom of their condition, followed by diarrhea and incontinence. They also commented that these symptoms had broad impacts. As one participant noted, "gas is extraordinarily painful if it's stuck"; this comment resonated with other participants who also correlated gas and flatulence to other GI-related symptoms, such as constipation, diarrhea, and incontinence.

Three-fourths of the participants indicated in the same polling question that constipation was a major symptom of their condition. One participant shared that "it [stool] feels like I'm passing razor blades." Many participants also observed that constipation is often a side effect of their prescription medicines. This was especially emphasized by webcast participants diagnosed with gastroparesis.

## Overall impact of a functional GI disorder on daily life

Participants also described the physical, social, and emotional impact that their functional GI disorder has had on their lives, including:

- **Inability to eat.** Participants highlighted their difficulty eating or inability to eat as a major impact of living with a functional GI disorder. Most participants shared that the inability to eat had significant physical, social, and emotional impacts. One web participant commented, "The smell of food makes me really sick." Another participant noted, "You can't eat because you're in pain [and] you're nauseous." A web participant commented on how their disease and inability to eat makes other people uncomfortable. As one participant summarized, "your life will do nothing but revolve around food and what you can't have"; this comment resonated with many in the audience. Participants also commented on the feeling of fullness after eating only a small amount.

- **Caring for self or family.** Some participants shared their perspectives on having to rely on caregivers for daily activities, including getting dressed or exercise due to the lack of strength. One participant noted that she is unable to take normal showers because of the "weakness and blackout spells that the water instigates." Another participant shared that she is "very limited on what I can and can't do," and that her husband had to alter his work schedule to help care for their children.

- **Job and school performance.** Participants shared that pain, nausea, bloating, and fatigue have made it difficult or impossible to be effective in the workplace or classroom. For example, a participant described the impact of nausea on her classwork as so debilitating that it felt like being "sick all the time." Another participant commented that she did not want to leave the house because of her symptoms, which led to her lagging behind on work. Participants also commented on the difficulty of concentrating at work, or attending meetings where they could not "afford to have an episode."

- **Emotional and social impacts.** Participants emphasized the many emotional and social impacts of living with functional GI disorders, including daily frustration and emotional distress. The majority of participants shared their difficulties in socializing and maintaining the sense of a "normal life" for themselves and their families. Several web participants commented that gas and flatulence were embarrassing and made it difficult to go out in social situations. Another participant explained how her condition impacted the social relationships of her children by sharing, "my kids don't get invited to that birthday party or that meeting at school because they know I can't make it or I'm not going to be able to eat the food." Another participant said she lost most of her friends because she cannot "go out with friends and be able to keep up." Other participants shared comments that their family and friends did not often understand the physical and emotional impacts of living with a functional GI disorder.

## Topic 2: Patient Perspectives on Treatments for Functional GI Disorders

The second main topic of discussion focused on patients' experiences with therapies used to treat their or their loved ones' condition. Four in-person panelists and one panelist via telephone provided their comments to start the conversation. They included:

- Panelist 1: a 56-year old woman born with Hirschsprung's disease and diagnosed with gastroparesis and dysmotility of her entire digestive tract
- Panelist 2: a 45-year old woman diagnosed with gastroparesis
- Panelist 3: a woman diagnosed chronic unexplained nausea and vomiting
- Panelist 4: a 55-year old woman diagnosed with GERD, chronic constipation, and idiopathic gastroparesis
- Panelist 5: a woman diagnosed 26 years ago with diarrhea-predominant IBS

Panelists shared their experiences with a variety of treatment regiments, including prescription medications, non-drug therapies, dietary management, and other lifestyle changes. They described a process of trial and error to find an effective approach to fit their specific needs. In the large-group facilitated discussion that followed, nearly all patients in the audience indicated by a show of hands that their experiences were reflected in the panelists' comments.

Throughout the dialogue, participants detailed the benefits and downsides they have experienced from various therapies and modifications (including lifestyle changes and diet management) used to manage their condition. This section ends with participants' perspectives on ideal treatments and broader consideration regarding treatments for functional GI disorders, including the need for better understanding of the disorders for proper diagnosis (e.g., through gastric emptying studies) and treatment.

### Perspectives on medical treatments for functional GI disorders

According to a polling question (*Appendix 3, Q10*), most participants reported taking or having taken drug therapies to help reduce their functional GI disorder symptoms. Prescription drug therapies were described as having widely varying degrees of effectiveness, and many participants noted they often switched therapies because they were unable to tolerate treatment side effects. Most participants also indicated that they rely on multiple therapies to help manage or treat their functional GI disorder. Their comments on experiences with specific drugs are summarized below.

The most commonly discussed treatment was Reglan (metoclopramide). One participant with gastroparesis noted that after being put on Reglan, she was able to start eating regularly and "suffered less nausea and dizziness"; however, she continued to suffer from severe fatigue. Another participant commented that Reglan was a promising treatment for her when she first started the treatment, but she "quickly started developing some early tardive dyskinesia-type symptoms." Other participants shared significant downsides to Reglan including more frequent vomiting, restless leg syndrome, and neurological side effects. A few participants also shared experiences where Reglan did not improve their symptoms at all.

Several participants commented that domperidone[3] was a part of their treatment regimen. One participant with gastroparesis commented that upon taking domperidone, she had "immediate, complete, reliable relief," with no adverse effects. Some participants noted that higher dosages of domperidone resulted in higher hormone levels (such as prolactin); these participants shared that their physicians would make dosage adjustments accordingly. Finally, other participants commented that they were unable, unwilling, or afraid to take domperidone, since it is not an FDA-approved drug.

Participants also shared their experiences with other therapies they were using to manage their GI symptoms. Several participants shared mixed experiences with Linzess (linaclotide). One participant commented on her daily reliance on Linzess for relief, while a web participant expressed that it did not work and caused "intense pain." Similarly, participants shared their experiences with Amitiza (lubiprostone) and included increased nausea and pain as resulting side effects. Participants also commented on their experiences with Imodium (loperamide). One participant shared that she would go back on Imodium in between alternative treatments, and that it is the "most reliable for short-term relief."

Participants mentioned a range of other drug therapies to address their GI symptoms. These included: pain medications, a range of anti-nausea drugs (e.g., Zofran (ondansetron), promethazine), antibiotics (e.g., erythromycin, rifaximin), antipsychotics (e.g., Zyprexa (olanzapine)), antidepressants (e.g., desipramine) and Botox (onabotulinumtoxinA) injections. Several participants also described taking acid reflux medications (such as Prilosec) to treat their acid reflux.

**Non-drug therapies**

*Gastric Electrical Stimulation*

Several participants shared mixed experiences with gastric electrical stimulation. One participant commented that it was a "lifesaver;" however, she also commented on "getting shocks" as a downside of the device. Another participant noted that while the device signals the stomach to help reduce nausea and vomiting, it would be more useful if it, "actually assists the stomach in contracting." One participant described the constant need to visit an emergency room to have the battery replaced, but that the device is "worth investigating" for those "who are having a terrible time, because any relief can be better than nothing."

*Dietary management*

Various dietary controls were identified as an essential component of treatment by many participants. One participant shared that her diet cannot include any fats or oils, while another web participant commented on eliminating genetically modified foods from the diet. Participants noted that the strict dietary restrictions placed a significant burden on their daily lives. A wide variety of vitamins, herbs and dietary supplements were mentioned as being used to treat specific symptoms, including Vitamin D, fish oil, mint, glutamine, deactivated charcoal, probiotics and digestive enzymes.

---

[3] Domperidone is not currently approved for marketing in the U.S. Patients 12 years of age and older with certain gastrointestinal (GI) conditions may be able to receive treatment with domperidone through an expanded access investigational new drug application (IND). For more information, please see http://www.fda.gov/Drugs/DevelopmentApprovalProcess/HowDrugsareDevelopedandApproved/ApprovalApplications/InvestigationalNewDrugINDApplication/ucm368736.htm.

*Other non-drug therapies*

Several participants mentioned that medical marijuana was effective in treating their pain and nausea. Other non-drug or physical therapies were also mentioned including acupuncture, massage, heating pads, homeopathic remedies, and visiting a chiropractor. Overall, participants noted some level of relief from these treatments.

**Treatment downsides**

Below is a summary of the challenging aspects of various treatments participants shared during this meeting.

- Many participants described the significant impact of treatment side effects. One participant stated, "I have not found a medication which I could take which does not make me tired or make my head foggy." One participant, whose treatment regime includes a patient-controlled analgesia (PCA) pump for her total parenteral nutrition (TPN), commented, "I've had multiple episodes of sepsis...I've lost a lot of functional ability."
- Some participants commented that side effects of a treatment can worsen symptoms of the underlying disease or introduce new bothersome GI effects. For example, a web participant commented that trying to manage her pain with pain medications resulted in slowed digestion, which was "equally debilitating."
- Some participants shared that weight gain is the most visible of their treatment side effects, but expressed concerns on the long-term effects of their treatments and how the side effects worsened with prolonged use. Participants also commented on the balance between being underweight due to the symptoms and then experiencing unwanted weight gain due to the side effects of their treatments.
- Some participants commented that their therapies worked well initially, but became less effective with time. One participant commented on how she went back on Imodium (loperamide), but "it didn't work completely and I was getting a rebound effect." The same participant also noted that she developed a tolerance for Immodium, and as a result kept having to take "more and more."
- Participants commented on the burden of their treatment regimes, including one participant who stated, "Every day I take over ten different medications to treat my symptoms, including four medications specifically for nausea." Another participant commented that in the process of trying different medications, "you just feel like a lab rat."
- Participants commented on the burden of treatment, including out-of-pocket costs for treatments not covered by insurance.

**Perspectives on an ideal treatment for functional GI disorders**

Participants were asked to identify specific attributes they would look for in an ideal treatment for their functional GI disorder. They provided a range of perspectives, which are summarized below.

- Participants commented on the need for increased awareness and medical knowledge of functional GI disorders by medical professionals. Participants stressed that proper diagnosis is critical to successful management and treatment of their condition. Many participants described their own difficulty in receiving a diagnosis (including being misdiagnosed), highlighting the lack of appropriate diagnostic tools. For example, one participant currently diagnosed with chronic unexplained nausea and vomiting shared that she had previously been diagnosed with gastroparesis because "sometimes I pass and sometimes I fail the gastric emptying studies."

- Short of a cure, many participants expressed the need for effective treatments that can better address the underlying cause of their disease, with less burdensome side effects. One participant reiterated that patients with a functional GI disorder often are unable to tolerate the side effects of their treatments and expressed that an ideal treatment would be a "gentle medication or supplement... that would not lead to tolerance."

- Several participants noted the need for fast-acting therapies that could control nausea, gas, or incontinence, and in turn provide them with the confidence that they would not have "accidents" in public. One participant shared that a fast-acting therapy would help to "gain some security wherever I am."

- Participants stressed the need for a treatment regimen that would enable them to have a more nutritious diet and also reduce their susceptibility to other diseases due to lack of nutrition. One web participant commented, "I need to be able to eat more than 500 calories daily so I can improve my quality and participation in life."

## Summary of Comments Submitted to the Public Docket

FDA received approximately 40 comment submissions to the public docket that supplemented the Patient-Focused Drug Development meeting on functional GI disorders. The majority of these comments were submitted by participants living with a functional GI disorder or their caregivers. FDA also received comments from advocacy organizations, including Gastroparesis Patient Association for Cures and Treatments, Critical Path Institute's Patient-Reported Outcome Consortium's Irritable Bowel Syndrome Working Group, International Foundation for Functional GI Disorders, Professional Compounding Centers for America, and the Celiac Disease Foundation.

The docket comments echoed the experiences and perspectives shared by participants of the meeting on the symptoms that affected their lives the most, the impacts of their disease on daily life, and their experiences with treatments for functional GI disorders. In the summaries that follow, particular focus is placed on experiences or perspectives that were not raised or addressed in detail at the public meeting.

### Submitted comments on symptoms of functional GI disorders

The symptoms of functional GI disorders mentioned on the docket reflected those discussed during the meeting. The most commonly mentioned symptoms included nausea, vomiting, abdominal pain, bloating, and fatigue. Other symptoms mentioned included acid reflux, colon spasms, cramping, insomnia, heartburn, and chronic dehydration. One commenter shared that her functional GI disorder resulted in pre-cancerous polyps in her stomach and intestines.

Several commenters expanded on the triggers for their GI-related symptoms. One participant shared that eating throughout the day significantly worsened her symptoms. She elaborated, "I must choose between eating and pain every single day." Other commenters noted that stress and hormone fluctuations significantly exacerbated their GI-related symptoms.

**Submitted comments on the overall impact of functional GI disorders on daily life**

The docket comments reflected the input received during the meeting related to the impact of functional GI disorders on patients' daily lives, and its significant toll on patients and their families. Most commenters shared that participating in physical activity has become very limited due to their conditions. As one commenter reiterated, "There are a limited number of things I can do with a group since I tend to have a reaction so easily." Commenters also echoed the impact of living with a functional GI disorder on family life, school and job performance and their inability to eat. One participant described her disorder as an "invisible illness" where "nothing makes you feel back to 100%."

**Submitted comments on current treatments for functional GI disorders**

The submitted comments reiterated the challenges of managing the many symptoms of functional GI disorders. The range of commenters' experiences was similar to the experiences shared at the public meeting. The prescription drug therapies mentioned most frequently were Reglan and domperidone. Non-drug therapies, such as dietary modifications, were also frequently mentioned. Commenters' experiences with prescription and non-drug therapies emphasized the variability of benefits and side effects from different patients. More detail is provided below.

- **Drug therapies:** One commenter shared that they had severe side effects while on Reglan, including high blood pressure and tachycardia. One commenter whose treatment regime includes domperidone stated that without her medications she is "completely bedridden," however, she commented that her medications don't improve her condition "to do much of anything except get out of bed." Another commenter reported that Linzess (linaclotide) does allow bowel movements, but is associated with "bloating and cramping/pain/discomfort ... [and] diarrhea for 2 to 3 hours after taking Linzess." A range of other drug therapies were mentioned, including Wellbutrin (bupropion), pain medications, anti-spasm medications, anti-psychotic medications and over-the-counter laxatives (such as MiraLax).

- **Medical devices or surgical treatments:** Medical devices or surgical treatments (such as a feeding tube) and IV therapy (such as TPN) were also mentioned. However, commenters also shared the downsides to medical procedures; one commenter shared that with TPN therapy, there was always a "fear of central line sepsis and liver failure." One commenter living with IBS shared that they had fecal microbiome transplants.

- **Non-drug therapies:** Discussion on non-drug therapies closely resembled input received during the meeting. In addition to various dietary controls, commenters also mentioned L-Glutamine, magnesium, probiotics, a gluten-free diet, essential oils, Capsicol, Seacure, Vitamin C, Vitamin B and Calcium.

**Submitted comments on ideal treatments for functional GI disorders**

Several perspectives were provided on ideal treatment for functional GI disorders, which reiterated the perspectives heard during the public meeting. Commenters identified the need for medications that addressed specific symptoms, including reducing nausea and increasing the ability to eat. Some stressed the need for "palatable, high-nutritive, high-protein, concentrates, wholesome, inexpensive liquid and non-solid foods," that were easy to digest for people living with functional GI disorders.

## Conclusion

Functional GI disorders encompass a spectrum of diseases with highly variable symptoms that significantly affect a patient's day-to-day functioning and way of life. Misunderstanding of functional GI disorders, even in the medical community, often leads to misdiagnosis, misguided treatment, and worse outcomes. This Patient-Focused Drug Development meeting provided FDA with the opportunity to hear from patients first-hand of the emotional, social, and physical toll that their condition has on their lives and the lives of their loved ones. Considering the distinct manifestation of functional GI disorders and the often overlap of multiple conditions in each patient, FDA is grateful to have heard the patients' voice on what symptoms, impacts, and aspects of treatments matter most to them, in addition to what factors are considered in making treatment decisions.

FDA recognizes that patients have a unique ability to contribute to our understanding of the broader context of this disease, which is important to our role, and that of others, in the drug development process. We are thankful to all of the participants who so thoughtfully and courageously shared such personal stories and perspectives. FDA shares the patient community's desire and commitment to furthering the development of safe and effective drug therapies.

A TREATMENT IMPROVEMENT PROTOCOL

# Addressing Viral Hepatitis in People With Substance Use Disorders

# TIP 53

Substance Abuse and Mental Health Services Administration
SAMHSA
www.samhsa.gov • 1-877-SAMHSA-7 (1-877-726-4727)

# 1 Overview of Viral Hepatitis

IN THIS CHAPTER



*You come in here to stop drinking and using drugs; I don't want to die no more. I don't want to go, to live in a box. I don't want to eat out of the garbage. I don't want to go to jail. I want to change. And 2 weeks, 3 weeks into this thing, I'm just starting to feel right, and I get news that I got hepatitis C.*

**—A Client's Perspective (Strauss, Astone, Munoz-Plaza, Hagan, & Des Jarlais, 2005, pp. 1821–1822)**

## Introduction

An estimated 3.5–5.3 million people in the United States live with chronic viral hepatitis (Institute of Medicine [IOM], 2010). Viral hepatitis is often a silent disease whose symptoms and signs become evident only after the disease has caused severe liver damage. The symptoms of hepatitis can take decades to manifest, so many people who are infected with hepatitis are unaware that they have the disease and therefore do not seek treatment. As a result, between 2010 and 2020, an estimated 150,000 people in the United States could die of liver cancer or other hepatitis-related liver disease (IOM, 2010). For many of these people, substance use will be a major factor that contributes to or worsens their hepatitis-related outcomes.

All people who use or have used illicit substances are at risk of contracting viral hepatitis. Injection drug use (IDU) is the primary way of contracting hepatitis C, and people who use substances are at risk for contracting other forms of viral hepatitis. Substance use disorders (SUDs) do not cause viral hepatitis, but people can contract or spread some types of viral hepatitis by sharing needles and other drug paraphernalia. In people who have chronic hepatitis, continued use of alcohol contributes to and frequently accelerates liver damage (Bhattacharya & Shuhart, 2003), increasing the likelihood that the individuals will develop cirrhosis or liver cancer.

In 2010, the U.S. Department of Health and Human Services (HHS) convened an interagency working group on viral hepatitis, comprised of experts throughout HHS to develop a comprehensive strategy for addressing the prevention, screening, and treatment of viral hepatitis, and for improving the coordination of care and treatment of individuals infected with viral hepatitis. The working group broadened the scope of expertise even further by soliciting information from other government agencies, professional organizations, community organizations, and members of the general public. As a result of many months of work by this diverse group of experts, HHS recently released *Combating the Silent Epidemic of Viral Hepatitis: U.S. Department of Health and Human Services Action Plan for the Prevention, Care and Treatment of Viral Hepatitis* (also called the Viral Hepatitis Action Plan) (HHS, 2011). This TIP supports the goals and objectives of the Viral Hepatitis Action Plan by providing information on the prevention and treatment of viral hepatitis and by encouraging behavioral health professionals to recommend hepatitis screening for their clients who might be at risk for hepatitis infection.

Viral hepatitis can be prevented and treated. Counselors, health professionals, and administrators in SUD treatment settings play an important role in promoting the prevention and treatment of viral hepatitis among their clients.

## Purpose of and Audience for the TIP

The main objective of this Treatment Improvement Protocol (TIP) is to improve care for clients with SUDs by increasing knowledge of viral hepatitis among staff in behavioral health programs that provide substance abuse treatment. Some surveys have shown that substance abuse treatment providers are not well informed about viral hepatitis (Strauss et al., 2006). Clients often perceive that counselors do not have the information they need (Munoz-Plaza, Strauss, Astone, Des Jarlais, & Hagan, 2004). With up-to-date information, counselors, health professionals, and administrators in SUD treatment settings can encourage clients to understand the serious nature of hepatitis, risk factors, the importance of liver wellness, screening, treatment options, and ways to avoid spreading—or contracting—hepatitis.

Other behavioral health treatment providers (e.g., counselors in mental health treatment settings, nurses, mid-level providers) will also find useful information in this TIP. Information is provided in lay terms so that it can be understood by readers who do not have medical training.

## Terminology

Terminology in the medical field may differ from that used in the substance abuse treatment field. This TIP uses terms from both disciplines. Appendix B contains a glossary of terms used in this TIP.

Because the TIP is primarily focused on care for clients with SUDs, *counselor* refers to *substance abuse treatment counselor*. *Client* refers to people seeking services at behavioral health programs providing substance abuse treatment. Occasionally, the TIP refers to people seeking services at a medical facility; in these instances, the term *patient* is used. *People* refers to adults, unless otherwise indicated.

*Treatment program* refers to a behavioral health program providing treatment for SUDs. *Medical care* refers to care for the body (e.g., treatment for hepatitis) as distinct from *behavioral health care*, which is the subset of medical care that addresses mental, emotional, and behavioral issues. *Co-occurring* is used to refer to health conditions (e.g., SUDs, mental disorders, hepatitis) that appear together in sequence or simultaneously; wherever this term is used, the pertaining conditions are indicated. *Hepatitis* refers to viral hepatitis infection.

*Relapse*, when used alone, refers to relapse to substance use. Virologists sometimes use relapse to refer to the return of hepatitis after antiviral treatment, which here is referred to as *virologic relapse*.

## The Liver

To appreciate the impact of hepatitis, it is essential to understand the liver—the organ predominantly affected in people with hepatitis. The liver, located on the upper right side of the abdomen just beneath the rib cage (Exhibit 1-1), performs numerous functions essential to human life.

**Exhibit 1-1 The Liver**

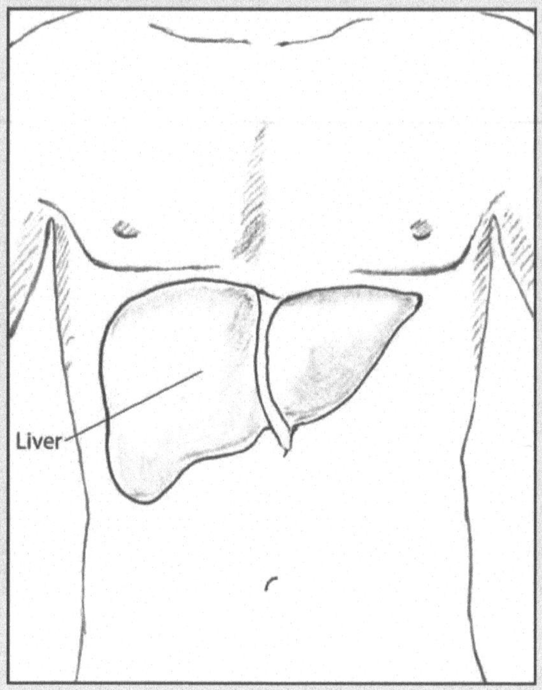


Blood passes from the intestines to the liver. Blood from the intestines contains nearly everything absorbed by the intestines, including nutrients and harmful or toxic substances (*toxins*). The liver breaks down toxins found in the blood and excretes them as harmless byproducts into the bile (a greenish yellow, thick, sticky fluid that aids in digestion) or back into the blood. Bile enters the intestine and leaves the body in stool. Byproducts excreted by the liver into blood are filtered out by the kidneys, then leave the body in urine. The liver also metabolizes drugs, alcohol, and prescription and over-the-counter medications, often making them inactive or easier to excrete from the body. If a person has a severely damaged liver, these substances build up in the body.

The liver manufactures several physiological products necessary for the body to function: cholesterol, bile, and other substances (e.g., clotting factors that are needed to stop bleeding). The liver also stores sugar, fats, and vitamins for later use. Sugar is stored in the liver as glycogen, transformed into glucose, and released into the bloodstream when needed.

## What Is Viral Hepatitis?

*Hepatitis* is inflammation of the liver. It can be caused by viruses, alcohol or substance use, exposure to toxins, and certain diseases. *Viral hepatitis* refers to liver inflammation caused by one of several types of viruses that attack the liver. In the United States, these are primarily hepatitis A virus (HAV), hepatitis B virus (HBV), and hepatitis C virus (HCV) (Exhibit 1-2), but other types of hepatitis viruses do exist. The body can rid itself of infection in some cases. In others, the body cannot get rid of the infection by itself and the infection becomes chronic (continues indefinitely).

**Exhibit 1-2 Overview of the Most Common Types of Viral Hepatitis**

| Category | Hepatitis A | Hepatitis B | Hepatitis C |
|---|---|---|---|
| Transmission route | Fecal–oral route | Blood and body fluids | Blood |
| Percentage of adults infected who develop chronic infection | 0% | 6%–10% | 75%–85% |
| Immunity after infection | Yes | Yes | No |
| Vaccine available | Yes | Yes | No |

Hepatitis can be acute, which means that the infection does not last longer than 6 months. If the body's immune system cannot fight off the virus within 6 months, the disease is considered chronic. In the United States, three to five times more people are living with chronic hepatitis B or C than with human immunodeficiency virus (HIV). Chronic hepatitis can lead to very serious health consequences—even death—because of liver failure or related medical conditions.

Most people who have chronic hepatitis do not know it (IOM, 2010). In most cases, people with infection have no symptoms of the disease, or their symptoms are so mild they do not see a medical care provider about them. Symptoms of hepatitis include the following:

- Fatigue (tiredness)
- General feeling of being unwell (malaise)
- Flu-like symptoms (e.g., headaches, muscle aches, low-grade fever)
- Lack of appetite, weight loss
- Nausea and vomiting, abdominal pain
- Jaundice (new or uncharacteristic yellow tinge to skin and mucus membranes)
- Diarrhea
- Itching of the skin
- Tea- or dark-colored urine
- Pale bowel movements

A person with chronic hepatitis can remain symptom free for decades while the liver is silently damaged. As hepatitis progresses and causes more liver damage, the liver may become scarred, referred to as *fibrosis*. Fibrosis sometimes leads to *cirrhosis*, which is profuse scarring of liver tissue. When cirrhosis develops, changes in the liver's structure compromise its ability to function. The *spleen* (an organ that fights infections and regulates the flow of blood in the body) may also be affected. Muscle wasting can occur, resulting from lack of appetite and the liver's inability to produce crucial proteins that build muscles. Sometimes the abdomen and ankles swell because of the body's increased difficulty with sodium handling and removing fluids and toxins. The person may develop jaundice. When liver damage is this extensive, serious complications are likely, including bleeding from the esophagus (varices) or stomach, abdominal swelling (ascites), and difficulty thinking and making decisions (encephalopathy). By the time these symptoms occur, liver damage is extensive, and the individual is at risk of liver failure or liver cancer—a condition that almost always has a poor prognosis.

## Hepatitis A

Hepatitis A never becomes chronic, and most individuals recover within 6 months. Once recovered, a person is no longer contagious and is immune to reinfection with HAV.

### Modes of Transmission

HAV is spread by the oral transmission of fecal matter (stool) of a person who is infected with HAV and it is extremely contagious. Minute amounts of fecal matter containing the virus left on a person's hands can contaminate water, food, or utensils, and a person who ingests this material can develop hepatitis A. HAV can survive outside the body for several days and in water for several months. People are most infectious during the 2 weeks before the onset of symptoms. HAV is not spread through casual contact. The virus is not present in semen.

### Disease Burden

An estimated one-third of U.S. residents have had HAV infection (Bell et al., 2005). The number of new HAV cases has declined by 92 percent since a vaccine became available in 1995. Nevertheless, approximately 3,000 new infections were investigated and reported in 2007, representing an estimated 25,000 infections during that year (Daniels, Grytdal, & Wasley, 2009). The primary risk factor in the United States for contracting hepatitis A is traveling to areas where HAV is endemic, followed by contact with someone who is infected with HAV, or having anal intercourse with an infected person. However, many people who contract hepatitis A do not report any risk factors (Klevens et al., 2010; Daniels et al., 2009).

### Disease Course

HAV infection is rarely life threatening, although severity and mortality may increase with age and underlying chronic liver disease. Signs and symptoms include fatigue, fever, loss of appetite, dark urine, and jaundice. When symptoms occur, they usually appear suddenly and generally disappear within a month. Hepatitis A can be serious when coupled with other forms of hepatitis or HIV.

### Hepatitis A and Substance Use

People who use drugs are at risk for acquiring hepatitis A. Outbreaks occur among people who inject drugs (Daniels et al., 2009; Wells, Fenaughty, Cagle, & Jaffe, 2006) and are associated with poor hygiene and low socioeconomic status (Crowcroft, 2003; Quaglio, Lugoboni, Messelani, Des Jarlais, & Lechi, 2006).

### Prevention

Hepatitis A is preventable. The most effective way to prevent HAV infection is through vaccination. The vaccine is given in two doses, 6 months apart. A combined HAV and HBV vaccine is also available.

The Centers for Disease Control and Prevention (CDC, 2010a) recommends hepatitis A vaccination for the following adults:

- People who use injection drugs
- Men who have sex with men (MSM)
- People with chronic liver disease
- People who receive blood clotting-factor concentrates
- People who travel to countries that have high rates of hepatitis A
- People with occupational risks of infection (e.g., workers in daycare centers, laboratories)

Despite recommendations for vaccination, many people are not vaccinated. Vaccination rates in high-risk groups range from 8 percent to 13 percent (Carey & Perlman, 2005; Chen & Cantrell, 2006). Moreover, half of those who had been vaccinated received only one dose instead of the two doses required for full protection. However, hepatitis A vaccination in the United States among children has been increasing since May 2006, when the universal vaccination of children (aged 12–23 months) was recommended. By 2008, coverage was estimated to be 40 percent in young children (CDC, 2010b).

Contraindications to receiving the hepatitis A vaccine include having a severe allergy to vaccine components and being moderately or severely ill at the time the vaccination is offered. All clients, especially pregnant women, should consult their medical care provider to determine whether they should get vaccinated against hepatitis A.

Washing hands frequently—especially after using the bathroom, changing a diaper, and before preparing food—helps prevent the spread of HAV.

## Hepatitis B

Hepatitis B can be acute or chronic. More than 90 percent of infants and 30 percent of children ages 1–5 years who have been exposed to HBV will remain chronically infected with HBV. By contrast, approximately 90 percent of adults with HBV infection alone (i.e., without co-infection) recover completely from HBV infection and do not become chronically infected (CDC, 2010c). For those with chronic infection, compromise of the immune system (e.g., by chemotherapy or HIV co-infection) places the person at risk for reactivation (Luetkemeyer, 2010; CDC, 2009).

### *Modes of Transmission*

HBV is very contagious; it is much more infectious than HIV (World Health Organization, 2009). HBV is spread through infected blood and other body fluids (e.g., semen) and can live outside the body for more than 7 days. Modes of transmission include:

- Sharing IDU equipment (e.g., needles, syringes, cookers, filters).
- Accidental needle sticks or other breaches of the skin, especially among those whose occupations expose them to blood (e.g., medical care workers, dentists).
- Unprotected sex with a partner who is infected with HBV.
- An infected mother passing the virus to her infant during delivery.
- Receipt of a blood transfusion or transplantation surgery from an infectious donor. (This is rare in the United States since mandatory screening was implemented in 1972.)

### *Disease Burden*

Hepatitis B is a major cause of liver disease worldwide. In 2007, there were approximately 43,000 new infections in the United States. Between 800,000 and 1.4 million people in the United States live with chronic hepatitis B (Wasley et al., 2010; Daniels et al., 2009). In the United States, Asian and Pacific Islanders and MSM are disproportionately infected with HBV.

### *Disease Course*

Approximately 35 percent of those infected exhibit symptoms. Usually, acute HBV infection alone is not life threatening.

Up to 10 percent of people with acute hepatitis B will develop chronic hepatitis after 6 months (Exhibit 1-3). Most of those with chronic infection remain symptom free, although they can infect other people. Some experience serious illness. HBV infections become chronic more frequently in people with compromised immune systems (e.g., people with HIV infection). Worldwide, hepatitis B is the most likely form of hepatitis to cause liver cancer, particularly hepatocellular carcinoma. Chronic hepatitis B can also result in cirrhosis of the liver, liver failure, and death. Daniels et al. (2009) estimate 3,000 people die in the United States per year from chronic HBV infection.

**Exhibit 1-3 Disease Course of Hepatitis B**

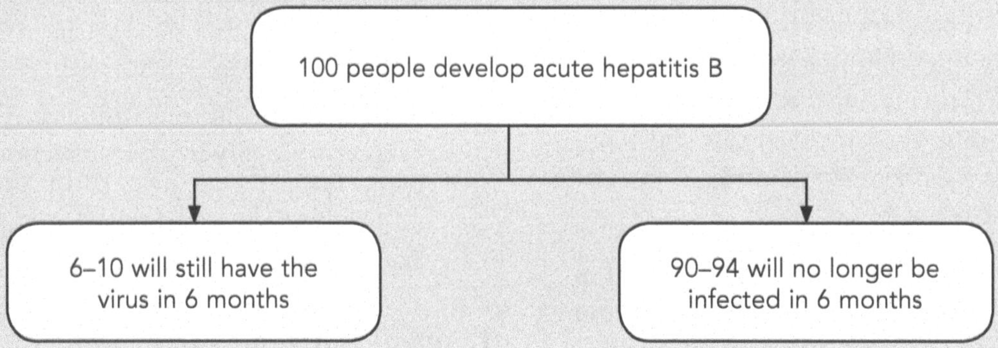


### *Hepatitis B and Substance Use*

Three percent to 11 percent of people who inject drugs have chronic hepatitis B (Weinbaum et al., 2008). One study suggests that rates of asymptomatic HBV infection among clients on methadone maintenance may be as high as 25 percent (Bart et al., 2008). Alcohol use by people with hepatitis B damages the liver, which is already compromised with the hepatitis infection.

### *Prevention*

Vaccination is the most effective way to prevent HBV infection. The consensus panel recommends HBV vaccination for the following adults:

- People who are infected with HCV
- People who are sexually active with or who share a household with a person with infectious HBV
- Men who have sex with men (MSM)
- People who inject drugs
- People with occupational exposure to blood (e.g., medical care workers, dentists)
- People who attend or work at institutions for people with developmental disabilities
- Hemodialysis patients or those with end-stage renal disease
- People who are infected with HIV
- Anyone with liver disease
- Anyone who lives in or travels to countries with high rates of HBV
- Adults in correctional settings

The HBV vaccine is given in three doses within a 6-month period. However, the most convenient way to provide immunization is with the combined hepatitis A/hepatitis B vaccine (sold under the brand name, Twinrix). It is administered in three intramuscular injections on a 0-, 1-, and 6-month schedule, or may be given on an accelerated schedule of four doses, given on days 0, 7, and 21–30 with a booster dose at 12 months (FDA, 2010a). Despite the availability of the HBV vaccine, many at-risk individuals have not been vaccinated. A study of people age 30 and younger who inject drugs found that only 22 percent had been vaccinated against HBV (Lum et al., 2008). Contraindications to getting the hepatitis B vaccine include having had a severe allergic reaction to a previous dose or to a component of the vaccine. Clients should discuss the vaccination with a medical care provider.

## Hepatitis C

Hepatitis C can be acute or chronic, but it starts as an acute infection (that may go unrecognized). Unlike people with hepatitis

A and B, people who have hepatitis C and clear the virus do not develop immunity; they can become reinfected with the virus at a later date.

### *Modes of Transmission*

Hepatitis C is a blood-borne disease. IDU is the most common risk factor for acquiring hepatitis C. The virus can enter the body through any puncture in the skin (e.g., cuts, burns, sores), and travels, via the blood, to the liver. Risks of sexual transmission are unclear but appear to be low, especially compared with sexual transmission rates of HIV or HBV. Nonetheless, HCV infection rates are higher in people who have multiple sex partners. Infections have been reported in individuals with no known risk factors.

### *Disease Burden*

HCV infection is the most prevalent chronic, blood-borne infection in the United States (Alter et al., 1999). Approximately 3.2 million U.S. residents have chronic HCV infection (CDC, 2010c). Forty percent of chronic liver disease—the 10th leading cause of death in the United States—is caused by HCV. Hepatitis C is most prevalent among people born between 1945 and 1965, the majority of whom were likely infected during the 1970s and 1980s, when infection rates were the highest. CDC (2010c) estimated 17,000 new infections in 2007, and people who inject drugs account for more than half of the new cases.

### *Disease Course*

HCV can be detected in the blood within 1–3 weeks of transmission. However, the majority of people with hepatitis C are asymptomatic.

Of people who contract hepatitis C, 15 percent to 25 percent clear the infection, but 75 percent to 85 percent do not and the infection becomes chronic (CDC, 2010c) (Exhibit 1-4). Chronic HCV is insidious, usually progressing very slowly and with few or no symptoms for the first 20–30 years after infection. Symptoms often do not occur until the liver damage has advanced. As the disease progresses, the liver may develop fibrosis, which can progress to cirrhosis. Approximately 12,000 people die each year from HCV-related liver disease (IOM, 2010).

**Exhibit 1-4 Disease Course of Hepatitis C**

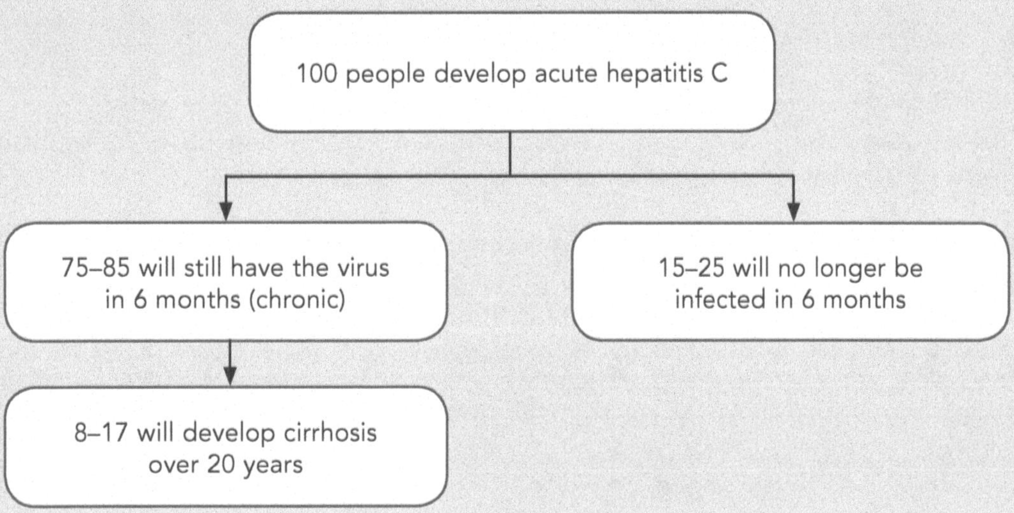

HCV infection appears to progress more quickly in men, people older than 50 at the time of infection, and people with concurrent HBV or HIV (Hézode et al., 2005). Mortality is high in people with HCV/HIV co-infection.

### Hepatitis C and Substance Use

HCV is highly contagious; people who inject drugs are more likely to contract hepatitis C than HIV (Garfein, Vlahov, Galai, Doherty, & Nelson, 1996). People who inject drugs are at high risk for becoming infected with HCV from sharing needles and drug use paraphernalia. Up to 91 percent of people who inject drugs and share needles or other paraphernalia over a prolonged period will eventually acquire HCV infection (Abou-Saleh & Foley, 2008; Macias et al., 2008; Maxwell, Shinderman, Miner, & Bennet, 2002; Tseng et al., 2007). Liver disease progresses more quickly in people who have HCV and abuse alcohol than in people with only one of the conditions (Bhattacharya & Shuhart, 2003; Felsen, Fishbein, & Litwin, 2010).

### Prevention

There is no vaccine against hepatitis C. It can be prevented only by avoiding contact with contaminated blood.

#### HCV—True or False?

***You can get HCV infection by using the razor of a person who is infected with HCV.***

**True.** HCV is spread through contact with infected blood, such as may be found on a razor or toothbrush.

***You'll probably get HCV infection if you eat food from a plate that wasn't cleaned well.***

**False.** You can only get HCV infection through contact with infected blood.

***Hepatitis C is mostly spread through unprotected sex.***

**False.** The greatest risk factor is IDU. Sexual transmission of HCV is rare, except in people who are infected with HIV. However, some evidence suggests that HCV might be passed through sex, if the sex includes the possibility of blood exposure (Tohme & Holmberg, 2010).

***A vaccine has been developed to protect against HCV.***

**False.** There is no vaccine against HCV.

***Hepatitis C can be spread when people who inject drugs share their rinse water.***

**True.** When people who are infected with HCV use needles, drops of their blood are mixed with the rinse water. Anyone who uses the same rinse water could contract HCV.

***Most people who have HCV infection will become seriously ill and die from liver disease.***

**False.** One to five percent of people who have HCV will die from HCV-related diseases. People who have additional medical or substance use problems are at increased risk of developing serious liver disease, which can be fatal. People who have other types of viral hepatitis or HIV infection are also more likely to get serious liver disease. However, people who adhere to hepatitis C treatment and abstain from alcohol and drugs improve their chances for a healthy life.

Adapted from Strauss et al., 2006.

## Other Types of Viral Hepatitis

Hepatitis D virus (HDV) infects only people who are already infected with hepatitis B. HDV is transmitted the same way as HBV—through blood and other body fluids. Because hepatitis D can occur only in people with hepatitis B, vaccination against HBV infection also prevents HDV infection. When people who have hepatitis B contract hepatitis D, the result can be a *superinfection*, which has a poor prognosis.

Hepatitis E virus (HEV) was first identified in 1980, and little is known about it. Hepatitis E manifests only as an acute infection. It is most often transmitted through the fecal–oral route, with the highest rates in countries with poor sanitation. While vaccines are not available at this time, they are in development.

Hepatitis F virus (HFV) was identified in 1991, and researchers disagree on whether it is a discrete type of viral hepatitis. No diagnostic tests exist for HFV infection.

Little is known about Hepatitis G virus (HGV) infection, which was identified in 1995, but it does not appear to cause significant liver damage.

## Co-Infection with Different Types of Viral Hepatitis

Some people are infected with more than one type of hepatitis. Several studies (Cacopardo, Nunnari, & Nigro, 2008; Crockett & Keeffe, 2005; Wietzke-Braun, Manhardt, Rosenberger, Ramadori, & Mihm, 2007) indicate that when co-infection occurs, one of four scenarios is possible:

- No effect. In some cases, there is no known effect from the concurrent infections.
- More severe disease. In most cases, co-infection worsens the severity of one type of hepatitis.

### Clinical Scenario

| | |
|---|---|
| Sarah: | "I don't see what the big deal is about hepatitis. I feel fine." |
| Counselor: | "Hepatitis is a silent disease. You could go for years feeling fine while hepatitis damages your liver." |
| Sarah: | "So, I get a little liver damage. I know lots of people with hep who just live with it." |
| Counselor: | "Let's work together during our sessions to better understand what hepatitis is really all about. It's true that some people can live with degrees of liver damage, depending on their overall health, but if your liver gets damaged enough, it won't work anymore. When your liver doesn't work, you become very ill. Your liver performs hundreds of functions that keep you alive. Right now, your liver is removing toxins, storing the nutrients your body needs, producing the materials you need to digest food, and doing many other things. If your liver stops working properly, your quality of life can be seriously lowered. What kind of life do you want for yourself?" |
| Sarah: | "I want to feel good and to be able to do all the things I like to do. I didn't realize that when a disease is 'silent,' it can actually be doing a lot of damage. I guess I can't just ignore my hepatitis and hope that it will go away." |

- Activation of disease. To become an active disease, HDV infection depends on co-infection with HBV.
- Deactivation of disease. In rare cases, co-infection may suppress previously active disease.

## Co-Infection with Viral Hepatitis and HIV

### *HAV/HIV Co-Infection*

HIV treatment may need to be temporarily suspended if HAV infection is acquired. Most studies suggest that this delay does not affect HIV progression. However, hepatitis A may be more severe and last longer in people who have both infections than in people who do not have HIV (Ida et al., 2002).

### *HBV/HIV Co-Infection*

As many as 90 percent of people who have HIV infection have been infected with HBV (i.e., with prior resolved infections; Rodriguez-Mendez, Gonzalez-Quintela, Aguilera, & Barrio, 2000; Scharschmidt et al., 1992), and 10 percent to 15 percent of these people will become chronic carriers. Most studies suggest that this co-infection does not significantly change the likelihood that the HIV infection will progress to AIDS. However, the co-infection increases the likelihood that HBV infection will become chronic and progress quickly and that liver damage might be more severe (Alberti, Vario, Ferrari, & Pistis, 2005; Sulkowski, 2008).

### *HCV/HIV Co-Infection*

HIV infection may increase a person's risk of contracting HCV through sexual contact (Delwaide, Bourgeois, Colle, & Robaeys, 2002). Approximately 25 percent to 33 percent of people who are infected with HIV are co-infected with HCV (Alberti et al., 2005; Rockstroh & Spengler, 2004). Some studies (Eyster et al., 1993; Garcia-Samaniego et al., 2001; Lesens, Deschenes, Steben, Belanger, & Tsoukas, 1999; Pol et al., 1998) suggest that people who have HCV/HIV co-infection are more likely to develop cirrhosis, liver cancer, and liver failure than those with hepatitis only. The presence of both infections increases the risk of liver toxicity from HIV medications. However, liver damage slows when HIV medications are taken by preserving or restoring immune function and reducing HIV-related immune activation and inflammation. Therefore, the benefits of HIV medications may outweigh the risks (Panel on Antiretroviral Guidelines for Adults and Adolescents, 2011; Hammer et al., 2008; Sherman, 2007). If untreated, HCV infection progresses more quickly in people who are co-infected with HIV than in those who are infected with HCV alone.

# VACCINATION CARDS

GET VACCINATED FOR **HEPATITIS A** AND **HEPATITIS B**

| Vaccine + dose # | Date | Manufacturer/lot | Route/site | Vaccinator |
|---|---|---|---|---|
| | | | | |
| | | | | |
| | | | | |
| | | | | |
| | | | | |

GET VACCINATED FOR **HEPATITIS A** AND **HEPATITIS B**

| Vaccine + dose # | Date | Manufacturer/lot | Route/site | Vaccinator |
|---|---|---|---|---|
| | | | | |
| | | | | |
| | | | | |
| | | | | |
| | | | | |

GET VACCINATED FOR **HEPATITIS A** AND **HEPATITIS B**

| Vaccine + dose # | Date | Manufacturer/lot | Route/site | Vaccinator |
|---|---|---|---|---|
| | | | | |
| | | | | |
| | | | | |
| | | | | |
| | | | | |

GET VACCINATED FOR **HEPATITIS A** AND **HEPATITIS B**

| Vaccine + dose # | Date | Manufacturer/lot | Route/site | Vaccinator |
|---|---|---|---|---|
| | | | | |
| | | | | |
| | | | | |
| | | | | |
| | | | | |

GET VACCINATED FOR **HEPATITIS A** AND **HEPATITIS B**

| Vaccine + dose # | Date | Manufacturer/lot | Route/site | Vaccinator |
|---|---|---|---|---|
| | | | | |
| | | | | |
| | | | | |
| | | | | |
| | | | | |

GET VACCINATED FOR **HEPATITIS A** AND **HEPATITIS B**

| Vaccine + dose # | Date | Manufacturer/lot | Route/site | Vaccinator |
|---|---|---|---|---|
| | | | | |
| | | | | |
| | | | | |
| | | | | |
| | | | | |

# Preventing Erectile Dysfunction

## What steps can I take to prevent erectile dysfunction?

You can help prevent many of the causes of erectile dysfunction (ED).

### Quit smoking

If you smoke, get help quitting. Smoking is linked to heart and blood vessel disease NIH, which can lead to ED. Even when heart and blood vessel disease and other possible causes of ED are taken into account, smoking still increases the chances that you will have ED.

### Follow a healthy eating plan

To help maintain erectile function, choose whole-grain foods, low-fat dairy foods, fruits and vegetables, and lean meats. Avoid foods high in fat, especially saturated fat, and sodium. Follow a healthy eating plan to help aim for a healthy weight, and control your blood pressure and diabetes. Controlling your blood pressure and diabetes may help prevent ED.

Also, avoid drinking too much alcohol. If you are having trouble cutting out alcohol, see a counselor who has expert knowledge in treating people who drink too much NIH.

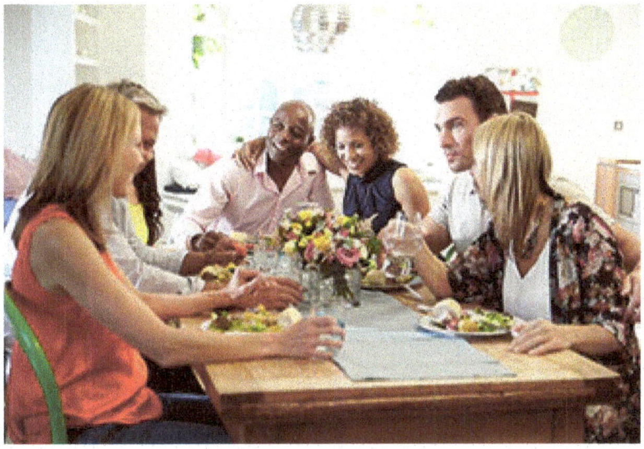

Take steps to prevent erectile dysfunction (ED): quit smoking, follow a healthy eating plan, maintain a healthy weight, and be physically active.

### Maintain a healthy weight to prevent diabetes and high blood pressure

Maintaining a healthy weight also can help delay the start of diabetes and keep your blood pressure down. Talk with your doctor about how to prevent diabetes—or manage the disease if you already have it. Get regular checkups to measure your blood pressure.

If you need to lose weight, talk with your health care provider about how to lose weight safely. Ask for a referral to a dietitian who can help you plan healthy meals to lose weight. Losing weight may help reduce inflammation, increase testosterone NIH levels, and increase self-esteem, all of which may help prevent ED. If you are at a healthy weight for your height, maintain that weight through healthy eating and physical activity.

## Be physically active

Physical activity increases blood flow through your body, including the penis. Talk with a health care professional before starting new activities. Beginners should start slow, with easier activities such as walking at a normal pace or gardening. You can gradually work up to harder activities, such as walking briskly or swimming. Aim for at least 30 minutes of activity most days of the week.

## Avoid using illegal drugs

Using illegal drugs may prevent you from getting or keeping an erection. For instance, some illegal drugs may prevent you from becoming aroused or feeling other sensations. Using illegal drugs may mask other psychological, emotional, or physical factors that may be causing your ED. Talk with your health care provider if you think you need help with drug abuse NIH.

**Last Reviewed July 2017**

URL of this page: //medlineplus.gov/ency/article/004024.htm

# Drugs that may cause erection problems

Many medicines and recreational drugs can affect a man's sexual arousal and sexual performance. What causes erection problems in one man may not affect another man.

Talk to your health care provider if you think that a drug is having a negative effect on your sexual performance. Never stop taking any medicine without first talking to your provider. Some medicines may lead to life-threatening reactions if you do not take care when stopping or changing them.

The following is a list of some medicines and drugs that may cause erectile dysfunction (ED) in men. There may be additional drugs other than those on this list that can cause erection difficulties.

Antidepressants and other psychiatric medicines:

- Amitriptyline (Elavil)
- Amoxapine (Asendin)
- Buspirone (Buspar)
- Chlordiazepoxide (Librium)
- Chlorpromazine (Thorazine)
- Clomipramine (Anafranil)
- Clorazepate (Tranxene)
- Desipramine (Norpramin)
- Diazepam (Valium)
- Doxepin (Sinequan)
- Fluoxetine (Prozac)
- Fluphenazine (Prolixin)
- Imipramine (Tofranil)

- Isocarboxazid (Marplan)
- Lorazepam (Ativan)
- Meprobamate (Equanil)
- Mesoridazine (Serentil)
- Nortriptyline (Pamelor)
- Oxazepam (Serax)
- Phenelzine (Nardil)
- Phenytoin (Dilantin)
- Sertraline (Zoloft)
- Thioridazine (Mellaril)
- Thiothixene (Navane)
- Tranylcypromine (Parnate)
- Trifluoperazine (Stelazine)

Antihistamine medicines (certain classes of antihistamines are also used to treat heartburn):

- Cimetidine (Tagamet)
- Dimenhydrinate (Dramamine)
- Diphenhydramine (Benadryl)
- Hydroxyzine (Vistaril)
- Meclizine (Antivert)
- Nizatidine (Axid)
- Promethazine (Phenergan)
- Ranitidine (Zantac)

High blood pressure medicines and diuretics (water pills):

- Atenolol (Tenormin)
- Bethanidine
- Bumetanide (Bumex)
- Captopril (Capoten)
- Chlorothiazide (Diuril)
- Chlorthalidone (Hygroton)

- Clonidine (Catapres)
- Enalapril (Vasotec)
- Furosemide (Lasix)
- Guanabenz (Wytensin)
- Guanethidine (Ismelin)
- Guanfacine (Tenex)
- Haloperidol (Haldol)
- Hydralazine (Apresoline)
- Hydrochlorothiazide (Esidrix)
- Labetalol (Normodyne)
- Methyldopa (Aldomet)
- Metoprolol (Lopressor)
- Nifedipine (Adalat, Procardia)
- Phenoxybenzamine (Dibenzyline)
- Phentolamine (Regitine)
- Prazosin (Minipress)
- Propranolol (Inderal)
- Reserpine (Serpasil)
- Spironolactone (Aldactone)
- Triamterene (Maxzide)
- Verapamil (Calan)

Thiazides are the most common cause of erectile dysfunction among the high blood pressure medicines. The next most common cause is beta blockers. Alpha blockers tend to be less likely to cause this problem.

Parkinson disease medicines:

- Benztropine (Cogentin)
- Biperiden (Akineton)
- Bromocriptine (Parlodel)
- Levodopa (Sinemet)
- Procyclidine (Kemadrin)

- Trihexyphenidyl (Artane)

Chemotherapy and hormonal medicines:

- Antiandrogens (Casodex, Flutamide, Nilutamide)
- Busulfan (Myleran)
- Cyclophosphamide (Cytoxan)
- Ketoconazole
- LHRH agonists (Lupron, Zoladex)
- LHRH antagonist (Firmagon)

Other medicines:

- Aminocaproic acid (Amicar)
- Atropine
- Clofibrate (Atromid-S)
- Cyclobenzaprine (Flexeril)
- Cyproterone
- Digoxin (Lanoxin)
- Disopyramide (Norpace)
- Dutasteride (Avodart)
- Estrogen
- Finasteride (Propecia, Proscar)
- Furazolidone (Furoxone)
- H2 blockers (Tagamet, Zantac, Pepcid)
- Indomethacin (Indocin)
- Lipid-lowering agents
- Licorice
- Metoclopramide (Reglan)
- Nonsteroidal anti-inflammatory drugs (NSAIDs, ibuprofen, etc.)
- Orphenadrine (Norflex)
- Prochlorperazine (Compazine)
- Pseudoephedrine (Sudafed)

- Sumatriptan (Imitrex)

Opiate analgesics (painkillers):

- Codeine
- Fentanyl (Innovar)
- Hydromorphone (Dilaudid)
- Meperidine (Demerol)
- Methadone
- Morphine
- Oxycodone (Oxycontin, Percodan)

Recreational drugs:

- Alcohol
- Amphetamines
- Barbiturates
- Cocaine
- Marijuana
- Heroin
- Nicotine

## Alternative Names

Impotence caused by medications; Drug-induced erectile dysfunction; Prescription medicines and impotence

## References

Berookhim BM, Mulhall JP. Erectile dysfunction. In: Sidawy AN, Perler BA, eds. *Rutherford's Vascular Surgery and Endovascular Therapy*. 9th ed. Philadelphia, PA: Elsevier; 2019:chap 191.

Burnett AL, Ramasamy R. Evaluation and management of erectile dysfunction. In: Partin AW, Dmochowski RR, Kavoussi LR, Peters CA, eds. *Campbell-Walsh-Wein Urology*. 12th ed. Philadelphia, PA: Elsevier; 2021:chap 69.

Waller DG, Sampson AP. Erectile dysfunction. In: Waller DG, Sampson AP, eds. *Medical Pharmacology and Therapeutics*. 5th ed. Philadelphia, PA: Elsevier; 2018:chap 16.

REVIEW

Open Access

# Smoke, alcohol and drug addiction and male fertility

Andrea Sansone[1*], Carla Di Dato[1], Cristina de Angelis[2,3], Davide Menafra[3], Carlotta Pozza[1], Rosario Pivonello[3], Andrea Isidori[1] and Daniele Gianfrilli[1]

**Abstract**

In recent decades, the decline in human fertility has become increasingly more worrying: while therapeutic interventions might help, they are vexing for the couple and often burdened with high failure rates and costs. Prevention is the most successful approach to fertility disorders in males and females alike. We performed a literature review on three of the most common unhealthy habits – tobacco, alcohol and drug addiction – and their reported effects on male fertility. Tobacco smoking is remarkably common in most first-world countries; despite a progressive decline in the US, recent reports suggest a prevalence of more than 30% in subjects of reproductive age – a disturbing perspective, given the well-known ill-effects on reproductive and sexual function as well as general health. Alcohol consumption is often considered socially acceptable, but its negative effects on gonadal function have been consistently reported in the last 30 years. Several studies have reported a variety of negative effects on male fertility following drug abuse – a worrying phenomenon, as illicit drug consumption is on the rise, most notably in younger subjects. While evidence in these regards is still far from solid, mostly as a result of several confounding factors, it is safe to assume that cessation of tobacco smoking, alcohol consumption and recreational drug addiction might represent the best course of action for any couple trying to achieve pregnancy.

## Background

Almost 15% of all couples trying to conceive are affected by infertility, and in almost half of these cases male infertility is the sole or a contributing factor [1]. The decline of male fertility is not an empty threat: evidence points at a steadily progressive decline of sperm concentration over the past 35 years [2]. These reports have rekindled the interest in the potential impact of environmental factors and lifestyle on fertility: in order to decrease the social costs of male infertility and the resulting burdens on public health, identifying preventable factors is of the utmost importance. Sedentary behavior and obesity have both been associated with impaired male fertility [3, 4] and have often been addressed as potentially preventable factors; a more detailed review on the effects of sports and physical activity on male fertility is included in this *Special Issue*. The role of other unhealthy lifestyles, such as smoking and alcohol consumption, and environmental stressors on general health is universally recognized, but their effects on male fertility are less known [5]. Indeed, male reproductive health may be a sensitive marker of pollution [6] and environmental exposures [7, 8]. For ethical reasons, interventional studies in regards to the effects of tobacco use, second-hand smoking, recreational drug abuse and alcohol consumption are generally not feasible in humans. The vast majority of studies on these topics are therefore retrospective [8]. Sadly, this leads to a wide array of confounders, for which control is limited. A partial solution comes from animal studies; however, exposure in these models is significantly higher than in humans, and as such results should be interpreted with caution.

In order to provide an up-to-date and reliable reference in regards to the possible role of alcohol, tobacco and recreational drugs on male fertility, we performed a thorough review of existing literature and gathered all necessary data.

* Correspondence: andrea.sansone@uniroma1.it
[1]Department of Experimental Medicine, Section of Medical Pathophysiology, Food Science and Endocrinology, Sapienza - University of Rome, Viale Regina Elena 324, 00161 Rome, Italy
Full list of author information is available at the end of the article

### Causes of male infertility

Couple infertility is defined by the failure to achieve pregnancy after at least 12 months of regular, unprotected intercourse. On the other hand, providing a fitting definition for male infertility is a more difficult task: diagnosis is traditionally based on semen analysis results, compared to the World Health Organization reference values [9].

Successful spermatogenesis is the result of the complex interaction between endocrine, paracrine and autocrine factors [10]. Unsurprisingly, several acquired and congenital conditions might impair the fine mechanisms involved in spermatogenesis (Table 1). Acquired testicular failure, as often observed following testicular torsion, orchitis, or administration of cytotoxic treatment is often associated with azoospermia. Varicocele, testicular trauma, and medications might affect fertility, although in most circumstances the spermatogenesis is impaired to a lesser extent. Genetic abnormalities, such as Klinefelter Syndrome or microdeletions in the AZF *(azoospermia factor)* region on the human male Y chromosome, usually manifest with azoospermia; however, small nucleotide polymorphisms are being investigated as a possible cause of "idiopathic" oligo-azoospermia. However, despite the recent discoveries in regards to the genetics of male infertility, to the present date most causes of oligozoospermia remain unknown.

Age is significantly associated with decline in semen quality, supposedly as a result of continued replications from mutated spermatogonial stem cells [11]. DNA fragmentation and chromatin condensation might also play a role in the pathogenesis of male infertility [12]. Among non-genetic causes of male infertility, oxidative stress resulting from exaggerated production of reactive oxygen species (ROS) is perhaps the most known factor. ROS are needed for capacitation, the acrosome reaction and ultimately fertilization; however, reduced clearance and excessive production are both able to induce DNA damage and defective membrane integrity in sperm cells, therefore resulting in reduced fertility potential [13]. Semen from fertile men has a more effective antioxidant capacity than that from infertile men; furthermore, immature teratozoospermic forms produce relatively more ROS than normal, mature sperm [13]. Inflammatory processes and vascular diseases, including varicocele, can supposedly increase ROS production: a thorough evaluation aimed to assess the presence of predisposing conditions is mandatory in the evaluation of any infertile male.

**Table 1** Possible acquired causes of male reproductive impairment

| |
|---|
| Hypothalamic-pituitary axis |
| Compressive effect (Pituitary or brain tumors) |
| Ablative effect (CNS surgery or radiotherapy) |
| Infiltrative effect (fungal infections, sarcoidosis, hemochromatosis) |
| Suppressive effect (exogenous AAS) |
| Quantitative alterations of spermatogenesis |
| Varicocele |
| Previous chemotherapy or radiotherapy |
| Testicular failure (torsion, orchitis, orchiectomy) |
| Comorbidities (liver and kidney disease) |
| Qualitative alterations of spermatogenesis |
| Oxidative stress |
| DNA damage |
| Ductal obstructions |
| Surgery (vasectomy, hernia repair, pelvic surgery) |
| Neurological disorders (Multiple Sclerosis, Spinal Cord Injury, neural tube defects) |
| Erectile or ejaculatory dysfunction |

*Abbreviations: CNS* central nervous system, *AAS* anabolic-androgenic steroid. Edited from H Tournaye, C Krausz and RD Oates [10]

### Tobacco smoking and male fertility

More than 60% of noncommunicable diseases list smoking among their risk factors, and every year more than six million deaths result from tobacco consumption and second-hand smoke [14]. Despite the growing body of evidence supporting its deleterious effects, smoking is still a widespread phenomenon, as proven by recent reports from the World Health Organization. More than one-third of all male adults worldwide use tobacco [15]; similarly, approximately 30% of women of reproductive age smoke cigarettes [16]. Europe is still the leading continent in regards to tobacco use, whereas smoking rates have gradually declined in the United States in recent years [17].

### Clinical studies

The deleterious effects of smoking on fertility have been described since 1983: Olsen and colleagues identified tobacco use as one of the causes of otherwise unexplained infertility in more than 1000 females [18]. To the present date, more than 4700 different chemicals have been identified in tobacco smoke [19], ranging from heavy metals to polycyclic aromatic hydrocarbons to mutagenic chemicals. A significant association between seminal plasma lead levels and lifetime smoking estimate has been reported [20]; likewise, smoking is considered the most common source of lead and cadmium exposure [21]. Some metal micronutrients involved in the pathogenesis of oxidative stress and male infertility, including arsenic and the aforementioned cadmium and lead, are routinely inhaled during combustion of tobacco or cigarette paper [21]. These metals all have mutagenic properties and are similarly associated with increased risk of male infertility, despite no significant differences in semen volume, concentration, and motility [22, 23]. On the other hand, impairments in sperm parameters have been observed in many studies in the last decades [24, 25]: in most of them, alterations in morphology and decreased concentration, motility and viability have been observed among smokers. A significant decrease in sperm concentrations of current smokers compared with those who had never smoked has been observed in a meta-analysis of more than 2500 men from five separate studies [26]. Similarly, Kunzle and colleagues have found a significant association between smoking and reduced sperm concentration in 2100 men presenting for fertility evaluation [27].

Mechanisms resulting in impaired sperm parameters have been investigated, but definite evidence is still missing. Ultra-structural abnormalities, mostly affecting axonemal microtubules and tail alterations, have been reported in heavy smokers [28, 29]; similarly, smoking impairs the acrosome reaction [30] and capacitation [31], two processes ultimately needed for fertilization. Increased oxidative stress has been suggested as a possible mechanism resulting in impaired sperm functions. Hypoxia resulting from cigarette smoking might also be responsible for impaired spermatogenesis, even more dramatically in patients with varicocele [8, 32]. Mitochondrial activity and chromatin structure in human sperm might be impaired by several toxins, therefore negatively affecting fertilization capacity both in vivo and in vitro [17, 33, 34].

Hypothetically, chronic cigarette smoking increases liver metabolism of testosterone, while at the same time inducing secretory dysfunction of Leydig and Sertoli cells [24]. However, there seems to be no general consensus on the effects of smoking on FSH and LH production: some studies have shown lower levels of both gonadotropins among smokers, whereas different researchers have observed increased concentration of LH and/or FSH following tobacco consumption [35, 36]. Considering all the possible confounding factors, testosterone concentration is remarkably difficult to ascertain among smokers: some studies have reported increased serum testosterone and dehydroepiandrosterone levels in smokers [35, 37], whereas others have suggested that mean levels of testosterone are not significantly different [38] between smokers and non-smokers.

The American Society of Reproductive Medicine in 2012 stated that "semen parameters and results of sperm function tests are 22% poorer in smokers than in non-smokers and the effects are dose-dependent" [16]. More recently, a meta-analysis study on a grand total of 5865 subjects has concluded that moderate and heavy smokers are more likely to have reduced sperm count and motility [17]. Evidence suggests a significant role for cigarette smoking on spermatogenesis, but on the other hand the impact of smoking on male fertility has yet to be fully elucidated. A preventive approach to infertility, suggesting smoking cessation and reduction of second-hand smoking in both women and men, should be suggested.

### Experimental studies

#### *Animal studies*

Cigarette smoking results in accumulation of benzo(a)pyrene (B[a]P) and cotinine, ultimately leading to DNA damage and testicular cytotoxicity in rodent models. In a recent study, Esakky and colleagues [39] reported significantly decreased expression of aryl hydrocarbon receptor (*Ahr*), and enhanced expression of Fas, FasL, BCL2, and activated caspase-3 proteins in testes exposed to cigarette smoke condensate. The reduced expression of Ahr increases susceptibility of germ cells to polycyclic aromatic hydrocarbons, while the remaining proteins all induce apoptosis via extrinsic (FAS, FASL) or mitochondrial processes (BCL, caspase-3). Tobacco use is also closely associated to reduced antioxidant activity, therefore worsening the effects of oxidative stress [40].

Exposure to cigarette smoke also impairs the activity of sorbitol dehydrogenase and lactate dehydrogenase, reflecting the effects on spermatogenesis and sperm maturation in rats [41]. Most importantly, histomorphological alterations of testes, significantly increased abnormalities in epidydimal spermatozoa and sperm DNA damage have been observed in rats exposed to cigarette smoke [41, 42]. In both in vitro and in vivo studies, nicotine resulted involved in direct impairment of sperm motility and in apoptosis induction in rat Leydig cells [43]. Mice exposed to cigarette smoke also underwent alterations in cell signal pathway networks, including ERK1/2, nuclear factor-κB and several protein kinases involved in spermatogenesis; furthermore, modified DNA methylation patterns were observed near transcriptional start sites for the *PEBP1* gene. Expression of *PEBP1* results in production of phosphatidylethanolamine-binding protein 1, a protein that in humans has been shown to interact with C-Raf, MAP2K1 and MAPK1 [44].

High doses of nicotine induce a significant decrease in sperm count and motility in prepubertal and adult rats exposed to progressively increasing concentrations of nicotine [45]. Impaired testicular function is also reflected in significantly decreased testosterone levels [45, 46], although as previously suggested it's still unclear whether these findings are valid for humans as well as rodents.

Smoking cessation, on the other hand, improves indices of sexual health for long-term male smokers [47] and, based on finding in animal models, might improve sperm parameters [48]. However, to the present date, no conclusive evidence on the real improvements in male fertility following smoking cessation has been obtained.

#### *Studies in humans*

Recent genome-wide studies have identified alterations in the methylation profile of 95 sites in smokers [49]. Smoking-related DNA damage and methylation patterns are observed in several human tissues - even those who are not directly exposed to it because of indirect systemic exposure [50]. DNA adducts and DNA damage are inversely associated with sperm parameters, mostly concentration and motility, and both are transmitted to the zygote with little chance of repair by the ovum [51]. Sperm DNA fragmentation is also linked with increased rates of spontaneous abortion [52] and should therefore be carefully assessed in subjects undergoing assisted reproduction techniques. Oxidative DNA damage [53] and higher cadmium levels [54] resulting from tobacco consumption are similarly associated to impaired fertility, resulting in longer time to pregnancy for couples.

Smoking also reduces sperm creatine kinase activity, therefore impairing sperm motility and energy homeostasis [55]. In vitro studies have shown nicotine, cotinine and cadmium as possible culprits; in vivo, both smoking duration and amount of cigarettes smoked per day seem able to reduce creatine kinase activity in sperm [56, 57].

### Alcohol consumption and male fertility

Clinical and experimental studies have examined alcohol consumption as a potential risk factor for male infertility, exerting a direct effect on both testosterone metabolism and spermatogenesis.

#### Clinical studies

The link between alcohol and fertility was investigated in 1985 for the first time. The analysis of seminal fluid samples and the hormonal evaluation of 20 men with alcohol dependence syndrome revealed a significant decrease in testosterone levels, seminal fluid volume and sperm concentration in chronic alcoholics than in controls [58]. Subsequently, a prospective autopsy study showed that a significant percentage of heavy drinkers (52.3%) had partial or complete spermatogenic arrest, and that the mean testicular weight of heavy drinkers was slightly but significantly lower compared with that of controls [59]. Muthusami et al., in 2005, found in chronic alcoholics a significant increase of FSH, LH, and E2 levels, while testosterone was significantly decreased. Semen volume, sperm count, motility, and number of morphologically normal sperm were significantly decreased [60]. In 2011 one meta-analysis including 57 studies and 29,914 subjects found a significant association between alcohol, semen volume, sperm morphology and sperm motility [61].

Therefore, chronic and excessive alcohol intake seem to have a detrimental effect on male reproductive hormones and on semen quality. Conversely, the effect of moderate alcohol intake is still under debate.

A cross sectional study from Jensen et al. on 8344 healthy men suggest that moderate alcohol intake (median weekly intake 8 units) is not adversely associated with semen quality in healthy men, whereas it was associated with higher serum testosterone levels [62]. Furthermore, chronic alcohol consumption seem to influence fertility more than acute alcohol consumption. Hansen et al. evaluated the association between last 5 days of alcohol intake, semen quality and reproductive hormones in a cross-sectional study among 347 men [63]. Alcohol intake was associated with impairment of most semen characteristics but without a coherent dose–response pattern. There was a tendency towards lower semen characteristics at higher intake of alcohol past 5 days and a hormonal shift towards higher estradiol/testosterone ratio. The importance of the timing of alcohol consumption was also established from Condorelli et al. The Authors retrospectively evaluated semen and hormonal parameters of moderate alcohol users, comparing occasional drinkers with daily drinkers. Within each group, a further comparison was made between the fertile subjects (pregnancy over the past 12 months) and the infertile patients (no evidence of pregnancy or fertilisation for at least 12 months). The results showed that infertile patients belonging to group of 'daily drinkers' have a semen quality and hormonal characteristics significantly worse compared with the other groups [64]. Time-to-pregnancy for was significantly longer in couples in which the male partner consumed more than 20 units of alcohol on a weekly basis [65], but literature is severely lacking concerning more moderate consumption of alcoholic beverages.

The mechanisms underlying the damage of alcohol on fertility are not yet fully clarified. Close and colleagues reported that current heavy alcohol users have significantly higher leukocyte concentrations in the seminal fluid compared with nonusers. After controlling for past sexually transmitted diseases and multiple substance exposures in a multivariate model, alcohol users had only a trend towards increased leukocytes in the seminal fluid [66]. Some Authors hypothesized that also maternal alcohol consumption during pregnancy can influence semen quality in the male offspring. From a cohort of Danish pregnant women established in 1984–1987, 347 young adult sons were selected for a follow-up study conducted in 2005–2006. The results of this study showed that the sperm concentration decreased with increasing prenatal alcohol exposure. No associations were found for sperm motility, sperm morphology, or any of the reproductive hormones, including testosterone [67].

### Experimental studies

#### *Animal studies*

Alcohol consumption has often been associated with an increase in β-endorphin levels that could be involved in testicular damage, inducing sperm apoptosis. In 1999 Yin and colleagues showed that morphine induces the expression of the protein Fas (also known as CD95 or APO-1), a receptor on the cell surface that triggers the cell's suicide by apoptosis when it binds to its ligand, FasL [68]. Furthermore, an experimental study demonstrated that treatment with naloxone and naltrexone in adult and pubertal male rats could prevent alcohol-induced testosterone inhibition [69].

Apoptosis is one of the responsible factors for spermatozoal chromatin disorders. Several studies showed that ethanol consumption disturb nuclear maturity and DNA integrity of spermatozoa. Talebi and colleagues evaluated the effect of ethanol consumption on sperm parameters and chromatin integrity of spermatozoa aspirated from cauda epididymis of rats. Results revealed that sperm progressive and non progressive motility of ethanol-consuming rats were significantly decreased compared with control animals and an alteration of nuclear maturity and DNA integrity [70].

Therefore, spermatogenic cells undergo apoptosis when treated with ethanol but the mechanism remain unclear. In the study of Jana and colleagues, intraperitoneal injection of ethanol induced apoptotic spermatogenic cell death with a decrease in the plasma and intra-testicular testosterone in adult male mice. In this study, western blot analysis revealed that repeated ethanol treatment decreased the expression of steroidogenic acute regulatory protein (StAR), 3b-hydroxysteroid dehydrogenase (3b-HSD) and 17b-hydroxysteroid dehydrogenase (17b-HSD); increased the expression of active caspase-3, p53, Fas and Fas-L; and led to up-regulation of Bax/Bcl-2 ratio and translocation of cytochrome c from mitochondria to cytosol in testis. Moreover, repeated ethanol treatment led to upregulation of caspase-3, p53, Fas and Fas-L transcripts; increase in caspase-3 and caspase-8 activities; diminution of 3b-HSD, 17b-HSD and GPx activities; decrease in the mitochondrial membrane potential along with ROS generation and depletion of glutathione pool in the testicular tissue [71].

#### *Studies in humans*

Polycyclic aromatic hydrocarbons (PAH) are ubiquitous pollutants in the environment, which are able to form DNA adducts when they are activated to DNA reactive metabolites. Measurement of DNA adducts is a widely used marker of DNA damage induced by environmental pollutants. Gaspari and colleagues evaluated data on (PAH)-DNA adducts in 182 men with morphological abnormalities in the sperm, finding a significant negative association was between daily alcohol consumption and PAH-DNA adducts in sperm [72]; similarly, Rossi and colleagues reported that increased alcohol consumption was associated with fertilization failure and reduced live birth rates [73], with a 21% decline in couples in which both partners drank more than 4 units per week. On the contrary, in the study of Horak et al., no correlation between alcohol and sperm DNA adducts was found [74]. Finally, Loft evaluated the level of oxidative DNA damage in terms of 7-hydro-8-oxo-20-deoxyguanosine (8-oxodG) in sperm DNA among 225 first-pregnancy planners and the 8-oxodG level was not significantly associated with consumption of alcohol [53].

Finally, the genetic background may modulate the impact of alcohol on spermatogenesis. The glutathione S-transferase (GST)-M1 genotype may be associated with a greater susceptibility to develop, via direct mechanism at testicular level, alcohol-induced spermatogenesis disorders. An autopsy study comprising 271 subjects showed that among 50 moderate drinking men, 48% had partial and 10% complete spermatogenic arrest. Among the 21 men with normal spermatogenesis, 42.9% had GST M1 genotype with a frequency similar to that found in men with partial or complete spermatogenic arrest (44.8%). Among the 212 heavy-drinking men, 21.2% of the subjects had normal spermatogenesis, 36.3% had partial spermatogenic arrest, 38.2% showed complete arrest spermatogenic arrest and 4.2% showed Sertoli cell-only syndrome. Interestingly, 27 of the 45 heavy drinkers with normal spermatogenesis (60%) men had the GST M1 genotype. The finding that >20% of heavy drinkers had normal spermatogenesis suggests that the GST M1 genotype exerts a protective effects on alcohol-induced spermatogenesis disorders [75].

### Drugs addiction and male fertility

Up to almost one in four men under the age of 35 years uses recreational drugs [76]. Several studies have suggested that these drugs might have adverse effects on human reproduction. Cannabis smoking has been shown to negatively impact male fertility, with an effect on hypothalamus-pituitary-gonadal axis, spermatogenesis, and sperm function, as cannabinoid receptors are expressed in the anterior pituitary, Leydig cells, Sertoli cells and in testicular tissues [77]. Similarly, negative effects on male fertility have been reported in subjects using cocaine, MDMA (ecstasy) and opioids. Cocaine use has been associated with other high-risk behaviors, such as tobacco smoking and sexually transmitted diseases, and might lead to testicular cell apoptosis; opioids act on the HPG axis, possibly resulting in hypogonadal hypogonadism; DNA damage and tubular degeneration have been described in rats treated with MDMA. Prevention of male infertility might be achieved by identifying and addressing the consequences of the "illicit drug epidemic".

### Clinical studies

In literature, human data on hormone levels following marijuana exposure are conflicting. Referring to animal studies it could be possible that consuming cannabis decrease serum luteinizing hormone and testosterone levels, but in clinical studies a univocal interpretation is lacking.

A study from Kolodny et al. on 20 men who used marijuana chronically showed significantly lower levels of plasma testosterone in this group than that in the control-group. Decreased testosterone was dose related. Abstention from marijuana use or stimulation with human chorionic gonadotropin during continued marihuana use produced marked increases in testosterone [78]. These results have been later contradicted. In 66 males neither chronic nor acute intake of marijuana had a significant effect on plasma testosterone levels, but also subjects who drank cannabis as a tea were included [79]. In a study of 27 men, no statistically significant changes in plasma testosterone levels were observed during and after the smoking period as compared with the pre-smoking base-line levels [80]. In four healthy males subjects, cannabis smoking significantly depressed plasma LH, while cortisol significantly increased [81]. On the contrary, in the study from Gundersen et al. on 1215 Danish healthy young men, of whom 45% had smoked marijuana during the past 3 months, marijuana use was associated with increased serum testosterone to the same level as cigarette smoking [82].

Conversely, regarding the effect of cannabis on spermatogenesis, clinical studies showed an effect on volume, number morphology, motility, and fertilization capacity.

In the study from Gundersen et al. regular use of marijuana was found to be associated with an impairment in semen quality, while irregular use seems to be irrelevant [82]. A study from Hembree et al. showed an association between marijuana use and decreased sperm count, which persisted in the following 4-week recovery period [83]. These data were confirmed also by a case study on a multidrug addict, in which semen abnormalities were detected before and 2 years after cessation of the abuse [84]. In a recent unmatched case-referent study with 1700 participants, it was clearly reported that cannabis exposure is a risk factor for poor sperm morphology [85]. Only one study on 159 men attending an infertility clinic demonstrated a positive correlation between marijuana use and percentage of motile sperm [66].

There are no studies on the effect of cannabis on the reproductive organs of men. Only Kolodny et al. reported no change in testicular size and texture in chronic marijuana users [78]. The differing results of these reports may in part be due to study design, the ingestion of other pharmacological agents, such as narcotics, alcohol and cigarette smoking.

Cocaine intake during pregnancy severely affects fetal development; however, little is known in regards to its effects on male fertility. The same applies to MDMA (Ecstasy): animal models might help understand the specific effects of both substances on male fertility. Bracken et al. [86] reported increased use of cocaine among subjects with lower sperm counts and motility; Samplaski et al. [87] more recently suggested that the higher rates of concurrent substance abuse, tobacco use and infections among cocaine users might lead to biased results.

Opioids act on the hypothalamic-pituitary axis by inhibiting the pulsatility of GnRH secretion: the resulting suppression of FSH and LH release consequently leads to impaired spermatogenesis and reduced testosterone concentrations [76]. Vuong et al. [88] performed a lengthy review of the effects of opioids on endocrine parameters, and concluded that there is still insufficient information on the long-term effects of opioids in regards to fertility despite concrete evidence of opioid-induced hypogonadism. Recent reports suggest that both sperm concentration and quality are impaired in opioid abusers: increased rates of DNA fragmentation and reduced expression of catalase-like and superoxide dismutase-like activity were observed in addict men compared to age-matched healthy volunteers [89].

### Experimental studies

#### *Animal studies*

Acute treatments with cannabinoids can decrease the fertilising capacity of sea urchin sperm [90]. In rodent studies, high THC doses caused a modest increase in abnormally formed sperm. Moreover, long-term cannabinoid exposure in male mice disrupted spermatogenesis and induced aberrations in sperm morphology [91].

Wenger and colleagues showed that THC alters pituitary LH release by inhibiting the release of LHRH, injecting THC into the third cerebral ventricle of male rats [92]. Smith et al. [93] found a significant decrease in serum testosterone concentration following acute doses of THC in rhesus monkeys. A study on adult male mice showed regressive changes in the testes and suppressed sperm count, viability and motility, caused by chronic intake of bhang. Bhang intake also caused significant

**Table 2** Effects of tobacco smoking, alcohol consumption and drug addiction on spermatogenesis and sperm parameters

| | Studies in humans | Animal studies |
|---|---|---|
| Tobacco smoking | Reduction of sperm concentration [26, 27]<br>Impairment of sperm motility [17]<br>Increase in ultra-structural abnormalities (axonemal microtubules and tail alterations) [28, 29]<br>Impairment of mitochondrial activity and chromatin structure [17, 33, 34]<br>Impairment of acrosome reaction and capacitation [30, 31]<br>Increase of DNA methylation patterns [49]<br>Alterations in ERK1/2, nuclear factor-κB signal pathway [44]<br>Reduction of creatine kinase activity in sperm [55–57] | Increase in apoptosis via extrinsic (FAS, FASL) or mitochondrial processes (BCL, caspase-3) in rats [39, 40]<br>Reduction of antioxidant activity in rats [40]<br>Increase in DNA damage in sperm rats [41, 42]; of DNA methylation patterns *PEBP1* gene in rats [44]<br>Reduction of sperm count and motility in rats [45] |
| Alcohol consumption | Reduction of seminal volume and sperm concentration [58, 61, 62]<br>Impairment of sperm motility and morphology [60, 61]<br>Increased sperm polycyclic aromatic hydrocarbon DNA adducts [72] | Increase in apoptosis (by upregulation of Fas) of spermatogenic cells in rats [68]<br>Alteration of nuclear maturity and DNA integrity in sperm cells of rats [70]<br>Increase in ROS generation and depletion of glutathione pool in testicular tissue of rats [71]<br>Impairment of sperm motility in rats [70] |
| Drug addiction | | |
| Marijuana | Decrease in sperm count [82–84]<br>Impairment of sperm morphology and motility [85, 102, 103]<br>Reduction of spontaneous acrosome reactions [102, 103] | Impaired sperm concentration and morphology in rats [91]<br>Inhibition of sperm ATP production in rats [104]<br>Reduction of fructose and citric acid contents in testis and prostate of male rats [95] |
| Cocaine | Impairment of sperm counts and motility [86] | Vasoconstriction of testicular blood vessels in rats resulting in ischemic and reperfusion injuries [96]<br>Reduction of diameter of seminiferous tubules [97]<br>Decrease in number of total germ cells [97]<br>Increase in oxidative stress in mice [98] |
| Opioids | Impaired spermatogenesis [76]<br>Increased rates of DNA fragmentation in humans [89]<br>Reduced expression of catalase-like and superoxide dismutase-like activity [89] | Increase of rates of DNA damage and tubular degeneration in rats [100, 101] |
| Amphetamines and Ecstasy | No data available | Vasoconstriction of testicular blood vessels in rats [96]<br>Increase in rates of DNA damage and tubular degeneration in rats [99] |

**Table 3** Effects of tobacco smoking, alcohol consumption and drug addiction on hormone levels

| | Studies in humans | Animal studies |
|---|---|---|
| Tobacco smoking | Increase in liver metabolism of testosterone [24]<br>Reduction of LH and/or FSH levels [34]<br>Increase in concentration of LH and/or FSH [35]<br>Increase in serum testosterone and DHEA levels [35, 37] | Reduction of testosterone levels in rats [45, 46] |
| Alcohol consumption | Decrease in testosterone levels [58, 59]<br>Increase in FSH, LH, and E2 levels [60] | Decrease in plasma and intra-testicular testosterone in rats [71] |
| Drug addiction | | |
| Marijuana | Decrease in levels of plasma testosterone [78]<br>Decreased levels of plasma LH, and increased levels of plasma cortisol [81]<br>Increased serum testosterone [82] | Inhibition of LHRH release in rats [92]<br>Decrease in testosterone levels in monkeys [93] |
| Cocaine | Increase in LH levels without modifying testosterone following acute administration [97] | Increase in LH levels; No effects on testosterone and estradiol in rats [97] |
| Opioids | Inhibition of the pulsatility of GnRH secretion; reduction of LH, FSH and testosterone levels [76] | Reduction of LH, without effect on FSH and testosterone levels in rats [101] |
| Amphetamines and Ecstasy | No data available | No effects on LH, FSH, Testosterone levels in male rats [99] |

decline in circulating testosterone level due to decline in testicular 3b HSD enzyme activity, a significant variation in the CB1 and CB2 receptors and FAAH protein levels (Fatty Acid Amide Hydrolase) in testes of mice exposed to bhang [94]. Finally, repeated subcutaneous administration of cannabis extract and delta-9-tetrahydrocannabinol reduced significantly fructose and citric acid contents of male reproductive organs of prepubertal as well as adult albino rats in a dose-related manner in the testis, prostate as well as in the epididymis [95].

Effects of cocaine and MDMA on fertility have been evaluated in animal models: in rodents, cocaine is able to induce prolonged vasoconstriction of testicular blood vessels, resulting in ischemic and reperfusion injuries [96]. In 1996, George et al. reported that in rats long-term exposure to cocaine resulted in reduced diameter of seminiferous tubules and similarly decreased number of total germ cells [97]. More recently, increased oxidative stress has been observed in mice following chronic administration of cocaine [98], suggesting a possible mechanism for testicular damage. Similar findings have been reported for Ecstasy and opioids: Barenys et al. described significantly decreased sperm concentration and motility, together with increased rates of DNA damage and tubular degeneration, in rats treated with varying dosages of MDMA [99], and similar findings have been described in mice treated with either tramadol [100] or morphine [101].

### *Studies in humans*

Whan et al. investigated the effects of delta-9-tetrahydrocannabinol (THC) on human sperm function in vitro. Both therapeutic and recreational levels of THC determined a dose dependent reduction of sperm motility and of spontaneous acrosome reactions [102]. Subsequent studies confirmed these results [103], but the mechanism still remained not fully understood. Morgan et al. investigated the effects of WIN 55,212-2, a CB1 cannabinoid receptor agonist, and D9-tetrahydracannabinol (D9-THC) on the ATP levels and motility of murine sperm in vitro. High concentrations of WIN 55,212-2 or D9-THC inhibit ATP production in sperm; this effect of WIN 55,212-2 is CB1 receptor dependent whereas that of D9-THC is not [104].

## Conclusions

Despite the lack of solid evidence from interventional studies, which are for the most part not feasible in humans, it is clear that smoking, alcohol use and recreational drug consumption are somehow able to impair male fertility, with possible synergistic, rather than addictive, effects. Impairments in spermatogenesis and sperm parameters as well as increased DNA methylation and oxidative stress have been observed in humans and animal models alike; similarly, effects on endocrine control of reproductive and sexual function have been reported in clinical and

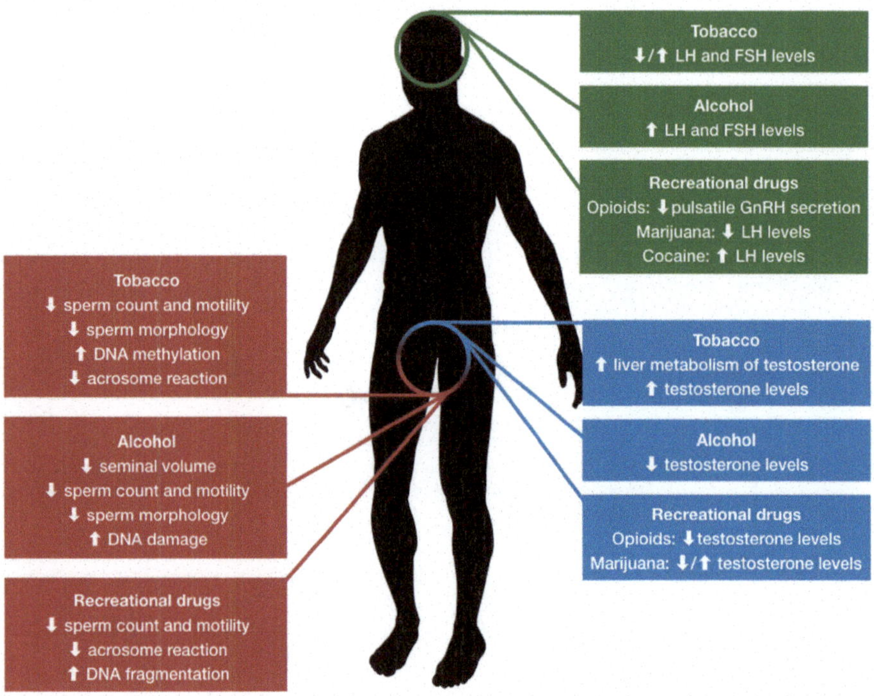


**Fig. 1** Effects of smoking, alcohol and drug abuse on spermatogenesis (left) and hormonal parameters (right) in males

experimental studies (Tables 2 and 3, Fig. 1). Discontinuation of all these habits should be suggested in all patients undergoing investigation for infertility in order to provide the best outcomes, although little is known in regards to the time needed for cessation of negative effects.

**Acknowledgements**
None

**Funding**
No funding was requested for this review.

**Availability of data and materials**
Literature research results are available from the authors on reasonable request.

**Declarations**
Since Prof. Pivonello served as Guest Editor of the thematic series "The Influence of Environment and Lifestyle on Human Fertility", peer review of the present manuscript was handled by another member of the *Reproductive Biology and Endocrinology* editorial board.

**Authors' contributions**
AMI and DG conceived the idea. AS and CdD were involved in literature collection. All authors independently and critically reviewed the selected manuscripts. AS and CdD were involved in drafting the early manuscript and equally contributed to the first draft, which was then expanded and improved by all authors. All authors reviewed and approved the completed manuscript.

**Ethics approval and consent to participate**
Not applicable.

**Consent for publication**
Not applicable.

**Competing interests**
The authors declare that they have no competing interests.

## Publisher's Note

Springer Nature remains neutral with regard to jurisdictional claims in published maps and institutional affiliations.

**Author details**
[1]Department of Experimental Medicine, Section of Medical Pathophysiology, Food Science and Endocrinology, Sapienza - University of Rome, Viale Regina Elena 324, 00161 Rome, Italy. [2]I.O.S.& COLEMAN Srl, Naples, Italy. [3]Dipartimento di Medicina Clinica e Chirurgia, Sezione di Endocrinologia, Università "Federico II" di Napoli, Naples, Italy.

Received: 30 October 2017 Accepted: 2 January 2018
Published online: 15 January 2018

**References**

1. Sharlip ID, Jarow JP, Belker AM, Lipshultz LI, Sigman M, Thomas AJ, Schlegel PN, Howards SS, Nehra A, Damewood MD, et al. Best practice policies for male infertility. Fertil Steril. 2002;77(5):873–82.
2. Sengupta P, Dutta S, Krajewska-Kulak E. The disappearing sperms: analysis of reports published between 1980 and 2015. Am J Mens Health. 2017;11(4): 1279–304.
3. Gaskins AJ, Afeiche MC, Hauser R, Williams PL, Gillman MW, Tanrikut C, Petrozza JC, Chavarro JE. Paternal physical and sedentary activities in relation to semen quality and reproductive outcomes among couples from a fertility center. Hum Reprod. 2014;29(11):2575–82.
4. Eisenberg ML, Kim S, Chen Z, Sundaram R, Schisterman EF, Buck Louis GM. The relationship between male BMI and waist circumference on semen quality: data from the LIFE study. Hum Reprod. 2014;29(2):193–200.
5. Barazani Y, Katz BF, Nagler HM, Stember DS. Lifestyle, environment, and male reproductive health. The Urologic clinics of North America. 2014;41(1): 55–66.
6. Moline JM, Golden AL, Bar-Chama N, Smith E, Rauch ME, Chapin RE, Perreault SD, Schrader SM, Suk WA, Landrigan PJ. Exposure to hazardous substances and male reproductive health: a research framework. Environ Health Perspect. 2000;108(9):803–13.
7. Nordkap L, Joensen UN, Blomberg Jensen M, Jorgensen N. Regional differences and temporal trends in male reproductive health disorders: semen quality may be a sensitive marker of environmental exposures. Mol Cell Endocrinol. 2012;355(2):221–30.
8. Gabrielsen JS, Tanrikut C. Chronic exposures and male fertility: the impacts of environment, diet, and drug use on spermatogenesis. Andrology. 2016; 4(4):648–61.
9. Cooper TG, Noonan E, von Eckardstein S, Auger J, Baker HW, Behre HM, Haugen TB, Kruger T, Wang C, Mbizvo MT, et al. World Health Organization reference values for human semen characteristics. Hum Reprod Update. 2010;16(3):231–45.
10. Tournaye H, Krausz C, Oates RD. Novel concepts in the aetiology of male reproductive impairment. Lancet Diabetes Endocrinol. 2017;5(7):544–53.
11. Johnson SL, Dunleavy J, Gemmell NJ, Nakagawa S. Consistent age-dependent declines in human semen quality: a systematic review and meta-analysis. Ageing Res Rev. 2015;19:22–33.
12. Valenti D, La Vignera S, Condorelli RA, Rago R, Barone N, Vicari E, Calogero AE. Follicle-stimulating hormone treatment in normogonadotropic infertile men. Nat Rev Urol. 2013;10(1):55–62.
13. Lombardo F, Sansone A, Romanelli F, Paoli D, Gandini L, Lenzi A. The role of antioxidant therapy in the treatment of male infertility: an overview. Asian J Androl. 2011;13(5):690–7.
14. Yao DF, Mills JN. Male infertility: lifestyle factors and holistic, complementary, and alternative therapies. Asian J Androl. 2016;18(3):410–8.
15. Prevalence of tobacco use [http://www.who.int/topics/tobacco/en/].
16. Practice Committee of the American Society for Reproductive. M: smoking and infertility: a committee opinion. Fertil Steril. 2012;98(6): 1400–6.
17. Sharma R, Harlev A, Agarwal A, Esteves SC. Cigarette smoking and semen quality: a new meta-analysis examining the effect of the 2010 World Health Organization Laboratory methods for the examination of human semen. Eur Urol. 2016;70(4):635–45.
18. Olsen J, Rachootin P, Schiodt AV, Damsbo N. Tobacco use, alcohol consumption and infertility. Int J Epidemiol. 1983;12(2):179–84.
19. Borgerding M, Klus H. Analysis of complex mixtures–cigarette smoke. Exp Toxicol Pathol. 2005;57(Suppl 1):43–73.
20. Benoff S, Centola GM, Millan C, Napolitano B, Marmar JL, Hurley IR. Increased seminal plasma lead levels adversely affect the fertility potential of sperm in IVF. Hum Reprod. 2003;18(2):374–83.
21. Jurasovic J, Cvitkovic P, Pizent A, Colak B, Telisman S. Semen quality and reproductive endocrine function with regard to blood cadmium in Croatian male subjects. Biometals. 2004;17(6):735–43.
22. Wang X, Zhang J, Xu W, Huang Q, Liu L, Tian M, Xia Y, Zhang W, Shen H. Low-level environmental arsenic exposure correlates with unexplained male infertility risk. Sci Total Environ. 2016;571:307–13.
23. de Angelis C, Galdiero M, Pivonello C, Salzano C, Gianfrilli D, Piscitelli P, Lenzi A, Colao A, Pivonello R. The environment and male reproduction: the effect of cadmium exposure on reproductive functions and its implication in fertility. Reprod Toxicol. 2017;73:105–27.
24. Dai JB, Wang ZX, Qiao ZD. The hazardous effects of tobacco smoking on male fertility. Asian J Androl. 2015;17(6):954–60.
25. Asare-Anane H, Bannison SB, Ofori EK, Ateko RO, Bawah AT, Amanquah SD, Oppong SY, Gandau BB, Ziem JB. Tobacco smoking is associated with decreased semen quality. Reprod Health. 2016;13(1):90.
26. Ramlau-Hansen CH, Thulstrup AM, Aggerholm AS, Jensen MS, Toft G, Bonde JP. Is smoking a risk factor for decreased semen quality? A cross-sectional analysis. Hum Reprod. 2007;22(1):188–96.
27. Kunzle R, Mueller MD, Hanggi W, Birkhauser MH, Drescher H, Bersinger NA. Semen quality of male smokers and nonsmokers in infertile couples. Fertil Steril. 2003;79(2):287–91.
28. Zavos PM, Correa JR, Karagounis CS, Ahparaki A, Phoroglou C, Hicks CL, Zarmakoupis-Zavos PN. An electron microscope study of the axonemal ultrastructure in human spermatozoa from male smokers and nonsmokers. Fertil Steril. 1998;69(3):430–4.

29. Yeung CH, Tuttelmann F, Bergmann M, Nordhoff V, Vorona E, Cooper TG. Coiled sperm from infertile patients: characteristics, associated factors and biological implication. Hum Reprod. 2009;24(6):1288–95.
30. Zalata AA, Ahmed AH, Allamaneni SS, Comhaire FH, Agarwal A. Relationship between acrosin activity of human spermatozoa and oxidative stress. Asian J Androl. 2004;6(4):313–8.
31. Shrivastava V, Marmor H, Chernyak S, Goldstein M, Feliciano M, Vigodner M. Cigarette smoke affects posttranslational modifications and inhibits capacitation-induced changes in human sperm proteins. Reprod Toxicol. 2014;43:125–9.
32. Taha EA, Ezz-Aldin AM, Sayed SK, Ghandour NM, Mostafa T. Smoking influence on sperm vitality, DNA fragmentation, reactive oxygen species and zinc in oligoasthenoteratozoospermic men with varicocele. Andrologia. 2014;46(6):687–91.
33. Calogero A, Polosa R, Perdichizzi A, Guarino F, La Vignera S, Scarfia A, Fratantonio E, Condorelli R, Bonanno O, Barone N, et al. Cigarette smoke extract immobilizes human spermatozoa and induces sperm apoptosis. Reprod BioMed Online. 2009;19(4):564–71.
34. Sharma R, Biedenharn KR, Fedor JM, Agarwal A. Lifestyle factors and reproductive health: taking control of your fertility. Reproductive biology and endocrinology : RB&E. 2013;11:66.
35. Blanco-Munoz J, Lacasana M, Aguilar-Garduno C. Effect of current tobacco consumption on the male reproductive hormone profile. Sci Total Environ. 2012;426:100–5.
36. Ochedalski T, Lachowicz-Ochedalska A, Dec W, Czechowski B. Examining the effects of tobacco smoking on levels of certain hormones in serum of young men. Ginekol Pol. 1994;65(2):87–93.
37. Lotti F, Corona G, Vitale P, Maseroli E, Rossi M, Fino MG, Maggi M. Current smoking is associated with lower seminal vesicles and ejaculate volume, despite higher testosterone levels, in male subjects of infertile couples. Hum Reprod. 2015;30(3):590–602.
38. Pasqualotto FF, Sobreiro BP, Hallak J, Pasqualotto EB, Lucon AM. Cigarette smoking is related to a decrease in semen volume in a population of fertile men. BJU Int. 2006;97(2):324–6.
39. Esakky P, Hansen DA, Drury AM, Felder P, Cusumano A, Moley KH. Paternal exposure to cigarette smoke condensate leads to reproductive sequelae and developmental abnormalities in the offspring of mice. Reprod Toxicol. 2016;65:283–94.
40. Pasqualotto FF, Umezu FM, Salvador M, Borges E, Jr., Sobreiro BP, Pasqualotto EB: Effect of cigarette smoking on antioxidant levels and presence of leukocytospermia in infertile men: a prospective study. Fertil Steril 2008, 90(2):278-283.
41. Abdul-Ghani R, Qazzaz M, Dabdoub N, Muhammad R, Abdul-Ghani AS. Studies on cigarette smoke induced oxidative DNA damage and reduced spermatogenesis in rats. J Environ Biol. 2014;35(5):943–7.
42. La Maestra S, De Flora S, Micale RT. Effect of cigarette smoke on DNA damage, oxidative stress, and morphological alterations in mouse testis and spermatozoa. Int J Hyg Environ Health. 2015;218(1):117–22.
43. Kim KH, Joo KJ, Park HJ, Kwon CH, Jang MH, Kim CJ. Nicotine induces apoptosis in TM3 mouse Leydig cells. Fertil Steril. 2005;83(Suppl 1):1093–9.
44. Yeung K, Janosch P, McFerran B, Rose DW, Mischak H, Sedivy JM, Kolch W. Mechanism of suppression of the Raf/MEK/extracellular signal-regulated kinase pathway by the raf kinase inhibitor protein. Mol Cell Biol. 2000;20(9): 3079–85.
45. Aprioku JS, Ugwu TC. Tobacco smoke exposure induces irreversible alteration of testicular function in prepubertal rats. J Basic Clin Physiol Pharmacol. 2016;27(6):577–84.
46. Oyeyipo IP, Raji Y, Bolarinwa AF. Nicotine alters male reproductive hormones in male albino rats: the role of cessation. J Hum Reprod Sci. 2013; 6(1):40–4.
47. Harte CB, Meston CM. Association between smoking cessation and sexual health in men. BJU Int. 2012;109(6):888–96.
48. Oyeyipo IP, Raji Y, Emikpe BO, Bolarinwa AF. Effects of nicotine on sperm characteristics and fertility profile in adult male rats: a possible role of cessation. J Reprod Infertil. 2011;12(3):201–7.
49. Shenker NS, Ueland PM, Polidoro S, van Veldhoven K, Ricceri F, Brown R, Flanagan JM, Vineis P. DNA methylation as a long-term biomarker of exposure to tobacco smoke. Epidemiology. 2013;24(5):712–6.
50. Cui X, Jing X, Wu X, Wang Z, Li Q. Potential effect of smoking on semen quality through DNA damage and the downregulation of Chk1 in sperm. Mol Med Rep. 2016;14(1):753–61.
51. Harlev A, Agarwal A, Gunes SO, Shetty A, du Plessis SS. Smoking and male infertility: an evidence-based review. The world journal of men's health. 2015;33(3):143–60.
52. Agarwal A, Majzoub A, Esteves SC, Ko E, Ramasamy R, Zini A. Clinical utility of sperm DNA fragmentation testing: practice recommendations based on clinical scenarios. Transl Androl Urol. 2016;5(6):935–50.
53. Loft S, Kold-Jensen T, Hjollund NH, Giwercman A, Gyllemborg J, Ernst E, Olsen J, Scheike T, Poulsen HE, Bonde JP, Oxidative DNA. Damage in human sperm influences time to pregnancy. Hum Reprod. 2003;18(6):1265–72.
54. Sapra KJ, Barr DB, Maisog JM, Sundaram R, Buck Louis GM. Time-to-pregnancy associated with Couples' use of tobacco products. Nicotine Tob Res. 2016;18(11):2154–61.
55. Ghaffari MA, Rostami M. The effect of cigarette smoking on human sperm creatine kinase activity: as an ATP buffering system in sperm. Int J Fertil Steril. 2013;6(4):258–65.
56. Sofikitis N, Takenaka M, Kanakas N, Papadopoulos H, Yamamoto Y, Drakakis P, Miyagawa I. Effects of cotinine on sperm motility, membrane function, and fertilizing capacity in vitro. Urol Res. 2000;28(6):370–5.
57. Oyeyipo IP, Maartens PJ, du Plessis SS. In vitro effects of nicotine on human spermatozoa. Andrologia. 2014;46(8):887–92.
58. Kucheria K, Saxena R, Mohan D. Semen analysis in alcohol dependence syndrome. Andrologia. 1985;17(6):558–63.
59. Pajarinen JT, Karhunen PJ. Spermatogenic arrest and 'Sertoli cell-only' syndrome–common alcohol-induced disorders of the human testis. Int J Androl. 1994;17(6):292–9.
60. Muthusami KR, Chinnaswamy P. Effect of chronic alcoholism on male fertility hormones and semen quality. Fertil Steril. 2005;84(4):919–24.
61. Li Y, Lin H, Li Y, Cao J. Association between socio-psycho-behavioral factors and male semen quality: systematic review and meta-analyses. Fertil Steril. 2011;95(1):116–23.
62. Jensen TK, Gottschau M, Madsen JO, Andersson AM, Lassen TH, Skakkebaek NE, Swan SH, Priskorn L, Juul A, Jorgensen N. Habitual alcohol consumption associated with reduced semen quality and changes in reproductive hormones; a cross-sectional study among 1221 young Danish men. BMJ Open. 2014;4(9):e005462.
63. Hansen ML, Thulstrup AM, Bonde JP, Olsen J, Hakonsen LB, Ramlau-Hansen CH. Does last week's alcohol intake affect semen quality or reproductive hormones? A cross-sectional study among healthy young Danish men. Reprod Toxicol. 2012;34(3):457–62.
64. Condorelli RA, Calogero AE, Vicari E, La Vignera S. Chronic consumption of alcohol and sperm parameters: our experience and the main evidences. Andrologia. 2015;47(4):368–79.
65. Hassan MA, Killick SR. Negative lifestyle is associated with a significant reduction in fecundity. Fertil Steril. 2004;81(2):384–92.
66. Close CE, Roberts PL, Berger RE. Cigarettes, alcohol and marijuana are related to pyospermia in infertile men. J Urol. 1990;144(4):900–3.
67. Ramlau-Hansen CH, Toft G, Jensen MS, Strandberg-Larsen K, Hansen ML, Olsen J. Maternal alcohol consumption during pregnancy and semen quality in the male offspring: two decades of follow-up. Hum Reprod. 2010; 25(9):2340–5.
68. Yin D, Mufson RA, Wang R, Shi Y. Fas-mediated cell death promoted by opioids. Nature. 1999;397(6716):218.
69. Gianoulakis C. Characterization of the effects of acute ethanol administration on the release of beta-endorphin peptides by the rat hypothalamus. Eur J Pharmacol. 1990;180(1):21–9.
70. Talebi AR, Sarcheshmeh AA, Khalili MA, Tabibnejad N. Effects of ethanol consumption on chromatin condensation and DNA integrity of epididymal spermatozoa in rat. Alcohol. 2011;45(4):403–9.
71. Jana K, Jana N, De DK, Guha SK. Ethanol induces mouse spermatogenic cell apoptosis in vivo through over-expression of Fas/Fas-L, p53, and caspase-3 along with cytochrome c translocation and glutathione depletion. Mol Reprod Dev. 2010;77(9):820–33.
72. Gaspari L, Chang SS, Santella RM, Garte S, Pedotti P, Taioli E. Polycyclic aromatic hydrocarbon-DNA adducts in human sperm as a marker of DNA damage and infertility. Mutat Res. 2003;535(2):155–60.
73. Rossi BV, Berry KF, Hornstein MD, Cramer DW, Ehrlich S, Missmer SA. Effect of alcohol consumption on in vitro fertilization. Obstet Gynecol. 2011;117(1): 136–42.
74. Horak S, Polanska J, Widlak P. Bulky DNA adducts in human sperm: relationship with fertility, semen quality, smoking, and environmental factors. Mutat Res. 2003;537(1):53–65.

75. Pajarinen J, Savolainen V, Perola M, Penttila A, Karhunen PJ. Polymorphism in the cytochrome P450 2E1 gene and alcohol-induced disorders of human spermatogenesis. Int J Androl. 1996;19(5):314–22.
76. Fronczak CM, Kim ED, Barqawi AB. The insults of illicit drug use on male fertility. J Androl. 2012;33(4):515–28.
77. du Plessis SS, Agarwal A, Syriac A. Marijuana, phytocannabinoids, the endocannabinoid system, and male fertility. J Assist Reprod Genet. 2015; 32(11):1575–88.
78. Kolodny RC, Masters WH, Kolodner RM, Toro G. Depression of plasma testosterone levels after chronic intensive marihuana use. N Engl J Med. 1974;290(16):872–4.
79. Friedrich G, Nepita W, Andre T. Serum testosterone concentrations in cannabis and opiate users. Beitr Gerichtl Med. 1990;48:57–66.
80. Mendelson JH, Kuehnle J, Ellingboe J, Babor TF. Plasma testosterone levels before, during and after chronic marihuana smoking. N Engl J Med. 1974; 291(20):1051–5.
81. Cone EJ, Johnson RE, Moore JD, Roache JD. Acute effects of smoking marijuana on hormones, subjective effects and performance in male human subjects. Pharmacol Biochem Behav. 1986;24(6):1749–54.
82. Gundersen TD, Jorgensen N, Andersson AM, Bang AK, Nordkap L, Skakkebaek NE, Priskorn L, Juul A, Jensen TK. Association between use of marijuana and male reproductive hormones and semen quality: a study among 1,215 healthy young men. Am J Epidemiol. 2015;182(6):473–81.
83. Hembree WC 3rd, Nahas GG, Zeidenberg P, Huang HF. Changes in human spermatozoa associated with high dose marihuana smoking. Adv Biosci. 1978;22-23:429–39.
84. Singer R, Ben-Bassat M, Malik Z, Sagiv M, Ravid A, Shohat B, Livni E, Mamon T, Segenreich E, Servadio C. Oligozoospermia, asthenozoospermia, and sperm abnormalities in ex-addict to heroin, morphine, and hashish. Arch Androl. 1986;16(2):167–74.
85. Pacey AA, Povey AC, Clyma JA, McNamee R, Moore HD, Baillie H, Cherry NM, Participating Centres of Chaps-UK. Modifiable and non-modifiable risk factors for poor sperm morphology. Hum Reprod. 2014;29(8):1629–36.
86. Bracken MB, Eskenazi B, Sachse K, McSharry JE, Hellenbrand K, Leo-Summers L. Association of cocaine use with sperm concentration, motility, and morphology. Fertil Steril. 1990;53(2):315–22.
87. Samplaski MK, Bachir BG, Lo KC, Grober ED, Lau S, Jarvi KA. Cocaine use in the infertile male population: a marker for conditions resulting in subfertility. Current urology. 2015;8(1):38–42.
88. Vuong C, Van Uum SH, O'Dell LE, Lutfy K, Friedman TC. The effects of opioids and opioid analogs on animal and human endocrine systems. Endocr Rev. 2010;31(1):98–132.
89. Safarinejad MR, Asgari SA, Farshi A, Ghaedi G, Kolahi AA, Iravani S, Khoshdel AR. The effects of opiate consumption on serum reproductive hormone levels, sperm parameters, seminal plasma antioxidant capacity and sperm DNA integrity. Reprod Toxicol. 2013;36:18–23.
90. Schuel H, Chang MC, Berkery D, Schuel R, Zimmerman AM, Zimmerman S. Cannabinoids inhibit fertilization in sea urchins by reducing the fertilizing capacity of sperm. Pharmacol Biochem Behav. 1991;40(3): 609–15.
91. Zimmerman AM, Zimmerman S, Raj AY. Effects of cannabinoids on spermatogenesis in mice. Adv Biosci. 1978;22-23:407–18.
92. Wenger T, Rettori V, Snyder GD, Dalterio S, McCann SM. Effects of delta-9-tetrahydrocannabinol on the hypothalamic-pituitary control of luteinizing hormone and follicle-stimulating hormone secretion in adult male rats. Neuroendocrinology. 1987;46(6):488–93.
93. Smith C, Moore C, Besch N, Besch P. Effect of marihuana (delta-9 tetrahydrocannabinol) on secretion of sex-hormones in mature male rhesus-monkey. In: Clinical Chemistry: 1976: AMER ASSOC CLINICAL CHEMISTRY 2101 L STREET NW, SUITE 202, WASHINGTON, DC 20037-1526; 1976. p. 1184.
94. Banerjee A, Singh A, Srivastava P, Turner H, Krishna A. Effects of chronic bhang (cannabis) administration on the reproductive system of male mice. Birth Defects Res B Dev Reprod Toxicol. 2011;92(3):195–205.
95. Chakravarty I, Ghosh JJ. Influence of cannabis and delta-9-tetrahydrocannabinol on the biochemistry of the male reproductive organs. Biochem Pharmacol. 1981;30(4):273–6.
96. Li H, George VK, Crawford SC, Dhabuwala CB. Effect of cocaine on testicular blood flow in rats: evaluation by percutaneous injection of xenon-133. J Environ Pathol Toxicol Oncol. 1999;18(1):73–7.
97. George VK, Li H, Teloken C, Grignon DJ, Lawrence WD, Dhabuwala CB. Effects of long-term cocaine exposure on spermatogenesis and fertility in peripubertal male rats. J Urol. 1996;155(1):327–31.
98. Li H, Jiang Y, Rajpurkar A, Tefilli MV, Dunbar JC, Dhabuwala CB. Lipid peroxidation and antioxidant activities in rat testis after chronic cocaine administration. Urology. 1999;54(5):925–8.
99. Barenys M, Gomez-Catalan J, Camps L, Teixido E, de Lapuente J, Gonzalez-Linares J, Serret J, Borras M, Rodamilans M, Llobet JM. MDMA (ecstasy) delays pubertal development and alters sperm quality after developmental exposure in the rat. Toxicol Lett. 2010;197(2):135–42.
100. Abdellatief RB, Elgamal DA, Mohamed EE. Effects of chronic tramadol administration on testicular tissue in rats: an experimental study. Andrologia. 2015;47(6):674–9.
101. Ahmadnia H, Akhavan Rezayat A, Hoseyni M, Sharifi N, Khajedalooee M, Akhavan Rezayat A. Short-period influence of chronic morphine exposure on serum levels of sexual hormones and spermatogenesis in rats. Nephrourol Mon. 2016;8(4):e38052.
102. Whan LB, West MC, McClure N, Lewis SE. Effects of delta-9-tetrahydrocannabinol, the primary psychoactive cannabinoid in marijuana, on human sperm function in vitro. Fertil Steril. 2006;85(3):653–60.
103. Amoako AA, Marczylo TH, Marczylo EL, Elson J, Willets JM, Taylor AH, Konje JC. Anandamide modulates human sperm motility: implications for men with asthenozoospermia and oligoasthenoteratozoospermia. Hum Reprod. 2013;28(8):2058–66.
104. Morgan DJ, Muller CH, Murataeva NA, Davis BJ, Mackie K. Delta9-Tetrahydrocannabinol (Delta9-THC) attenuates mouse sperm motility and male fecundity. Br J Pharmacol. 2012;165(8):2575–83.

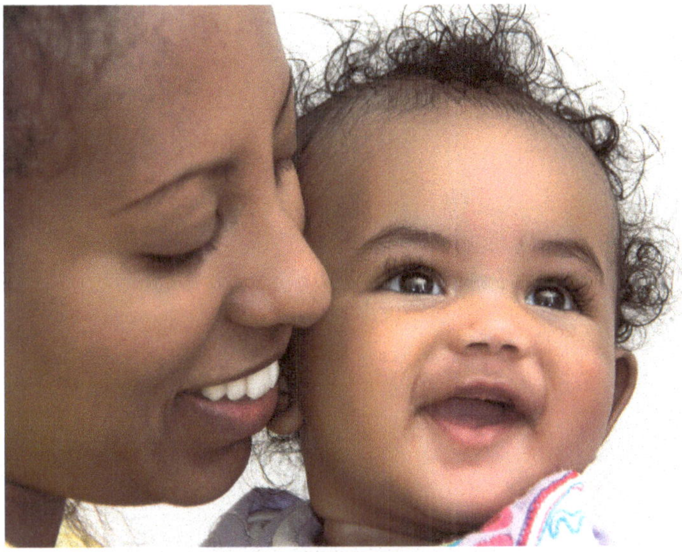

# A COLLABORATIVE APPROACH TO THE TREATMENT OF PREGNANT WOMEN WITH OPIOID USE DISORDERS

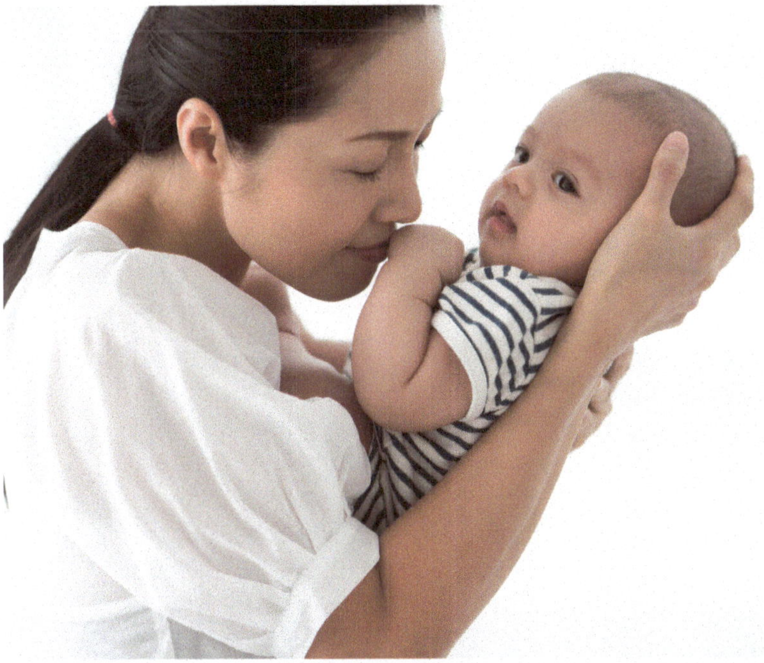

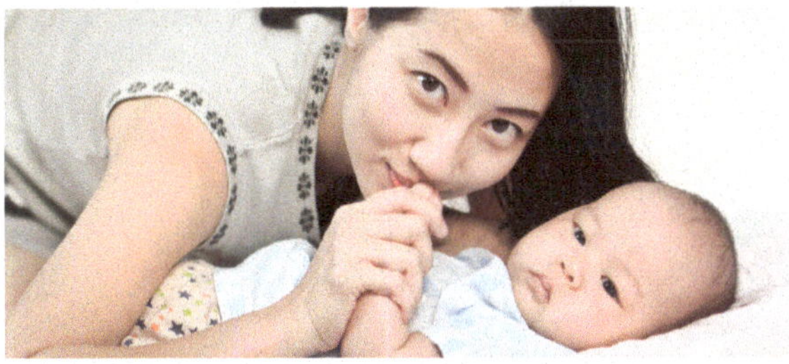

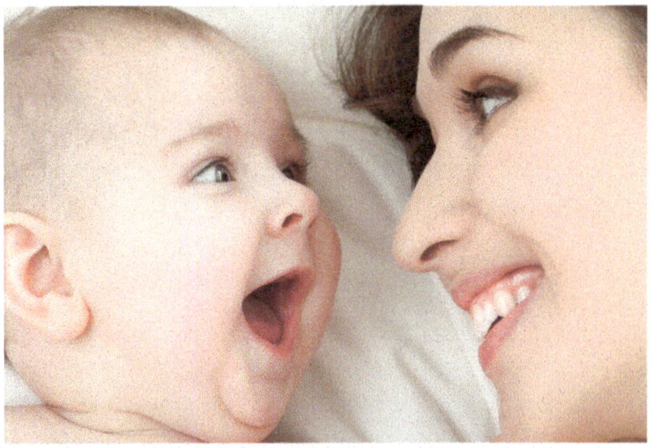

## Practice and Policy Considerations for Child Welfare, Collaborating Medical, and Service Providers

DEPARTMENT OF HEALTH & HUMAN SERVICES USA

ACF

Children's Bureau

Substance Abuse and Mental Health Services Administration

SAMHSA

www.samhsa.gov • 1-877-SAMHSA-7 (1-877-726-4727)

# Introduction

This guidance publication is intended to support the efforts of states, tribes, and local communities in addressing the needs of pregnant women with opioid use disorders and their infants and families.[1] National data show that from 2000 to 2009 the use of opioids during pregnancy increased from 1.19 to 5.63 per 1,000 hospital births (Patrick, Schumacher, Benneyworth, Krans, McAllister, & Davis, 2012). Because of the high rate of opioid use and misuse among all women, including pregnant women, medical, social service, and judicial agencies are having to confront this concern more often and, in some communities, at alarming rates.

Opioids are drugs that reduce the intensity of pain signals. The term "opiates" refers only to natural opium derivatives, and the term "opioids" refers to drugs that activate opioid receptors, including opiates, heroin, and synthetic opioids (e.g., certain prescription painkillers, such as oxycodone) (CSAT, 2004).

Data from SAMHSA's National Survey on Drug Use and Health show that between 2007 and 2014, the numbers of past-year heroin initiates, heroin users, and people with heroin dependence increased significantly (SAMHSA, 2015). The pattern of initiating heroin use has changed over the past decade. Approximately three-quarters of persons who use heroin report prior non-medical use of prescription opioids, as well as current abuse or dependence on additional substances such as stimulants, alcohol, and marijuana. Conversely a small percentage, approximately four percent, of persons with non-medical use of prescription drugs initiate heroin use. However given the 10.3 million persons who reported non-medical use of prescription drugs in 2014, this small percentage of conversion to heroin generates several hundred thousand new heroin users (Compton, Jones & Baldwin, 2016).

When pregnant women use opioids, their infants may be affected. Neonatal abstinence syndrome (NAS) is the common term used to represent the pattern of clinical findings typically associated with opioid withdrawal in newborns (Hudak & Tan, 2012). However, the U.S. Food and Drug Administration (FDA) now uses the term "neonatal opioid withdrawal syndrome" on warning labels when referring to the maternal use of opioids during pregnancy.[2] Most newborns of mothers who used opioids during pregnancy develop symptoms of NAS, a postnatal drug withdrawal syndrome, primarily caused by maternal opioid use (Patrick et al., 2012). The range and severity of the symptoms experienced by the infant depends on a variety of factors, including the type of opioid the infant was exposed to and whether the infant was exposed to multiple substances. Treatment of NAS includes non-pharmacological and pharmacological methods.

Abrupt discontinuation of opioid use during pregnancy can result in premature labor, fetal distress, and miscarriage. Medical withdrawal from opioids should be conducted under the supervision of physicians experienced in perinatal addiction (Kaltenbach, Berghella, & Finnegan, 1998). However, pregnant women who stop using opioids and subsequently relapse are at greater risk of overdose death. There is also an increased risk of harm to the fetus. Because NAS is treatable, medication-assisted treatment (MAT) is typically recommended instead of withdrawal or abstinence (Jones, O'Grady, Malfi, & Tuten, 2008).

[1] According to the U.S. National Library of Medicine, the term "infant" is used to describe a child from newborn to 1 year (http://www.nlm.nih.gov/medlineplus/ency/article/002004.htm), and the term "newborn" (neonate) is used to describe an infant who is 4 weeks old or younger (http://www.nlm.nih.gov/medlineplus/ency/article/002271.htm). For the purpose of this document, these definitions are applied.

[2] "What is the Federal Government Doing to Combat the Opioid Abuse Epidemic?" Statement of Douglas C. Throckmorton, M.D., Deputy Director for Regulatory Programs, Center for Drug Evaluation and Research, Food and Drug Administration, Department of Health and Human Services before the Subcommittee on Oversight and Investigations, Committee on Energy and Commerce, U.S. House of Representatives on May 1, 2015. http://www.fda.gov/newsevents/testimony/ucm446076.htm

The use of MAT during pregnancy is a recommended best practice for the care of pregnant women with opioid use disorders[3] (American College of Obstetricians and Gynecologists Committee on Health Care for Underserved Women, & American Society of Addiction Medicine, 2012). MAT is the use of medications in combination with counseling and behavioral therapies to provide a whole-patient approach to the treatment of substance use disorders (SAMHSA, 2014a). Research shows that a combination of medication and behavioral therapies is most successful for substance use disorder treatment. MAT is clinically driven and focuses on individualized patient care.

Medications used to treat opioid use disorders include methadone and buprenorphine. Both of these medications stop and prevent opioid withdrawal and reduce opioid cravings, allowing the person to focus on other aspects of recovery.

Like any medication given during pregnancy, the use of MAT in pregnant women has both risks and benefits to the mother and fetus. Therefore, MAT needs careful consideration by the pregnant women themselves as well as coordination by the providers and agencies that have influence and authority over this population of pregnant women and their infants.

To inform this guidance document, the National Center on Substance Abuse and Child Welfare (NCSACW), the Substance Abuse and Mental Health Services Administration (SAMHSA), and the Administration on Children and Families (ACF) formed a national panel of experts (listed in *Appendix 6: Additional Acknowledgments*). This panel identified the practice and policy considerations that each partner agency or organization needs to consider when working with, and on behalf of, pregnant women with opioid use disorders and their children. These experts met several times over six months in 2014.

Panel members agreed that building knowledge, skills, and expertise within the healthcare (including obstetrics, pediatrics, substance abuse treatment, and mental health), child welfare, and judicial systems and tribal communities will enable these entities to better deliver coordinated services to this population of pregnant women and their families. This guidance document is designed to assist these systems in improving their collaborative practice and to provide information about additional resources that will strengthen their capacity to provide coordinated, best-practice care and services.

The overarching message of this guide is that a coordinated, multi-system approach best serves the needs of pregnant women with opioid use disorders and their infants. Collaborative planning and implementation of services that reflect best practices for treating opioid use disorders during pregnancy are yielding promising results in communities across the country. Advance planning for the treatment of pregnant women with opioid use disorders that addresses safe care for mothers and their newborns can help prevent unexpected crises at the time of delivery. This guidance document provides background information on the treatment of pregnant women with opioid use disorders, summarizes key aspects of guidelines that have been adopted by professional organizations across many of the disciplines, presents a comprehensive framework to organize these efforts in communities, and provides a collaborative practice guide for community planning to improve outcomes for these families. A set of appendices provides details on implementing the recommendations in the guide as well as a summary of lessons from one community's experience over the past decade.

[3] The fifth edition of the *Diagnostic and Statistical Manual of Mental Disorders* ([DSM-5] American Psychiatric Association, 2013) uses the term "opioid use disorder" to include abuse of or dependence on opioids. Previous editions of the DSM differentiated between the two categories. The DSM-5 combines abuse and dependence into a single disorder, measured on a continuum from mild to severe.

# Background

Opioid medications used to relieve pain are beneficial to many people but are often overprescribed.[4] The overuse and misuse of these medications in the United States over the past decade has contributed to thousands of overdose deaths. According to the Centers for Disease Control and Prevention (CDC), from 1999 to 2010, yearly prescription opioid overdose deaths among women increased from 1,287 to 6,631 (CDC, 2013). These numbers represent a 400 percent increase over 10 years (see *Scope of the Problem* on page 5 for additional information). The use of heroin has also increased greatly over the last decade. Between 2007 and 2014, the numbers of past-year heroin initiates, heroin users, and people with heroin dependence has increased significantly (SAMHSA, 2015).

The use of MAT, in combination with counseling and behavioral therapies, and access to a range of supportive services, such as housing and employment services, assists the mother in achieving a more stable life (Newman & Kagen, 1973; Finnegan, 1991; CSAT, 2005). In turn, it also stabilizes the intrauterine environment and avoids subjecting the fetus to repeated episodes of withdrawal, which places the fetus at higher risk for morbidity and mortality (Kaltenbach & Finnegan, 1998; Jones et al., 2005; CSAT, 2005). According to the National Institute on Drug Abuse (NIDA):

---

"Methadone maintenance therapy (MMT) enhances an opioid-dependent woman's chances for a trouble-free pregnancy and a healthy baby. Compared with continued opioid [use], MMT lowers her risk of developing infectious diseases, including hepatitis and HIV; of experiencing pregnancy complications, including spontaneous abortion and miscarriages; and of having a child with challenges including low birth weight and neurobehavioral problems.

Along with these benefits, MMT may also produce a serious adverse effect. Like most drugs, methadone enters fetal circulation via the placenta. The fetus becomes dependent on the medication during gestation and typically experiences withdrawal when it separates from the placental circulation at birth. The symptoms of withdrawal, known as neonatal abstinence syndrome (NAS) include hypersensitivity and hyperirritability, tremors, vomiting, respiratory difficulties, poor sleep, and low-grade fevers. Newborns with NAS often require hospitalization and treatment, during which they receive medication (often morphine) in tapering doses to relieve their symptoms while their bodies adapt to becoming opioid-free." (Whitten, 2012).

---

Methadone has been accepted as a treatment for opioid use disorders during pregnancy since the late 1970s (Kaltenbach & Finnegan, 1998; Kandall et al., 1999; CSAT, 2005). In 1998, a National Institutes of Health consensus panel recommended methadone maintenance as the standard of care for pregnant women with opioid use disorders (National Consensus Development Panel on Effective Medical Treatment of Opiate Addiction, 1998). However, the use of buprenorphine for the management of opioid use disorders is becoming more widely used, with the emergence of data from randomized clinical

[4] The Office of Disease Prevention and Health Promotion has developed Pathways to Safer Opioid Use, a training resource that uses the principles of health literacy and a multimodal, team-based approach to promote the appropriate, safe, and effective use of opioids to manage chronic pain. http://www.health.gov/hcq/training.asp#pathways

trials that demonstrate its safety and efficacy (Jones et al., 2005; Fischer et al., 2006; Jones et al., 2010). Between 2005 and 2008, A National Institute on Drug Abuse (NIDA)-supported clinical trial, the Maternal Opioid Treatment: Human Experimental Research (MOTHER) study, examined the use of both methadone and buprenorphine maintenance therapy during pregnancy. Both medications are widely used to help individuals with opioid use disorders achieve stability and decrease illicit opioid use. The study also found that infants exposed to buprenorphine required shorter treatment duration and less medication to treat the symptoms of NAS and experienced shorter hospital stays when compared to infants exposed to methadone. No significant difference was found with respect to any serious maternal or neonatal adverse events (e.g., abnormal fetal health, neurological symptoms; Jones et al., 2010).

Methadone and buprenorphine are classified as Pregnancy Category C[5] drugs by the FDA, meaning that adequate, well-controlled studies of how these drugs affect pregnant women are lacking. However, prescribing methadone or buprenorphine during pregnancy is not considered "off-label." Choosing to proceed with methadone or buprenorphine treatment during pregnancy is an individual decision that women should make with their health care providers.

Another medication used to treat opioid use disorders is naltrexone. Naltrexone functions as a pure opioid blocker; however, withdrawal can be induced if naltrexone is administered to an individual who is engaged in current opioid use. Thus, induction to naltrexone requires detoxification and an opioid-free period, which may lead to relapse vulnerability, re-establishment of physical dependence, increased risk behaviors, treatment dropout, and possible opioid overdose and death. There is insufficient research to support the use of naltrexone during pregnancy. When considering naltrexone use during pregnancy, the potential risk to the fetus should be given due consideration. Before research is conducted to determine the safety of naltrexone use during pregnancy, the benefits and risks must be carefully weighed (Jones, Chisolm, Jansson, & Terplan, 2013). Additional information on the use of methadone, buprenorphine, and naltrexone appears in *Appendix 4: Key Features of Medications Approved for Treating Opioid Use Disorders*. As more women using MAT during pregnancy give birth to newborns, the field is gaining knowledge about the typical withdrawal course that newborns experience, based on the types and doses of medications mothers are given to treat opioid use disorders as well as other aspects of their prenatal obstetrical care.

Some distinctions among women who use opioids during pregnancy are paramount to understand because of care coordination for both mothers and infants. Although women who use opioids during pregnancy test positive for opioid use at the birth of their newborn, the supports and system responses should differ depending on whether or not the mother's opioid use is medically managed. Generally, women who use opioids during pregnancy and/or at delivery can be categorized within one of the following groups:

- Are receiving pain management with medications under the care of a physician.
- Are under the care of a physician and undergoing treatment for an opioid use disorder with medications, such as methadone or buprenorphine.
- Are misusing or abusing opioid pain medications with or without a prescription (e.g., obtaining pills illegally for a non-medical use, "doctor shopping," obtaining a prescription illegally).
- Are using or abusing illicit opioids, particularly heroin.

[5] In December 2014, the FDA published the Requirements for Pregnancy and Lactation Labeling Rule. The nomenclature is not used in the final rule, which requires the removal of the Pregnancy Categories A, B, C, D, and X from all human prescription drug and biological product labeling. Labeling is based on descriptive subsections for pregnancy exposure and risk, lactation, and effects to reproductive potential for females and males. Retrieved from http://www.gpo.gov/fdsys/pkg/FR-2014-12-04/pdf/2014-28241.pdf (accessed August 19, 2015).

Women with opioid use disorders often face a host of complex and entwined issues. Although they may come from all socioeconomic backgrounds, their lives are complicated by psychosocial and environmental factors. Often, there is a history of sexual abuse and/or interpersonal violence, inadequate social supports, unpredictable parenting models, poor nutrition, unstable housing, and co-occurring psychiatric conditions. Pregnant women with opioid use disorders are likely to use multiple substances during pregnancy, including tobacco and alcohol. Fetal Alcohol Spectrum Disorders (FASD) is a term used to describe the range of conditions, including physical, mental, and behavioral conditions as well as learning disabilities, that can be experienced by an individual prenatally exposed to alcohol.[6] Infants prenatally exposed to multiple substances are at risk for developing a wide spectrum of physical, emotional, and developmental problems. Exposure to multiple substances can affect an infant's withdrawal symptoms. Other factors that can affect the infant's withdrawal symptoms include the type of opioid that the mother used, whether the mother's opioid use disorder was medically managed, and whether she received routine prenatal care. The hospital environment itself, such as the methodology used to treat the infant's withdrawal symptoms is also an important factor that can reduce or exacerbate the infant's withdrawal (see the section on *Neonatal Abstinence Syndrome* for additional information).

Growing concerns about the substantial increase in the number of pregnant women and newborns who test positive for opiates, coupled with the overwhelmingly inaccurate and alarmist reporting by the popular media regarding this issue, prompted more than 50 leading national and international researchers and experts to release an open letter to the media and policy makers in March 2013. In an effort to counter misinformation about pregnant women and prescription opioid use, these experts noted the following:

Newborn babies are NOT born "addicted" and referring to newborns with NAS as "addicted" is inaccurate, incorrect, and highly stigmatizing.

Portraying NAS babies as "victims" results in the vilification of their mothers, who are then viewed as perpetrators, and further perpetuates the criminalization of addiction.

Using pejorative labels such as "oxy babies," "oxy tots," "victims," "tiny addict," or "born addicted" places these children at substantial risk of stigma and discrimination and can lead to inappropriate child welfare interventions.

NAS is treatable and has not been associated with long-term adverse consequences.

Mischaracterizing MAT as harmful and unethical contradicts the efficacy of MAT and discourages the appropriate and federally recommended treatment for opioid use disorder.

— International Drug Policy Consortium, 2013

# Scope of the Problem

## Opioid Use Trends

Rates of prescription opioid pain medication use vary across regions of the country and among subpopulations. From 2000 through 2013, the rate of overdose deaths related to heroin increased across all regions—11-fold in

[6] Resources for FASD include (1) the CDC website (http://www.cdc.gov/ncbddd/fasd/facts.html) and (2) the FASD Center for Excellence (http://fasdcenter.samhsa.gov).

the Midwest, more than 4-fold in the Northeast, more than 3-fold in the South, and doubled in the West (Hedegaard, Chen, & Warner, 2015). As the opioid crises emerged, by 2008 the states with the highest rates of opioid-related morbidity and mortality were concentrated in the Appalachian region (e.g., Kentucky, West Virginia, and Ohio) (Behavioral Health Coordinating Committee [BHCC], 2013). States vary a great deal in rates of: (1) non-medical use of opioid pain medications, (2) prescriptions for opioid pain medications, and (3) drug overdose deaths (Centers for Disease Control and Prevention, 2013). States with lower rates of non-medical use of and prescriptions for opioid pain medications also had lower rates of drug overdose deaths (Centers for Disease Control and Prevention, 2011).

Opioid use and related consequences also vary by several key demographics. For example, the Medicaid patient population is more likely to receive prescriptions for opioid pain medications and to have opioids prescribed at higher doses and for longer periods of time than the non-Medicaid patient population. Opioid medication overdose deaths are also more common among Medicaid-eligible populations (BHCC, 2013).

The overall rate of first time heroin use increased among all women, from 0.06 percent in 2002–2004 to 0.10 percent in 2009–2011, estimated to be an increase from 43,000 women to 77,000 women (SAMHSA, 2013). Among women, the number of overdose deaths due to the use of prescription opioid pain medications has increased significantly since 2007, surpassing deaths from motor vehicle-related injuries. Overdose deaths due to opioid medication increased among women more than 5-fold between 1999 and 2010, totaling 47,935 during that period (CDC, 2013).

From 1992 to 2012, treatment admissions for pregnant women among all female admissions remained stable at four percent. However, the proportion of pregnant women entering treatment who reported any prescription opioid misuse increased substantially from two percent in 1992 to 28 percent in 2012, an increase from 351 to 6,087 women. The proportion of pregnant women who entered treatment and reported prescription opioids as their primary substance increased from one percent in 1992 to 19 percent in 2012, an increase from 124 to 4,268 women (Martin, Longinaker, & Terplan, 2014).

## Neonatal Abstinence Syndrome

Among infants, the incidence of NAS increased from 1.20 per 1,000 hospital births in 2000 to 3.39 in 2009 (Patrick et al., 2012) and 5.80 in 2012 (Patrick, Davis, Lehmann & Cooper, 2015). In a study of 299 neonatal intensive care units (NICU) across the country, the rate of NICU admissions for infants with NAS increased from 7 cases per 1,000 admissions in 2004 to 27 cases per 1,000 admissions in 2013 (Tolia, Patrick, Bennett, Murthy, Sousa, Smith, Clark & Spitzer, 2015). The study by Patrick et al. (2012) did not distinguish between NAS that resulted from illicit opioids, prescription opioid pain medications, or MAT. Between 2006 and 2012, the rate of infant and maternal hospitalizations related to substance use increased substantially, from 5.1 to 8.7 per 1,000 infant hospitalizations and from 13.4 to 17.9 per 1,000 maternal hospitalizations, resulting in a total cost of $944 million in 2012 (Fingar, Stocks, Weiss & Owens, 2015). In 2012, among the neonatal stays with a substance-related condition, approximately 60% were related to neonatal drug withdrawal or NAS. Among maternal stays related to substance abuse, almost one-fourth involved opioids (Finger et al., 2015).

As previously discussed, NAS is the term used to represent the pattern of effects that are associated with opioid withdrawal in newborns (Hudak & Tan, 2012). NAS symptoms are affected by a variety of factors, including the type of opioid the infant was exposed to, the point in gestation when the mother used the opioid, genetic factors, and exposure to multiple substances (Wachman, Hayes, Brown, Paul, Harvey-Wilkes, Terrin, Huggins, Aranda, & Davis, 2013). To assess the severity of the infant's symptoms, a scoring system, such as the Finnegan Neonatal Abstinence Scoring System or the Lipsitz Neonatal Drug-Withdrawal Scoring System is used. The results of the scoring system are used in conjunction with an assessment of other factors, including the infant's gestational age, overall health, medical history, exposure to other substances, and tolerance or response to medications, to determine the course of treatment (Jansson, Velez, & Harrow, 2009).

Non-pharmacological treatment is the standard of care for the infant with NAS and should start at birth and continue throughout the infant's hospitalization and beyond (Velez & Jansson, 2008). Non-pharmacological treatment seeks to soothe the infant's symptoms, while also encouraging the mother–infant bond. Some of the symptoms associated with NAS can be challenging and disruptive to the attachment between the mother and infant, particularly for women who have substance use disorders and may have difficulty responding to an infants' cues. Non-pharmacological methods include rooming together post-delivery and modification of the environment to support attachment and provide a soothing environment for the infant. Environmental modifications include swaddling the infant and reducing his or her exposure to light and excessive noise.

Pharmacological treatment is primarily intended to relieve NAS symptoms and its associated complications, such as fever, weight loss, and seizures. Pharmacological treatment typically entails using a neonatal morphine solution or methadone (Hudak & Tan, 2012). Supports are necessary to address the challenges and risk factors that mothers and infants may face following discharge from the hospital. As previously described, women with opioid use disorders often face complex psychosocial, environmental, and cultural factors that can impact treatment, recovery, and parenting. Post-discharge supportive services can include identifying family or others for social support and participating in ongoing support groups, counseling, housing services, and follow-up services for the infant. See *Appendix 5: Children and Recovery Mothers (CHARM) Collaborative in Burlington, Vermont: A Case Study*, for information on post-discharge supportive services.

The advent of new medications used in treating opioid use disorders during pregnancy calls for additional studies on the long-term impact of prenatal exposure to opioids to better understand the best course of treatment for affected children (Wahlsten & Sarman, 2013; Hamilton, McGlone, MacKinnon, Russell, Bradnam, & Mactier, 2010; Farid, Dunlop, Tait, & Hulse, 2008).

**Treatment considerations for newborns with prenatal substance exposure are available in a 2012 clinical report from the American Academy of Pediatrics. The Academy recommends that staff with training in identifying signs of withdrawal monitor these infants and initiate therapy when indicated.**

**"Each nursery that cares for infants with neonatal withdrawal should develop a protocol that defines indications and procedures for screening for maternal substance abuse. In addition, each nursery should develop and adhere to a standardized plan for the evaluation and comprehensive treatment of infants at risk for or showing signs of withdrawal."**

**—Hudak & Tan, 2012**

# Guidelines for Supporting Collaborative Policy and Practice

This guidance is intended to support the development of collaborative, interagency policies and practices that can assist communities to develop approaches that support the health, safety, well-being, and recovery of pregnant women with opioid use disorders and their infants. These approaches begin with prevention strategies designed to help all women of childbearing age, as well as their health care providers, to understand both the implications of opioid use during pregnancy and the interventions in the prenatal period that extend through—and ideally beyond—the postpartum time frame. This guidance highlights key decision points and recommended strategies based on the research literature as well as evidence from innovative strategies being implemented around the country.

Any response to the many barriers facing the families of pregnant women with opioid use disorders must be grounded in solutions within the community that reflect best practices (e.g., evidence-based practices) as well as perspectives, resources, and policies that address the needs of the community. A number of communities across the United States have developed collaborative initiatives to make systems and processes work more effectively for women with opioid use disorders and their infants. Although these approaches vary, they share a focus on coordinating the goals and efforts of an array of partners. In particular, efforts focus on effective screening and linkages to treatment in the prenatal period, as well as efficient communication between hospitals and community partners. One of these well-developed initiatives is described in the case study in *Appendix 5: Children and Recovery Mothers (CHARM) Collaborative in Burlington, Vermont: A Case Study.*

## Existing Guidelines

Research shows that a combination of medication and behavioral therapies is the most successful way to treat opioid use disorders and increases the likelihood of cessation of opioid abuse (CSAT, 2005). Similarly, the literature summarizing the most current research offers best-practice guidance for developing efficacious practices and policies for women with opioid use disorders and their infants.

Recommendations have been published in the last several years by national and international organizations, such as the American College of Obstetricians and Gynecologists (ACOG), World Health Organization (WHO), US HHS, SAMHSA, American Society of Addiction Medicine (ASAM), Legal Action Center, and American Academy of Pediatrics. Although this publication is not intended to provide an exhaustive literature review, some of the key recommendations from these organizations are cited throughout, and select highlights are presented in the section that follows. Links to these publications are provided in *Appendix 3: Training Needs and Resources*.

### American College of Obstetricians and Gynecologists and American Society of Addiction Medicine

The following excerpt from the 2012 ACOG and ASAM Committee Opinion on Opioid Abuse, Dependence, and Addiction in Pregnancy summarizes the current knowledge of the risks and benefits of MAT for opioid use during the prenatal and postpartum period.

Opioid use in pregnancy is not uncommon, and the use of illicit opioids during pregnancy is associated with an increased risk of adverse outcomes. The current standard of care for pregnant women with opioid use disorders is referral for opioid-assisted therapy with methadone, but. . . evidence suggests that buprenorphine also should be considered. Medically supervised tapered doses of opioids during pregnancy often result in relapse to former use.[7] Abrupt discontinuation of opioids in an opioid-dependent pregnant woman can result in preterm labor, fetal distress, or fetal demise. During the intrapartum and postpartum period, special considerations are needed for women who are opioid dependent to ensure appropriate pain management, to prevent postpartum relapse and a risk of overdose, and to ensure adequate contraception to prevent unintended pregnancies. Patient stabilization with opioid-assisted therapy is compatible with breastfeeding. Neonatal abstinence syndrome is an expected and treatable condition that follows prenatal exposure to opioid agonists. All infants born to women who use opioids during pregnancy should be monitored for neonatal abstinence syndrome and be treated if indicated.

---

### World Health Organization

**The WHO's *Guidelines for the identification and management of substance use and substance use disorders in pregnancy* (2014) provide technical guidance primarily for health care professionals who work with women and their infants from conception to birth as well as during the postnatal period. The publication also offers guidelines on identifying and managing alcohol and other substance use in pregnant women, with the goal of ensuring healthy outcomes for both pregnant women and their infants. While developing the recommendations, WHO established the following overarching principles to provide guidance in planning, implementing, and evaluating the most relevant recommendations, based on regional contexts and available resources.**

---

PRIORITIZING PREVENTION. Preventing, reducing and ceasing the use of alcohol, tobacco and illicit drugs before and during pregnancy and in the postpartum period for breastfeeding mothers are essential for optimizing the health and well-being of women and their children. Ensure that women who are receiving opioid treatment for a medical condition understand the risks of prenatal exposure and have access to highly effective birth control methods.

ENSURING ACCESS TO PREVENTION AND TREATMENT SERVICES. All pregnant women and their families affected by substance use disorders should have access to affordable prevention and treatment services and interventions delivered with special attention to confidentiality, legal and human rights; women should not be excluded from accessing health care because of their substance use. Treatment, especially residential programs, for postpartum women should incorporate consideration for the infant and siblings.

RESPECTING PATIENT AUTONOMY. The autonomy of pregnant and breastfeeding women should always be respected; each woman with a substance use disorder needs to be fully informed

[7] The optimal methadone dosage for pregnant women generally increases throughout pregnancy, and this increase does not necessarily increase fetal exposure to methadone. See John Drozdick, III, et al., *Methadone Trough Levels in Pregnancy*, 187 American Journal of Obstetrics and Gynecology, 1184 (2002); John J. McCarthy, *Addiction Treatment Forum, Methadone Dosing During Pregnancy: Does Anyone Have a Clue?* (Oct. 2012).

about the risks and benefits, for herself and for her fetus or infant, of available treatment options, when making decisions about her health care and the care of her infant.

**PROVIDING COMPREHENSIVE CARE.** Services for pregnant and breastfeeding women with substance use disorders should have a level of comprehensiveness that matches the complexity and multifaceted nature of substance use disorders and their antecedents in this population.

**SAFEGUARDING AGAINST DISCRIMINATION AND STIGMATIZATION.** Interventions should be provided to pregnant and breastfeeding women in ways that prevent stigmatization, discrimination, criminalization, and marginalization of women seeking treatment to benefit themselves and their infants. Prevention and treatment should promote and facilitate family, community and social support as well as social inclusion by fostering strong links with available childcare, economic supports, education, housing, and relevant services.

In addition to these principles, WHO makes specific practice recommendations. One recommendation suggests that pregnant women should be advised to continue or begin opioid maintenance therapy with methadone or buprenorphine.

## American Society of Addiction Medicine

ASAM's *National Practice Guideline for the Use of Medications in the Treatment of Addiction Involving Opioid Use* (2015) provides information on evidence-based treatment of opioid use disorder, including guidelines for the treatment of pregnant women. The publication discusses recommendations on assessment and diagnosis, treatment, and the use of psychosocial treatment in conjunction with medications. ASAM's recommendations for the treatment of opioid use disorders in pregnant women include:

---

**ASSESSMENT OF OPIOID USE DISORDER IN PREGNANT WOMEN.** A comprehensive assessment, including medical examination and psychosocial assessment is recommended in evaluating opioid use disorder in pregnant women. The clinician should ask questions in a direct and nonjudgmental manner to elicit a detailed and accurate history.

**OPIOID AGONIST TREATMENT IN PREGNANCY.** Decisions to use opioid agonist medications in pregnant women with opioid use disorder revolve around balancing the risks and benefits to maternal and infant health. Opioid agonist treatment is thought to have minimal long-term impacts on children relative to harms resulting from maternal use of heroin and prescription opioids. Therefore, women with opioid use disorder who are not in treatment should be encouraged to start opioid agonist treatment with methadone or buprenorphine monotherapy (without naloxone) as early in the pregnancy as possible. Pregnancy in women with opioid use disorder should be co-managed by an obstetrician and an addiction specialist physician.

**OPIOID AGONISTS VERSUS WITHDRAWAL MANAGEMENT.** Pregnant women who are physically dependent on opioids should receive treatment using agonist medications rather than withdrawal management or abstinence as these approaches may pose a risk to the fetus. Furthermore, withdrawal management has been found to be inferior in effectiveness over pharmacotherapy with opioid agonists and increases the risk of relapse without fetal or maternal benefit.

INDUCTION AND DOSING OF OPIOID AGONISTS. Treatment with methadone should be initiated as early as possible during pregnancy.

BREASTFEEDING. Mothers receiving methadone and buprenorphine monoproduct for the treatment of opioid use disorders should be encouraged to breastfeed.

---

In addition to these aforementioned organizations, state and local jurisdictions have developed guidelines for hospitals, child welfare agencies, treatment providers, and other care providers regarding MAT, NAS treatment, and responses to pregnant women with opioid dependency. These guidelines may help ensure a more consistent approach among communities within a given state or region. Addressing disparities in treatment related to resource shortages and geographic and financial barriers to accessing health care and other services is another vital consideration in meeting the needs of pregnant women with opioid use disorders.

One example of a regional approach that incorporates best practice guidelines is the CHARM Collaborative in Burlington, Vermont—a multidisciplinary group of agencies serving women with opioid use disorders and their families during pregnancy and through infancy. The CHARM Collaborative focuses on meeting the needs of pregnant and postpartum women who have a history of opioid use and their infants. This group emerged in the late 1990s in response to the increasing need for MAT resources for pregnant women with opioid use disorders. Today, the CHARM Collaborative includes 11 organizations that collectively provide this population of women with coordinated comprehensive care from child welfare, medical (including obstetrics and pediatrics) and substance abuse treatment professionals across Vermont. Their efforts have ensured that the vast majority of pregnant women are identified and provided treatment during the prenatal period. They jointly develop plans for the infant and family's safety and well-being prior to the baby's birth. Additional information on the approach and practices of the CHARM Collaborative is provided in *Appendix 5: Children and Recovery Mothers (CHARM) Collaborative in Burlington, Vermont: A Case Study*.

## Need for Collaboration Among Multiple Agencies

Professionals in the child welfare, judicial, medical (including obstetrics, pediatrics, substance abuse treatment, and mental health), and addiction treatment systems generally share significant concerns about pregnant women who misuse opioids and newborns with NAS and other problems related to in utero drug or alcohol exposure. However, this is often where the consensus ends. At times, the responses of various systems to the needs of these families diverge, resulting in apparent conflicts among treatment practices, medical recommendations, and the policies and oversight provided by courts and child welfare services.

The types of agencies and professionals that provide treatment and other services to pregnant women with opioid use disorders and their infants can vary widely from one community to another. A considerable range and mix of approaches, settings, programs, and professionals can be involved, and health and social service systems typically operate and intersect in ways that are unique to each community. This mixture of participating systems and relationships among them affects service coordination. For example, several different professionals and specialty providers within the medical care system (i.e., an obstetrician, neonatologist, pediatrician, and addiction specialist) might provide care to a woman and her infant during the prenatal and postpartum periods. Within the substance abuse treatment system, treatment is delivered in a variety of settings (e.g., residential facilities, outpatient clinics, and offices of physicians who provide MAT), using a combination of therapeutic approaches (e.g., medications, individual and group counseling, and self-help groups). In the child welfare system, services are delivered along a continuum, based on risk and safety factors that range from supports to children remaining in the custody of their parents (often referred to as in-home services) to out-of-home care (e.g., foster or kinship care).

Different systems and provider communities also have different policies, priorities, and perspectives. For example, hospitals—even those in the same state or county—often have inconsistent protocols for screening infants for prenatal substance exposure and sometimes have seemingly inconsistent practices for contacting child welfare agencies if substance use is detected or NAS is diagnosed. Even when hospitals have clear policies in place, adherence to these policies depends largely on the relationships between hospital staff and child welfare workers. Adherence to policies also varies by medical team members' perceptions of whether a positive toxicology screen for the newborn is likely to trigger legal consequences for the mother, which may be perceived to not be in the best interest of the mother and infant (National Abandoned Infants Assistance Resource Center, 2012).

> "Medication-Assisted Treatment (MAT) is an evidence-based practice that combines pharmacological interventions with substance abuse counseling and social support. Although not for everyone, it is an essential part of the comprehensive array of services available to people struggling with addiction to alcohol or other drugs.
>
> A paradox in our field is that although we recognize addiction as a chronic, relapsing disease, some substance abuse counselors and administrators have been reluctant to embrace new technologies for its treatment. At the same time, most physicians and other health care professionals receive little or no training in the treatment of addiction. As a result, adoption of MAT has been slow in some areas."
>
> — Mark G. Stringer, Director
> Missouri Department of Health,
> Division of Behavioral Health

The fact that many non-medical professionals can potentially affect treatment decisions for pregnant women with opioid use disorders further exacerbates the care of women and their infants. These professionals may include judges (if the woman is involved in the criminal justice system) or residential substance abuse treatment providers that do not offer MAT. If a woman is already involved in the child welfare system as a result of a case related to her older children, child welfare social workers and judicial representatives related to this separate case also influence decisions regarding her care, and these decisions might not be consistent with her treatment plan or best practice recommendations. If a woman is receiving MAT in an opioid treatment program (OTP) or buprenorphine from her doctor, she is likely to experience conflict if she also participates in a substance abuse treatment program or a mutual aid support group that does not embrace the use of MAT. It is essential to recognize that each mutual aid support group is autonomous and self-directed; and group members may have their own views on the use of MAT. Despite this potential conflict, each professional and the organizations or systems that they represent are responding to the directives issued from their respective fields of practice. If no such directives exist, they must rely on their best professional judgment when making critical decisions that affect women and their infants and that have the potential to impact entire families.

Every professional involved needs to understand the different contexts of opioid use by a pregnant woman to accurately assess her distinct needs and those of her family members in order to implement the most appropriate and comprehensive plan of care. In addition to being familiar with effective and evidence-based addiction treatment, treatment counselors, social workers, health care providers, and legal system professionals need to be aware of the primary risk and protective factors that promote or inhibit resiliency in women and their children. These factors have a direct impact on the types and intensities of support and supervision that a woman requires throughout pregnancy as well as during the critical first year of parenting a newborn.

For example, child welfare agencies have the complicated dual role of supporting families while monitoring them to prevent child maltreatment. These agencies have risk and safety assessment policies and practices that are intended to identify immediate safety concerns for children, while evaluating the risk and protective factors of each family. When making decisions about whether to intervene and how to do so in the most supportive manner, staff must take into account the distinctions related to a woman's history, motivation, and pattern of opioid use (and other drug use).

The Child Abuse and Prevention Treatment Act (CAPTA) Reauthorization Act of 2010 require states to have policies and procedures for hospitals to notify child protective services (CPS) of all children born who are affected by illegal substance use or withdrawal symptoms resulting from prenatal drug exposure or

The privacy provisions in the U.S. Code of Federal Regulations (C.F.R.), Title 42, Part 2, describe the limited circumstances in which information about a patient's treatment for a substance use disorder may be disclosed with and without the patient's consent. The regulations are available at http://www.ecfr.gov/cgi-bin/text-idx?c=ecfr&sid=b7e8d29be4a2b815c404988e29c06a3e&rgn=div5&view=text&node=42:1.0.1.1.2&idno=42

42 C.F.R. 2 applies to all clinicians who use a controlled substance (i.e., methadone and buprenorphine) for detoxification or maintenance treatment of a substance use disorder. Such physicians must register with the federal Drug Enforcement Agency (DEA), and their DEA license, along with representations concerning their status as opioid treatment providers, makes them subject to the regulations.

With limited exceptions, 42 C.F.R. 2 requires patient consent for disclosures of protected health information, even for the purposes of treatment, payment, or health care operations. Consent for disclosure must be in writing.

42 C.F.R. 2 does not apply to information on substance use treatment maintained in connection with the Veterans' Administration or the Armed Forces (42 CFR § 2.12 (c)).

Most substance-abuse treatment programs are also subject to the Health Insurance Portability and Accountability Act of 1996 Privacy Rule. In 2004, SAMHSA issued a guidance document that summarizes the differences between the two rules and implementation solutions, which is available at http://www.samhsa.gov/sites/default/files/part2-hipaa-comparison2004.pdf

Frequently asked questions (FAQs) about substance abuse confidentiality regulations are available on the SAMHSA website. The FAQs include information on exceptions to 42 C.F.R. 2 (e.g. medical emergencies) and guidance on which entities or individuals are subject to the regulations. http://www.samhsa.gov/about-us/who-we-are/laws/confidentiality-regulations-faqs

indications of FASD (CAPTA, 2010). CAPTA requires CPS agencies to develop a plan of safe care for every such infant referred to their agency and address the health and substance use disorder treatment needs of the infant. The 2016 Title V, *Section 503, "Infant Plan of Safe Care"* of S. 524, "Comprehensive Addiction and Recovery Act of 2016" requires the plan of safe care to also address the treatment needs of affected family or caregivers and requires states to develop a monitoring system to determine whether and how the local entities are providing referrals to and delivery of appropriate services for the infant and affected family or caregiver. The Comprehensive Addiction and Recovery Act of 2016 was signed into law on July 22, 2016. CAPTA also requires that all children who are younger than three years who are substantiated victims of child maltreatment are referred to early intervention agencies that provide developmental disabilities services (Office on Child Abuse and Neglect, 2003). However, state, tribal, and local agency policies determine how newborns with prenatal substance exposure are identified, whether notice to CPS constitutes a report alleging child abuse or neglect, and the level and type of proof needed to warrant further investigation (Young et al., 2009 ). For these reasons, CPS agencies handle referrals of infants with prenatal substance exposure in ways that vary greatly by state and community. A February 2015 analysis by the Guttmacher Institute showed that four states require health care professionals to test newborns for prenatal drug exposure when drug use is suspected, while 15 states require providers to report women to CPS for suspected drug use during pregnancy (Guttmacher Institute, 2015). Different CPS agencies also make very different decisions regarding whether an infant remains in the custody of the mother. These decisions determine how infants are evaluated for early intervention service needs and whether they receive these services when needed. These inconsistencies in policy and practice result in differing approaches across communities to identify pregnant women in need of treatment and different responses for the infant's care and safety considerations.

In addition to these practice and policy concerns, there are often knowledge gaps about the risk and safety of a newborn who tests positive for opioids. For example, professionals need to understand distinctions in risk and safety between infants exposed to opioids as a result of the mother's opioid use or misuse versus infants exposed to opioids as a result of the mother's treatment for opioid dependency with medications under a doctor's care. In addition, in the well-meaning effort to maintain child safety, child welfare agencies may establish uninformed requirements on minimal dosing of MAT medications or withdrawal from MAT for women as a condition for keeping custody of their newborns[8] and may use a positive toxicology result for methadone or buprenorphine at birth as a presumptive cause for child removal.

These decisions often have negative and sometimes irrevocable consequences for families, including interference with the critical mother–infant attachment process. In addition, many Family Treatment Drug Courts (FTDCs) around the country treat a woman's use of MAT as a criterion for excluding her from participating in or graduating from the program until she is no longer taking medications. The National Association of Drug Court Professionals (NADCP) resolved that drug courts should not impose blanket prohibitions against the use of MAT for their participants and further suggests that drug courts attain reliable expert consultation on the appropriate use of MAT for their participants, including partnering with substance abuse treatment programs (NADCP, 2013). In addition, recognizing that MAT may be an essential part of a comprehensive treatment plan, SAMHSA Treatment Drug Court grantees were encouraged, beginning in 2015, to use a percentage of the annual grant award to pay for FDA-approved medications.

State laws vary regarding legislation on the use of substances during pregnancy. The variance includes whether there is criminal prosecution or if substance use is considered maltreatment and grounds for termination of parental rights under civil statutes. The 2013 National Drug Control Strategy states that criminal justice professionals should include the use of MAT

[8] Minimal dosing may in fact *increase* the likelihood of relapse as well as *increase* risks to both the mother and infant. Important health issues are associated with proper dosing. (Kaltenbach et al., 1998)

as appropriate treatment for an opioid use disorder for those individuals involved in the judicial system (Office of National Drug Control Policy, 2013). The previously described analysis by the Guttmacher Institute showed that one state allows assault charges to be filed against pregnant women who use certain substances and that 18 states consider evidence of substance use during pregnancy (often only evidence of use and not a diagnosis of dependency or addiction or findings of harm) to indicate child abuse and provide grounds for termination of parental rights (Guttmacher Institute, 2015). On the other hand, some states have begun to implement Safe Harbor legislation to facilitate access to treatment for pregnant women. Safe Harbor laws provide a provision in a law or agreement that protects against liability or penalty as long as set conditions have been met. Two states have implemented or introduced Safe Harbor laws in which pregnant women who seek treatment for opioid and other substance use disorders, in the absence of other risk or safety factors, will not have to fear risking loss of custody of their infant or termination of parental rights.

As amended in 2010, the Child Abuse Prevention and Treatment Act (CAPTA) requires states to include the following in their state plans.

An assurance in the form of a certification by the Governor of the State that the State has in effect and is enforcing a State law, or has in effect and is operating a statewide program relating to child abuse and neglect that includes:

A) policies and procedures (including appropriate referrals to child protection service systems and for other appropriate services) to address the needs of infants born with and identified as being affected by illegal substance abuse or withdrawal symptoms resulting from prenatal drug exposure, or a Fetal Alcohol Spectrum Disorder, including a requirement that health care providers involved in the delivery or care of such infants notify the child protective services system of the occurrence of such condition in such infants, except that such notification shall not be construed to: (I) establish a definition under Federal law of what constitutes child abuse or neglect; or (II) require prosecution for any illegal action;

B) the development of a plan of safe care for the infant born and identified as being affected by illegal substance abuse or withdrawal symptoms, or a Fetal Alcohol Spectrum Disorder.

The CAPTA Reauthorization Act of 2010 is available at: http://www.gpo.gov/fdsys/pkg/BILLS-111s3817enr/pdf/BILLS-111s3817enr.pdf

— Section 106(b)(2)(B)(ii-iii) of the Child Abuse Prevention and Treatment Act [42 U.S.C. 5106a(b)(2)(B)(ii-iii)]

Title V, Section 503, "Infant Plan of Safe Care," of S. 524, "Comprehensive Addiction and Recovery Act of 2016" was signed into law on July 22, 2016. The bill amends CAPTA to address the health and substance use disorder treatment needs of the infant and affected family or caregiver; and to ensure the development and implementation by the State of monitoring systems regarding the implementation of plans to determine whether and in what manner local entities are providing, in accordance with State requirements, referrals to and delivery of appropriate services for the infant and affected family or caregiver.

The 2016 changes also provide monitoring and oversight changes for HHS.

The Comprehensive Addiction and Recovery Act of 2016 is available at: https://www.congress.gov/bill/114th-congress/senate-bill/524

The various configurations and approaches in each discipline can exacerbate the challenges in coordinating services among providers, agencies, and organizations. The many differences that exist need to be reconciled to facilitate a coordinated cross-disciplinary approach. The purpose of this document is to assist communities in assessing their current practice and to develop practice and policy improvements to better meet the needs of these families.

# Comprehensive Framework for Intervention

As discussed in the previous section, many professionals may be involved in decisions related to the treatment, care, and supervision of pregnant women with opioid use disorders. These decision makers might include health care providers, substance abuse treatment providers, child welfare workers, and judicial system representatives (e.g., judges, parents' lawyers, and children's lawyers or advocates). Each of these professionals and the systems they represent are responding to directives that stem from a combination of federal regulations, state legislation, ethics, and system-specific guidelines.

Ideally, these directives are aligned to ensure the best possible outcomes for both mothers and infants. Unfortunately, however, this is not usually the case, particularly when state laws or agency policies are silent on or conflict with best practices, or are driven by misinformation. When directives are unclear, conflicting, or missing, workers must rely on their professional judgment to determine the best approach and course of action.

Without proper training and knowledge about best practices, professionals might not serve the best interests of mothers, children, and families. To surmount this risk, professionals must establish mechanisms for working together across systems, agencies, and providers to develop a coordinated and cohesive approach. Such an approach has the highest likelihood of achieving successful outcomes related to maternal and child health, newborn care, mother–infant attachment, positive parenting practices, child safety, and family well-being.

Strategies to help are typically most effective when designed to address needs beyond substance abuse treatment, such as for co-occurring mental health issues, trauma, housing, child care, employment, parenting, and a range of other personal supports. A family-centered and gender-responsive approach addresses many of these needs in a culturally responsive[9] manner (Werner, Young, Dennis, & Amatetti, 2007; King, Duan, & Amaro, 2014). When states, tribes, and communities recognize the positive and often cost-effective impact of a collaborative approach, public agencies and private providers have a powerful incentive to work together in alternative and innovative ways.

## Overview of Substance-Exposed Infants (SEI) Framework

This guidance leverages and is informed by the five-point intervention framework developed by the NCSACW and funded by SAMHSA and the Administration on Children, Youth, and Families. This framework, which was the organizing foundation for the SAMHSA report *Substance-Exposed Infants: State Responses to the Problem*, serves as a comprehensive model that identifies five major time frames when intervention in the life of an infant can help reduce the potential harm of prenatal substance exposure (Young et al., 2009).

[9] For more information on cultural competence, see SAMHSA's Treatment Improvement Protocol (TIP) 59 – *Improving Cultural Competence* (http://store.samhsa.gov/shin/content//SMA14-4849/SMA14-4849.pdf).

The five points of intervention are:

1. Pre-pregnancy: During this time, interventions can include promoting awareness among women of child-bearing age and their family members of the effects that prenatal substance use can have on infants.
2. Prenatal: During this time, health care providers have the opportunity to screen pregnant women for substance use as part of routine prenatal care and to make referrals that facilitate access to treatment and related services for the women who need these services.
3. Birth: Interventions during this time include health care providers testing newborns for prenatal substance exposure at the time of delivery.
4. Neonatal: During this time, health care providers can conduct a developmental assessment of the newborn and ensure access to services for the newborn as well as the family.
5. Throughout childhood and adolescence: During this time, interventions include the ongoing provision of coordinated services for both child and family.

The framework also illustrates the following key issues:

- The birth event is only one of several opportunities to affect outcomes. Therefore, it is important to understand the extent of those opportunities and which interventions are most needed and most likely to be effective at each point in time.
- Cross-system linkages are necessary to ensure services are coordinated across the spectrum of prevention, intervention, and treatment.

The NCSACW's five-point framework emerged from a multi-year review and analysis of existing policies and practices in 10 states regarding prenatal exposure to alcohol and other drugs. This effort was designed to help state, tribal, and local governments to identify opportunities for strengthening interagency efforts that address prevention, intervention, identification, and treatment of complications related to prenatal substance exposure. The framework focuses on immediate and ongoing services for infants, mothers, and families. The NCSACW reviewed states' policies regarding:

> ACOG's 2015 legislative priorities include promoting public health efforts to reduce maternal opioid dependence and NAS as well as opposing punitive legislation against women with opioid dependence whose babies are born with NAS (ACOG, 2015).

- Pre-pregnancy efforts to engage women with substance use disorders in treatment to prevent prenatal substance exposure in the women's future infants.
- Screening and assessment during pregnancy to ensure that women have access to treatment and needed supports.
- Health care, supportive services at birth, and notification of CPS when infants are identified as having been prenatally affected by illegal substances, as consistent with CAPTA.
- Services to infants with prenatal substance exposure or infants who require care (along with their parents and siblings) during the neonatal period.
- Ongoing coordinated services for this population of children and their families throughout childhood and adolescence (Young et al., 2009).

This review showed a wide variation in state policies and practices related to meeting the needs of infants with prenatal substance exposure, thus highlighting the need for guidance based on best practices and current literature in the field. This guidance also needs to provide recommendations that can be adapted and customized to benefit women and children within the context of each community's unique mix of resources, challenges, and perspectives.

Compared to efforts by individual agencies and systems, collaboration across multiple agencies and systems, coupled with strong leadership and consistent communication, offers a more effective approach, a more efficient way of doing business, and ultimately leads to better outcomes.

This five-point intervention framework highlights opportunities for cross-system collaboration and policy development at each critical point in time, from pre-pregnancy throughout an infant's early years. The framework also integrates recommendations for best practices related to outreach, engagement, treatment, and support for mothers and their infants along the five-point continuum. The framework shows that no single system has the necessary resources, information, or influence needed to adequately serve this vulnerable mother–infant dyad and other involved family members who are likely to need services. All those who have a role in improving outcomes for such families need to collaborate in order to put the necessary policies and practices in place. These collaborations can set the stage for maternal recovery from substance use disorders, child safety, and the well-being of all those involved.

## A Guide for Collaborative Planning

The opportunity for practice and policy improvement exists largely because so many different agencies, organizations, and providers have a legal or professional responsibility to act or address the needs of pregnant women with opioid use disorders and their infants. Without a comprehensive coordinated response that includes child welfare and healthcare, including obstetrics, pediatrics, substance abuse treatment, and mental health professionals, families are not well served. Cross-system initiatives lead to better results by facilitating better communication, clearly defining the roles of the various professionals who serve these families, and maximizing the resources of multiple stakeholders who have a vested interest in accomplishing shared goals.

Efforts that specify the roles and responsibilities of each partner help ensure that efforts from multiple systems to support individuals, families, and communities have a stronger cumulative impact and are sustained over time to address the full range of practice and policy considerations (Young, Nakashian, Yeh, & Amatetti, 2006). However, collaborative practice can be difficult to establish and implement for a number of reasons, including competing priorities, rules in agencies or organizations that conflict with the approaches of others, lack of leadership, confusion about roles, unmet training needs, use of different terminologies, limits on time and resources, information gaps, and mistrust. Communities are often unprepared to provide services to the large number of pregnant women who misuse prescription medications and heroin, and these agencies have not yet organized a coordinated response. In other communities, all of the involved parties might not know the rules, regulations, and practice standards that operate in the various systems. In fact, partner agencies often need to understand what services are available and who the providers are in each system.

To understand the array of local services and overcome the barriers to coordinating services to meet the needs of this population of pregnant woman and their infants, prospective collaborative partners from each of the primary systems of health care, substance abuse treatment, mental health, child welfare, and dependency and Family Drug Courts need to know what questions to ask when they begin their joint planning. These questions must be identified regardless of whether the potential partners' intent is to initiate, expand, or truly integrate their services and systems.

# Building the Collaborative Team[10]

To build and foster cross-system collaboration, building an effective coordinating team is of paramount importance. This section presents a description of a collaborative team. Ideally, collaborative teams include a steering committee, a core team, and work groups.

## The Collaborative Team

Preferably, the state, tribe, or local government creates the collaborative team and endows it with the capacity and resources needed to support and sustain its major initiatives. A well-designed collaborative team can support the plans set in motion and ensure goals are met, especially if the team convenes on a regular and predictable basis and keeps its focus on systems change, improved outcomes, and sustainability.

One way to organize the team is as follows:

- **Steering Committee**—This committee oversees and designates the members of the core team (defined below); facilitates necessary cabinet, council, commission, and legislative policy changes;[11] and works to remove system barriers. The committee consists of multidisciplinary top executives, directors, and leaders across each of the collaborating entities. Participation and presence of key decision makers will increase the efficiency and effectiveness of the meetings.

  **TIP:** *Keep steering committee leaders engaged by informing members of the collaborative team's progress so that they are prepared to pave the way for necessary change.*

- **Facilitator**—Guides the team in decision making. The facilitator role can be fulfilled by bringing in an outside facilitator, appointing representatives from the different systems to conjointly fulfill the role, or appointing representatives from the different systems to rotate in the facilitator role. These strategies can help the systems share responsibility, while also avoiding the perception that the initiative is being "run" by one agency. Having system representatives fulfill the facilitator role requires the representative to be aware and understand his or her multiple and potentially conflicting roles. In the facilitator role, system representatives must diligently maintain the distinction between their role as the facilitator and as the system representative. When the boundaries of these roles are delineated and respected, others will be more inclined to trust and respect the boundaries as well. Ideally, the facilitator role, or the various configurations that can fulfill the facilitator role, requires familiarity with the subject matter and how the systems operate (Pennsylvania State University, 2015).

  **TIP:** *Facilitate decision making among multiple systems by appointing a formal facilitator. Facilitating a multidisciplinary team requires skills that differ from those required to direct single-agency work groups; stakeholders from different disciplines do not have jurisdiction over each other, and decision making by decree or majority rule will not work in these situations.*

- **Core Team**—Responsible for implementing policy changes at each organization. The core team is multidisciplinary and consists of mid-management representatives from each

---

[10] For more information on developing a collaborative team and structure, see Screening and Assessment for Family Engagement, Retention, and Recovery (SAFERR) https://www.ncsacw.samhsa.gov/resources/SAFERR.aspx

[11] If using federal funding, these actions must be taken in compliance with Section 503(b) of the Departments of Labor, Health and Human Services, and Education, and Related Agencies Appropriations Act, 2016 (S. 1695). Section 503(b) provides that no federal funds from the HHS annual appropriations act may be used to pay the "salary or expenses of any grant or contract recipient, related to any activity designed to influence legislation or appropriations pending before the Congress or any State legislature." https://www.congress.gov/bill/114th-congress/senate-bill/1695

collaborating entity in addition to consumers, advocates, and representatives of other organizations, as appropriate.

**TIP:** *Include no more than six to eight individuals in the core team. Core Team members should have sufficient authority and flexibility to approve agency-level practice and policy changes to sustain the collaborative team's momentum by achieving "quick wins."*

- **Work Groups**—Created by the steering committee to address priorities of the collaborative initiative. Work groups include members of the core team and additional key stakeholders, such as providers and practitioners, consumers and advocates.

**TIP:** *Give your work groups specific challenges they can address by using first-hand knowledge from key stakeholders regarding effective tools and strategies, such as devising a communication protocol.*

This type of structure can be used at the state, tribal, and local levels. At the local level, for example, the health department might convene the collaborative team. Ideally, all of these entities work closely together to accomplish jointly identified goals and shared priorities for improving practice and policy.

This structure helps ensure:

- Sustainability of the initiative through the authority and endorsement of the steering committee;
- Communication through accountability in the hierarchical and peer-to-peer relationships of the core team;
- Regional broad-level buy-in through the participation and investment of the diverse stakeholders who make up the work groups; and
- Internally supported change through the investment and commitment of multiple systems to achieve collaboratively defined outcomes.

Cross-system teams must consider several steps as they prepare to engage in collaborative planning. These steps, (1) setting the stage for collaboration, (2) engage key stakeholders and establish work groups, (3) define shared goals, and (4) identify strategies and jointly monitor outcomes, are discussed below. Questions are posed to guide the purpose and outcome of each step. *Appendix 1: Facilitators Guide* includes a facilitator's guide and a set of tools to help the development of a work plan, based on prioritization of identified goals. The tools include a Cross-System Guide, to develop a baseline understanding of areas of strength and opportunities for improvement, and five System-Specific Guides, to understand the context of the initiative from multiple points of view. For instance, each system's perspective of the "primary" client (e.g., mother, infant, or family) differs. The identified "primary" client often drives the system's response and goal. For example, the MAT provider may consider the mother as the primary client, with interventions targeted solely at her. In comparison, the infant's neonatologist or pediatrician may identify the infant as the primary client. Although each service provider must provide services within their scope of practice, understanding the impact of opioid use disorders on the mother and infant as well as what services and supports are needed for optimal outcomes requires a mutual understanding of the involved systems. The guides can provide the necessary background for teams before making decisions about—and committing valuable resources to—statewide practice and policy changes.

## STEP 1: Setting the Stage for Collaboration

Once the core team has been formed, some general fact gathering and sharing by all team members is necessary so that each member understands:

- What practices and policies are in place in each team member's service system and in the other service systems;
- Partner mandates and priorities that are likely to affect, and possibly limit, their level of involvement;

- The terminology that each team member's organization uses most frequently and how the organizations define these terms (e.g., "treatment");
- The baseline resources, resource gaps, and barriers in each system; and
- What needs to be addressed and improved, particularly from the perspective of mothers, children, and family members, to provide the necessary care.

## STEP 2: Engage Key Stakeholders and Establish Work Groups

To determine which partners should be involved in the initiative, an assessment of the current level of collaboration is helpful. Questions to answer include: Who is currently working on the issue being tackled? What does each of these individuals or organizations contribute? And, significantly, which key stakeholders are missing from the conversation?

Core team members on the collaborative team should, at a minimum, include child welfare professionals, key dependency court and family drug court professionals, mental health providers, Medicaid officials, and healthcare providers. Healthcare providers include office- and hospital-based obstetricians, pediatricians, neonatologists, primary care providers, hospitalists, medical social workers, and opioid treatment and other substance abuse treatment providers (including residential, intensive outpatient, and outpatient treatment providers).[12, 13] Other stakeholders, including lead staff from agencies such as Temporary Assistance for Needy Families, maternal and child health agencies, and housing authorities, may also play key roles in the collaborative team.

Other potential participants include organizations that are unique to the community and provide services for this population of families, such as women's or children's health resource centers; early child intervention organizations; and clinical, financial, or legal resource centers as well as representation from tribes in communities with American Indian populations and/or tribal leadership. Finally, it is critical to ensure that pregnant women or mothers representing the target population have a voice in the process and are active participants in planning, informing, communicating, and collaborating.

Key stakeholder participation in the collaborative team is likely to be determined by existing partnerships and whether the overall effort is intended to provide new services, expand existing services, or increase levels of service integration across systems.

## STEP 3: Define Shared Goals

Every state, tribe, and community is supported and challenged by its own systems, issues, beliefs, and ideals. On occasion, the existing protocols, culture, and financial constraints may affect the collaborative team's ability to be successful in coordinating their approach and share accountability for the outcomes. Therefore, each team member needs to evaluate how their system-specific and individual principles and values will lead practice and policy change and understand the perspectives that are influencing the positions and decisions of the other partners.

To create principles for their work together, the team should collectively examine and discuss fundamental questions, such as:

- What is each represented agency's role in achieving shared priorities and outcomes (e.g., How does child welfare services support parent recovery? How do treatment providers for parents support child safety and permanency and family well-being?)

---

[12] Dependency courts refer to courts that handle dependency cases involving children and youth under 18, including child maltreatment (see https://www.childwelfare.gov/pubPDFs/cwandcourts.pdf).

[13] Family Drug Courts (also referred to as Family Dependency Treatment Courts, Family Treatment Courts, Dependency Drug Courts, and Family Treatment Drug Courts) use a multidisciplinary approach, recognizing that their clients (i.e., parents, children, and families who enter the Family Drug Court) often face a range of challenges in addition to a substance use disorder (see http://www.cffutures.org/files/publications/FDC-Guidelines.pdf).

- What does each team member believe about the nature of substance use and substance use disorders?
- Do team members agree on the markers of effective practice and service delivery? What are those markers?
- How is "best interest" defined for infants? For mothers? For families? Do mothers have sufficient input in determining this?
- What do team members or policy leaders believe about the use of MAT for women who are pregnant or breastfeeding?
- What do team members believe constitutes recovery?

### STEP 4: Identify Strategies and Jointly Monitor Outcomes

A crucial component of developing a coordinated response is the ongoing transfer of knowledge across professionals, agencies, and organizations. This knowledge transfer enables the team to establish and maintain a shared understanding of evidence-based practices for pregnant women with opioid use disorders and their infants from a multi-system perspective. To facilitate this knowledge transfer, the team needs to:

- Review the desired outcomes for each system by, for example, determining how success is defined and measured, identifying baseline levels for clients, and finding out whether better (or additional) indicators are available to demonstrate progress. For example, hospitals may be focused on positive birth outcomes, child welfare focused on child safety, and substance use disorder treatment agencies may be focused on measures of recovery.
- Determine the metrics (e.g., number of pregnant women treated with MAT) that need to be developed and tracked to effectively measure success over time. This can include assessing what technology is available to track outcomes. Recent developments, such as electronic health records and Health Information Exchanges, can help facilitate communication across systems and, ultimately, be an avenue to measure outcomes.
- Create a method for communicating progress related to key indicators (e.g., a report card or dashboard) to ensure transparency and promote accountability for results.
- Review the plan for sustaining change and determine, for example, how the team will document, maintain, and build on the collaboration's institutional knowledge.

To facilitate the development of a work plan that addresses the needs of pregnant women with opioid use disorders and their infants, see *Appendix 1: Facilitator's Guide* for the tools.

## Concluding Thoughts

This report provides practical, evidence-informed guidance to help collaborative, cross-disciplinary teams support effective, healthy outcomes for pregnant women with opioid use disorders and their infants. This guide underscores the potential impact of opioid use during pregnancy and the importance of a systems-level approach that is driven and endorsed by state and tribe leadership to mobilize resources and facilitate cross-system practice and policy changes. It also provides a framework for communities to take stock of their current policies and identify areas for improvement. It is the view of the national panel of experts that informed this guide that top-down approaches that do not include the views of local practitioners, other professionals, and families will likely lead to resistance and uneven implementation. For collaborative practices to be successful, all parties involved must witness and experience the benefits.

It is beyond the scope of this guidance to adequately address the entire range of topics related to pregnant women with opioid use disorders and their families; however, it is important to highlight some additional focus areas that states, tribes, and communities might want to factor into their planning and policy development.

**Value of Prevention.** For the vast majority of women, drug use or misuse begins long before they become pregnant. Therefore, key drivers for achieving healthier pregnancies and births and better child safety outcomes is ensuring women of childbearing age have better access to effective birth control methods[14] and engaging women of childbearing age who have substance use disorders to seek treatment before they become pregnant. Broad community approaches to preventing opioid use disorders are underway in many states and should be expanded to target opioid use during pregnancy. Current community approaches include SAMHSA's Strategic Prevention Framework Partnerships for Success, which seeks to target the use and misuse of prescription medications and heroin among persons ages 12–25 (SAMHSA, 2014b).

**Improved Data Collection, Management, and Reporting.** Improved data collection is urgently needed to better illuminate the challenges these families face and to be able to measure the success and effectiveness of different interventions and approaches. The prevalence of substance use during pregnancy is often underreported, mostly because pregnant women feel shame and guilt, aggravated by the societal stigma which is so pervasive in most communities. Most health care systems do not use universal screening for substance use during pregnancy or delivery, contributing to the lack of data. Community responses to infant prenatal exposure, child welfare referrals, and case dispositions are also unevenly tracked. Identifying crucial indicators, such as referrals to child welfare agencies, as part of the CAPTA requirements and developing ways to collect information would strengthen responses to families and the use of community resources.

As we seek to learn more about how to respond successfully to the unique needs of pregnant women with opioid use disorders, we can draw from and build on lessons from the past. In this guidance document, we have focused on the unique needs of pregnant women with opioid use disorders. However, much of the guidance and principles provided are applicable to all women with substance use disorders and their infants. We hope that strengthening collaborative relationships to respond to this need will ensure that those relationships endure and offer a ready resource for addressing other challenges in the future.

[14] Visit the ACOG website for information on contraception, including guidance on which forms of birth control are most appropriate, based on each woman's needs: http://www.acog.org/Womens-Health/Birth-Control-Contraception.

# Chronic Kidney Disease in the United States, 2021

Accessible Version: https://www.cdc.gov/kidneydisease/publications-resources/CKD-national-facts.html

When people develop **chronic kidney disease (CKD)**, their kidneys become damaged and over time may not clean the blood as well as healthy kidneys. If kidneys do not work well, toxic waste and extra fluid accumulate in the body and may lead to high blood pressure, heart disease, stroke, and early death. However, people with CKD and people at risk for CKD can take steps to protect their kidneys with the help of their health care providers.

## CKD Is Common Among US Adults

### Fast Stats

- More than 1 in 7, that is 15% of US adults or 37 million people, are estimated to have CKD.†
- As many as 9 in 10 adults with CKD **do not know** they have CKD.
- About 2 in 5 adults with severe CKD **do not know** they have CKD.

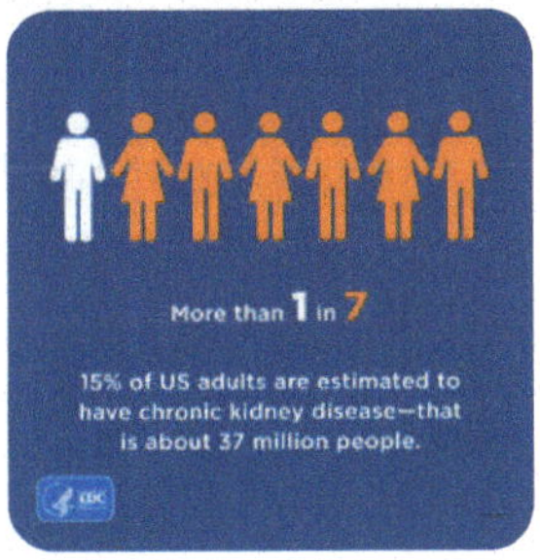


## CKD Risk Factors

Diabetes and high blood pressure are the more common causes of CKD in adults. Other risk factors include heart disease, obesity, a family history of CKD, inherited kidney disorders, past damage to the kidneys, and older age.

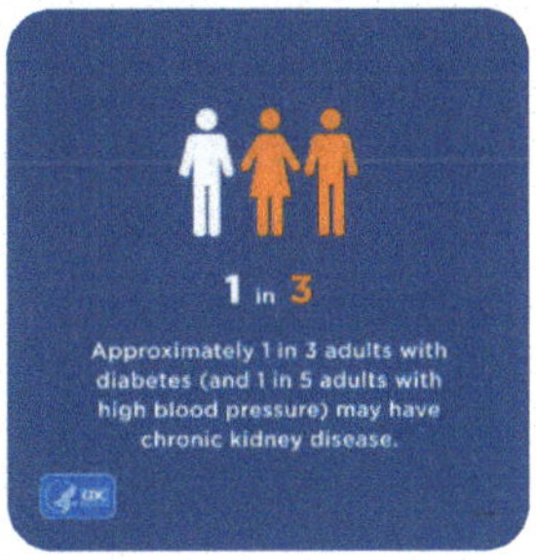


**Managing blood sugar and blood pressure can help keep kidneys healthy.**

## CKD by Age, Sex, and Race/Ethnicity

### According to current estimates:†

- CKD is more common in people aged 65 years or older (38%) than in people aged 45–64 years (12%) or 18–44 years (6%).
- CKD is slightly more common in women (14%) than men (12%).
- CKD is more common in non-Hispanic Black adults (16%) than in non-Hispanic White adults (13%) or non-Hispanic Asian adults (13%).
- About 14% of Hispanic adults have CKD.

**Percentage of US Adults Aged 18 Years or Older With CKD,† By Age, Sex, and Race/Ethnicity**

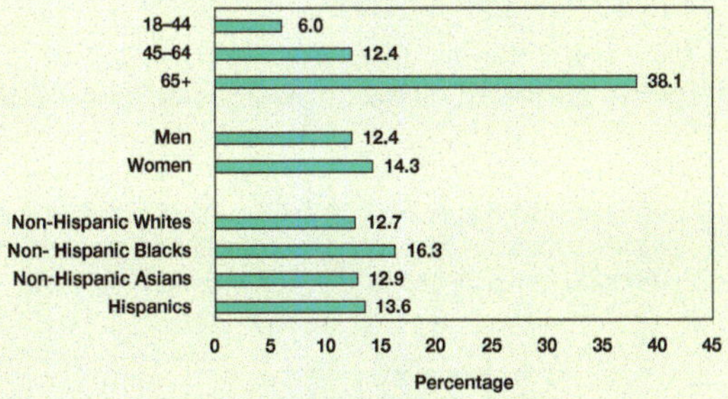


†CKD stages 1–4 using data from the 2015–2018 National Health and Nutrition Examination Survey and the CKD Epidemiology Collaboration (CKD-EPI) equation. For more details on the methods, see 'How the Estimates Were Calculated.'

†**How the estimates were calculated:** Percentage of CKD stages 1–4 among US adults aged 18 years or older using data from the 2015–2018 National Health and Nutrition Examination Survey and the CKD Epidemiology Collaboration (CKD-EPI) equation. CKD stage 5 (that is, kidney failure) was not included. These estimates were based on a single measure of albuminuria or serum creatinine; they do not account for persistence of albuminuria or levels of creatinine that are higher than normal as indicated by the Kidney Disease Improving Global Outcomes recommendations. Thus, CKD in this report might be overestimated. Estimates by sex and race/ethnicity were age-standardized using the 2000 US census population; the overall percentage is unadjusted. The number of adults with CKD stages 1–4 was estimated by applying the overall percentage to the 2019 US Census population aged 18 years or older. Blood pressure-lowering medications included angiotensin-converting enzyme inhibitors or angiotensin II receptor blockers; diagnosed diabetes was self-reported.

U.S. Department of Health and Human Services
Centers for Disease Control and Prevention

322964-A March 04, 2021

## Ways to Prevent CKD

- *Manage* risk factors for CKD:
  - High blood pressure.
  - High blood sugar levels.

Keeping a healthy body weight through a balanced diet and physical activity may help manage blood pressure and blood sugar levels in people with diabetes or in people at risk of developing type 2 diabetes.

**Preventing type 2 diabetes can help prevent CKD and kidney failure.**

## Treatment to Lower Blood Pressure

- Blood pressure–lowering medications are recommended for people with diabetes and CKD. However, the percentage of adults with CKD and diagnosed diabetes who are prescribed blood pressure–lowering medications is less than ideal.
  - Prescription of blood pressure–lowering medications is higher in people with CKD and diagnosed diabetes aged 45 years or older (about 70%) than in those aged 18–44 years (30%).
  - Prescription of blood pressure–lowering medications is similar in adult women and men with CKD and diagnosed diabetes (about 50%).
  - Prescription of blood pressure–lowering medications is higher in non-Hispanic Black adults with CKD and diagnosed diabetes (63%) than in non-Hispanic White adults (37%) or non-Hispanic Asian adults (32%).
  - About 47% of Hispanic adults with CKD and diagnosed diabetes are prescribed blood pressure–lowering medications.

**Percentage of US Adults Aged 18 Years or Older With CKD and Diagnosed Diabetes Who Were Prescribed Blood Pressure–Lowering Medications,† by Age, Sex, and Race/Ethnicity**

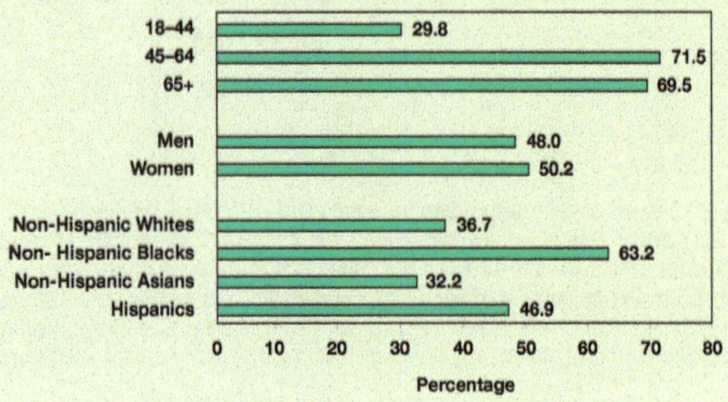


†Angiotensin-converting enzyme inhibitors or angiotensin II receptor blockers using data from the 2015–2018 National Health and Nutrition Examination Survey. For more details on the methods, see 'How the Estimates Were Calculated.'

## Testing and Treatment: Find it Early, Treat it Early

- *Test* for CKD regularly in people who have diabetes, high blood pressure, or other risk factors for CKD. People with CKD may not feel ill or notice any symptoms until CKD is advanced.
- The only way to find out if people have CKD is through simple blood and urine tests. The blood test checks for the level of creatinine, a waste product produced by muscles, to see how well the kidneys work. The urine test checks for protein, which may indicate kidney damage.
- Following a healthy diet and taking medicine for diabetes, medicine for high blood pressure, and other medications to protect the kidneys may keep CKD from getting worse and may prevent other health problems such as heart disease.

## CKD-Related Health Problems

As CKD worsens over time, related health problems become more likely. However, CKD-related health problems can improve with treatment.

### Heart Disease and Stroke

- Having CKD increases the chances of having heart disease and stroke.
- Managing high blood pressure, blood sugar, and cholesterol levels—all factors that increase the risk for heart disease and stroke—is very important for people with CKD.

### Early Death

Adults with CKD are at a higher risk of dying earlier than adults of similar age without CKD.

### Health Problems Due to Low Kidney Function

- Anemia or low red blood cell count, which can cause fatigue and weakness.
- Extra fluid in the body, which can cause high blood pressure, swelling in the legs, or shortness of breath.
- A weakened immune system, which make it easier to develop infections.
- Loss of appetite or nausea.
- Decreased sexual response.
- Confusion, problems with memory and thinking, or depression.
- Low calcium levels and high phosphorus levels in the blood, which can cause bone disease and heart disease.
- High potassium levels in the blood, which can cause an irregular or abnormal heartbeat and lead to death.

## Kidney Failure

Kidney failure happens when kidney damage is severe and kidney function is very low. Dialysis or a kidney transplant is then needed for survival. Kidney failure treated with dialysis or a kidney transplant is called **end-stage renal disease (ESRD)**. CKD is more likely to lead to kidney failure, especially in older adults, if the kidneys are damaged by the inability to manage risk factors, repeated kidney infections, or drugs or toxins that are harmful to the kidneys. Social factors such as lower income and related factors of food insecurity and poorer access to quality health care are also associated with worsening CKD. However, not everyone with CKD develops kidney failure. If CKD is detected early, treatment may slow the decline in kidney function and delay kidney failure. In some cases, kidney failure develops even with treatment.

**Renal is a medical term meaning "having to do with the kidneys."**

**Talk to a kidney doctor about treatment options if CKD is severe and kidney function is very low.**

## Facts About ESRD

- In 2018, about 131,600 people in the United States started treatment for ESRD.
- Nearly 786,000 people in the United States, or 2 in every 1,000 people, are currently living with ESRD: 71% are on dialysis and 29% are living with a kidney transplant.
- For every 2 women who develop ESRD, 3 men develop ESRD.
- For every non-Hispanic White person who develops ESRD, 3 non-Hispanic Black people develop ESRD.
- For every 3 non-Hispanic people who develop ESRD, 4 Hispanic people develop ESRD.
- Among adults aged 18 years or older in the United States, diabetes and high blood pressure are the main causes of ESRD.
- Among children and adolescents younger than 18 years in the United States, polycystic kidney disease and glomerulonephritis (inflammation of the kidneys) are the main causes of ESRD.

**Reported Causes of End-Stage Renal Disease in the United States**

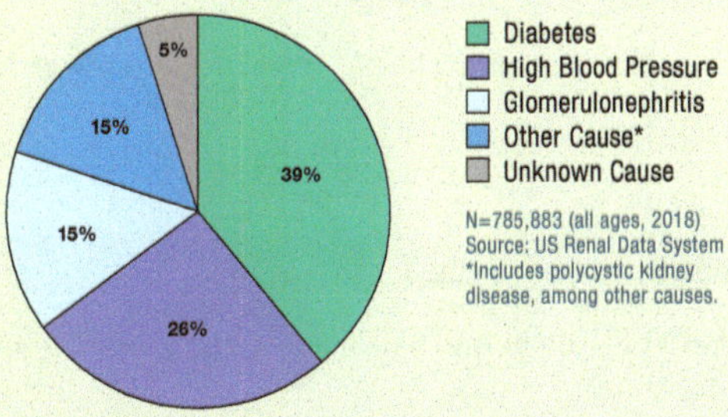


N=785,883 (all ages, 2018)
Source: US Renal Data System
*Includes polycystic kidney disease, among other causes.

## People with CKD Can Lower Their Risk for Kidney Failure

- *Learn* about CKD from a primary care doctor or a kidney doctor (nephrologist) to better understand treatment options and protect the kidneys. People with glomerulonephritis, polycystic kidney disease, or other kidney disease should talk about specific treatment options with a kidney doctor.
- *Monitor and manage* blood sugar and blood pressure.
  - Have blood sugar and blood pressure checked regularly.
  - Use medicines if prescribed to lower blood sugar and blood pressure.
- *Manage* CKD:
  - Make lifestyle changes (e.g., healthy eating, physical activity) to prevent more kidney damage. Meet with a dietitian to create a kidney-healthy eating plan that is low in salt and fat and has the right amount and source of protein. As CKD gets worse, the plan may also include limiting phosphorus and potassium.
  - Use medicines as directed to slow the decline in kidney function.
  - Stop smoking or do not start smoking.
  - Avoid exposures that can harm the kidneys or cause kidney function to suddenly get worse:
    - Certain medicines:
      - Over-the-counter pain medicines like ibuprofen and naproxen, which are also called non-steroidal anti-inflammatory drugs.
      - Some antibiotics.
    - Certain herbal supplements.
    - Excessive alcohol intake.
  - Review with health care providers all prescription and over-the-counter medications to make sure they are safe for the kidneys. Always talk to a doctor before taking any supplements.
  - Check with a doctor about other behaviors or substances that can harm the kidneys or about special precautions to take when doing medical tests or procedures, such as imaging studies or colonoscopies.

**People with diabetes, high blood pressure, or CKD need to talk to their doctor about how to protect their kidneys.**

## What Happens If You Have Kidney Damage?

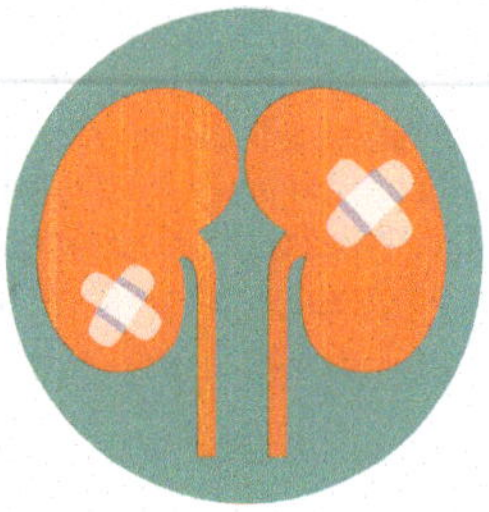

Changes or damage to your kidneys may cause your kidneys to fail. If your kidneys fail, your blood must be filtered (dialysis treatments) several times a week.

You may also need to have a kidney transplant.

## How Will You Know If You Have Kidney Problems?

- Ask your doctor to test your blood and your pee.
- If the doctor finds protein (albumin) in your pee, it is a sign of the start of kidney disease caused by diabetes.
- Get tested yearly.
- Get tested more often if:
  - » Your test shows protein in your pee or;
  - » Your kidneys are not working as they usually do.

## If You Have Diabetes, Take These Steps:

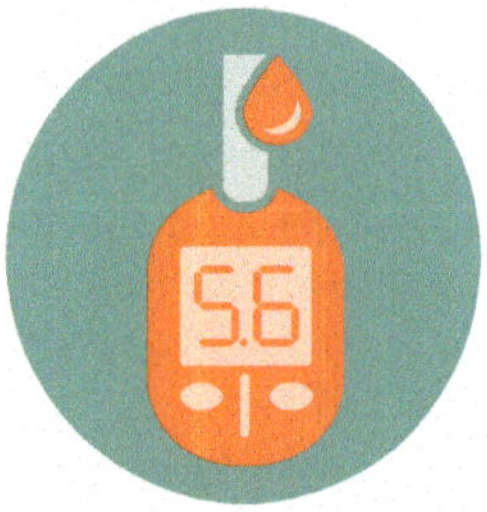


- Meet blood sugar targets as often as you can.
- Get tested for your average level of blood sugar over the past three months (A1C test).
- Get your A1C test at least twice a year, but ideally up to four times a year.
- If your blood pressure is high, check it regularly and get it under control to make sure your kidneys stay healthy.
- Talk to your doctor about medicines that harm your kidneys and other ways to lower your blood pressure.

## What is the Best Way to Keep Your Kidneys Healthy?

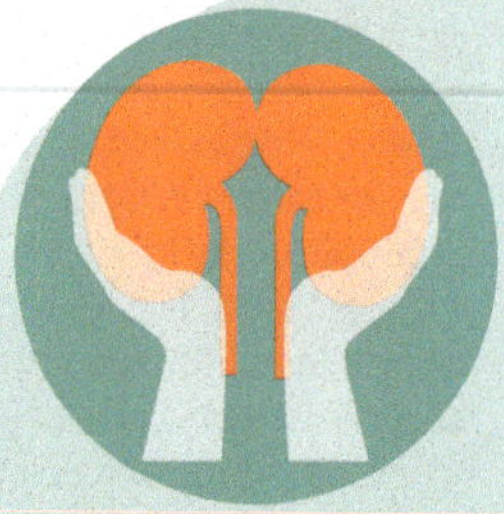

- Keep your blood pressure below 140/90, or ask your doctor what the best blood pressure target is for you.
- Stay in your target cholesterol range.
- Eat foods lower in salt.
- Eat more fruits and vegetables.
- Stay active.
- Take your medications as directed.

## Who is More Likely to Develop Kidney Disease?

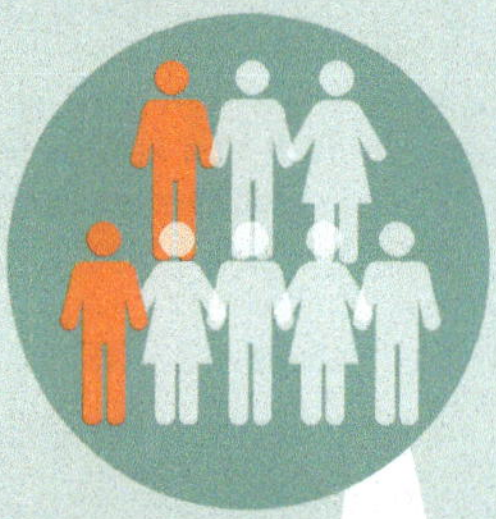

- Approximately 1 of 3 adults with diabetes and 1 of 5 adults with high blood pressure may have CKD.
- In addition to diabetes and high blood pressure, other problems that put you at greater chance of kidney disease include: heart disease, obesity (being overweight), and a family history of CKD. Kidney infections and a physical injury can also cause kidney disease.

## What Can You Do to Prevent Kidney Failure?

- Get tested for CKD regularly if you are at risk.
- Find it early. Treat it early.
- Ask your doctor to test your blood or pee. If you have diabetes, get tested yearly.
- If you have diabetes, stay in your target blood sugar range as much as possible.
- Lose weight if you are overweight.
- Get active. Physical activity helps control blood sugar levels.
- Quit smoking.
- Getting a checkup? Make sure to get your kidneys checked too.
- Take medications as directed.
- If you have CKD, meet with a dietitian to make a kidney-healthy eating plan.

Learn more: www.cdc.gov/ckd

October 2021

# NIH News in Health

National Institutes of Health · Department of Health and Human Services · **newsinhealth.nih.gov**



## Fighting Fatty Liver

### Steps Against a Silent Disease

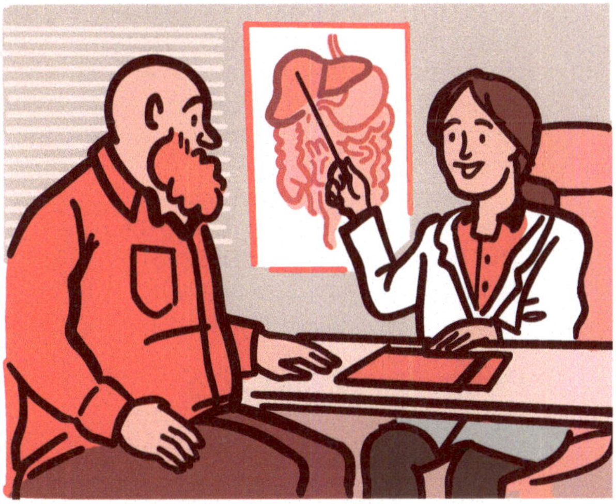

You may not give your liver much thought. But it performs essential functions every day. Like other parts of the body, fat can build up in your liver. That may damage the liver and lead to serious health problems.

It's normal to have some fat in your liver cells. But too much can interfere with your liver's normal functioning. The liver acts as a filter to remove toxins from your blood. It helps digest your food. And it also helps keep your blood sugar constant, among other activities.

Fatty liver disease has become increasingly common. But it often has no symptoms. If you have symptoms, they may include fatigue and discomfort in the upper right side of your abdomen.

"There are an awful lot of people walking around with liver disease, and most of them don't know it," says Dr. Matt Cave, a liver specialist at the University of Louisville. "It's important to be aware of the disease so people can get screened by their doctors."

**Fat Build Up** • Certain health conditions, your genes, your diet, and your digestive system can make you more likely to develop fatty liver disease. When this happens, it is called nonalcoholic fatty liver disease.

"About one-third of U.S. adults have nonalcoholic fatty liver disease," says Dr. Rohit Loomba, a liver disease expert at UC San Diego Health.

People with obesity or type 2 diabetes are at greater risk of nonalcoholic fatty liver disease. It affects about 75% of people who carry excess weight and 90% of people with severe obesity.

Heavy alcohol consumption can also cause fatty liver disease. This is called alcohol-associated fatty liver disease.

"Alcohol is **metabolized** in the liver. And if you drink high amounts, it basically acts as a toxin," explains Dr. Laura Nagy, who studies alcohol's effects on the liver at the Cleveland Clinic.

It's long been known that obesity and alcohol contribute to fatty liver disease. But more recently, scientists have learned that some toxins around us may also play a role.

"The new kid on the block, so to speak, is the role of chemical pollution in fatty liver disease," Cave says. His research was among the first to link chemicals to the disease.

His team discovered a high rate of the disease among workers at a chemical manufacturing plant. All worked heavily with a chemical called vinyl chloride. This chemical is mainly used for making the PVC in plastic products.

Since then, many more chemicals have been linked to fatty liver disease. Some are found in common household products and stick around in the environment. Chemical exposures may work together with other risk factors to worsen the disease.

"We're finding that these things probably serve as double whammies," Cave explains. "Say you eat a bad diet and have a chemical exposure. The chemical may make the effects of the diet worse."

**Finding Fatty Liver** • Most people who have fatty liver disease don't

*continued on page 2*

### Definitions

**Metabolize**
To change a food or drug in the body into another form through chemical reactions.

*continued from page 1*

end up with liver damage. But some develop **inflammation** and damage in their liver cells. This stage of fatty liver disease is known as nonalcoholic steatohepatitis, or NASH.

If NASH gets worse, it can cause permanent scarring and liver hardening. Liver disease at this stage is called cirrhosis. It can lead to liver failure or liver cancer.

Researchers are still trying to understand why liver disease worsens in some people but not others. But you can take steps to reverse this damage. The liver has the ability to repair itself. That's why it's important to find fatty liver disease in an early stage.

Often, a doctor will discover fatty liver disease when running blood tests for other reasons. If you have symptoms or are at higher risk, your health care provider may want to run blood or imaging tests. These tests can help look for a fatty liver and determine how severe it is.

The only test to determine whether the disease has progressed to NASH is a liver biopsy. During a biopsy, your doctor will take a small piece of tissue from your liver. The sample is then examined for signs of inflammation or scarring.

"A biopsy can be painful, and it can lead to bleeding, perforation, or infection," Loomba says. And many of the people who undergo biopsy don't end up having NASH. So Loomba's research team is focused on noninvasive tests for fatty liver disease. They're also looking at new ways to test for advanced liver disease.

His team has developed advanced imaging techniques that reduce the need for biopsies. They're able to painlessly measure how much fat and scarring is present in the liver.

**Undoing Early Damage** • The most effective fatty liver treatment involves a change in lifestyle. Weight loss is helpful.

"But the weight loss has to be pretty significant," says Loomba. You have to lose about 7% of your body weight to resolve NASH. You'll need to lose at least 10% to reduce fibrosis, or scarring.

Losing weight can also help reduce your risk of heart attack and stroke. Heart disease is the leading cause of death in people with nonalcoholic fatty liver disease.

Better nutrition can help, too. Try to avoid weight gain and increase your exercise. And limit your alcohol use. Alcohol can have harmful effects on liver disease.

You might also consider washing your fruits and vegetables before eating. This can lower your exposure to pesticides.

Right now, there are no FDA-approved treatments for fatty liver disease. Studies have shown that vitamin E and diabetes medications that also cause weight loss may help patients with NASH. Several promising drugs are being tested in clinical trials.

To prevent fatty liver disease, aim for a healthy weight and drink alcohol in moderation. Understanding what counts as one drink can help you keep track, says Nagy. To learn about the different sizes of drinks, visit www.rethinkingdrinking.niaaa.nih.gov. For more tips to protect your liver, see the Wise Choices box. ■

## Definitions

**Inflammation**
Heat, swelling, and redness caused by the body's protective response to injury or infection.

## Wise Choices
### Protect Against Fatty Liver Disease

- **Try to maintain a healthy weight and eat sensible portions.**
- **Try to lose weight gradually if you're overweight.**
- **Limit how much fat you eat.** Replace saturated fats with healthier unsaturated fats, like those in fish, flaxseeds, and walnuts.
- **Eat more fruits, vegetables, and whole grains.**
- **Avoid foods and drinks with large amounts of sugars, especially fructose.** These include sweetened soft drinks, sports drinks, sweetened tea, and juices.
- **Avoid heavy alcohol use.** Drinking too much alcohol can have harmful effects on the liver.
- **Quit smoking.** Smoking may increase the chances of developing nonalcohol fatty liver disease. Get free help to quit smoking at smokefree.gov, 1-800-QUIT-NOW (1-800-784-8669), or by texting QUIT to 47848.

**NIH News in Health**
**ISSN 2375-6993** (Print) **ISSN 1556-3898** (Online)
**Editor** Harrison Wein, Ph.D.
**Managing Editor** Tianna Hicklin, Ph.D.
**Graphics** Alan Defibaugh (illustrations), Bryan Ewsichek (design)
**Contributors** Erin Bryant and Sharon Reynolds



newsinhealth.nih.gov

NIH National Institutes of Health
*NIH...Turning Discovery Into Health®*

Office of Communications & Public Liaison
Building 31, Room 5B52
Bethesda, MD 20892-2094
email: nihnewsinhealth@od.nih.gov
phone: 301-451-8224

## Web Links

For more about fatty liver disease, see "Links" in the online article: newsinhealth.nih.gov/2021/10/fighting-fatty-liver

# Recognizing Jaundice

## Signs That Your Liver Isn't Delivering

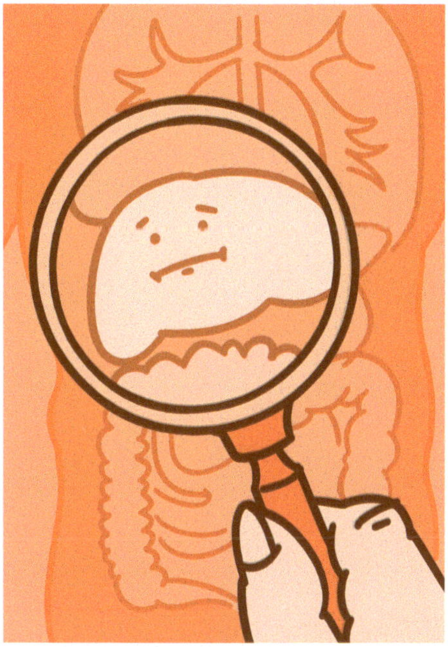

Some babies have a yellowish tint to their skin or the whites of their eyes right after birth. This is called jaundice. It can happen to adults, too. For adults, it can be a sign of a serious health condition.

Your liver helps rid your body of natural waste products and other harmful substances. If something interferes with this process, toxic compounds can build up in your body.

Jaundice happens when you have too much of a compound called bilirubin. Bilirubin forms when your body breaks down old or damaged red blood cells. The most common symptom is a yellow tint to your skin, the whites of your eyes, or the inside of your mouth. You may also have dark urine or pale stools.

Babies become jaundiced when their livers can't break down all the bilirubin that is produced the first few days after birth. Jaundice in babies usually goes away on its own in a week or two. If it goes on longer than this, they should be evaluated by a doctor.

In adults, many health conditions can lead to jaundice. One of the more common causes is when bile ducts get blocked. Bile ducts drain bilirubin from the liver into the intestines. They can get blocked by hard, pebble-like pieces of material that form in the gallbladder, called gallstones. Gallstones are usually made of bilirubin or cholesterol (a waxy, fat-like substance). Cancers of the bile duct or pancreas can also cause a blockage.

Jaundice can also be a sign of liver disease. Some liver diseases are caused by drinking too much alcohol or taking drugs. Others are caused by too much fat buildup in the liver.

Misusing certain medications, like acetaminophen, can damage the liver and lead to jaundice. So can hepatitis, or inflammation of the liver. Viruses are the most common cause of hepatitis. But the condition can be caused by other things, like toxins and certain diseases.

If a liver disease lasts for only a short time, the liver may be able to heal. But if the disease becomes chronic, meaning it lasts for a long time, it can lead to scarring of the liver. This scarring is called cirrhosis. Cirrhosis can impair the liver's ability to function and may eventually lead to liver failure.

Not everyone who has jaundice has a serious health condition. Some people are born with a condition called Gilbert syndrome. This condition slows the liver's ability to break down bilirubin. It can lead to short periods of high bilirubin levels and, sometimes, jaundice. But it doesn't lead to further complications and doesn't need special treatment.

If you have any symptoms of jaundice, see a health care provider right away. "Your provider will need to do liver tests to figure out what type of jaundice it is," says Dr. David Goldberg, a liver specialist at the University of Miami Health System.

Treatment depends on the cause. Gallstones are most commonly treated with surgery to remove the gallbladder. Liver damage that's caused by medications will often heal once you stop taking the medication. Antiviral drugs can treat hepatitis virus infections. People with a chronic liver disease should limit alcohol use to prevent further liver damage.

Goldberg is one of several NIH-funded researchers studying whether cholesterol-lowering drugs called statins can slow or prevent the progression of liver disease.

You can take steps to protect yourself from things that damage the liver. See the Wise Choices box for tips on keeping your liver healthy. ■

### Wise Choices

#### Take Care of Your Liver

- **Eat a healthy diet and maintain a healthy weight.**
- **Take steps to prevent hepatitis infections.** Get vaccinated against hepatitis A and B. Always wash your hands after using the toilet, changing diapers, and before and after handling or preparing food. Learn more at bit.ly/3U4xptL.
- **Limit alcohol use.** Drinking too much alcohol harms the liver.
- **Quit smoking.** You can get free help quitting at 1-800-QUIT-NOW or smokefree.gov.
- **Take medications only as directed.**
- **Tell your provider about all the medicines you take,** including over-the-counter drugs and supplements.

### Web Links

For more about jaundice, see "Links" in the online article: newsinhealth.nih.gov/2022/10/recognizing-jaundice

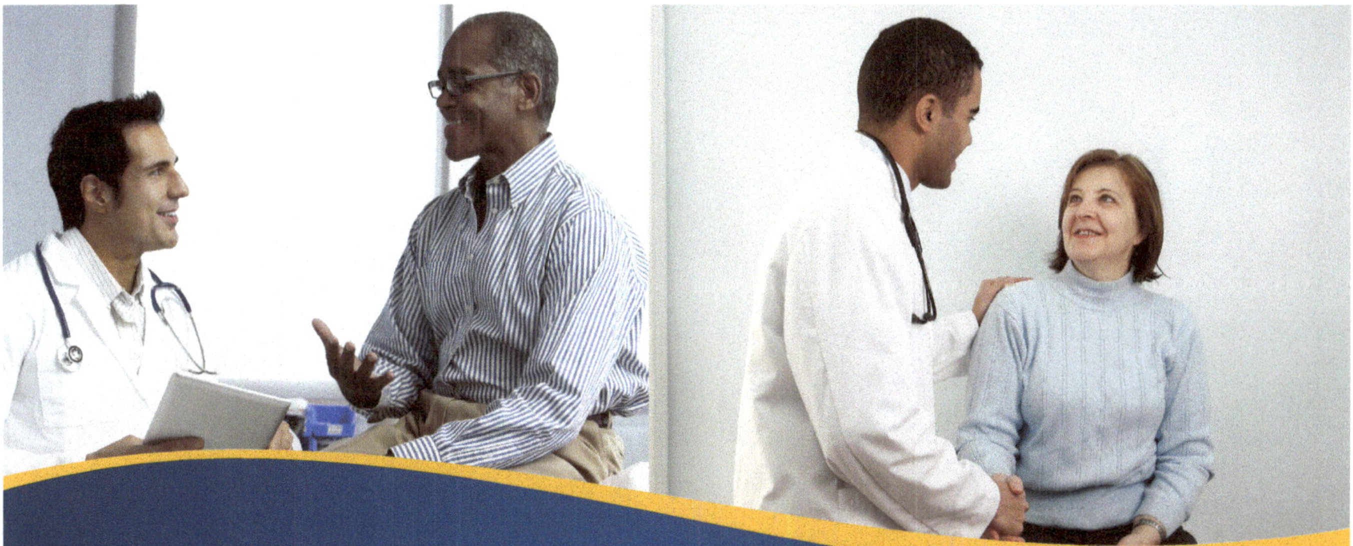

A QUICK GUIDE ON

# Chronic Obstructive Pulmonary Disease

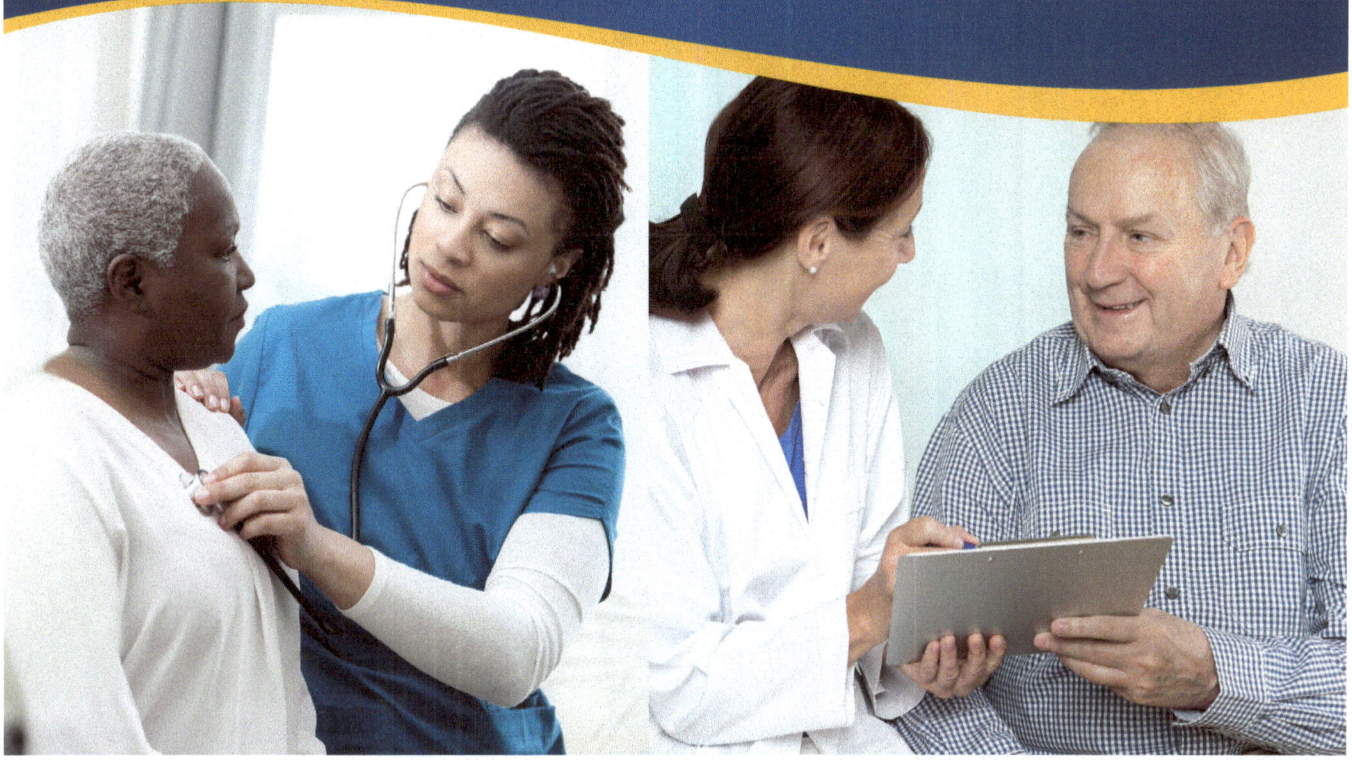

**U.S. Department of Health and Human Services**
National Institutes of Health
National Heart, Lung, and Blood Institute

LEARN MORE
BREATHE BETTER®

**COPD, or chronic obstructive pulmonary disease, is a serious lung disease that over time makes it hard to breathe.** Other names for COPD include chronic bronchitis or emphysema.

COPD, a leading cause of death, affects millions of Americans and causes long-term disability.

Most often, COPD occurs in people age 40 and over who...

- Have a history of smoking
- Have had long-term exposure to lung irritants such as air pollution, chemical fumes, or dust from the environment or workplace
- Have a rare genetic condition called alpha-1 antitrypsin (AAT) deficiency
- Have a combination of any of the above

## MAJOR COPD RISK FACTORS

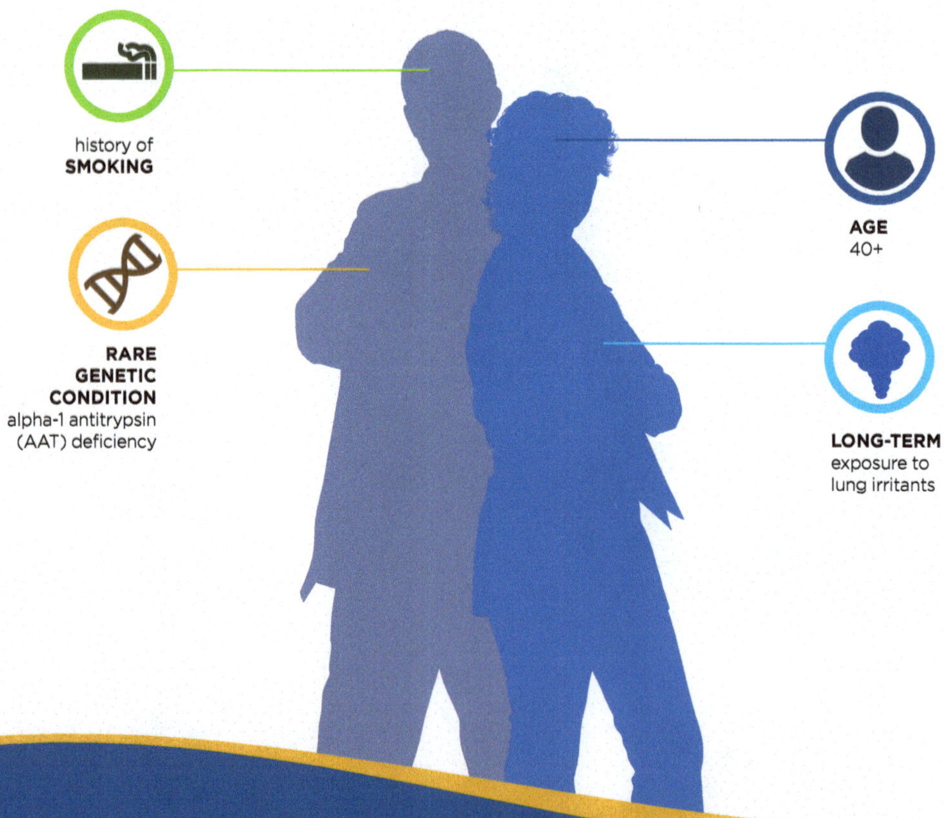


# WHAT IS COPD?

## To understand what COPD is, we first need to understand how respiration and the lungs work:

**When air is breathed in**, it goes down the windpipe into tubes in the lungs called bronchial tubes or airways. Within the lungs, bronchial tubes branch into thousands of smaller, thinner tubes called bronchioles. These tubes end in bunches of tiny round air sacs called alveoli.

Small blood vessels called capillaries run through the walls of the air sacs. When air reaches the air sacs, oxygen passes through the air sac walls into the blood in the capillaries. At the same time, carbon dioxide (the respiration waste gas) moves from the capillaries into the air sacs. This process is called **gas exchange**.

The airways and air sacs are elastic (stretchy). When breathing in, each air sac fills up with air like a small balloon. When breathing out, the air sacs deflate and the air goes out.

**In COPD, less air flows in and out of the airways because of one or more of the following:**

- The airways and air sacs lose their elastic quality.
- The walls between many of the air sacs are destroyed.
- The walls of the airways become thick and inflamed.
- The airways make more mucus than usual, which can clog them.

**GAS EXCHANGE IN A LUNG**

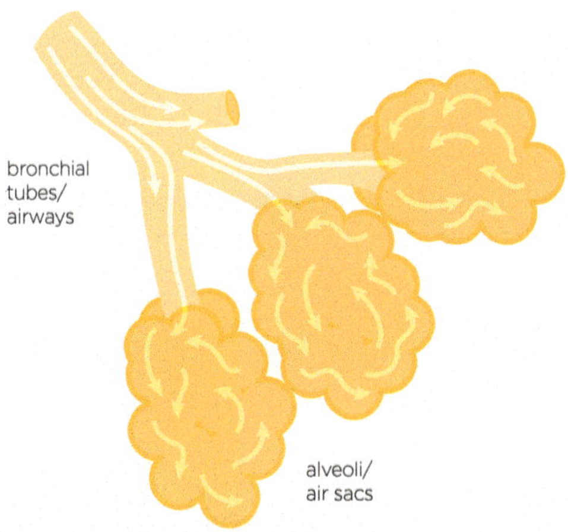


**COPD DECREASES AIR FLOW AND GAS EXCHANGE IN THE LUNGS**

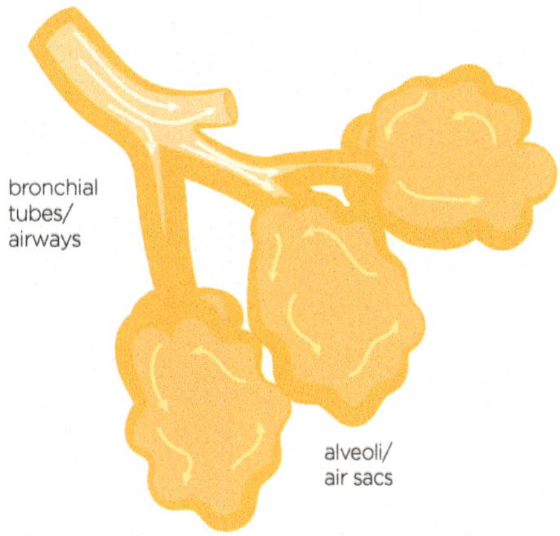


## HOW DOES COPD AFFECT BREATHING?

**In emphysema,** the walls between many of the air sacs are damaged. As a result, the air sacs lose their shape and become floppy. This damage also can destroy the walls of the air sacs, leading to fewer and larger air sacs instead of many tiny ones. If this happens, the amount of gas exchange in the lungs is reduced.

**In chronic bronchitis,** the lining of the airways is constantly irritated and inflamed. This causes the lining to thicken. Lots of thick mucus forms in the airways, making it hard to breathe.

**Most people who have COPD have a variable combination of both emphysema and chronic bronchitis.** Thus, the general term "COPD" is more accurate.

Some people who have asthma can also develop COPD. Asthma is a chronic (long-term) lung disease that inflames and tightens the airways. Asthma treatments usually can reverse the inflammation and narrowing. However, in the presence of COPD, much of the reversibility is lost.

## At first, COPD may cause no symptoms or only mild symptoms.

As the disease gets worse, symptoms usually become more severe. When symptoms are mild, they may not be noticed right away and people may adjust their lifestyle to make breathing easier. For example, taking the elevator instead of the stairs.

### COMMON SIGNS AND SYMPTOMS OF COPD INCLUDE:

- CONSTANT COUGH
- SHORTNESS OF BREATH doing everyday activities
- CAN'T BREATHE DEEP
- EXCESS SPUTUM
- WHEEZING

### CHRONIC OBSTRUCTIVE PULMONARY DISEASE

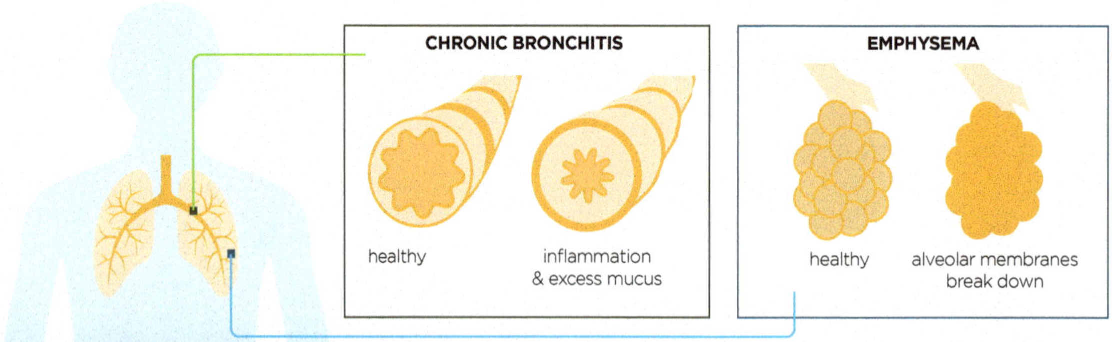


# COPD: EMPHYSEMA, CHRONIC BRONCHITIS, AND SYMPTOMS

## COPD diagnosis is based on:

- **Signs and symptoms:** chronic cough, excess sputum
- **Personal and medical history:** smoking history or exposure to lung irritants, such as secondhand smoke, air pollution, chemical fumes, or dust
- **Test results:** lung function tests, spirometry

Lung function tests measure how much air is breathed in and out, how fast air is breathed out, and how well lungs deliver oxygen to the blood.

The main lung function test for COPD is spirometry but other tests, such as a lung diffusion capacity test, also might be used. Spirometry can detect COPD before symptoms become severe. It is a simple, non-invasive breathing test that measures the amount of air a person can blow out of the lungs (volume) and how fast he or she can blow it out (flow). The test helps detect COPD and its severity and can also find out whether other conditions, such as asthma or heart failure, are causing the symptoms.

**Other tests may include:**

- Chest x-ray or chest CT scan
- Arterial blood gas test

There currently is no cure for COPD. Lifestyle changes and treatments can greatly improve a patient's quality of life and allow them to stay more active and slow the progression of the disease.

**Treatment options may include:**

- Medications: bronchodilators, inhaled steroids, anti-inflammatory agents
- Pulmonary rehabilitation
- Physical activity training
- Oxygen supplementation
- Surgery

**Lifestyle changes may include:**

- Avoiding lung irritants, such as smoke and pollutants
- Getting ongoing care, including:
  - Visiting a healthcare provider regularly
  - Taking medications as directed
  - Getting flu (influenza), pneumococcal, and COVID-19 vaccines as recommended by a healthcare provider
- Monitoring activities and symptoms
- Preparing for disease flare-ups

## COPD: DIAGNOSIS AND TREATMENT OPTIONS

# STI

**Sexually Transmitted Infections**

# National Strategic Plan

for the United States | **2021–2025**

DEPARTMENT OF HEALTH & HUMAN SERVICES · USA

# EXECUTIVE SUMMARY

Over the past decade, the United States has witnessed alarming increases in rates of sexually transmitted infections (STIs) including syphilis, chlamydia, and gonorrhea, amounting to a public health crisis. From 2014 to 2018, the rates of reported cases of primary and secondary syphilis, congenital syphilis, gonorrhea, and chlamydia rose 71%, 185%, 63%, and 19%, respectively. Human papillomavirus (HPV), the most common STI, accounts for 14 million new infections each year.

The consequences of the STI epidemic are enormous. When left untreated, STIs can lead to long-term, irreversible health outcomes such as chronic pelvic pain, infertility, adverse pregnancy outcomes, neonatal death, and congenital abnormalities, and can facilitate HIV acquisition. HPV can cause numerous forms of cancer, although most HPV types associated with cancer are preventable through vaccination. HPV vaccination rates are lower than for other routinely recommended childhood and adolescent vaccinations in the United States despite evidence that the vaccine has a substantial impact on reducing HPV infections, HPV-associated pre-cancers, cancers, and genital warts. Many Americans largely underestimate the risk of STIs and for myriad reasons may not proactively seek care. In addition, racial and ethnic disparities contribute to an unequal burden of STIs in the United States.

As recognized by several national reports and authorities, efforts to date to address STIs have been fragmented and insufficient. Despite actions to reverse the trend, resources are often strained in many state and local public health settings. In addition, STIs cost Americans billions of dollars each year in direct medical expenses. Combined, the health and economic toll can affect the quality of life and prosperity of millions of people. Coordinated, innovative approaches and sustained efforts are needed to reverse this increasing trajectory and to curtail the ever-growing burden of STIs.

This inaugural STI National Strategic Plan (STI Plan) sets forth a vision for the nation with goals, objectives, and strategies to meaningfully prevent and control STIs in the United States. It is intended to serve as a roadmap for federal and nonfederal stakeholders at all levels to reverse the upward trends in STI rates. The STI Plan focuses on four of the STIs with the highest morbidity rates, the most persistent and pervasive STI inequalities according to national data, and the greatest impact on the health of the nation: chlamydia, gonorrhea, syphilis, and HPV. HIV, another significant STI, is the focus of a separate HIV National Strategic Plan. Hepatitis B and hepatitis C, which can also be transmitted sexually, are the focus of a separate Viral Hepatitis National Strategic Plan.

The STI Plan also includes indicators to measure progress and quantitative targets for each indicator. The components of the STI Plan are contained and discussed in Section III.

The STI Plan establishes the following vision:

**VISION**

*The United States will be a place where sexually transmitted infections are prevented and where every person has high-quality STI prevention, care, and treatment while living free from stigma and discrimination.*

*This vision includes all people, regardless of age, sex, gender identity, sexual orientation, race, ethnicity, religion, disability, geographic location, or socioeconomic circumstance.*

This vision is accompanied by five high-level goals, which frame the STI Plan's more specific objectives. The order of goals and objectives does not indicate any prioritization, and many are intertwined. The five goals and associated objectives are as follows:

### Goal 1: Prevent New STIs

1.1 Increase awareness of STIs and sexual health

1.2 Expand implementation of quality, comprehensive STI primary prevention activities

1.3 Increase completion rates of routinely recommended HPV vaccination

1.4 Increase the capacity of public health, health care delivery systems, and the health workforce to prevent STIs

### Goal 2: Improve the Health of People by Reducing Adverse Outcomes of STIs

2.1 Expand high-quality affordable STI secondary prevention, including screening, care, and treatment, in communities and populations most impacted by STIs

2.2 Work to effectively identify, diagnose, and provide holistic care and treatment for people with STIs by increasing the capacity of public health, health care delivery systems, and the health workforce

### Goal 3: Accelerate Progress in STI Research, Technology, and Innovation

3.1 Support research and investments to develop STI vaccines and bring them to market

3.2 Support the development and uptake of STI multipurpose prevention technologies, antimicrobial prophylaxis regimens, and other preventive products and strategies

3.3 Support the development and uptake of innovative STI diagnostic technologies, therapeutic agents, and other interventions for the identification and treatment of STIs, including new and emerging disease threats

3.4 Identify, evaluate, and scale up best practices in STI prevention and treatment, including through translational, implementation, and communication science research

### Goal 4: Reduce STI-Related Health Disparities and Health Inequities

4.1 Reduce stigma and discrimination associated with STIs

4.2 Expand culturally competent and linguistically appropriate STI prevention, care, and treatment services in communities disproportionately impacted by STIs

4.3 Address STI-related social determinants of health and co-occurring conditions

### Goal 5: Achieve Integrated, Coordinated Efforts That Address the STI Epidemic

5.1 Integrate programs to address the syndemic of STIs, HIV, viral hepatitis, and substance use disorders

5.2 Improve quality, accessibility, timeliness, and use of data related to STIs and social determinants of health

5.3 Improve mechanisms to measure, monitor, evaluate, report, and disseminate progress toward achieving national STI goals

The vision, goals, objectives, and other components of the STI Plan were developed and approved by a dedicated Steering Committee, composed of subject matter experts from across the federal government, with public comment from numerous and varied stakeholders. The STI Plan is designed to be accessible to a broad audience, including people working in public health, health care, government, community-based organizations, private industry, research, and academia. It serves as a roadmap for all stakeholders at all levels to guide development of policies, initiatives, and actions for STI prevention and control. Because certain demographic groups and areas are disproportionately impacted by STIs, the STI Plan also identifies populations and geographic regions with higher rates of STIs (i.e., priority populations) so that federal agencies and other stakeholders can focus their resources to realize the greatest impact. The priority populations were identified based on national-level data. Stakeholders are encouraged to review the data for the populations they serve to help focus their efforts.

Interwoven throughout the STI Plan are approaches to address the individual, community, and structural factors and inequities that contribute to the spread of STIs, such as stigma and social determinants of health. The STI Plan highlights opportunities to integrate STI prevention and control into HIV, viral hepatitis, substance use disorders, and other public health efforts by leveraging capacity and infrastructure across the domains and breaking down operational and funding silos.

A recurring theme is the need for innovative solutions and approaches to address the ongoing and emerging challenges to STI prevention and control, including expanding the types of community and clinical sites that address STIs and developing vaccines, point-of-care diagnostic tools, and therapeutics. The plan is designed to facilitate a whole-of-nation response to the STI epidemic in the United States and to successfully prevent and reduce STI-associated morbidity and mortality.

The STI Plan includes indicators for measuring progress and quantitative targets for each indicator. There are seven core indicators, some of which are stratified to measure progress in addressing disparities in STIs (i.e., disparities indicators). Although focused on the years 2021–2025, the STI Plan includes annual targets through 2030 because STIs will continue to pose a threat to the public's health. To ensure implementation and accountability, a Federal Implementation Plan that documents the specific actions that federal partners will take to achieve the STI Plan's goals and objectives will be released subsequent to the STI Plan. Progress toward meeting the STI Plan's goals will be monitored and reported annually.

Substance Abuse and Mental Health Services Administration
SAMHSA
www.samhsa.gov • 1-877-SAMHSA-7 (1-877-726-4727)

IN BRIEF
Fall 2014 • Volume 8 • Issue 2

# Treating Sleep Problems of People in Recovery From Substance Use Disorders

Sleep problems are a common complaint among people with substance use disorders (SUDs). They can occur during withdrawal, but they can also last months and years into recovery[1] and can be associated with relapse to substance use.[2] This *In Brief* alerts healthcare providers to the relationship between sleep disturbances and SUDs and provides guidance on how to assess for and treat sleep problems in patients in recovery.

## Sleep Disturbances and Substance Use

Many Americans suffer from unhealthy sleep-related behaviors. The prevalence of insomnia symptoms (difficulty initiating or maintaining sleep) in the general population is estimated at 33 percent, with an estimated 6 percent having a diagnosis of insomnia.[3] According to a 12-state survey conducted by the Centers for Disease Control and Prevention:[4]

- 35.3 percent of survey respondents obtain less than 7 hours of sleep on average during a 24-hour period.
- 48.0 percent snore.
- 37.9 percent unintentionally fall asleep during the day.

Substance/medication-induced sleep disorder is recognized in the *Diagnostic and Statistical Manual of Mental Disorders,* Fifth Edition.[5] Substance use can exacerbate sleep difficulties, which in turn present a risk factor for substance use or relapse to use.[6] The types of sleep problems vary by substance used and can include insomnia, sleep latency (the time it takes to fall asleep), disturbances in sleep cycles and sleep continuity, or hypersomnia (excessive daytime sleepiness).[5] Specific findings on the relationship between sleep disturbances and substance use are presented below.

### Alcohol Abuse

Insomnia and other sleep disturbances are common symptoms of alcohol dependence.[1,7] Many people with alcohol use disorder (AUD) have insomnia before entering treatment.[7] Reported rates of sleep problems among people with AUD in treatment range from 25 to 72 percent.[8] Some people in recovery from AUD may continue to have sleep problems, including insomnia or sleep-disordered breathing (such as sleep apnea), for weeks, months, or sometimes years after initiating abstinence.[9,10,11]

### Illicit Drug Use

Sleep disturbances are common among people abstaining from chronic substance use. People stopping marijuana use can experience sleep problems in the first days of withdrawal,[12] and these problems can last for weeks.[13,14] People in detoxification from opioids often report symptoms of insomnia.[15,16] A study that objectively measured sleep in people who chronically use cocaine found that sleep quality deteriorated during a period of abstinence, even though the subjects perceived their sleep to be improving.[17] Another study of people in withdrawal from cocaine found that three-quarters experienced poor sleep quality.[18] In a study of college students, those who reported a history of nonmedical psychostimulant use or current use reported worse subjective and overall sleep quality and more sleep disturbance compared with those who had not used such substances.[19]

## The Effects of Sleep Loss During Recovery

Sleep loss can have significant negative effects on the physical, mental, and emotional well-being of people in recovery. It can also interfere with substance abuse treatment. Persistent sleep complaints after withdrawal are associated with relapse to alcohol use.[20,21] Poor sleep quality before a quit attempt from cannabis use is a risk factor for lapsing back into use within 2 days.[22]

### Medication-Assisted Treatment and Sleep Disorders

Disrupted sleep, including central sleep apnea and related daytime sleepiness, is prevalent in people on methadone maintenance therapy for opioid dependence.[23,24] Methadone dose and duration of opioid use prior to treatment correlate linearly with sleep problems.[23] The prevalence of sleep problems is attributable to the methadone, which is a full μ-opioid agonist, and to concurrent factors that often affect patients in recovery from opioid addiction, such as mental disorders, benzodiazepine abuse, and chronic pain. Buprenorphine, a partial μ-opioid agonist, at routine therapeutic doses has also been found to induce significant alterations of breathing during sleep.[25]

## Assessing Sleep Disorders

If a patient initiating withdrawal from a substance or recovering from an SUD complains of a sleep disturbance, the healthcare provider should assess for causes by doing the following:[26]

- Determine the duration of recovery and medications used for SUD treatment.
- Ask questions about difficulty falling asleep, waking during the night, amount of sleep per night, snoring, sleep apnea, excessive movements during sleep, uncontrollable movements that are relieved by getting up and walking, and excessive daytime sleepiness. If possible, ask significant others the same questions about the patient.
- Rule out other causes of the sleep problem, such as stress, a life crisis, or side effects of medications the patient is taking.
- Ask the patient to write in a sleep diary or log immediately on awakening. The patient should record total time in bed, time of sleep onset, number of times awakened, and total time spent awake.
- Determine the frequency and duration of symptoms of insomnia. If difficulties occur two or three nights per week and last for 1 month or more, the patient warrants a diagnosis of insomnia.

Note that some patients tend to overestimate the quality and duration of their sleep on self-report questionnaires and in sleep logs.[27,28] If warranted, a referral for an objective sleep study in a sleep laboratory can be made.

## Treatments

The association between insomnia and relapse calls for treatment that addresses insomnia during recovery. The first step in treating insomnia should focus on the status of the patient's recovery. Patients should be receiving treatment from an appropriate substance abuse treatment program. It is important to address other psychological, social, and medical problems that may contribute to insomnia, such as co-occurring mental and medical disorders, use of medications that disturb sleep, and nicotine use.[29,30]

### Nonpharmacological Treatments

Nonpharmacological treatments are preferred because many pharmacological treatments for insomnia have the potential for abuse and can interfere with SUD recovery. Research on cognitive–behavioral therapy (CBT) to treat insomnia has shown positive results, generally[26,31,32] and

### What Healthcare Providers Can Do

- Screen for insomnia among people in recovery from SUDs.
- Include questions about sleep during the routine patient history.
- Rule out other causes of sleep problems (e.g., stress, medications).
- Educate patients about sleep hygiene, and make referrals to a specialist if necessary.
- Conduct a careful evaluation, and consider risk factors, before prescribing sedative–hypnotic medications to treat insomnia.
- Monitor patients for signs of abuse or diversion of scheduled medications prescribed to treat insomnia and other sleep disorders.

### Exhibit 1. Nonpharmacological Treatments

- **Mindfulness meditation.** The patient moves into a state of restful, present-moment alertness, which reduces stress and improves self-control.[33,34]
- **Progressive muscle relaxation.** The patient concentrates on tensing and relaxing groups of muscles.[8,35]
- **Biofeedback.** The patient becomes aware of physiologic stress responses and how to control them.[26]
- **CBT for insomnia.** The patient's dysfunctional beliefs and behaviors are modified to improve his or her emotional state.[26,36]
- **Stimulus control.** The patient reassociates the bedroom with the rapid onset of sleep.[37]
- **Exercise.** Regular physical activity relieves stress and tires the patient.[26]
- **Sleep restriction therapy.** The patient limits sleep to a few hours and progressively increases it until the desired amount of sleep time is achieved.[26]
- **Bright-light therapy.** Exposure to a natural bright light while awake helps promote normal sleep patterns.[38]
- **Dental devices and continuous positive airway pressure machines.** These devices help the patient with obstructive sleep apnea breathe more easily during sleep.[39]

also in patients who are alcohol dependent.[40] Exhibit 1 lists several nonpharmacological interventions that have shown some degree of effectiveness. Combining approaches may be more effective than using one approach.[38]

Healthcare providers can educate patients about simple nonpharmacological techniques that can improve sleep[41] (see Exhibit 2). Sleep education includes teaching about sleep, the effects of recovery from substance use on sleep, and health practices and environmental factors that affect sleep.[38] Sleep can be improved by limiting bedroom activities to sleeping (e.g., refraining from activities such as reading the newspaper, paying bills, or working on electronic devices) and going to bed only when sleepy and at about the same time each day. These activities help reassociate the bed and bedroom with going to sleep.[37] Establishing a relaxing presleep routine, which can include progressive muscle relaxation,[35] imagery,[42] or a warm bath,[41] also promotes sleep. Some patients may benefit from referral to a sleep medicine specialist.

## Pharmacological Treatments

### Over-the-counter medications and dietary supplements

Some people who have trouble sleeping have tried over-the-counter sleep medications or dietary supplements to help them sleep. Patients may ask about these, and care should be taken to explain their safety and efficacy. Many over-the-counter sleep medications contain antihistamines that cause sedation.[38] They are not recommended as a long-term treatment for insomnia because they negatively affect the natural sleep cycle and have side effects such as morning grogginess, daytime sleepiness, and impaired alertness and judgment.[43,44] Furthermore, evidence supporting their long-term effectiveness is insufficient.[43]

Popular dietary supplements taken with the intent to promote sleep include valerian and melatonin. Valerian, an herb, is thought to have sedative effects.[45,46] However, studies of valerian offer mixed results,[47,48] and evidence supporting the supplement's efficacy is insufficient to warrant its use.[49,50] In addition, valerian could damage the liver.[47] Melatonin is a brain hormone that helps regulate sleep patterns.[51] Limited evidence shows that it can treat chronic insomnia in some people and, to date, there is no evidence that it is harmful.[52]

### Prescription medications without known abuse potential

Medications without known abuse potential should be the first treatment option when pharmacotherapy is necessary to treat insomnia during recovery. Ramelteon and doxepin are the only unscheduled prescription medications approved by the U.S. Food and Drug Administration (FDA) for the treatment of insomnia. Ramelteon decreases the amount of time it takes to fall asleep.[53,54] Doxepin, originally FDA approved as an antidepressant, has been approved for treating insomnia typified by problems staying asleep. These medications may be suitable for treating insomnia in patients in recovery, because they do not appear to have potential for abuse.[55,56,57]

### Exhibit 2. Promoting Sleep Hygiene: Tips for a Good Night's Sleep[58,59]

- Go to bed and get up at the same times each day.
- Use natural light (that comes through a window) to remind yourself of when it's time to be asleep and awake. This can help you set a healthy sleep–wake cycle.
- Exercise regularly.
- If you take naps, keep them short and before 5 p.m.
- Don't eat or drink too much when it is close to bedtime.
- Avoid caffeine (in coffee, tea, chocolate, cola, and some pain relievers) and nicotine for several hours before bedtime.
- Wind down before going to bed (e.g., take a warm bath, do light reading, practice relaxation exercises).
- Keep the bedroom a relaxing place—avoid working or paying bills in bed.
- Sleep in a dark, quiet room that isn't too hot or too cold.
- Don't lie in bed awake. If you can't fall asleep within 20 minutes, get up and do something relaxing.

### Off-label medications

Other medications are often prescribed off label (for purposes other than the medication's FDA-approved use) to treat insomnia. According to a survey of addiction medicine physicians, the sedating antidepressant trazodone is the medication most often prescribed for the management of sleep disorders in patients in early recovery from AUD.[60] One study found that its use among people in recovery from AUD improved sleep efficiency.[61] Studies of its effects on abstinence and relapse in persons with AUD are conflicting. A 2008 study comparing trazodone with placebo for people after detoxification from alcohol showed that the trazodone group had improved sleep quality but had less improvement in the proportion of days abstinent while taking the medication. Furthermore, when the medication was discontinued, the trazodone group experienced less improvement in abstinence days and an increase in the number of drinks per drinking day.[62] In contrast, a study published in 2011 of patients discharged from residential treatment did not find an association between trazodone use and relapse or return to heavy drinking.[63] A study of patients on methadone maintenance treatment found that trazodone use provided no improvement in sleep.[64]

Other sedating antidepressants that have been used to treat insomnia include amitriptyline, mirtazapine, nefazodone, and nortriptyline.[65] In a study of the use of mirtazapine on subjects with cocaine dependence and co-occurring depression, the medication decreased sleep latency; however, it had no measurable effect on treatment for cocaine dependence and depressive symptoms.[66]

Gabapentin, an anticonvulsant with sedative properties, also has evidence of efficacy for treating insomnia.[50,67] It has been found to be more effective in promoting sleep than lorazepam (an anxiolytic commonly prescribed to treat insomnia) among people withdrawing from alcohol.[67] It has also been found to be more effective than trazodone in promoting sleep among those in early recovery.[68] Acamprosate, a medication used to maintain alcohol abstinence, may also improve sleep during withdrawal from alcohol.[21,69]

### Prescription medications with known abuse potential

Sedative–hypnotic medications, such as benzodiazepines and nonbenzodiazepines, are commonly prescribed to treat sleep problems. However, these medications should be avoided by people with histories of SUDs, who are at increased risk for abusing them.[44,70] Benzodiazepines, such as alprazolam, diazepam, and triazolam, are especially risky for use with people with SUDs because they are potentially addicting. They can also cause residual daytime sedation, cognitive impairment, motor incoordination, and rebound insomnia.[50] Long-term treatment of insomnia with benzodiazepines may lead to withdrawal symptoms (e.g., anxiety, irritability, seizures) when patients stop taking the medications. A careful clinical evaluation is needed to ensure appropriate prescribing. Measures to prevent abuse include the following:[71]

- Observe closely and perform ongoing evaluations.
- Prescribe a few tablets at a time.
- Schedule frequent office visits.
- Conduct occasional urine screenings.
- Use one source to dispense the medication.
- Occasionally taper the medication.
- Be attentive to risk factors such as antisocial personality disorder and dependence on multiple substances.

Alternatives to benzodiazepines include sedative–hypnotic medications such as zaleplon, eszopiclone, and zolpidem. These medications all have the same mechanism of action as benzodiazepines but lack some of the negative side effects. However, some research indicates that at high doses they may have the same side effects as benzodiazepines.[72] The three medications are Schedule IV controlled substances, indicating abuse potential. For these reasons, these medications should be used only for short-term treatment of insomnia in people with a history of SUDs.

## Web Resources

**American Academy of Sleep Medicine**
http://www.aasmnet.org

**National Center on Sleep Disorders Research**
http://www.nhlbi.nih.gov/about/org/ncsdr

**National Sleep Foundation**
http://www.sleepfoundation.org

## Notes


1 Teplin, D., Raz, B., Daiter, J., Varenbut, M., & Tyrrell, M. (2006). Screening for substance use patterns among patients referred for a variety of sleep complaints. *American Journal of Drug and Alcohol Abuse, 32,* 111–120.

2 Brower, K. J., & Perron, B. E. (2010). Prevalence and correlates of withdrawal-related insomnia among adults with alcohol dependence: Results from a national survey. *American Journal on Addictions/American Academy of Psychiatrists in Alcoholism and Addictions, 19*(3), 238–244.

3 Ohayon, M. M. (2002). Epidemiology of insomnia: What we know and what we still need to learn. *Sleep Medicine Reviews, 6*(2), 97–111.

4 Centers for Disease Control and Prevention. (2011). Unhealthy sleep-related behaviors—12 States, 2009. *Morbidity and Mortality Weekly Report, 60,* 233–238.

5 American Psychiatric Association. (2013). *Diagnostic and statistical manual of mental disorders* (5th ed.). Arlington, VA: American Psychiatric Publishing.

6 Hasler, B. P., Smith, L. J., Cousins, J. C., & Bootzin, R. R. (2012). Circadian rhythms, sleep, and substance abuse. *Sleep Medicine Reviews, 16,* 67–81.

7 Brower, K. J., Krentzman, A., & Robinson, E. A. R. (2011). Persistent insomnia, abstinence, and moderate drinking in alcohol-dependent individuals. *American Journal on Addictions/American Academy of Psychiatrists in Alcoholism and Addictions, 20*(5), 435–440.

8 Stein, M. D., & Friedmann, P. D. (2005). Disturbed sleep and its relationship to alcohol use. *Substance Abuse, 26*(1), 1–13.

9 Brower, K. J. (2003). Insomnia, alcoholism and relapse. *Sleep Medicine Reviews, 7*(6), 523–539.

10 Colrain, I. M., Turlington, S., & Baker, F. C. (2009). Impact of alcoholism on sleep architecture and EEG power spectra in men and women. *SLEEP, 32*(10), 1341–1352.

11 Currie, S. R., Clark, S., Rimac, S., & Malhotra, S. (2003). Comprehensive assessment of insomnia in recovering alcoholics using daily sleep diaries and ambulatory monitoring. *Alcoholism: Clinical and Experimental Research, 27*(8), 1262–1269.

12 Vandrey, R., Smith, M. T., McCann, U. D., Budney, A. J., & Curran, E. M. (2011). Sleep disturbance and the effects of extended-release zolpidem during cannabis withdrawal. *Drug and Alcohol Dependence, 117,* 38–44.

13 Bolla, K. I., Lesage, S. R., Gamaldo, C. E., Neubauer, D. N., Wang, N.-Y., Funderburk, F. R., et al. (2010). Polysomnogram changes in marijuana users who report sleep disturbances during prior abstinence. *Sleep Medicine, 11*(9), 882–889.

14 Vandrey, R. G., Budney, A. J., Moore, B. A., & Hughes, J. R. (2005). A cross-study comparison of cannabis and tobacco withdrawal. *American Journal on Addictions/American Academy of Psychiatrists in Alcoholism and Addictions, 14,* 54–63.

15 Hillhouse, M., Domier, C. P., Chim, D., & Ling, W. (2010). Provision of ancillary medications during buprenorphine detoxification does not improve treatment outcomes. *Journal of Addictive Diseases, 29*(1), 23–29.

16 Wallen, M. C., Lorman, W. J., & Gosciniak, J. L. (2006). Combined buprenorphine and clonidine for short-term opiate detoxification: Patient perspectives. *Journal of Addictive Diseases, 25*(1), 23–31.

17 Morgan, P. T., Pace-Schott, E. F., Sahul, Z. H., Coric, V., Stickgold, R., & Malison, R. T. (2006). Sleep, sleep-dependent procedural learning and vigilance in chronic cocaine users: Evidence for occult insomnia. *Drug and Alcohol Dependence, 82*(3), 238–249.

18 Sofuoglu, M., Dudish-Poulsen, S., Poling, J., Mooney, M., & Hatsukami, D. K. (2005). The effect of individual cocaine withdrawal symptoms on outcomes in cocaine users. *Addictive Behaviors, 30,* 1125–1134.

19 Clegg-Kraynok, M. M., McBean, A. L., & Montgomery-Downs, H. E. (2011). Sleep quality and characteristics of college students who use prescription psychostimulants nonmedically. *Sleep Medicine, 12,* 598–602.

20 Hornyak, M., Haas, P., Veit, J., Gann, H., & Riemann, D. (2004). Magnesium treatment of primary alcohol-dependent patients during subacute withdrawal: An open pilot study with polysomnography. *Alcoholism: Clinical and Experimental Research, 28*(11), 1702–1709.

21 Staner, L., Boeijinga, P., Danel, T., Gendre, I., Muzet, M., Landron, F., & Luthringer, R. (2006). Effects of acamprosate on sleep during alcohol withdrawal: A double-blind placebo-controlled polysomnographic study in alcohol-dependent subjects. *Alcoholism: Clinical and Experimental Research, 30*(9), 1492–1499.

22 Babson, K. A., Boden, M. T., Harris, A. H., Stickle, T. R., & Bonn-Miller, M. O. (2013). Poor sleep quality as a risk factor for lapse following a cannabis quit attempt. *Journal of Substance Abuse Treatment, 44,* 438–443.

23 Peles, E., Schreiber, S., & Adelson, M. (2006). Variables associated with perceived sleep disorders in methadone maintenance treatment (MMT) patients. *Drug and Alcohol Dependence, 82*(2), 103–110.

24 Wang, D., Teichtahl, H., Drummer, O., Goodman, C., Cherry, G., Cunnington, D., & Kronborg, I. (2005). Central sleep apnea in stable methadone maintenance treatment patients. *Chest, 128,* 1348–1356.

25 Farney, R. J., McDonald, A. M., Boyle, K. M., Snow, G. L., Nuttall, R. T., Coudreaut, M. F., et al. (2013). Sleep disordered breathing in patients receiving therapy with buprenorphine/naloxone. *European Respiratory Journal, 42,* 394–403.

26 Schutte-Rodin, S., Broch, L., Buysse, D., Dorsey, C., & Sateia, M. (2008). Clinical guideline for the evaluation and management of chronic insomnia in adults. *Journal of Clinical Sleep Medicine, 4,* 487–504.

27 Conroy, D. A., Arnedt, J. T., Brower, K. J., Strobbe, S., Consens, F., Hoffmann, R., & Armitage, R. (2006). Perception of sleep in recovering alcohol-dependent patients with insomnia: Relationship with future drinking. *Alcoholism: Clinical and Experimental Research, 30*(12), 1992–1999.

28 Currie, S. R., Malhotra, S., & Clark, S. (2004). Agreement among subjective, objective, and collateral measures of insomnia in postwithdrawal recovering alcoholics. *Behavioral Sleep Medicine, 2*(3), 148–161.

29 Stein, M. D., Herman, D. S., Bishop, S., Lassor, J. A., Weinstock, M., Anthony, J., & Anderson, B. J. (2004). Sleep disturbances among methadone maintained patients. *Journal of Substance Abuse Treatment, 26,* 175–180.

30 Zhang, L., Samet, J., Caffo, B., & Punjabi, N. M. (2006). Cigarette smoking and nocturnal sleep architecture. *American Journal of Epidemiology, 164*(6), 529–537.

31 Babson, K. A., Feldner, M. T., & Badour, C. L. (2010). Cognitive behavioral therapy for sleep disorders. *Psychiatric Clinics of North America, 33*(3), 629–640.

32 Mitchell, M. D., Gehrman, P., Perlis, M., & Umscheid, C. A. (2012). Comparative effectiveness of cognitive behavioral therapy for insomnia: A systematic review. *BMC Family Practice, 13:*40. doi:10.1186/1471-2296-13-40

33 Britton, W. B., Bootzin, R. R., Cousins, J. C., Hasler, B. P., Peck, T., & Shapiro, S. L. (2010). The contribution of mindfulness practice to a multicomponent behavioral sleep intervention following substance abuse treatment in adolescents: A treatment-development study. *Substance Abuse, 31*(2), 86–97.

34 Tang, Y.-Y., Tang, R., & Posner, M. I. (2013). Brief meditation training induces smoking reduction. *Proceedings of the National Academy of Sciences of the United States of America, 110*(34), 13971–13975.

35 McCallie, M. S., Blum, C. M., & Hood, C. J. (2006). Progressive muscle relaxation. *Journal of Human Behavior in the Social Environment, 13*(3), 51–66.

36 Verbeek, I. H., Konings, G. M., Aldenkamp, A. P., Declerck, A. C., & Klip, E. C. (2006). Cognitive behavioral treatment in clinically referred chronic insomniacs: Group versus individual treatment. *Behavioral Sleep Medicine, 4*(3), 135–151.

37 Passarella, S., & Duong, M.-T. (2008). Diagnosis and treatment of insomnia. *American Journal of Health-System Pharmacy, 65*(10), 927–934.

38 Neubauer, D. N. (2009). Current and new thinking in the management of comorbid insomnia. *American Journal of Managed Care, 15*(Suppl.), S24–S32.

39 Wolkove, N., Elkholy, O., Baltzan, M., & Palayew, M. (2007). Sleep and aging: 2. Management of sleep disorders in older people. *Canadian Medical Association Journal, 176*(10), 1449–1454.

[40] Arnedt, J. T., Conroy, D. A., Armitage, R., & Brower, K. J. (2011). Cognitive-behavioral therapy for insomnia in alcohol dependent patients: A randomized controlled pilot trial. *Behaviour Research and Therapy, 49*(4), 227–233.

[41] Currie, S. R., Clark, S., Hodgins, D. C., & el-Guebaly, N. (2004). Randomized controlled trial of brief cognitive–behavioural interventions for insomnia in recovering alcoholics. *Addiction, 99,* 1121–1132.

[42] Schmidt, R. E., Harvey, A. G., & Van der Linden, M. (2011). Cognitive and affective control in insomnia. *Frontiers in Psychology, 2:*349. doi:10.3389/fpsyg.2011.00349

[43] American Academy of Sleep Medicine. (2006). *AASM position statement: Treating insomnia with over-the-counter sleep aids.* Westchester, IL: Author.

[44] Jones, E. M., Knutson, D., & Haines, D. (2003). Common problems in patients recovering from chemical dependency. *American Family Physician, 68*(10), 1971–1978.

[45] Bent, S., Padula, A., Moore, D., Patterson, M., & Mehling, W. (2006). Valerian for sleep: A systematic review and meta-analysis. *American Journal of Medicine, 119*(12), 1005–1012.

[46] Morin, A. K., Jarvis, C. I., & Lynch, A. M. (2007). Therapeutic options for sleep-maintenance and sleep-onset insomnia. *Pharmacotherapy, 27*(1), 89–110.

[47] Taibi, D. M., Landis, C. A., Petry, H., & Vitiello, M. V. (2007). A systematic review of valerian as a sleep aid: Safe but not effective. *Sleep Medicine Reviews, 11*(3), 209–230.

[48] Taibi, D. M., Vitiello, M. V., Barsness, S., Elmer, G. W., Anderson, G. D., & Landis, C. A. (2009). A randomized clinical trial of valerian fails to improve self-report, polysomnographic, and actigraphic sleep in older women with insomnia. *Sleep Medicine, 10*(3), 319–328.

[49] Buscemi, N., Vandermeer, B., Friesen, C., Bialy, L., Tubman, M., Ospina, M., et al. (2005). *Manifestations and management of chronic insomnia in adults* [Summary of Evidence Report/ Technology Assessment Number 125]. AHRQ Pub. No. 05-E021-1. Rockville, MD: Agency for Healthcare Research and Quality.

[50] National Institutes of Health. (2005, June 13–15). NIH State-of-the-Science Conference Statement on manifestations and management of chronic insomnia in adults. *NIH Consensus Science Statements, 22*(2), 1–30.

[51] Pandi-Perumal, S. R., Srinivasan, V., Maestroni, G. J., Cardinali, D. P., Poeggeler, B., & Hardeland, R. (2006). Melatonin: Nature's most versatile biological signal? *FEBS Journal, 273*(13), 2813–2838.

[52] Lemoine, P., Garfinkel, D., Laudon, M., Nir, T., & Zisapel, N. (2011). Prolonged-release melatonin for insomnia—An open-label long-term study of efficacy, safety, and withdrawal. *Therapeutics and Clinical Risk Management, 7,* 301–311.

[53] Borja, N. L., & Daniel, K. L. (2006). Ramelteon for the treatment of insomnia. *Clinical Therapeutics, 28*(10), 1540–1555.

[54] Roth, T., Seiden, D., Wang-Weigand, S., & Zhang, J. (2007). A 2-night, 3-period, crossover study of ramelteon's efficacy and safety in older adults with chronic insomnia. *Current Medical Research and Opinion, 23*(5), 1005–1014.

[55] Johnson, M. W., Suess, P. E., & Griffiths, R. R. (2006). Ramelteon: A novel hypnotic lacking abuse liability and sedative adverse effects. *Archives of General Psychiatry, 63*(10), 1149–1157.

[56] Roth, T., Seiden, D., Sainati, S., Wang-Weigand, S., Zhang, J., & Zee, P. (2006). Effects of ramelteon on patient-reported sleep latency in older adults with chronic insomnia. *Sleep Medicine, 7,* 312–318.

[57] U.S. Food and Drug Administration. (2010). FDA approved labeling text 3.17.10 NDA 22036: Highlights of prescribing information. Retrieved August 18, 2014, from http://www.accessdata.fda.gov /drugsatfda_docs/label/2010/022036lbl.pdf

[58] Harvard Medical School, Division of Sleep Medicine. (2007). *Twelve simple tips to improve your sleep.* Retrieved August 18, 2014, from http://healthysleep.med.harvard.edu/healthy/getting /overcoming/tips

[59] National Sleep Foundation. (n.d.). *Sleep hygiene.* Retrieved August 18, 2014, from http://www.sleepfoundation.org /ask-the-expert/sleep-hygiene

[60] Friedmann, P. D., Herman, D. S., Freedman, S., Lemon, S. C., Ramsey, S., & Stein, M. D. (2003). Treatment of sleep disturbance in alcohol recovery: A national survey of addiction medicine physicians. *Journal of Addictive Diseases, 22*(2), 91–103.

[61] Le Bon, O., Murphy, J. R., Staner, L., Hoffmann, G., Kormoss, N., Kentos, M., et al. (2003). Double-blind, placebo-controlled study of the efficacy of trazodone in alcohol post-withdrawal syndrome: Polysomnographic and clinical evaluations. *Journal of Clinical Psychopharmacology, 23*(4), 377–383.

[62] Friedmann, P. D., Rose, J. S., Swift, R., Stout, R. L., Millman, R. P., & Stein, M. D. (2008). Trazodone for sleep disturbance after alcohol detoxification: A double-blind, placebo-controlled trial. *Alcoholism: Clinical and Experimental Research, 32*(9), 1652–1660.

[63] Kolla, B. P., Schneekloth, T. D., Biernacka, J. M., Frye, M. A., Mansukhani, M. P., Hall-Flavin, D. K., et al. (2011). Trazodone and alcohol relapse: A retrospective study following residential treatment. *American Journal on Addictions/American Academy of Psychiatrists in Alcoholism and Addictions, 20,* 525–529.

[64] Stein, M. D., Kurth, M. E., Sharkey, K. M., Anderson, B. J., Corso, R. P., & Millman, R. P. (2012). Trazodone for sleep disturbance during methadone maintenance: A double-blind, placebo-controlled trial. *Drug and Alcohol Dependence, 120*(1–3), 65–73.

[65] Conroy, D., Arnedt, J. T., & Brower, K. J. (2008). Insomnia in patients with addictions: A safer way to break the cycle. *Current Psychiatry, 7*(5), 97–109.

[66] Afshar, M., Knapp, C. M., Sarid-Segal, O., Devine, E., Colaneri, L. S., Tozier, L., et al. (2012). The efficacy of mirtazapine in the treatment of cocaine dependence with comorbid depression. *American Journal of Drug and Alcohol Abuse, 38,* 181–186.

[67] Malcolm, R., Myrick, L. H., Veatch, L. M., Boyle, E., & Randall, P. K. (2007). Self-reported sleep, sleepiness, and repeated alcohol withdrawals: A randomized, double blind, controlled comparison of lorazepam vs gabapentin. *Journal of Clinical Sleep Medicine, 3*(1), 24–32.

[68] Karam-Hage, M., & Brower, K. J. (2003). Open pilot study of gabapentin versus trazodone to treat insomnia in alcoholic outpatients. *Psychiatry and Clinical Neurosciences, 57,* 542–544.

[69] Perney, P., Lehert, P., & Mason, B. J. (2012). Sleep disturbance in alcoholism: Proposal of a simple measurement, and results from a 24-week randomized controlled study of alcohol-dependent patients assessing acamprosate efficacy. *Alcohol and Alcoholism, 47*(2), 133–139.

[70] Hajak, G., Müller, W. E., Wittchen, H. U., Pittrow, D., & Kirch, W. (2003). Abuse and dependence potential for the non-benzodiazepine hypnotics zolpidem and zopiclone: A review of case reports and epidemiological data. *Addiction, 98,* 1371–1378.

[71] Ciraulo, D. A., & Nace, E. P. (2000). Benzodiazepine treatment of anxiety or insomnia in substance abuse patients. *American Journal on Addictions/American Academy of Psychiatrists in Alcoholism and Addictions, 9*(4), 276–284.

[72] Liappas, I. A., Malitas, P. N., Dimopoulos, N. P., Gitsa, O. E., Liappas, A. I., Nikolaou, C. K., & Christodoulou, G. N. (2003). Zolpidem dependence case series: Possible neurobiological mechanisms and clinical management. *Journal of Psychopharmacology, 17*(1), 131–135.

## *In Brief*

This *In Brief* was written and produced under contract numbers 270-04-7049 and 270-09-0307 by the Knowledge Application Program, a Joint Venture of JBS International, Inc., and The CDM Group, Inc., for the Substance Abuse and Mental Health Services Administration (SAMHSA), U.S. Department of Health and Human Services (HHS). Christina Currier served as the Contracting Officer's Representative.



**Electronic Access and Copies of Publication:** This publication may be ordered or downloaded from SAMHSA's Publications Ordering Web page at http://store.samhsa.gov. Or, please call SAMHSA at 1-877-SAMHSA-7 (1-877-726-4727) (English and Español).

**Recommended Citation:** Substance Abuse and Mental Health Services Administration. (2014). Treating Sleep Problems of People in Recovery From Substance Use Disorders. *In Brief,* Volume 8, Issue 2.

**Originating Office:** Quality Improvement and Workforce Development Branch, Division of Services Improvement, Center for Substance Abuse Treatment, Substance Abuse and Mental Health Services Administration, 1 Choke Cherry Road, Rockville, MD 20857.

**HHS Publication No. (SMA) 14-4859**
**Printed 2014**

Substance Abuse and Mental Health Services Administration
SAMHSA
www.samhsa.gov • 1-877-SAMHSA-7 (1-877-726-4727)

Brain and Behavior

Open Access

REVIEW

# Epidemic of illicit drug use, mechanisms of action/addiction and stroke as a health hazard

Katherine Esse[1,2], Marco Fossati-Bellani[1], Angela Traylor[1,3] & Sheryl Martin-Schild[1,2]

[1]Stroke Program, Department of Neurology, Tulane University School of Medicine, 1440 Canal Street, TB-52, Suite 1000, New Orleans, Louisiana 70112-2715

[2]Department of Internal Medicine, Tulane University School of Medicine, 1440 Canal Street, TB-52, Suite 1000, New Orleans, Louisiana 70112-2715

[3]Department of Psychiatry & Behavioral Sciences, Tulane University School of Medicine, 1440 Canal Street, TB-52, Suite 1000, New Orleans, Louisiana 70112-2715

**Keywords**

Acute ischemic stroke, illicit drugs, intracerebral hemorrhage, subarachnoid hemorrhage, substance abuse.

**Correspondence**

Sheryl Martin-Schild, M.D., Ph.D., Stroke Program at Tulane University School of Medicine, Department of Neurology, 1440 Canal Street, TB-52, Suite 1000, New Orleans, LA 70112-2715. Tel: (504) 988-0972, Fax: (504) 988-6263. E-mail: smartin2@tulane.edu

Received: 18 April 2011; Accepted: 02 May 2011.

doi: 10.1002/brb3.7

## Abstract

Drug abuse robs individuals of their jobs, their families, and their free will as they succumb to addiction; but may cost even more: a life of disability or even life lost due to stroke. Many illicit drugs have been linked to major cardiovascular events and other comorbidities, including cocaine, amphetamines, ecstasy, heroin, phencyclidine, lysergic acid diethylamide, and marijuana. This review focuses on available epidemiological data, mechanisms of action, particularly those leading to cerebrovascular events, and it is based on papers published in English in PubMed during 1950 through February 2011. Each drug's unique interactions with the brain and vasculature predispose even young, healthy people to ischemic or hemorrhagic stroke. Cocaine and amphetamines have the strongest association with stroke. However, the level of evidence firmly linking other drugs to stroke pathogenesis is weak. Large epidemiological studies and systematic evaluation of each drug's action on the brain and cardiovascular system are needed to reveal the full impact of drug use on the population.

## Introduction

Approximately 2.2 million people reported current illicit drug use in the 2009 United States National Health Survey (Substance Abuse and Mental Health Services Administration 2010). Almost one million emergency department (ED) visits in the United States involved illicit drugs in 2007 (Drug Abuse Warning Network 2010). Though it is difficult to clearly associate deaths directly to drug exposure, an estimated 17,000 deaths were attributed to illicit drug use in 2000 (Mokdad et al. 2004). The major causes of death from drugs are overdose, suicide, AIDS, and accidents; however, cerebrovascular disease is a significant source of morbidity from drug use. Drug use may be the most common predisposing condition for stroke among patients under 35 years of age. In fact, drug abusers aged 15 to 44 years were 6.5 times more likely to have a stroke than nondrug users (Kaku and Lowenstein 1990). Of 422 patients aged 15–44 with acute ischemic stroke (AIS), 12.1% were found to have recent drug use and 4.7% had drug abuse as the likely cause of stroke (Sloan et al. 1998). Lastly, a large population-based study of 1935 patients with stroke diagnoses revealed that 14.4% of intracerebral hemorrhages (ICH) and 14.4% of AISs were associated with drug use (Westover et al. 2007). Despite this obvious connection between illicit drugs and stroke, epidemiologic data are hard to find. Most evidence that illegal drugs are risk factors for stroke is anecdotal (Brust 2002). Using the data from a number of case studies and a limited number of population studies, this article will outline various illicit drugs and their association to AIS, ICH, and subarachnoid hemorrhage (SAH).

The main illicit drugs associated with stroke are cocaine, amphetamines, Ecstasy, heroin/opiates, phencyclidine (PCP), lysergic acid diethylamide (LSD), and cannabis/marijuana. Tobacco and ethanol are also associated with stroke, but will not be discussed here. This article will outline current epidemiology, pharmacology, evidence related to strokes, and mechanisms of action related to stroke risk for each drug listed above. The table summarizes proposed stroke mechanisms for each reviewed drug and stroke subtype.

## Search strategy and selection criteria

References for this review were identified by searches of PubMed from 1950 until February 2011 with the terms "ischemic stroke," "intracerebral hemorrhage," "subarachnoid hemorrhage," "illicit drugs," "substance abuse," "cocaine," "amphetamines," "heroin," "marijuana," "phencyclidine," "lysergic acid diethylamide," and "Ecstasy." Articles were also identified through searches of the authors' own manuscripts and relevant publications. Only papers published in English were reviewed.

## Associated Drugs

### Cocaine

In the 1970s, recreational use of cocaine became widespread due to the production of crack cocaine, a purer and cheaper form of cocaine. The late 1980s saw an epidemic of cocaine: 30 million people of all socioeconomic backgrounds were cocaine users and 6 million were cocaine addicts (Agarwal and Sen 2010). In 2009, cocaine was the second-most commonly used illicit drug in the United States after marijuana. Of one million illicit drug-related ED visits yearly in the United States, nearly half are related to cocaine, making cocaine the most frequent cause of illicit drug-related ED visits (The DAWN report 2010).

#### Pharmacology

Cocaine comes in two chemical forms: the hydrochloride salt, which is the powdered form of cocaine that is water soluble, and cocaine alkaloid, a free base that is lipid soluble. The effects of cocaine include local anesthesia, vasoconstriction, and central nervous system stimulation. Cocaine prevents neurotransmitter (dopamine, norepinephrine, serotonin, and acetylcholine) reuptake at presynaptic nerve terminals, thereby increasing the amounts of neurotransmitters available for stimulation of sympathetic nerves. The euphoria related to cocaine use is a result of accumulation of dopamine and serotonin in the mesolimbic and mesocortical areas of the brain (Treadwell and Robinson 2007). These reward circuits are related to drug-seeking behavior, addiction, and dependence, making cocaine one of the most potent and highly addictive chemicals (Goforth et al. 2010).

#### Cocaine and stroke

As crack cocaine use increased in the 1970s and 1980s, case reports of cocaine-associated AIS, ICH, and SAH became more prevalent, which is especially striking given the young age at which strokes occurred. A review article in the late 1980s found that the mean age of patients with cocaine-related stroke was 32.5 years (Klonoff et al. 1989).

Case series characterizing the brain location and etiology of each type of cocaine-related stroke have been performed. Cocaine-associated AISs have been reported in nearly every vascular territory in the brain; anterior circulation, posterior circulation, spinal cord, brainstem, and retina have been affected (Brust 2002). Both cortical and subcortical strokes can occur (Daras et al.; Jacobs et al. 1989). The etiology of ischemic infarcts varies as well; large artery, small artery, and cardioembolic strokes all appear to be of relatively equal incidence (Martin-Schild et al. 2009).

While AIS is far more common than ICH or SAH overall, the frequency of hemorrhagic stroke is disproportionately high in cocaine-related strokes (Treadwell and Robinson 2007). Intracerebral hemorrhages are found throughout the brain, including basal ganglia, thalamus, lobar, brainstem, and cerebellar locations. While one study found mostly lobar locations (73% of 34 patients) (Kaku and Lowenstein 1990), a recent study of 45 cocaine users with ICH found predominantly ICH in the basal ganglia (Martin-Schild et al. 2010). This may depend on the prevalence of underlying hypertension in different populations. The prevalence of underlying vascular lesions in patients with cocaine-related ICH has been variable, ranging from 10% (Martin-Schild et al. 2010) to nearly 50% related to ruptured aneurysms or arteriovenous malformations (AVMs) (Brust 2002; Enevoldson 2004).

#### Mechanisms of strokes

The main etiologies that have been suggested include hypertensive surges, vasospasm, enhanced platelet aggregation, cerebral vasculitis, accelerated atherosclerosis, and cardioembolism (Treadwell and Robinson 2007).

Chronic uncontrolled hypertension is a major risk factor for stroke. Repeated use of cocaine can raise blood pressure, increasing the risk for stroke, even in patients who do not have baseline hypertension. Hypertensive surges may be responsible for the majority of hemorrhagic strokes associated with cocaine use.

Vasospasm is a fascinating mechanism for cocaine-induced stroke. Defined as sudden and usually reversible changes in vascular caliber due to vascular smooth muscle changes, vasospasm is more commonly encountered as a complication of SAH. A case study of cocaine users, however, found tunica media and elastic lamina damage in vessels in multiple locations in the brain possibly due to chronic vasospasm (Konzen

Stroke Mechanisms by Drug and Stroke Type

| | Acute Ischemic Stroke | Intracerebral Hemorrhage | Subarachnoid Hemorrhage |
|---|---|---|---|
| Cocaine | • Vasospasm<br>• Enhanced platelet aggregation<br>• Vasculitis<br>• Accelerated atherosclerosis<br>• Cardioembolism<br>○ Arrhythmia<br>○ Cardiomyopathy<br>○ Septic embolism | • Hypertensive surges<br>• Mycotic aneurysm rupture from cardioembolic event<br>• Hemorrhagic transformation of embolism | • Aneurysm rupture from hypertensive surges<br>• Facilitation of aneurysm formation |
| Amphetamines | • Cardioembolism<br>○ Arrhythmias with thrombosis<br>○ Cardiomyopathy<br>• Vasculitis<br>• Microinfarcts from blood vessel injury and accelerated atherosclerosis | • Hypertensive surge | • Aneurysms |
| Ecstasy | • Cardioembolism from:<br>○ Arrhythmias<br>○ Cardiomyopathy<br>• Vasospasm → Vessel wall damage<br>• Direct vasoconstrictive effect of Serotonin<br>• Hyperthermia→Clotting cascade/DIC → microinfarcts | • Hypertensive surge<br>• Vasodilation from decreased serotonin from chronic use<br>• Consumptive coagulopathy = spontaneous bleed | • Aneurysm formation and rupture |
| Heroin/Opiates | • Cardioembolism·<br>○ Endocarditis<br>○ Foreign bodies<br>• Arteritis/Vasculitis<br>• Hypotension/Hypoxemia | None | None |
| PCP | • Vasospasm? (only in vitro) | • Hypertensive effect | • Weakened arterial walls |
| LSD | • Vasospasm<br>• Direct vasoconstrictive effect of Serotonin | None | None |
| Marijuana | • Hypotension?<br>• Vasospasm?<br>• Cardioembolism from arrhythmias? | None | None |

et al. 1995). Radiographic studies (Kaufman et al. 1998) confirmed animal studies (He et al. 1994) that demonstrated a dose-dependent vasoconstriction of cerebral vessels on magnetic resonance angiography in response to cocaine.

The pathophysiology of vasospasm in cocaine use is multifactorial. Cocaine has effects on the calcium channels in smooth muscle cells in vascular walls. It promotes the release of calcium from the sarcoplasmic reticulum and also may allow influx of external calcium into the smooth muscle cells, causing contraction of the vessel walls. Accumulation of catecholamines caused by prevention of reuptake may result in smooth muscle contraction by an effect on several receptors in the vessel walls. This latter mechanism is supported by dopamine antagonist (haloperidol) and calcium channel blocker (verapamil) prevention of vasospasm in cocaine-exposed smooth muscle cells (He et al. 1994). Endothelin-1, an endogenous vasoactive peptide, has been implicated in the development of atherosclerosis and vasoconstriction. Endothelin-1 has been detected in the urine and serum of cocaine users. An endothelin-1 antagonist reversed cocaine-induced vasospasm in animal models (Fandino et al. 2003). Vasoconstriction may play a role in cocaine-related stroke even days after last cocaine use. Metabolized by the liver, cocaine has a half-life of approximately 1 hour, but major provasoconstrictive metabolites can last for days. There is also large variation among individuals, with metabolites lingering in chronic users for up to 3 weeks (Enevoldson 2004).

Vasospasm may cause endothelial injury, resulting in intimal hyperplasia and platelet activation and aggregation, ultimately occluding vessels (Treadwell and Robinson 2007). This may be why microvascular white matter changes are found on MRI in chronic cocaine users (Volkow et al. 1988; Goforth et al. 2010). Cocaine administration activates platelets resulting in $\alpha$-granule release and the formation of platelet-rich microaggregates (Heesch et al. 2000). It also increases platelet responsiveness to arachidonic acid, and causes the release of thromboxane $\beta 2$ and plasminogen activating factor-1 inhibitor (PAI-1). All of these factors promote platelet aggregation (Togna et al. 1985; Kolodgie et al. 1995) and facilitation of thrombus formation.

Very few cases of biopsy-proven vasculitis associated with cocaine exposure have been reported. These cases describe a hypersensitivity-type vasculitic morphology that differs from the typical inflammatory central nervous system vasculitis. Supporting this is the fact that in cases of presumed cocaine-induced vasculitis, steroids failed to improve the patient's symptoms in the short term (Merkel et al. 1995). Most studies have failed to demonstrate these findings on autopsy (Brust 2002; Enevoldson 2004).

Cocaine may promote accelerated atherosclerosis, leading to longer term increased risk for AIS in cocaine users. Rabbits with high cholesterol that were exposed to cocaine demonstrated a greater extent of cholesterol plaque in the proximal thoracic aorta than control rabbits (Kolodgie et al. 1993). In the presence of cocaine, cell membranes are more permeable to atherogenic lipoproteins (Kolodgie et al. 1993, 1995, 1999).

Cardioembolism is a well-known cause of cocaine-related stroke. Mechanisms of embolism and ischemic stroke include infective endocarditis in patients who inject cocaine hydrochloride, arrhythmia, acute and chronic dilated cardiomyopathy, and myocardial infarction (Sloan and Mattioni 1992). Cocaine use is highly associated with infective endocarditis: in one study of drug users with endocarditis, 79% were cocaine users (Chambers et al. 1987). In addition to embolization, endocarditis can cause a septic cerebral arteritis. Endocarditis provokes ICH from rupture of mycotic aneurysms and hemorrhagic transformation of embolic stroke (Hart et al. 1987; Enevoldson 2004; Hagan and Burney 2007).

Hypertensive surge with or without an underlying vascular malformation is the most common implicated etiology for ICH and SAH. The indirect sympathomimetic effects of cocaine transiently raise the systolic blood pressure, which can cause spontaneous bleeding in existing AVMs, aneurysms, or areas of old ischemic strokes, or may actually facilitate aneurysm formation (Nolte et al. 1995). Cocaine users with ICH have very high blood pressure on admission (Martin-Schild et al. 2009), and have blood in classic hypertensive locations. Brainstem hemorrhages were over-represented in patients with cocaine-associated ICH. Cocaine users with ICH have worse short-term functional outcome compared to patients with hemorrhage who are not cocaine users. In fact, cocaine users with ICH were nearly five times more likely to be dependent and three times more likely to die than patients with ICH who did not use cocaine (Martin-Schild et al. 2010). When SAH occurs in cocaine users, aneurysms are often detected on angiography (Oyesiku et al. 1993; Fessler et al. 1997).

## Amphetamines

Widespread amphetamine abuse began during World War II, when it was offered to soldiers to fight fatigue and improve morale. By the 1950s, there was an upswing in legal prescription of amphetamines in the United States. The manufacture and distribution of amphetamines was greatly reduced after the passage of the Controlled Substances Act in 1970. In the late 1980s and 1990s, however, amphetamines were back in vogue, due to the ease and low expense of synthesizing methamphetamines in amateur laboratories. As of 2000, an estimated 35 million people abused amphetamines worldwide, as compared with 15 million cocaine abusers (Albertson et al. 2007).

### Pharmacology

Amphetamines constitute a group of drugs with chemical similarity to the natural neurotransmitters epinephrine and dopamine. Synthetic modifications result in differing effects and properties. Each is a weak base and can be absorbed via multiple routes. Depending on the particular drug and dosage, the half-life can range from 10 to 30 hours. Methamphetamine (meth) is the most potent of amphetamines and is most commonly abused; it has a half-life of 12 hours, is metabolized through the liver, and has an active metabolite which is a potent hallucinogen.

Amphetamines block the presynaptic reuptake of the catecholamines dopamine, norepinephrine, and serotonin, allowing these neurotransmitters to remain in the synapse to trigger and saturate the postsynaptic receptors. The user feels euphoric and experiences increased motor movements, increased productivity, decreased appetite, and increased libido (Albertson et al. 1999; Winslow et al. 2007; Freye and Levy 2009). Amphetamines create strong effects of addiction, craving, and tolerance in chronic users (Freye and Levy 2009). Amphetamines have wide-ranging effects on nearly every organ system. Amphetamines have been linked to myocardial infarction, cardiomyopathy, renal failure, liver failure, respiratory failure, stroke, memory loss, confusion, and a many psychiatric symptoms.

### Amphetamines and stroke

Amphetamine use increases the odds of stroke by almost four times that of nonusers (Petitti et al. 1998) and results in greater disability and mortality rates (Westover et al. 2007). AIS, ICH, and SAHs have been reported in the literature. Most case series report a disproportionate rate of hemorrhagic stroke with amphetamine use, up to twice the risk of cocaine (odds ratio 4.95 vs. 2.33) (Westover et al. 2007).

### Mechanisms of stroke

Amphetamines, like cocaine, are sympathomimetic. Therefore, the mechanisms of stroke in amphetamine users are similar to those of cocaine-related strokes. Up to 75% of patients with methamphetamine-related stroke have significantly elevated blood pressures on arrival (Perez et al. 1999). Amphetamines may accelerate hypertensive heart disease with myocardial hypertrophy and interstitial fibrosis and cause direct myocardial toxicity with contraction-band necrosis (Yeo et al. 2007; Yi et al. 2008; Ito et al. 2009). Cardiomyopathy is a well-established complication of amphetamine abuse. Methamphetamine use is associated with a 3.7-fold increase in the odds of detecting cardiomyopathy (95% confidence interval: 1.8–7.8) (Yeo et al. 2007). Methamphetamine users with cardiomyopathy have lower left ventricular ejection fractions and higher end-diastolic and left atrial volumes than heart failure patients without methamphetamine use (Ito et al. 2009). Cardiomyopathy results in arrhythmias and thrombosis, leading directly to cardio-embolic strokes.

Unlike cocaine, an association between chronic amphetamine use, stroke and vasculitis have been reported. Angiography in multidrug abusers detected findings consistent with necrotizing periarteritis in multiple organs on angiography, and confirmed those findings, specifically in the central nervous system on autopsy of select cases. Amphetamines were the most commonly abused drug in these studies (Citron et al. 1970; Halpern and Citron 1971; Margolis and Newton 1971; Stafford et al. 1975; Wooten et al. 1983; Salanova and Taubner 1984; Shibata et al. 1991; Brust 1997; Ho et al. 2009).

Acute increase in systolic blood pressure during amphetamine use leads to spontaneous ICH (McGee et al. 2004). In fact, hemorrhagic strokes have been observed after only a single use of amphetamines (Stoessl et al. 1985). Most cases of ICH involve brain regions commonly affected in hypertensive ICH (Ho et al. 2009). Histopathological evidence support that repeated amphetamine abuse can result in blood vessel injury, leading to vessel wall necrosis, microinfarcts in small vessels, and atherosclerosis (McGee et al. 2004; Ho et al. 2009). Amphetamine-related SAHs mostly frequently report underlying aneurysms (Ho et al. 2009; Kaku and Lowenstein 1990).

### Ecstasy

Ecstasy is a nonspecific name for a variety of "designer drugs" used mainly by young adults. They are derivatives of amphetamine. The majority of Ecstasy in use is 3,4-methylenedioxymeth-amphetamine, or MDMA, N-ethyl-3,4-methylenedioxyamphetamine or MDEA (sometimes called "Eve"), or 3.4-methylenedioxyamphetamine (MDA). Recent epidemiological data indicate that Ecstasy use is increasing among college students (Strote et al. 2002).

### Pathophysiology

Though Ecstasy is derivative of amphetamine, the drug more closely resembles the hallucinogen mescaline, rendering it to be a blend of hallucinogenic and catecholaminergic effects. Ecstasy increases the release of, and inhibits the reuptake of, serotonin and norephinephrine, with lesser effects on dopamine. The toxicity, time course, and intensity of reaction can differ significantly between preparations. The drug is usually ingested in pill form, metabolized by the liver, and generally achieves peak concentration in the blood approximately two hours after ingestion.

### Ecstasy and stroke

There are no epidemiological studies specifically studying the incidence of Ecstasy-related strokes. There are a small number of case studies of both ischemic and hemorrhagic strokes occurring within hours of ingestion of Ecstasy (Hughes et al. 1993; Harries and De Silva 1992; Gledhill et al. 1993; Manchanda and Connolly 1993; Hanyu et al. 1995; Kalant 2001; Auer et al. 2002).

### Mechanisms of stroke

The vascular distribution of AISs related to Ecstasy use is variable. The possible etiologies of MDMA-induced stroke are similar to those of cocaine- and amphetamine-related strokes. Cardiac arrhythmias, have been implicated in Ecstasy-related cardiac death, and are potential causes of Ecstasy-related stroke via cardioembolism (Hughes et al. 1993). Cardiomyopathy has also been described in Ecstasy users and is associated with congestive heart failure, arrhythmia, and stroke.

After exposure to Ecstasy, vasospasm and necrosis have been observed in the vasculature of the globus pallidus and occipital cortex, making damage from AIS most likely in these areas (Reneman et al. 2000; Rojas et al. 2005; Hagan and Burney 2007). Damage to the vessel walls over time from chronic vasospasm and necrosis may also lead to both thrombosis and aneurysmal dilatation of cerebral vessels. This can then lead to AIS, ICH, or SAH (Kalant 2001; Auer et al. 2002). Ecstasy increases the bioavailability of serotonin, a potent vasoconstrictive amine, which decreases cerebral blood flow and can lead to cerebral infarction (Hanyu et al. 1995). Long-term use of Ecstasy results in decreased overall serotonin availability and vasodilation, and even ICH in the setting of hypertension (Reneman et al. 2000).

High fever, provoked by Ecstasy's activation of the hypothalamus, may trigger the clotting cascade, resulting in disseminated intravascular coagulation and microinfarcts throughout the body, including the brain, as well as bleeding due to consumptive coagulopathy (Kalant 2001; Freye and Levy 2009). Very little evidence supports vasculitis as a complication of Ecstasy use (Manchanda and Connolly 1993).

Hypertensive surge may lead to small-vessel ICH or large-vessel hemorrhage via rupture of an underlying cerebrovascular malformation. Esctasy-related ICH occurs in regions commonly affected by hypertension, and SAH is usually associated with an underlying aneurysm.

## Opiates/Heroin

Heroin is a semi-synthetic derivative of opium. Heroin addiction became a problem around the turn of the 20th century. The United States Department of Health and Human Services' National Household Survey on Drug Abuse Study estimated that in 2008, 3.8 million people over the age of 12 had used heroin during their lifetime. In 2009, 180,000 people in the United States used heroin for the first time, representing a significant increase from prior years (Substance Abuse and Mental Health Services Administration 2010).

### Pharmacology

Heroin binds to endogenous opiate receptors (mu, kappa, and delta) located throughout the body, including the brain and the spinal cord. The mu receptor is responsible for analgesia, euphoria, nervous system depression, respiratory depression, and constipation. Heroin, unlike morphine, is able to cross the blood–brain barrier very easily. Heroin tends to cause hypotension from decreased peripheral vascular resistance, bradycardia by inhibiting the baroreceptor reflex, and respiratory depression by slowing the brain's response to high $CO_2$ and low oxygen levels. When heroin is injected, the initial effect, or "rush," occurs within a few minutes and peaks at around 10 minutes. After this, sedation ensues and lasts about one hour.

### Stroke and heroin

Heroin and other opiates are known to cause severe morbidity and death from violence, overdose, AIDS, suicide, and sepsis. However, strokes associated with heroin/opiate use are rarely reported. Despite this scarce reporting, opiates were 16 times less likely to cause hemorrhagic strokes and five times less likely to cause ischemic stroke than amphetamines (Westover et al. 2007). Most reported strokes associated with heroin use are ischemic (Hagan and Burney 2007).

### Mechanisms of stroke

Heroin-associated stroke is most often due to cardioembolism in the setting of infective endocarditis (Hagan and Burney 2007). Another source for embolic disease from heroin use is foreign bodies that have been added to the heroin. Foreign bodies (potentially including starch, sugar, Ajax, quinine, lactose, mannitol, caffeine, aspirin, lidocaine, strychnine, and talcum powder) enter the circulation and become lodged in the lungs. A granulomatous reaction leads to pulmonary hypertension, causing or exacerbating right-to-left pulmonary shunts predisposing to cardioembolic strokes (Brust 1989; Lucas 2005).

Arteritis and vasculitis have also been indirectly implicated as a cause of heroin-related strokes. "Beading" on angiography along with supporting laboratory studies has been reported, but pathological evidence supporting this theory is lacking (Brust 1997) and it is not known if the vessel changes are in response to the heroin itself or adulterants. Other potential causes of stroke include hypotension and hypoxemia induced by opiate overdose; these can result in global hypoxic-ischemic injury to classically vulnerable areas of the brain (Andersen and Skullerud 1999).

## Phencyclidine (PCP)

Phencyclidine, known as PCP, is classified as a dissociative anesthetic similar to ketamine. The drug was initially introduced as an anesthetic that did not paralyze the diaphragm or cause respiratory depression, but it was pulled from the market due to reports of adverse neuropsychiatric reactions after anesthesia. PCP use has declined over time (Lerner and Burns 1978; Gahlinger 2004). The lifetime prevalence of PCP use in the United States was estimated at approximately 6.6 million people over the age of 12 (Substance Abuse and Mental Health Services Administration 2010).

### Pharmacology

The full range of PCP effects on the brain are incompletely understood, due to effects on multiple neurotransmitter pathways and receptors including N-methyl D-aspartate (NMDA) (antagonist) nicotinic acetylcholine (antagonists) and dopamine (agonist). Complicating the picture further, PCP may have its *own* receptors on cerebral vessels (Altura et al. 1983). Since PCP is stored in the body's fat, re-mobilization from those stores can cause recurrent symptoms for days to months. PCP is metabolized by the liver, and has multiple metabolites. Ten percent of the dose of phencyclidine is excreted unchanged in the urine, and can be picked up by a urine drug screen (Domino 1978; Gahlinger 2004; West et al. 2011).

### PCP and Stroke

A total of five cases of PCP-associated stroke were found in the literature—all of them were hemorrhagic. PCP's sympathomimetic hypertensive effect may be the provoking factor. Hypertension is one of the primary clinical findings in PCP intoxication (McCarron et al. 1981). Spikes of severe hypertension can occur hours to days after use. PCP-related SAH has been reported and may result from weakening of arterial walls (Boyko et al. 1987). While vasospasm can be provoked in vitro by PCP (Altura et al. 1983) in a dose-dependent manner at concentrations paralleling those of patients who overdosed on the drug, there are no reported cases confirming vasospasm in association with stroke in PCP users.

## LSD

Lysergic acid diethylamide, or LSD, is a potent hallucinogen. During the 1950s to 1970s, the psychiatric community extensively explored the use of LSD to treat psychosis, alcohol addiction, autism, and criminal behavior. Its current popularity is declining: the number of new users dropped from 958,000 in 2000 to 337,000 in 2009 (Mechem and Hall 2008; Substance Abuse and Mental Health Services Administration 2010).

### LSD and Stroke

Only four cases of stroke related to LSD have been reported in the literature. All of the cases involved AIS in patients under the age of 25 (Sobel et al. 1971; Lieberman et al. 1974). The two cases in which LSD was the sole drug used by the patients were cases that involved large-artery occlusions. Similar to ergot alkaloids, LSD affects serotonin receptors and may cause vessel constriction. In vitro, LSD produces significant vasospasm of cerebral arteries; this effect is reversed by a 5-HT antagonist (methysergide) or a calcium channel blocker (verapamil) (Altura and Altura 1981). Given the apparent ability of LSD to cause vasospasm in vitro, it is more likely that a vasospastic process is responsible for LSD-related strokes (Altura and Altura 1981).

## Marijuana

Marijuana is the most commonly used recreational drug in the United States, and 15 states have approved marijuana for medical use (State Medical Marijuana Laws 2010). More than 16.7 million people reported marijuana use within the past month on a national survey conducted in 2009 (Substance Abuse and Mental Health Services Administration 2010).

### Marijuana and Stroke

Evidence supporting marijuana's role in stroke is scarce, considering its widespread use. One study demonstrated an odds ratio for AIS with marijuana use of 1.76 (95% confidence interval 1.15–2.71), even when controlling for other risk factors (Kaku and Lowenstein 1990). Twenty-one cases of imaging-positive stroke related to marijuana use have been reported (Cooles and Michaud 1987; Zachariah 1991; Barnes et al. 1992; Lawson and Rees 1996; McCarron and Thomas 1997; Mouzak et al. 2000; Mesec et al. 2001; Mathew et al. 2003; Finsterer et al. 2004; Geller et al. 2004; Moussouttas 2004; Mateo et al. 2005; Aryana and Williams 2007; Duchene et al. 2010; Renard et al. 2010). Twenty were ischemic infarcts in men; one was an ischemic infarct in a woman (Duchene et al. 2010). No consistent pattern of infarct distribution was identified.

Proposed mechanisms for marijuana-associated cerebral infarction include hypotension, vasospasm, and arrhythmia with resulting cardioembolism (Cooles and Michaud 1987; Mathew et al. 2003; Geller et al. 2004; Moussouttas 2004; Mateo et al. 2005; Aryana and Williams 2007). Since these phenomena are often transient, the direct role in stroke is elusive. Cannabinoids have a role in cerebral autoregulation, vascular tone, and cardiac pathology (Mittleman et al. 2001; Mathew et al. 2003; Moussouttas 2004) and may provoke the reversible vasoconstriction syndrome associated with thunderclap headache, SAH, ICH, and cerebral ischemia (Ducros et al. 2007).

## Conclusion

Illicit drugs are used by millions of people every day. Based on an extensive review of the medical literature, it is apparent that these illicit drugs are dangerous for many reasons, and some of them appear to increase a person's risk for both ischemic and hemorrhagic strokes. The evidence is fairly clear that cocaine and amphetamines are strongly linked to stroke, but Ecstasy, opiates, phencyclidine, LSD, and marijuana simply do not have the burden of evidence required to firmly link usage to stroke pathogenesis. Unfortunately, the lack of standardization and the propensity for many of these drugs to be mixed with adulterants has muddied the picture of how these drugs act in the body. Further, the study of illicit drugs is hampered by the need for patient or surrogate disclosure or reliance on urine toxicology for which commonly used medications may result in a falsely positive urine drug test (Brahm et al. 2010). Regardless, future studies are needed to systematically evaluate how each of these chemicals acts on the cerebrovascular system. In addition, the lack of epidemiological studies on drugs and stroke hinders the ability of researchers to gain perspective on the impact that drug use may have on the population. Going forward, research on illicit drugs and their relationship to stroke and other morbidities is a responsibility that cannot be denied by those devoted to reducing the burden of stroke and cardiovascular health on society.

## References


Agarwal, P. and S. Sen. 2010. Neurologic effects of cocaine: eMedicine neurology. [homepage on the Internet]. Available from: http://emedicine.medscape.com/article/1174408-overview

Albertson, T. E., R. W. Derlet, and B. E. Van Hoozen. 1999. Methamphetamine and the expanding complications of amphetamines. West J. Med. 170:214–219.

Albertson, T. E., N. J. Kenyon, and B. Morrissey. 2007. Amphetamines and Derivatives. In: M. Shannon, S. W. Borron, and M. Burns, editors. Haddad and Winchester's clinical management of poisoning and drug overdose [Internet]. 4th ed. Philadephia (PA): Saunders Elsevier. Available from MD Consult.

Altura, B. T. and B. M. Altura. 1981. Phencyclidine, lysergic acid diethylamide, and mescaline: cerebral artery spasms and hallucinogenic activity. Science 212:1051–1052.

Altura, B. T., R. Quirion, C. B. Pert, and B. M. Altura. 1983. Phencyclidine ("angel dust") analogs and sigma opiate benzomorphans cause cerebral arterial spasm. Proc. Natl. Acad. Sci. USA 80:865–869.

Andersen, S. N. and K. Skullerud. 1999. Hypoxic/ischaemic brain damage, especially pallidal lesions, in heroin addicts. Forensic Sci. Int. 102:51–59.

Aryana, A. and M. A. Williams. 2007. Marijuana as a trigger of cardiovascular events: speculation or scientific certainty? Int. J. Cardiol. 118:141–144.

Auer, J., R. Berent, T. Weber, E. Lassnig, and B. Eber. 2002. Subarachnoid haemorrhage with "ecstasy" abuse in a young adult. Neurol. Sci. 23:199–201.

Barnes, D., J. Palace, and M. D. O'Brien. 1992. Stroke following marijuana smoking. Stroke 23:1381.

Boyko, O. B., P. C. Berger, and E. R. Heinz. 1987. Pathological and radiological correlation of subarachnoid hemorrhage in phencyclidine abuse. Case report. J. Neurosurg. 67:446–448.

Brahm, N. C., L. L. Yeager, M. D. Fox, K. C. Farmer, and T. A. Palmer. 2010. Commonly prescribed medications and potential false-positive urine drug screens. Am. J. Health Syst. Pharm. 67:1344–1350.

Brust, J. C. 2002. Neurologic complications of substance abuse. J. Acquir. Immune Defic. Syndr. 31(Suppl 2):S29–S34.

Brust, J. C. 1997. Vasculitis owing to substance abuse. Neurol. Clin. 15:945–957.

Brust, J. C. M. 1989. Stroke and drugs. In: P. J. Vinken, G. W. Bruyn, H. L. Klawans, and J. F. Toole, editors. Handbook of clinical neurology: Vascular diseases, part III. Vol. 55. Amsterdam (The Netherlands): Elsevier Science Publishers.

Chambers, H. F., D. L. Morris, M. G. Täuber, and G. Modin. 1987. Cocaine use and the risk for endocarditis in intravenous drug users. Ann. Intern. Med. 106:833–836.

Citron, B. P., M. Halpern, M. McCarron, G. D. Lundberg, R. McCormick, I. J. Pincus, *et al.* 1970. Necrotizing angiitis associated with drug abuse. N. Engl. J. Med. 283:1003–1011.

Cooles, P. and R. Michaud. 1987. Stroke after heavy cannabis smoking. Postgrad. Med. J. 63:511.

Daras, M., A. J. Tuchman, and S. Marks. Central nervous system infarction related to cocaine abuse. Stroke 22:1320–1325.

Domino, E. F. 1978. Neurobiology of phencyclidine—an update. NIDA Res. Monogr. 18–43.

Drug Abuse Warning Network. 2010. DAWN emergency department publications: 2007: National estimates of drug-related emergency department visits. [homepage on the Internet]. [cited 2010 Oct 16]. Available from: United States, Substance Abuse and Mental Health Services Web site: http://dawninfo.samhsa.gov/pubs/edpubs/

Duchene, C., S. Olindo, N. Chausson, S. Jeannin, P. Cohen-Tenoudji, and D. Smadja. 2010. Cannabis-induced cerebral and myocardial infarction in a young woman. Rev. Neurol. (Paris) 166:438–442.

Ducros, A., M. Boukobza, R. Porcher, M. Sarov, D. Valade, and M-G. Bousser. 2007. The clinical and radiological spectrum of reversible vasoconstriction syndrome. A prospective series of 67 patients. Brain 130:3091–3101.

Enevoldson, T. P. 2004. Recreational drugs and their neurologic consequences. J. Neurol. Neurosurg. Psychiatry 75(Suppl 3): iii9–iii15.

Fandino, J., J. D. Sherman, M. Zuccarello, and R. M. Rapoport. 2003. Cocaine-induced endothelin-1-dependent spasm in rabbit basilar artery in vivo. J. Cardiovasc. Pharmacol. 41:158–161.

Fessler, R. D., C. M. Esshaki, R. C. Stankewitz, R. R. Johnson, and F. G. Diaz. 1997. The neurovascular complications of cocaine. Surg. Neurol. 47:339–345.

Finsterer, J., P. Christian, and K. Wolfgang. 2004. Occipital stroke shortly after cannabis consumption. Clin. Neurol. Neurosurg. 106:305–308.

Freye, E. and J. V. Levy. 2009. Pharmacology and abuse of cocaine, amphetamines, ecstasy and related designer drugs: A comprehensive review on their mode of action, treatment of abuse and intoxication [Internet]. Dordrecht, Heidelberg, London, New York: Springer Science + Business Media.

Gahlinger, P. M. 2004. Club drugs: MDMA, gamma-hydroxybutyrate (GHB), Rohypnol, and ketamine. Am. Fam. Physician 69:2619–2626.

Geller, T., L. Loftis, and D. S. Brink. 2004. Cerebellar infarction in adolescent males associated with acute marijuana use. Pediatrics 113:e365–370.

Gledhill, J. A., D. F. Moore, D. Bell, and J. A. Henry. 1993. Subarachnoid haemorrhage associated with MDMA abuse. J. Neurol. Neurosurg. Psychiatry 56:1036–1037.

Goforth, H. W., R. Murtaugh, and F. Fernandez. 2010. Neurologic aspects of drug abuse. Neurol. Clin. 28:199–215.

Hagan, I. G. and K. Burney. 2007. Radiology of recreational drug abuse. Radiographics 27:919–940.

Halpern, M. and B. P. Citron. 1971. Necrotizing angiitis associated with drug abuse. Am. J. Roentgenol. Radium Ther. Nucl. Med. 111:663–671.

Hanyu, S., K. Ikeguchi, H. Imai, N. Imai, and M. Yoshida. 1995. Cerebral infarction associated with 3,4-methylenedioxymethamphetamine ('ecstasy') abuse. Eur. Neurol. 35:173.

Harries, D. P. and R. N. De Silva. 1992. Misuse of ecstasy. Br. Med. J 305:310.

Hart, R. G., K. Kagan-Hallet, and S. E. Joerns. 1987. Mechanisms of intracranial hemorrhage in infective endocarditis. Stroke 18:1048–1056.

He, G. Q., A. Zhang, B. T. Altura, and B. M. Altura. 1994. Cocaine-induced cerebrovasospasm and its possible mechanism of action. J. Pharmacol. Exp. Ther. 268:1532–1539.

Heesch, C. M., C. R. Wilhelm, J. Ristich, J. Adnane, F. A. Bontempo, and W. R. Wagner. 2000. Cocaine activates platelets and increases the formation of circulating platelet containing microaggregates in humans. Heart 83:688–695.

Ho, E. L., S. A. Josephson, H. S. Lee, and W. S. Smith. 2009. Cerebrovascular complications of methamphetamine abuse. Neurocrit. Care 10:295–305.

Hughes, J. C., M. McCabe, and R. J. Evans. 1993. Intracranial haemorrhage associated with ingestion of 'ecstasy'. Arch. Emerg. Med. 10:372–374.

Ito, H., K. K. Yeo, M. Wijetunga, T. B. Seto, K. Tay, and I. J. Schatz. 2009. A comparison of echocardiographic findings in young adults with cardiomyopathy: with and without a history of methamphetamine abuse. Clin. Cardiol. 32:E18–E22.

Jacobs, I. G., M. H. Roszler, J. K. Kelly, M. A. Klein, and G. A. Kling. 1989. Cocaine abuse: Neurovascular complications. Radiology 170(1 Pt 1):223–227.

Kaku, D. A. and D. H. Lowenstein. 1990. Emergence of recreational drug abuse as a major risk factor for stroke in young adults. Ann. Intern. Med. 113:821–827.

Kalant, H. 2001. The pharmacology and toxicology of "ecstasy" (MDMA) and related drugs. Can. Med. Assoc. J. 165:917–928.

Kaufman, M. J., J. M. Levin, M. H. Ross, N. Lange, S. L. Rose, T. J. Kukes, *et al.* 1998. J. Am. Med. Assoc. 279:376–380.

Klonoff, D. C., B. T. Andrews, and W. G. Obana. 1989. Stroke associated with cocaine use. Arch. Neurol. 46:989–993.

Kolodgie, F. D., A. Farb, and R. Virmani. 1995. Pathobiological determinants of cocaine-associated cardiovascular syndromes. Hum. Pathol. 26:583–586.

Kolodgie, F. D., P. S. Wilson, J. F. Cornhill, E. E. Herderick, W. J. Mergner, and R. Virmani. 1993. Increased prevalence of aortic fatty streaks in cholesterol-fed rabbits administered intravenous cocaine: the role of vascular endothelium. Toxicol. Pathol. 21:425–435.

Kolodgie, F. D., P. S. Wilson, W. J. Mergner, and R. Virmani. 1999. Cocaine-induced increase in the permeability function of human vascular endothelial cell monolayers. Exp. Mol. Pathol. 66:109–122.

Konzen, J. P., S. R. Levine, and J. H. Garcia. 1995. Vasospasm and thrombus formation as possible mechanisms of stroke related to alkaloidal cocaine. Stroke 26:1114–1118.

Lawson, T. M. and A. Rees. 1996. Stroke and transient ischemic attacks in association with substance abuse in a young man. Postgrad. Med. J. 72:692–693.

Lerner, S. E. and R. S. Burns. 1978. Phencyclidine use among youth: history, epidemiology, and acute and chronic intoxication. NIDA Res. Monogr. 21:66–118.

Lieberman, A. N., W. Bloom, P. S. Kishore, and J. P. Lin. 1974. Carotid artery occlusion following ingestion of LSD. Stroke 5:213–215.

Lucas, C. E. 2005. The impact of street drugs on trauma care. J. Trauma 59(3 Suppl):S57–S60.

Manchanda, S. and M. J. Connolly. 1993. Cerebral infarction in association with ecstasy abuse. Postgrad. Med. J. 69:874–875.

Margolis, M. T. and T. H. Newton. 1971. Methamphetamine ("speed") arteritis. Neuroradiology 2:179–182.

Martin-Schild, S., K. C. Albright, H. Hallevi, A. D. Barreto, M. Philip, V. Misra, *et al.* 2010. Intracerebral hemorrhage in cocaine users. Stroke 41:680–684.

Martin-Schild, S., K. C. Albright, V. Misra, M. Philip, Ad. Barreto, H. Hallevi, *et al.* 2009. Intravenous tissue plasminogen activator in patients with cocaine-associated acute ischemic stroke. Stroke 40:3635–3637.

Mateo, I., A. Pinedo, M. Gomez-Beldarrain, J. M. Basterretxea, and J. C. Garcia-Monco. 2005. Recurrent stroke associated with cannabis use. J. Neurol. Neurosurg. Psychiatry 76:435–437.

Mathew, R. J., W. H. Wilson, and R. Davis. 2003. Postural syncope after marijuana: a transcranial Doppler study of the hemodynamics. Pharmacol. Biochem. Behav. 75:309–318.

McCarron, M. M., B. W. Schulze, G. A. Thompson, M. C. Conder, and W. A. Goetz. 1981. Acute phencyclidine intoxication: incidence of clinical findings in 1,000 cases. Ann. Emerg. Med. 10:237–242.

McCarron, M. O. and A. M. Thomas. 1997. Cannabis and alcohol in stroke. Postgrad. Med. J. 73:448.

McGee, S. M., D. N. McGee, and M. B. McGee. 2004. Spontaneous intracerebral hemorrhage related to methamphetamine abuse: autopsy findings and clinical correlation. Am. J. Forensic Med. Pathol. 25:334–337.

Mechem, C. C. and A. H. Hall. 2008. CBRNE—Incapacitating agents, LSD: eMedicine emergency medicine. [homepage on the Internet]. Available from: http://emedicine.medscape.com/article/833040-overview

Merkel, P. A., W. J. Koroshetz, M. C. Irizarry, and M. E. Cudkowicz. 1995. Cocaine-associated cerebral vasculitis. Semin. Arthritis Rheum. 25:172–183.

Mesec, A., U. Rot, and A. Grad. 2001. Cerebrovascular disease associated with marijuana abuse: a case report. Cerebrovasc. Dis. 11:284–285.

Mittleman, M. A., R. A. Lewis, M. Maclure, J. B. Sherwood, and J. E. Muller. 2001. Triggering myocardial infarction by marijuana. Circulation 103:2805–2809.

Mokdad, A. H., J. S. Marks, D. F. Stroup, and Jl. Gerberding. 2004. Actual causes of death in the United States, 2000. J. Am. Med. Assoc. 291:1238–1245.

Moussouttas, M. 2004. Cannabis use and cerebrovascular disease. Neurologist 10:47–53.

Mouzak, A., P. Agathos, E. Kerezoudi, A. Mantas, and E. Vourdeli-Yiannakoura. 2000. Transient ischemic attack in heavy cannabis smokers—how 'safe' is it? Eur. Neurol. 44:42–44.

Nolte, K. B., L. M. Brass, and C. F. Fletterick. 1995. Neurology 46:1291–1296.

Oyesiku, N. M., A. R. Colohan, D. L. Barrow, and A. Reisner. 1993. Cocaine-induced aneurysmal rupture: an emergent negative factor in the natural history of intracranial aneurysms? Neurosurgery 32:518–525.

Perez, J. A. Jr., E. L. Arsura, and S. Strategos. 1999. Methamphetamine-related stroke: four cases. J. Emerg. Med. 17:469–471.

Petitti, D. B., S. Sidney, C. Quesenberry, and A. Bernstein. 1998. Stroke and cocaine or amphetamine use. Epidemiology 9:596–600.

Renard, D., G. Taieb, G. Gras-Combe, and P. Labauge. Cannabis-related myocardial infarction and cardioembolic stroke. J. Stroke Cerebrovasc. Dis. 2010 Sep 10; [epub ahead of print].

Reneman, L., J. B. Habraken, C. B. Majoie, J. Booij, and G. J. den Heeten. 2000. MDMA ("Ecstasy") and its association with cerebrovascular accidents: preliminary findings. Am. J. Neuroradiol. 21:1001–1007.

Rojas, R., R. Riascos, D. Vargas, H. Cuellar, and J. Borne. 2005. Neuroimaging in drug and substance abuse part I: cocaine, cannabis and ecstasy. Top Magn. Reson. Imaging 16:231–238.

Salanova, V. and R. Taubner. 1984. Intracerebral haemorrhage and vasculitis secondary to amphetamine use. Postgrad. Med. J. 60:429–430.

Shibata, S., K. Mori, I. Sekine, and H. Suyama. 1991. Subarachnoid and intracerebral hemorrhage associated with necrotizing angiitis due to methamphetamine abuse—an autopsy case. Neurol. Med. Chir (Tokyo) 31:49–52.

Sloan, M. A., S. J. Kittner, B. R. Feeser, J. Gardner, A. Epstein, M. A. Wozniak, *et al.* 1998. Illicit drug-associated ischemic stroke in the Baltimore-Washington Young Stroke Study. Neurology 50:1688–1693.

Sloan, M. A. and T. A. Mattioni. 1992. Concurrent myocardial and cerebral infarctions after intranasal cocaine use. Stroke 23:427–430.

Sobel, J., O. E. Espinas, and S. A. Friedman. 1971. Carotid artery obstruction following LSD capsule ingestion. Arch. Intern. Med. 127:290–291.

Stafford, C. R., B. M. Bogdanoff, L. Green, and H. B. Spector. 1975. Mononeuropathy multiplex as a complication of amphetamine angiitis. Neurology 25:570–572.

State Medical Marijuana Laws. [homepage on the Internet]. 2010. Available from: National Conference of State Legislatures Web site: http://www.ncsl.org/default.aspx?tabid=19587

Stoessl, A. J., G. B. Young, and T. E. Feasby. 1985. Intracerebral haemorrhage and angiographic beading following ingestion of catecholaminergics. Stroke 16:734–736.

Strote, J., J. E. Lee, and H. Wechsler. 2002. Increasing MDMA use among college students: results of a national survey. J. Adolesc. Health 30:64–72.

Substance Abuse and Mental Health Services Administration (SAMHSA). NSDUH: Latest national survey on drug use and health, substance abuse data, SAMHSA, office of applied studies. [homepage on the Internet]. 2010. Available from: United States, Department of Health and Human Services Web site: http://www.oas.samhsa.gov/nsduhLatest.htm

The DAWN report: Highlights of the 2009 drug abuse warning network (DAWN) findings on drug-related emergency department visits. [homepage on the Internet]. 2010. Available from: United States, Substance Abuse and Mental Health Services Web site: http://dawninfo.samhsa.gov/files/SpecTopics/DAWN2010`SR034.pdf

Togna, G., E. Tempesta, A. R. Togna, N. Dolci, B. Cebo, and L. Caprino. 1985. Haemostasis 15:100–107.

Treadwell, S. D. and T. G. Robinson. 2007. Cocaine use and stroke. Postgrad. Med. J. 83:389–394.

Volkow, N. D., A. Valentine, and M. Kulkarni. 1988. Radiological and neurological changes in the drug abuse patient: a study with MRI. J. Neuroradiol. 15:288–293.

West, P. L., N. J. Mckeown, and R. S. Helman. 2011. Phencyclidine toxicity: eMedicine Emergency Medicine. [homepage on the Internet]. Available from: http://emedicine.medscape.com/article/816348-overview

Westover, A. N., S. Mcbride, and R. W. Haley. 2007. Stroke in young adults who abuse amphetamines or cocaine. Arch. Gen. Psychiatry 64:495–502.

Winslow, B. T., K. I. Voorhees, and K. A. Pehl. 2007. Methamphetamine abuse. Am. Fam. Physician 76:1169–1174.

Wooten, M. R., M. S. Khangure, and M. J. Murphy. 1983. Intracerebral hemorrhage and vasculitis related to ephedrine abuse. Ann. Neurol. 13:337–40.

Yeo, K. K., M. Wijetunga, H. Ito, J. T. Efird, K. Tay, T. B. Seto, *et al.* 2007. The association of methamphetamine use and cardiomyopathy in young patients. Am. J. Med. 120:165–171.

Yi, S. H., L. Ren, T. T. Yang, L. Liu, H. Wang, and Q. Liu. 2008. Myocardial lesions after long-term administration of methamphetamine in rats. Chin. Med. Sci. J. 23:239–243.

Zachariah, S. B. 1991. Stroke after heavy marijuana smoking. Stroke 22:406–409.

# SECTION TWO:
# ADDICTION & MENTAL HEALTH RESOURCES

# MENTAL ILLNESS (GENERAL)

*Taking responsibility for your mental health is an important part of your personal health care. Individuals with a substance use disorder (SUD) and a behavioral addiction may also have a co-occurring mental disorder. A substance use disorder is a mental disorder that impacts the individual's brain and behavior. This disorder coupled with a mental disorder may lead to an inability to control the use of substances such as alcohol, illegal or legal drugs and others. Co-occurring mental disorders may include, for example, depression, anxiety disorders, bipolar disorder, personality disorders and attention-deficit hyperactivity disorder (ADHD). Behavioral addictions often interact with depression and anxiety disorders in an attempt to elevate or calm mood.*

While SUDs and mental disorders commonly occur together, one does not cause the other. Both addiction risks and mental disorder risks tend to run in families (familial), suggesting genes may be a risk factor. People with a mental disorder may seek out substances to make them feel better. For example, anxiety and depression may lead to self-medicating with alcohol or illegal drugs, or prescription drug abuse. If these substances make the individual feel better, the usage often escalates. Substance use and SUD may alter the brain structure and function leading to a greater chance of developing a mental disorder. Some prescription drugs may cause depression and anxiety and prescriptions should be managed to minimize the risk of mental health issues.

Over 60 percent of adolescents in substance use disorder treatment programs also meet diagnostic criteria for another mental illness. Research has shown that people with mental, personality and substance use disorders are at increased risk for non-medical use of prescription painkillers. Behavioral addiction, such as internet gaming addiction or overuse of social media, may also contribute to mental disorders such as ADHD and depression. Withdrawal to internet activities may contribute to a variety of personality disorders and mental health issues.

Seeking early intervention for both addiction and mental disorders is key to managing both conditions. Clear, honest communication with healthcare providers is necessary to receive the targeted help needed for both addiction and mental issues. Only by discussing feelings and symptoms can the individual be provided appropriate care. Understanding the early warning signs of mental health issues, even absent a diagnosis of addiction, may provide the best opportunity to remission and recovery. Early warning signs of mental health issues may be evident and may include:

- Persistent, sad or anxious mood
- Irritability
- Feeling hopeless
- Abusing alcohol or other substances to feel better, even temporarily
- Loss of interest in formerly enjoyed activities
- Lack of energy, talking slowly or moving slowly
- Restlessness

- Poor concentration or difficulty making decisions
- Sleep problems, too little or too much
- Vague physical symptoms
- Changes in appetite or weight
- Thoughts of death or suicide

Behavioral health treatments and services will help individuals with both common mental illnesses and substance use disorders. Counseling, psychotherapies, outpatient and inpatient treatment programs and other interventions will help change behaviors, thoughts and emotions. Medications may be needed. Early treatment is the best approach to insuring remission and recovery. Understanding oneself is necessary to controlling substance use disorders and behavioral disorders such as a gambling addiction. Treatments must be individualized and tailored to the addiction and mental disorder being addressed.

Substance use, behavioral addictions and mental disorders respond to prevention and early intervention strategies. Education about use and misuse of chemical agents and escapist activities and provider training is critical. Only by discussing feelings and symptoms can the individual be directed to appropriate care. Clear and honest communication is necessary to receive the targeted help needed for both addiction and mental issues. Never be afraid to be open and honest with the healthcare provider. Taking the first step in sharing concerns will ultimately lead to a better quality of life.

## Agencies & Associations

1 **Action Autonomie**
3958 Rue Dandurand 514-525-5060
Montreal, Quebec, H1X-1P7 Fax: 514-525-5580
lecollectif@actionautonomie.qc.ca
www.actionautonomie.qc.ca
Community organization for individuals with mental illness who unite their efforts collectively in order to defend their rights. Action Autonomie educates others on their rights while navigating the mental health care system.

2 **American Academy of Child and Adolescent Psychiatry (AACAP)**
3615 Wisconsin Avenue NW 202-966-7300
Washington, DC 20016 Fax: 202-464-0131
communications@aacap.org
www.aacap.org
Promotes the healthy development of children, adolescents, and families through advocacy, education, and research.
*Warren Y.K. Ng, MD, MPH, President*
*Debra E. Koss, MD, Secretary*

3 **American Association on Intellectual and Developmental Disabilities**
8403 Colesville Road 202-387-1968
Silver Spring, MD 20910 Fax: 202-387-2193
www.aaidd.org
Promotes progressive policies, scientific research, effective practices, and universal human rights for people with intellectual and developmental disabilities.
*Margaret A. Nygren, EdD, Executive Director & CEO*

4 **American Psychiatric Association**
800 Maine Avenue SW 202-559-3900
Washington, DC 20024 apa@psych.org
www.psychiatry.org
A medical specialty society representing a growing membership of psychiatrists. Offers information for psychiatrists, medical students, patients and families.

5 **American Psychological Association**
750 First Street NE 202-336-5500
Washington, DC 20002 800-374-2721
TTY: 202-336-6123
www.apa.org
Advances the creation, communication, and application of psychological knowledge to benefit society and improve people's lives.
*Frank C. Worrell, PhD, President*
*Jean A. Carter, PhD, Treasurer*

6 **Association of Children's Residential & Community Services**
648 North Plankinton Avenue 877-332-2272
Milwaukee, WI 53203 info@togetherthevoice.org
togetherthevoice.org
A national organization focused on providing residential therapeutic treatment for children and adolescents with behavioral health disorders.
*Kari Sisson, Executive Director*

7 **Canadian Federation of Mental Health Nurses**
850 Mitchell St. administration@cfmhn.ca
Fredericton, N.B., E3B-6C5 www.cfmhn.ca
A national voice for psychiatric and mental health nurses in Canada, providing resources relevant to the field.
*Sarah Flogen, President*
*Stephanie Svensson, Secretary*

8 **Canadian Mental Health Association (CMHA)**
250 Dundas St. W. 416-646-5557
Toronto, Ontario, ON M5T-2Z5 info@cmha.ca
www.cmha.ca
Promotes the mental health of all and supports the recovery of people experiencing mental illness.
*Margaret Eaton, National CEO*
*Zainab Jibril-Babaita, National Operations Coordinator*

9 **Coalition of Behavioral Health**
14 Penn Plaza 212-742-1600
New York, NY 10122 thecoalition@coalitionny.org
www.coalitionny.org
An advocacy organization of New York's mental health community representing over 100 non-profit community health agencies that serve clients in the five boroughs of New York City.
*Amy Dorin, President & CEO*
*Marissa Williams, Policy & Advocacy Manager*

10 **Community Access, Inc.**
17 Battery Place 212-780-1400
New York, NY 10004 www.communityaccess.org
A non-profit agency providing housing and advocacy for people with disabilities.
*Christopher Alcazar, Chief Operating Officer*
*Justin Barron, Director, Community Engagement Services*

11 **Family Action Network**
P.O. Box 322 765-643-4357
Winnetka, IN 60093-0322 info@familyactionnetwork.net
www.familyactionnetwork.net
An organization that curates a high-quality speaker series. The program is free and open to the public.
*Lonnie Stonitsch, Executive Director*
*Annemarie Anderson, Director, Operations*

12 **Goodwill Industries International, Inc.**
15810 Indianola Drive contactus@goodwill.org
Rockville, MD 20855 www.goodwill.org
A nonprofit, community-based organization whose mission is to help people achieve self-sufficiency through the dignity and power of work, serving people who are disadvantaged, disabled or elderly. The mission is accomplished through providing independent living skills, affordable housing, and training and placement in community employment. The GoodWill Network includes 160 independent, local locations across the U.S. and Canada.
*Ned Helms, Chair*
*Steven C. Preston, President & CEO*

13 **Goodwill Industries-Suncoast, Inc.**
727-523-1512
888-279-1988
TTY: 727-579-1068
www.goodwill-suncoast.org
A nonprofit, community-based organization whose mission is to help people achieve self-sufficiency through the dignity and power of work, serving people who are disadvantaged, disabled or elderly. The mission is accomplished through providing independent living skills, affordable housing, and training and placement in community employment.
*Sandra Young, Chair*
*Deborah A. Passerini, President & CEO*

14 **JIMHO Affiliated Centers (Justice in Mental Health Organization)**
520 Cherry Street 517-371-2221
Lansing, MI 48933 Fax: 517-371-2221
brwellwood@yahoo.com
www.jimho.org
JIMHO advocates for the rights and dignity that all people suffering from mental or emotional illness deserve.

15 **Mental Health America**
500 Montgomery Street 703-684-7722
Alexandria, VA 22314 800-969-6642
Fax: 703-684-5968
mhanational.org
Mental Health America is a community-based nonprofit organization committed to enabling the mental wellness of all Americans. MHA advocates for greater access to quality health services and seeks to educate individuals on identifying symptoms, as well as intervention and prevention.
*Schroeder Stribling, President & CEO*

16 **Mentally Ill Kids in Distress**
2642 E. Thomas Road
Phoenix, AZ 85016
602-253-1240
800-35M-IKID
Fax: 602-253-1250
Phoenix@MIKID.org
www.mikid.org
MIKD offers support, education, and skills development to families and children experiencing mental health and behavior challenges in Arizona and Colorado.
*Erin Callinan, President*
*Sean Gunderson, Vice President*

17 **National Alliance for Hispanic Health**
www.healthyamericas.org
Members are Spanish-speaking mental health professionals and patients and those interested in services and decision-making that consider culture and community.
*Sheila E. Raviv, M.A., Secretary*
*Don Liebentritt, J.D., Treasurer*

18 **National Alliance on Mental Illness (NAMI)**
4301 Wilson Blvd.
Arlington, VA 22203
703-524-7600
800-950-6264
www.nami.org
Committed to building better lives for the millions of Americans affected by mental illness by raising awareness and offering community support.
*Joyce A. Campbell, President*
*Daniel H. Gillison, Jr., CEO*

19 **National Association of State Mental Health Program Directors (NASMPHD)**
675 N. Washington St.
Alexandria, VA 22314
703-739-9333
www.nasmhpd.org
Offers referrals to state mental health programs, services and physicians for persons with mental illness.
*Brian Hepburn, MD, Executive Director*
*Aaron J. Walker, MPA, Policy Director*

20 **National Council for Behavioral Health**
1400 K Street NW
Washington, DC 20005
202-684-7457
communications@thenationalcouncil.org
www.thenationalcouncil.org
Represents community mental health centers working on Capitol Hill to ensure funding for community mental health services. Offers technical support and guidance and serves as a liaison with state organizations and other mental health related organizations.
*Linda Rosenberg, MSW, President & CEO*
*Jeannie Campbell, Executive Vice President & COO*

21 **National Federation of Families**
15800 Crabbs Branch Way
Rockville, MD 20855
240-403-1901
ffcmh@ffcmh.org
www.ffcmh.org
Provides leadership to develop and sustain a nationwide network of family-run organizations.
*Joy Hogge, President*
*Lynda Gargan, PhD, Executive Director*

22 **National Institute of Mental Health**
6001 Executive Boulevard
Bethesda, MD 20892-9663
866-615-6464
nimhinfo@nih.gov
www.nimh.nih.gov
The National Institute of Mental Health works to transform the understanding and treatment of mental illnesses through basic and clinical research, paving the way for prevention, recovery, and cure.
*Joshua A. Gordon, M.D., Ph. D., Director*

23 **Option Institute**
2080 S. Undermountain Road
Sheffield, MA 01257
413-229-2100
800-714-2779
Fax: 413-229-8931
participantsupport@option.org
www.option.org
Self-defeating beliefs, along with attitudes and judgments, can lead to a host of physical and psychological challenges. The Option Institute offers programs designed to help people gain new perspectives on the attitudes and judgments that may be affecting their lives.
*Barry Kaufman, Co-Founder*
*Samahria Lyte Kaufman, Co-Founder*

24 **Parent Professional Advocacy League**
77 Rumford Avenue
Waltham, MA 02453
866-815-8122
Fax: 617-542-7832
info@ppal.net
www.ppal.net
An organization of families of children with mental, emotional or behavioral needs and concerned professionals. PPAL support groups are run in many areas across the country.
*Pam Sager, Executive Director*
*Meri Viano, Associate Director*

25 **United Advocates for Children and Families**
3133 Arden Way
Sacramento, CA 95825
916-692-8087
info@uacf4hope.org
www.uacf4hope.org
UACF education, training, and technical assistance programs and services to children and youth with mental, emotional, and behavioral challenges.

26 **World Federation for Mental Health**
wfmh.global
International organization dedicated to improving the care and treatment of individuals with mental disorders, and raising public awareness and understanding of mental health.
*Nasser Loza, President*
*Andrew Mohanraj, Treasurer*

## *Alaska*

27 **NAMI: Alaska**
P.O. Box 201753
Anchorage, AK 99520
907-272-0227
800-950-6264
info@namianchorage.org
namialaska.org
*Dick Fagnant, President*
*Ann Ringstad, Executive Director*

## *Arizona*

28 **NAMI: Arizona**
5025 E. Washington Street
Phoenix, AZ 85034
480-994-4407
namiarizona.org

## *Arkansas*

29 **NAMI: Arkansas**
1012 Autumn Road
Little Rock, AR 72211
501-661-1548
800-844-0381
Fax: 501-312-7540
help@namiarkansas.org
namiarkansas.org
*Chris Beckers, LPN, President*
*Buster Lackey, PhD, LPC, LADAC, Executive Director*

## *California*

30 **NAMI: California**
425 University Avenue
Sacramento, CA 95825
916-567-0163
info@namica.org
www.namicalifornia.org
*Joseph Farrow, President*
*Jessica Cruz, Chief Executive Officer*

## *Colorado*

31 **FFCMH: Colorado**
7475 W. 5th Ave.
Lakewood, CO 80226
888-429-3369
ian@leepetersoncpa.com
www.coloradofederation.org

32 **NAMI: Colorado**
3333 S. Bannock St.
Englewood, CO 80110
303-321-3104
info@namicolorado.org
www.namicolorado.org

*Babu George Mathew, President*
*Ray Merenstein, Executive Director*

## *Delaware*

33 **Mental Health Association in Delaware**
100 W. 10th St.
Wilmington, DE 19801-6604
302-654-6833
jlafferty@mhainde.org
www.mhainde.org

*Larence Kirby, Ph.D., LPCMH, President*
*Victoria Kim Chang, Ed.D., Vice President*

34 **NAMI: Delaware**
2400 W 4th Street
Wilmington, DE 19805
302-427-0787
Fax: 302-427-2075
namide@namide.org
www.namide.org

*Joshua Thomas, CEO & Executive Director*

## *District of Columbia*

35 **NAMI: District of Columbia**
1629 K. St. NW
Washington, DC 20006-1631
202-466-0972
namidc@namidc.org
www.namidc.org
*Jean Harris, MSN, RN, CNA, President & Interim Executive Director*

## *Florida*

36 **Federation of Families of Florida, Inc.**
101 Nw 1st Ave.
South Bay, FL 33493
561-518-7997
Fax: 813-974-7712
info@flfamilies.net
www.federationoffamilies.org

37 **NAMI: Florida**
P.O. Box 961
Tallahassee, FL 32302
850-671-4445
850-671-4445
Fax: 850-671-5272
info@namiflorida.org
www.namiflorida.org

*Ashley Grimes, President*
*Jarrod Strickland, Executive Director*

## *Georgia*

38 **NAMI: Georgia**
4120 Presidential Pkwy.
Atlanta, GA 30340-3776
770-234-0855
800-728-1052
Fax: 770-234-0237
namigeorgia@namiga.org
www.namiga.org

*Ron Koon, President*
*Kim H. Jones, Executive Director*

## *Hawaii*

39 **NAMI: Hawaii**
770 Kapiolani Boulevard
Honolulu, HI 96813-5240
808-591-1297
info@namihawaii.org
namihawaii.org

*6 pages*
*Kumi MacDonald, Executive Director*
*Anisa Wiseman, Program Director*

## *Idaho*

40 **FFCMH: Idaho**
704 North 7th Street
Boise, ID 83702
208-433-8845
800-905-3436
Fax: 208-433-8337
info@idahofederation.org
www.idahofederation.org

*Ruth York, Executive Director*
*Michelle Batten, Family Engagement Director*

41 **NAMI: Idaho**
P.O. Box 2256
Boise, ID 83701
idahonami@gmail.com
namiidaho.org
*Christina Cernansky, President*
*Beth Markley, CFRE, Executive Director*

## *Illinois*

42 **NAMI: Illinois**
101 North Wacker Dr.
Chicago, IL 60606
217-522-1403
nami@namiillinois.org
namiillinois.org

*John Schladweiler, President*
*Andy Wade, Executive Director*

## *Indiana*

43 **NAMI: Indiana**
921 E. 86th St.
Indianapolis, IN 46240-1841
317-925-9399
800-677-6442
info@namiindiana.org
www.namiindiana.org

*Barbara Thompson, Executive Director*
*Linda Williams, Program Director*

## *Iowa*

44 **NAMI: Iowa**
3839 Merle Hay Rd.
Des Moines, IA 50322
515-254-0417
info@namiiowa.org
www.namiiowa.com

*Jim Romar, President*
*Peggy Huppert, Executive Director*

## *Kansas*

45 **NAMI: Kansas**
1801 SW Wanamaker Rd.
Topeka, KS 66604
785-233-0755
resources@namikansas.org
namikansas.org

*David Schmitt, President*
*Sherrie Vaughn, Executive Director*

## *Kentucky*

46 **K.Y. Partnership for Families and Children**
600 Teton Trail
Frankfort, KY 40601
502-875-1320
800-369-0533
www.kypartnership.org

47 **NAMI: Kentucky**
201 Mechanic Street
Lexington, KY 40507
859-225-6264
888-338-4164
Fax: 859-423-1200
namiky.org

*Melony Cunningham, Executive Director*

## *Louisiana*

48 **NAMI: Louisiana**
P.O. Box 1509
Baton Rouge, LA 70821-1509
225-291-6262
866-851-6264
Fax: 225-291-6244
info@namilouisiana.org
www.namilouisiana.org

*Antonio P.D. Carriere, MPA, President*
*LaShonda G. Williams, Executive President*

## *Maine*

49 **NAMI: Maine**
52 Water Street
Hallowell, ME 04347
207-622-5767
800-464-5767
Fax: 207-621-8430
info@namimaine.org
www.namimaine.org

*Michael Pooler, President*
*Jennifer Thompson, Executive Director*

## Maryland

50 **The Arc Maryland**
8601 Robert Fulton Drive
Columbia, MD 21046
410-571-9320
Marge_Samels@umail.umd.edu
*Lori Scott, President*
*Guy Stephens, Vice Preisdent*

## Massachusetts

51 **NAMI: Massachusetts**
331 Montvale Ave.
Woburn, MA 01801-4675
617-580-8541
Fax: 617-580-8673
info@namimass.org
www.namimass.org
*Annabel Lane, President*
*Amanda Stone, Comms. & Public Policy Specialist*

## Michigan

52 **Association for Children's Mental Health**
6017 W Street Joseph Highway
Lansing, MI 48917
517-372-4016
888-226-4543
Fax: 517-372-4032
jshank@acmh-mi.org
www.acmh-mi.org
ACMH provides parent-to-parent support; education, networking, and leadership opportunities; and information dissemination to families across Michigan struggling with emotional, behavioral, or mental health challenges.
*Jane Shank, Executive Director*

53 **NAMI: Michigan**
401 S. Washington
Lansing, MI 48933
517-485-4049
info@namimi.org
namimi.org
*Steve Slayton, Board President*
*Kevin Fischer, Executive Director*

## Minnesota

54 **Minnesota Association for Children's Mental Health**
23 Empire Drive
St. Paul, MN 55103
651-644-7333
800-528-4511
Fax: 651-644-7391
info@macmh.org
www.macmh.org
MACMH promotes positive mental health and offers resources to communities across Minnesota, including as publications, events, and support groups.
*Brandon Jones, MD, Executive Director*
*Rachael Jacques, Director, Development & Programming*

55 **NAMI: Minnesota**
1919 University Avenue West
St. Paul, MN 55104
651-645-2948
Fax: 651-645-7379
namihelps@namimn.org
namims.org
*Mariah Owens, President*
*Sue Abderholden, Executive Director*

## Mississippi

56 **Mississippi Families as Allies**
840 E. River Place
Jackson, MS 39202
601-355-0915
800-833-9671
Fax: 601-355-0919
info@faams.org
www.faams.org
Families as Allies is a statewide organization that offers support, resources, and events for families of children with behavioral health challenges.
*Joy Hogge, PhD, Executive Director*
*Dominic Deleo, Communications Director*

57 **NAMI: Mississippi**
298 Commerce Park Drive
Jackson, MS 39206
601-899-9058
800-357-0388
Fax: 601-956-6380
stateoffice@namims.org
www.namims.org
*Sitaniel Johnson Wimbley, Executive Director*

## Missouri

58 **NAMI: Missouri**
3405 W. Truman Blvd.
Jefferson City, MO 65109
573-634-7727
info@namimissouri.org
namimissouri.org
*12 pages*
*Holly Miles, President*
*Gena Terlizzi, Executive Director*

## Montana

59 **Family Support Network**
1002 10th Street W
Billings, MT 59102
406-256-7783
Fax: 406-256-9879
info@mtfamilysupport.org
www.mtfamilysupport.org
Offers intervention, support, and assistance to children diagnosed with mental illness. Serves communities in the Yellowstone, Big Horn, Musselshell, Carbon, Sweet Grass, and Stillwater counties.
*Shawn Byrne, MSW, Executive Director*
*Nancy Farrar, Operations Director*

60 **NAMI: Montana**
P.O. Box 1021
Helena, MT 59624
406-443-7871
888-280-6264
Fax: 406-862-6352
colleen@namimt.org
namimt.org
*Matt Kuntz, Executive Director*

## Nevada

61 **NAMI: Nevada**
100 N. Arlington Ave.
Reno, NV 89501
775-470-5600
Fax: 775-329-1618
info@naminevada.org
naminevada.org
*Robin V. Reedy, Executive Director*

## New Hampshire

62 **NAMI: New Hampshire**
85 North State Street
Concord, NH 03301
603-225-5359
800-242-6264
Fax: 603-228-8848
info@naminh.org
www.naminh.org
*Todd E. Donovan, President*
*Susan Stearns, Executive Director*

## New Jersey

63 **All Access Mental Health**
819 Alexander Road
Princeton, NJ 08540
609-452-2088
Fax: 609-452-0627
info@aamh.org
www.aamh.org
This organization was founded to create a permanent community support system for mentally ill and developmentally disabled adults and their families. Serves the Greater Mercer County area of New Jersey.
*Cynthia Murphy, President*
*Suzanne Caimi Lynn, Treasurer*

64 **NAMI: New Jersey**
1562 Route 130
North Brunswick, NJ 08902
732-940-0991
866-626-4664
info@naminj.org
www.naminj.org

*Joyce A. Campbell, President*
*Daniel H. Gillison, Jr., CEO*

## *New Mexico*

65 **NAMI: New Mexico**
3900 Osuna Rd NE
Albuquerque, NM 87109
505-260-0154
naminewmexico.org
*Sherri Rhoten, President*
*Gabrielle Dietrich, Executive Director*

## *New York*

66 **Families Together in New York State**
737 Madison Avenue
Albany, NY 12208
518-432-0333
Fax: 518-434-6478
info@ftnys.org
www.ftnys.org

A family-run organization that serves children with social, emotional, behavioral and cross-systems challenges.
*Paige Pierce, Executive Director*
*Daphnne Brown, Deputy Director*

67 **Mental Health Association in Dutchess County**
253 Mansion Street
Poughkeepsie, NY 12601
845-473-2500
info@mhadutchess.org
mhadutchess.org

The Mental Health Association in Dutchess County promotes positive mental health, providing rehabilitation programs and support services for adults with a history of mental illness.
*Paul Ackermann, President*
*Michael Hawkins, Vice President*

68 **Mental Health Association in Orange County**
Mental Health Association of Orange County
73 James P. Kelly Way
Middletown, NY 10940
845-342-2400
Fax: 845-343-9665
www.mhaorangeny.com

Mental Health Association of Orange County/MHA is a private, not-for-profit organization seeking to promote the mental health and emotional well being of Orange County residents. Under the leadership of a volunteer Board of Directors, MHA's staff members, consultants and volunteers provide free mental health services to thousands of Orange County residents each year. Several volunteers answer several hotlines, provide companionship, public education, direct services and assist with fundraisers.
*Angela Jo Henze, Executive Director*
*Deborah de Jong, Associate Executive Director*

69 **NAMI: New York**
150 Broadway
Menands, NY 12204
518-462-2000
Fax: 518-462-3811
info@naminys.org
www.naminys.org

*Mary Bartlett, President*
*Ann Canastra, Treasurer*

## *North Dakota*

70 **FFCMH: North Dakota**
523 N. 4th St.
Bismarck, ND 58501
701-222-3310
877-822-6287
Fax: 701-222-3310
cmccleary@ndffcmh.com
ndffcmh.org

## *Ohio*

71 **NAMI: Ohio**
1225 Dublin Road
Columbus, OH 43215
614-224-2700
800-686-2646
Fax: 614-224-5400
TTY: 866-924-1478
namiohio@namiohio.org
www.namiohio.org

*Judge Judy Campbell, President*
*Luke Russell, Executive Director*

## *Oklahoma*

72 **NAMI: Oklahoma**
P.O. Box 1306
El Reno, OK 73036
405-601-8283
800-583-1264
info@namioklahoma.org
www.namioklahoma.org

*Kelly Willingham, President*
*Lorna Palmer, Executive Director*

## *Oregon*

73 **NAMI: Oregon**
147 SE 102nd Ave.
Portland, OR 97216
503-230-8009
800-343-6264
namioregon@namior.org
namior.org

*Andrew Grover, President*
*Chris Bouneff, Executive Director*

74 **Oregon Family Support Network**
7110 SW Fir Loop
Tigard, OR 97223
503-430-0917
info@ofsn.net
www.ofsn.org

*Melissa First, Supervisor*
*Sandy Bumpus, Executive Director*

## *Pennsylvania*

75 **NAMI Keystone: Pennsylvania**
105 Braunlich Drive
Pittsburgh, PA 15237
412-366-3788
888-264-7972
info@namikeystonepa.org
www.namikeystonepa.org

*Kathy Testoni, President*
*Charma D. Dudley, PhD, FPPR, Vice President*

## *Rhode Island*

76 **NAMI: Rhode Island**
154 Waterman St.
Providence, RI 02906
401-331-3060
Fax: 401-274-3020
info@namirhodeisland.org
www.namirhodeisland.org

*Stephen Duryea, President*
*Beth Lamarre, Executive Director*

## *South Carolina*

77 **NAMI: South Carolina**
1735 St. Julian Place
Columbia, SC 29204
800-788-5131
namisc@namisc.org
www.namisc.org

*Bill Lindsey, Executive Director*
*Sharyn Pittman, Program Coordinator*

## *South Dakota*

78 **NAMI: South Dakota**
1601 E. 69th Street
Sioux Falls, SD 57108
605-271-1871
800-551-2531
namisd@midconetwork.com
namisouthdakota.org

*Chritie Lueth, President*
*Sheri Nelson, Executive Director*

### Tennessee

79 **NAMI: Tennessee**
1101 Kermit Drive 615-361-6608
Nashville, TN 37217 800-467-3589
www.namitn.org

*Jeff Fladen, Executive Director*
*Roger Stewart, Deputy Director*

### Texas

80 **FFCMH: Texas**
7800 Shoal Creek Road 512-407-8844
Austin, TX 78752 866-893-3264
Fax: 512-407-8266
info@txffcmh.org
www.txffcmh.org

81 **NAMI: Texas**
P.O. Box 300817 512-693-2000
Austin, TX 78703 www.namitexas.org
*Greg Hansch, LMSW, Executive Director*
*Alyssa Lopez, Operations Manager*

### Utah

82 **NAMI: Utah**
1600 West 2200 South 801-323-9900
West Valley City, UT 84119 877-230-6264
Fax: 801-323-9799
www.namiut.org

*Rob Wesemann, Executive Director*
*Jayden Drake, State Programs Coordinator*

### Vermont

83 **FFCMH: Vermont**
P.O. Box 1577 802-876-7021
Williston, VT 05495 800-639-6071
Fax: 802-329-2135
vffcmh@vffcmh.org
www.vffcmh.org

*John Pierce, President*
*Sandi Yandow, Executive Director*

84 **NAMI: Vermont**
600 Blair Park Road 802-876-7949
Williston, VT 05495 800-639-6480
info@namivt.org
namivt.org

*Chip Siler, President*
*Laurie Emerson, Executive Director*

### Virginia

85 **NAMI: Virginia**
P.O. Box 8260 888-486-8264
Richmond, VA 23226-0260 info@namivirginia.org
www.namivirginia.org

*Tom Spurlock, President*
*Kathy Harkey, Executive Director*

### Washington

86 **NAMI: Washington**
1107 NE 45th Street 206-783-4288
Seattle, WA 98105 office@namiwa.org
www.namiwa.org
*Lauren B. Simonds, MSW, Executive Director & CEO*
*Anna Nepomuceno, Director, Public Policy*

### West Virginia

87 **Mountain State - Parents, Children & Adolescents Network**
2351 Garfield Avenue 304-428-0365
Parkersburg, WV 26101 800-244-5385
DonnaMoss@msp-can.org
www.mspcan.org

### Wisconsin

88 **NAMI: Wisconsin**
414 Atlas Ave. 608-268-6000
Madison, WI 53714 800-236-2988
nami@namiwisconsin.org
www.namiwisconsin.org
*Mary Kay Battaglia, Executive Director*
*Stacey Mohr-Johannsen, Associate Director*

89 **Wisconsin Family Ties**
16 N Carroll Street 608-267-6800
Madison, WI 53703 800-422-7145
Fax: 608-267-6801
info@wifamilyties.org
www.wifamilyties.org

### Wyoming

90 **NAMI: Wyoming**
P.O. Box 1883 307-265-2573
Casper, WY 82602 namiwyominginfo@gmail.com
www.namiwyoming.org

*Roy C. Walworth, President*
*Donna Sedey, Vice President*

## Foundations

91 **American Psychiatric Association Foundation**
800 Maine Ave. S.W. 202-559-3888
Washington, DC 20024 lcoffin@psych.org
apafdn.org
The APA Foundation administers public outreach programs to eliminate mental health stigma.
*Lilia Coffin, General Questions*
*Erin Connors, Sr. Media Relations Specialist*

92 **American Psychological Foundation (APF)**
750 First Street N.E. 202-336-5843
Washington, DC 20002-4242 202-336-5812
foundation@apa.org
www.apa.org/apf
APF provides funding opportunities for early career psychologists and graduate students.
*Michelle Quist Ryder, PhD, Interim CEO*
*Shalonta Bowman, Special Development Coordinator*

93 **Family Service Foundation, Inc.**
5301 76th Avenue 301-459-2121
Landover Hills, MD 20784 Fax: 301-459-0675
www.fsfinc.org
Offers mental health and developmental disability services to clients in the State of Maryland.
*Gordon A. Raley, MSW, Chief Executive Officer*
*Erika Jones, MS, Dir., Developmental Disability Services*

94 **Foundation for Children with Intellectual and Developmental Disabilities**
1001 Frederick Road fcidd1948@gmail.com
Catonsville, MD 21228 www.fcidd.org
The FCIDD provides grants to organizations that help individuals with intellectual and developmental disabilities. This includes camps, employment facilities, music therapy, therapeutic riding, and teacher training.
*Sly Bieler, President*
*Joe O'Toole, Executive Officer*

95 **Inclusion Canada Foundation**
1 University Avenue 416-661-9611
Toronto, ON, M5J-2P1 855-661-9611
Fax: 905-436-3587
inform@inclusioncanada.ca
inclusioncanada.ca
A registered Canadian Public Foundation that raises funds to support individuals and families with intellectual disabilities, through research, policy work, and training oppportunities.
*Krista Carr, Executive Vice President*
*Jason Carr, Exec. Dir., Community Engagement & Dev.*

## Libraries & Resource Centers

96 **Alta Bates Summit Medical Center**
2001 Dwight Way 510-204-4444
Berkeley, CA 94704 www.altabatessummit.org/
Alta Bates Summit Medical Center has made community healthcare a priority. Areas of clinical expertise include cardiovascular and behavioral health, orthopedics, rehabilitation, and oncology care.
*Carolyn McGee, Medical Librarian*

97 **Central Louisiana State Hospital Medical and Professional Library**
242 West Shamrock Street 318-484-6363
Pineville, LA 71360 Fax: 318-484-6284
bentonmcgee@hotmail.com
www.clmlc.org
The Consortium was established to increase and better utilize the health information resources of Central Louisiana. Information on psychiatry, psychology and mental health is offered.
*Carol Rogers, Director*

98 **National Mental Health Consumers' Self-Help Clearinghouse**
selfhelpclearinghouse@gmail.com
www.mhselfhelp.org
The National Mental Health Consumers' Self-Help Clearinghouse, the nation's first national consumer technical assistance center, has played a major role in the development of the mental health consumer movement. The consumer movement strives for dignity, respect, and opportunity for those with mental illnesses.
*Joseph Rogers, Founder & Executive Director*
*Susan Rogers, Director*

## Research Centers

99 **Anxiety Disorders Center**
University of Wisconsin
Department of Psychiatry 608-263-6100
Madison, WI 53719 www.psychiatry.wisc.edu/uwpFacilities.ht
Provides evaluation and treatment for individuals suffering from anxiety disorders as well as training and education for clinicians.
*Andy Alexander, PhD, Professor*
*Ruth Benca, MD, PhD, Professor*

100 **Institute of Psychiatry and Human Behavior: University of Maryland**
655 West Baltimore Street 410-706-7410
Baltimore, MD 21201 Fax: 410-706-0235
alehman@psych.umaryland.edu
www.medschool.umaryland.edu
Studies in psychiatric disorders.
*Anthony Lehm MD, Director*
*Craig Vantyke, Chief Executive Officer*

101 **Jane & Terry Semel Institute for Neuroscience & Human Behavior**
Neuropsychiatric Institute
760 Westwood Plaza 310-825-2631
Los Angeles, CA 90095 800-825-9989
www.semel.ucla.edu
Studies behaviorial and psychosocial disorders.
*Peter Whybrow, Director*
*Fawzy Fawzy, Associate Director*

102 **Langley Porter Psychiatric Institute**
University of California
401 Parnassus Avenue 415-476-7365
San Francisco, CA 94143 www.universityofcalifornia.edu
Conducts clinical studies on psychiatric disorders.
*Samuel Barno Faucher, Director*

103 **Medical College of Pennsylvania: Eastern Psychiatric Institute**
3200 Henry Avenue 215-842-6990
Philadelphia, PA 19129
Offers research into all aspects of mental illness.
*Michael Spohn, Director*

104 **Menninger Clinic: Department of Research**
12301 S. Main Street 713-275-5140
Houston, TX 77035 800-351-9058
Fax: 785-350-5392
www.menningerclinic.com
Focuses research on mental health issues.
*B. Christoph Frueh, PhD, Director of Clinical Research*
*Chris Fowler, PhD, Associate Director of Clinical Research*

105 **NIH Clinical Center**
National Institute of Health
9000 Rockville Pike 301-496-4000
Bethesda, MD 20892 800-411-1222
Fax: 301-402-2984
TTY: 866-411-1010
prpl@mail.cc.nih.gov
www.cc.nih.gov
Established in 1953 as the research hospital of the National Institutes of Health. Designed so that patient care facilities are close to research laboratories, so that new findings of basic and clinical scientists can be quickly applied to the treatment of patients. Upon referral by physicians, patients are admitted to NIH clinical studies.
*John I Gallin, MD, Clinical Center Director*
*David Henderson, MD, Deputy Director for Clinical Care*

106 **State University of New York at Stony Brook: Mental Health Research**
450 Clarkson Avenue 718-270-1270
Brooklyn, NY 11203 www.stonybrook.edu
*Benjamin S. Hsiao, PhD, Vice President for Research*

107 **Thresholds Psychiatric Rehabilitation**
2700 N Ravenswood Avenue 773-281-3800
Chicago, IL 60614 Fax: 773-818-90
thresholds@thresholds.org
www.luc.edu
A psychosocial rehabilitation agency serving persons with severe and persistent mental illness.
*Tom MD, Director*
*Peter Whybrow, Director*

108 **University of Michigan: Mental Health Research Institute**
205 Washtenaw Place 734-763-1817
Ann Arbor, MI 48109 UMresearch@umich.edu
www.umich.edu
Focuses on the diagnosis, treatment and prevention of mental illnesses and disorders.
*Dr. Bernard Schulz, Chair of Psychiatry*

109 **University of Minnesota Department of Psychiatry**
420 Delaware Street SE 612-624-2430
Minneapolis, MN 55455 Fax: 612-265-91
www.umn.edu
Behavior and mental illness research.

110 **University of Missouri: Columbia Missouri Institute of Mental Health**
5247 Fyler Avenue 573-634-8787
Saint Louis, MO 63139 Fax: 314-644-8834
Mental health policy and ethics studies.

111 **University of Pittsburgh: Western Psychiatric Institute & Clinic**
3811 Ohara Street 412-246-6356
Pittsburgh, PA 15213 Fax: 412-246-6350
reitzpm@msx.upmc.edu
www.pitt.edu
Advancement of basic and clinical knowledge in mental health and psychiatric care.

112 **Vanderbilt Kennedy Center**
Vanderbilt University
110 Magnolia Center 615-322-8240
Nashville, TN 37203 Fax: 615-228-36
kc@vanderbilt.edu
www.kc.vanderbilt.edu
Mental health research.
*Donna G. Eskind, Chair*
*Cathy S. Brown, Past Chair*

113 **Veterans Medical Center: Mental Health Clinical Research Center**
3801 Miranda Avenue 650-858-3941
Palo Alto, CA 94304 www.va.gov
*Jerome Gallin, Director*
*David Henderson, Deputy Director for Clinical Care*

114 **Yeshiva University: Soundview-Throgs Neck Community Mental Health Center**
2527 Glebe Avenue 718-904-4400
Bronx, NY 10461 Fax: 718-931-7307
Mental health mental illness and recovery from mental illness research.

## Support Groups & Hotlines

115 **Alabama Education of Homeless Children and Youth Program**
Alabama State Department of Education
5348 Gordon Persons Building 334-242-8199
Montgomery, AL 36130 Fax: 334-420-9633
www.alsde.edu/html/home.asp
The major responsibilities of the Federal Programs Section are to administer all federally funded education programs and to provide technical assistance to local education agencies and schools. These responsibilities include promoting, supervising, and coordinating statewide educational programs with federal programs in addition to assisting schools in developing, revising, and implementing their school wide plans.
*Maggie McDonald, Program/Education Director*
*Augusta Reimer, Leadership Project Coordinator*

116 **Allies with Families**
505 East 200 South 801-433-2595
Salt Lake City, UT 84102 877-477-0764
Fax: 801-521-0872
Allies@AlliesWithFamilies.org
www.allieswithfamilies.org
Allies with Families was created in 1991 to offer practical support and resources for parents and their children and youth who face serious emotional, behavioral and mental health challenges.
*Lori Cerar, Executive Director*
*Karen Greenwell, Project Director and Newsletter Editor*

117 **Child & Adolescent Behavioral Health**
919 2nd Street NE 330-454-7917
Canton, OH 44704 Fax: 330-452-8860
www.childandadolescent.org/
The Child and Adolescent Service Center (CASC) was founded and incorporated in 1976 by a standing committee of the Stark County Mental Health Foundation. CASC provides dynamic leadership through innovative service, training and evaluation and is committed to providing culturally-sensitive programs and services throughout the community.
*Lisa Warburton-Gregory, President*
*Michael Johnson, Chief Executive Officer*

118 **Common Voice for Pierce County Parents**
10402 Kline Street 253-537-2145
Lakewood, WA 98445 Fax: 253-537-2162
nrascon@dadsmove.org
www.ffcmh.org/find-local-chapter
A Common Voice for Pierce County Parents is affiliated with the Federation of Families for Children's Mental Health (FFCMH), a national organization dedicated exclusively to helping children with mental health needs and their families achieve a better quality of life.

119 **Emotional Health Anonymous**
P.O. Box 4245 651-647-9712
St. Paul, MN 55104 Fax: 651-647-1593
www.emotionsanonymous.org
A twelve-step organization, similar to Alcoholics Anonymous. Compsed of people who come together in weekly meetings for the purpose of working toward recovery from emotional difficulties.
*Karen Mead, Executive Director*

120 **Federation of Families of South Carolina**
810 Dutch Square Boulevard 803-772-5210
Columbia, SC 29210 866-779-0402
Fax: 803-772-5212
FedFamSC@yahoo.com
www.fedfamsc.org
*Kathleen Scharer, President*
*Roxann McKinnon, Vice President*

121 **Florida Institute for Family Involvement (FIFI)**
3927 Spring Creek Highway 305-293-7626
Crawfordville, FL 32327 877-926-3514
Fax: 863-582-9358
HewFLMOM@aol.com
www.fifionline.org
Florida Institute for Family Involvement (FIFI), an affiliate of Federation of Families for Children's Mental Health (FFCMH), enhances, facilitates, and supports family and consumer involvement in the development of responsive, family centered, and community based systems of care. FIFI works in collaboration with state, federal, and private programs to develop a resource and training information center to enable individuals to advocate for appropriate services and make wise service choices.
*Connie Hawke, Co-Director*
*Tara Bremer, Co-Director*

122 **Georgia Parent Support Network (GPSN)**
1381 Metropolitan Parkway 404-758-4500
Atlanta, GA 30310 Fax: 404-758-6833
rheba.smith@gpsn.org
www.gpsn.org/
Georgia Parent Support Network (GPNS) provides support, education, and advocacy for children and youth with mental illness, emotional disturbances, and behavioral differences and their families.
*Kathy Dennis, Board President*
*Sue L. Smith, Ed.D, Chief Executive Officer*

123 **Hawaii Families As Allies (HFAA)**
99-209 Moanalua Road 808-487-8785
Aiea, HI 96701 866-361-8825
Fax: 808-487-0514
hfaa@hfaa.net
www.hfaa.net/
Hawaii Families As Allies (HFAA) is a statewide parent-controlled family network organization that provides support, services and information for families of children and adolescents with emotional and/or behavioral challenges. HFAA is the Hawaii state chapter of the Federation of Families for Children's Mental Health, a national organization that advocates for service system change so that families are valued and treated as true partners.
*Linda Machado, Executive Director*
*Charlene Daraban, Family Resource Specialist*

124 **Iowa Federaion of Families for Children's Mental Health (FFCMH)**
106 South Booth 319-462-2187
Anamosa, IA 52205 888-400-6302
Fax: 319-462-6789
www.iffcmh.org
The mission of Iowa Federation of Families for Children's Mental Health is to link families to community, county and state partners for needed supports and services; and to promote systems change that will enable families to live in a safe, stable and respectful environment.
*Lori Reynolds, Executive Director*
*Heidi Reynolds, Program Director*

125 **KALEIDOSCOPE**
1340 S. Damen Avenue 773-278-7200
Chicago, IL 60608 Fax: 773-278-5663
TTY: 773-292-4086
info@kaleidoscope4kids.org
www.kaleidoscope4kids.org
*William J. Binder, Chair*
*Ivy Walker, Vice Chairman-Secretary*

126 **Laradon Services for Children and Adults with Developmental Disabilities**
5100 Lincoln Street 303-296-2400
Denver, CO 80216 866-381-2163
Fax: 303-296-4012
TDD: 7209746821
www.laradon.org
Laradon specializes in services to children and adults with developmental disabilities, operating 15 programs that are designed to help each individual develop to his or her fullest potential and maximize self-sufficiency.
*John Galvin, Chairman*
*Frank Lucero, PhD, Executive Director*

127 **National Health Information Center**
Office of Disease Prevention & Health Promotion
1101 Wootton Pkwy Fax: 240-453-8281
Rockville, MD 20852 odphpinfo@hhs.gov
www.health.gov/nhic
Supports public health education by maintaining a calendar of National Health Observances; helps connect consumers and health professionals to organizations that can best answer questions and provide up-to-date contact information from reliable sources; updates on a yearly basis toll-free numbers for health information, Federal health clearinghouses and info centers.
*Don Wright, MD, MPH, Director*

128 **Navajo Nation Office of Special Education & Rehabilitation Services (OSERS)**
P.O. Box 1420 928-871-6338
Window Rock, AZ 86515 866-341-9918
Fax: 928-871-7865
osers@navajo.org
www.osers.navajo-nsn.gov/
Navajo OSERS is a program within the Division of DINE Education, which offers vocational rehabilitation to people with disabilities. Vocational Rehabilitation includes an array of services, which are funded by a grant to the Navajo Nation from the U.S. Department of Education. The goal of vocational rehabilitation is to assist people with disabilities to obtain or maintain employment.
*Treva M. Roanhorse, Director*
*Paula S. Seanez, Assistant Director*

129 **Nevada PEP**
2101 S. Jones Boulevard 702-388-8899
Las Vegas, NV 89146 800-216-5188
Fax: 702-388-2966
KTaycher@nvpep.org
www.nvpep.org
A statewide non-profit helping families who have children with disabilities, and the professionals who work with them. Support groups, training, workshops, lending resource library. Services are provided at no cost.
*Karen Taycher, Executive Director*
*Stephanie Vrsnik, Community Development Director*

130 **PACER Center**
8161 Normandale Boulevard 952-838-9000
Bloomington, MN 55437 800-537-2237
Fax: 952-838-0199
TTY: 952-838-0190
pacer@pacer.org
www.pacer.org
*Paula F. Goldberg, Executive Director*
*Mary Schrock, Chief Operating and Development Officer*

131 **Parent Education Network (PEN) Project Health**
Family Network on Disabilities of Florida
2735 Whitney Road 727-523-1130
Clearwater, FL 33760 800-825-5736
Fax: 727-523-8687
wilbur@fndfl.org
www.fndfl.org/programs/pen-parent-educat
The PEN Project provides: information on specific disabilities; individual assistance by telephone, email, and in-person; referrals to local, state, and national resources; opportunities for youths with disabilities to be involved in training to parents and students; and, collaboration with Family Network on Disabilities Heart and Hope annual statewide conference for families.
*Wilbur Smith, Co-Chief Executive Officer*
*Anna M. McLaughlin, Co-Chief Executive Officer*

132 **Parent Support Network of Rhode Island**
1395 Atwood Avenue 401-467-6855
Johnston, RI 02919 800-483-8844
Fax: 401-467-53
c.ciano@psnri.org
www.psnri.org
Family-run organization whose mission is to provide support, education and advocacy to parents of children at risk for or who have emotional, behavioral, and/or mental health challenges.
*Linda Winfield, Board President*
*Cathy Ciano, Executive Director*

## Print Resources

133 **American Journal of Psychiatry**
American Psychiatric Association Publishing
800 Maine Avenue, S.W. 202-459-9722
Washington, DC 20024 800-368-5777
Fax: 202-403-3094
appi@psych.org
ajp.psychiatryonline.org
The American Journal of Psychiatry - "the most widely read psychiatric journal in the world" - publishes the latest research in the field of psychiatry.
*Monthly*
*Ned H. Kalin, MD, Editor-in-Chief*

134 **American Journal on Intellectual and Developmental Disabilities (AJIDD)**
Amer. Assoc. on Intellectual & Dev. Disabilities
8403 Colesville Road 202-387-1968
Silver Spring, MD 20910 Fax: 202-387-2193
www.aamr.org
A scientific, scholarly, and archival multidisciplinary journal that publishes current research in the intellectual and developmental disabilities field.
*Bimonthly*
*Frank Symons, PhD, Editor, 2019-2026*

135 **American Psychologist Journal**
American Psychological Association
750 First Street NE 202-336-5500
Washington, DC 20002-4242 800-374-2721
TTY: 202-336-6123
www.apa.org
Articles on current issues in psychology as well as empirical, theoretical and practical articles on broad aspects of psychology. Publishes nine times a year, beginning in January.
*Harris Cooper, PhD, Editor*

136 **Inclusion**
Amer. Assoc. On Intellectual & Dev. Disabilities
8403 Colesville Road 202-387-1968
Silver Spring, MD 20910 Fax: 202-387-2193
www.aamr.org
A peer-reviewed journal that promotes the full inclusion of people with intellectual and developmental disabilities in society.
*Quarterly*
*Colleen Thoma, PhD, Co-Editor*
*LaRon Scott, EdD, Co-Editor*

137 **Intellectual and Developmental Disabilities (IDD)**
Amer. Assoc. On Intellectual & Dev. Disabilities
8403 Colesville Road 202-387-1968
Silver Spring, MD 20910 Fax: 202-387-2193
www.aamr.org
A peer-reviewed, multidisciplinary journal of policy, practices, and perspectives in the intellectual and developmental disabilities field.
*Bimonthly*
*Amy Hewitt, PhD, Interim Editor*

138 **Psychiatric Services**
American Psychiatric Association Publishing

800 Maine Avenue, S.W. 202-459-9722
Washington, DC 20024 800-368-5777
Fax: 202-403-3094
ps.psychiatryonline.org

This peer-reviewed journal publishes research on mental health services.
*Monthly*
*Lisa Dixon, M.D., M.P.H., Editor*

139 **Psychopharmacology Bulletin**
2205 Rockefeller Lane 310-374-4200
Redondo Beach, CA 90278 support@medworksmedia.com
www.medworksmedia.com

Emphasizes rapid, informal dissemination of recent research findings that have not previously appeared in the more formal literature.
*James M. LaRossa Jr., Publisher*
*Michael E. Thase, MD, Editor*

## Digital Resources

140 **Advocate**
National Alliance on Mental Illness (NAMI)
4301 Wilson Boulevard 703-524-7600
Arlington, VA 22203 800-950-6264
www.nami.org

NAMI's Advocate magazine is available to members at least twice a year. Digital editions can be downloaded online. Publishes a variety of mental health topics.

141 **NAMI Now**
National Alliance on Mental Illness (NAMI)
4301 Wilson Boulevard 703-524-7600
Arlington, VA 22203 800-950-6264
www.nami.org

AMI's digital newsletter, available to members, features relevant news and information on mental illness.

142 **PsychiatryOnline.org**
American Psychiatric Association Publishing
800 Maine Avenue, S.W. 202-459-9722
Washington, DC 20024 800-368-5777
Fax: 202-403-3094
appi@psych.org
psychiatryonline.org

Hosts numerous psychiatry and mental health publications, including the journals The American Journal of Psychiatry, FOCUS, The Journal of Neuropsychiatry and Clinical Neurosciences, Psychiatric Services, Psychiatric Research and Clinical Practice, and The American Journal of Psychotherapy.

## Web Sites

143 **American Psychological Association**
www.apa.org

Advances the creation, communication, and application of psychological knowledge to benefit society and improve people's lives.

144 **Healing Well**
www.healingwell.com

An online health resource guide to medical news, chat, information and articles, newsgroups and message boards, books, disease-related web sites, medical directories, and more for patients, friends, and family coping with disabling diseases, disorders, or chronic illnesses.

145 **HealthlinkUSA**
www.healthlinkusa.com

Health information concerning treatment, cures, prevention, diagnosis, risk factors, research, support groups, email lists, personal stories and much more. Updated regularly.

146 **MedicineNet**
www.medicinenet.com

An online resource for consumers providing easy-to-read, authoritative medical and health information.

147 **Medscape**
www.medscape.com

Medscape offers specialists, primary care physicians, and other health professionals the Web's most robust and integrated medical information and educational tools.

148 **Mental Health America**
mhanational.org

Provides informational materials; lobbies for Federal mental health legislation; and stimulates funding of research on the causes and treatment of mental illnesses.

149 **MentalHealth.com**
www.mentalhealth.com

A site whose goal is to improve understanding, diagnosis, and treatment of mental illness throughout the world. Includes information on specific disorders, medications, diagnosis, research, news, and other internet links.

150 **MentalHealth.org**
www.mentalhealth.org

Leading the national system that delivers mental health services. Provides the treatment and support services neede by adults with mental disorders and children with serious emotional problems.

151 **MyHealthfinder**
www.healthfinder.gov

Searchable, carefully developed web site offering information on over 1000 topics. Developed by the US Department of Health and Human Services, the site can be used in both English and Spanish.

152 **National Alliance on Mental Illness (NAMI)**
www.nami.org

Offers support to members; supports research efforts; and educates the public to reduce the stigma attached to mental illnesses.

153 **National Federation of Families**
www.ffcmh.org

Providing leadership to develop and sustain a nationwide network of family-run organizations.

154 **WebMD**
www.webmd.com

Provides credible information, supportive communities, and in-depth reference material about health subjects. A source for original and timely health information, as well as material from well-known content providers.

155 **World Federation for Mental Health**
www.wfmh.com

Mission is to promote, among all people and nations, the highest possible level of mental health in its broadest biological, medical, educational, and social aspects.

# PERSONALITY DISORDERS

*Personality disorders (PDs) are a group of psychological disorders defined by the most recent version of the Diagnostic and Statistical Manual for Mental Disorders (DSM-5) as significant impairments in an individual in their environment and difficulties in interpersonal functions. Research indicates that both biological and environmental influences will shape personality. Behavior involves interaction between an individual's personality and the situation in which they find themselves. The situation influences how the individual may react at any given time. For those with substance use disorder or behavioral addiction, a personality disorder may influence how the individual responds to addiction. As many as 65-90 percent of patients evaluated for substance use disorder have at least one co-occurring personality disorder. PDs should not be considered as a direct result of substance use disorder or other medical condition.*

Addictive personality traits such as anxiety, impulsivity, depression and unnecessary risk taking, can be triggered by drugs and alcohol, a genetic predisposition or heredity, trauma or attention deficit disorder. The common, underlying factor in every addiction is a need for feeling reward. This reward comes from a chemical release in the brain that fulfills a craving. People who are addicted are usually the last to recognize the problem and the last to recognize that their self-medication does not work. Defining the core problem is the first step.

Personality disorders as defined in the DSM-5 manual may be labeled as:

- Antisocial personality disorder
- Avoidant personality disorder
- Borderline personality disorder
- Dependent personality disorder
- Histrionic personality disorder
- Narcissistic personality disorder
- Paranoid personality disorder
- Obsessive-compulsive disorder
- Schizoid personality disorder
- Schizotypal personality disorder

Personality is comprised of thinking, behaving and feeling, and this combination is considered part of an individual's personality. A person's mood, coping skills, attitudes and interactions with others and society influence personality. It is often difficult to diagnose personality disorders. In the clinical definition of PD, it is difficult to differentiate between normal or expected personality characteristics and a personality disorder.

Contemporary psychologists believe there are five basic dimensions of personality: extraversion (also deemed extroversion), agreeableness, openness, conscientiousness and neuroticism. Understanding personality traits and what they mean can provide insight into personality without significant testing. For example, extraversion is being social, agreeableness is kindness, openness is creativity, conscientiousness is being thoughtful and neuroticism is emotional instability and sadness.

Personality disorders may reflect extreme variants of these basic personality dimensions. PDs occur so frequently with other types of psychological disorders, including addictive behaviors, that it is challenging to sort through symptoms to determine what is evidence of each disorder. When an individual struggles with a personality disorder, seeking external means to cope, including abusing alcohol, chemical substances and other activities, may lead to addiction.

Prevention activities are crucial to preventing the use and misuse of drugs leading to the development of substance use disorders and behavioral addictions. Often, it requires the individual to reach out for help such as with a crisis help line or a help line to deal with gambling addiction. With a PD diagnosis, it is difficult for individuals as they may lack insight into their own behaviors. If the individual does seek help, it is usually for a secondary issue such as alcoholism or depression. The role of the family and healthcare providers is essential to recognizing PD and addiction and getting the individual the help needed to cope.

## Agencies & Associations

156 **American Psychiatric Association**
800 Maine Avenue S.W. 202-559-3900
Washington, DC 20024 apa@psych.org
www.psychiatry.org

A medical specialty society representing a growing membership of psychiatrists. Offers information for psychiatrists, medical students, patients and families.

157 **American Psychological Association**
750 First Street NE 202-336-5500
Washington, DC 20002 800-374-2721
TTY: 202-336-6123
www.apa.org

Advances the creation, communication, and application of psychological knowledge to benefit society and improve people's lives.

*Frank C. Worrell, PhD, President*
*Jean A. Carter, PhD, Treasurer*

158 **Association for Behavioral and Cognitive Therapies**
305 Seventh Avenue 212-647-1890
New York, NY 10001 Fax: 212-647-1865
abct.org

A multidisciplinary organization dedicated to utilizing and advancing scientific approaches in the understanding and prevention of human behavioral and cognitive problems.

*Mary Jane Eimer, CAE, Executive Director*
*David Teisler, CAE, Deputy Director/Dir., Communications*

159 **Association of Children's Residential & Community Services**
648 North Plankinton Avenue 877-332-2272
Milwaukee, WI 53203 info@togetherthevoice.org
togetherthevoice.org

A national organization focused on providing residential therapeutic treatment for children and adolescents with behavioral health disorders.

*Kari Sisson, Executive Director*

160 **Center for Family Support (CFS)**
333 Seventh Avenue 888-813-5014
New York, NY 10001 svernikoff@cfsny.org
www.cfsny.org

The Center for Family Support offers assistance to individuals with developmental and related disabilities, as well as their families, and provides support services and programs that are designed to accommodate individual needs. Offers services throughout New York City, Westchester County, Long Island, and New Jersey.

*Steven Vernikoff, Executive Director*
*Barbara Greenwald, Chief Operating Officer*

161 **Center for Mental Health Services (CMHS)**
Substance Abuse and Mental Health Services Admin.
5600 Fishers Lane 877-726-4727
Rockville, MD 20857 TTY: 800-487-4889
samhsa.gov

Promotes the treatment of mental illness and emotional disorders by increasing accessibility to mental health programs; supporting outreach, treatment, rehabilitation, and support programs and networks; and encouraging the use of scientifically-based information when treating mental disorders. CMHS provides information about mental health via a toll-free number and numerous publications.

*Anita Everett, M.D., DFAPA, Director*

162 **Depression and Bipolar Support Alliance**
Depression and Bipolar Support Alliance
55 East Jackson Boulevard 800-826-3632
Chicago, IL 60604 Fax: 312-642-7243
www.dbsalliance.org

DBSA provides support, information, and assistance to individuals living with mood disorders (depression and bipolar disorder).

*Michael Pollock, Chief Executive Officer*
*Maria Margaglione, Programs Director*

163 **Mental Health America**
500 Montgomery Street 703-684-7722
Alexandria, VA 22314 800-969-6642
Fax: 703-684-5968
mhanational.org

Mental Health America is a community-based nonprofit organization committed to enabling the mental wellness of all Americans. MHA advocates for greater access to quality health services and seeks to educate individuals on identifying symptoms, as well as intervention and prevention.

*Schroeder Stribling, President & CEO*

164 **National Alliance on Mental Illness (NAMI)**
4301 Wilson Boulevard 703-524-7600
Arlington, VA 22203 800-950-6264
nami.org

NAMI is an organization dedicated to raising awareness on mental health and providing support and education for Americans affected by mental illness. NAMI advocates for access to services and treatment and fosters an environment of awareness and understanding for those concerned with mental health.

*Joyce A. Campbell, President*
*Daniel H. Gillison, Jr., CEO*

165 **National Association for the Dually Diagnosed (NADD)**
321 Wall Street 845-331-4336
Kingston, NY 12401 info@thenadd.org
thenadd.org

NADD is a nonprofit organization designed to increase awareness of, and provide services for, individuals with developmental disabilities and mental illness. NADD emphasizes the importance of quality mental healthcare for people with mental health needs and offers conferences, information resources, educational programs, and training materials to professionals, parents, and organizations.

*Jeanne M. Farr, MA, Chief Executive Officer*
*Robert J. Fletcher, DSW, Founder & CEO Emeritus*

166 **National Institute of Mental Health**
6001 Executive Boulevard 866-615-6464
Bethesda, MD 20892-9663 nimhinfo@nih.gov
nimh.nih.gov

The National Institute of Mental Health conducts clinical research on mental disorders and seeks to expand knowledge on mental health treatments.

*Joshua A. Gordon, M.D., Ph. D., Director*

167 **Shulman Center for Compulsive Theft, Spending & Hoarding**
P.O. Box 250008 248-358-8508
Franklin, MI 48025 terrenceshulman@theshulmancenter.com
theshulmancenter.com

The Shulman Center provides counseling and professional services designed to help individuals with compulsive stealing, spending, and hoarding disorders. The Shulman Center supports individuals, families, companies, and communities through education, assessment, and treatment.

*Tina M. Shulman, CMT, Creative Director*

168 **TARA Association for Borderline Personality Disorder**
23 Greene Street 212-966-6514
New York, NY 10013 tara4bpd@gmail.com
tara4bpd.org

A not-for-profit organization promoting educational programs and research on the causes and treatment of personality disorders. TARA seeks to raise awareness on personality disorder and to eliminate the stigma attached to it.

*Valerie Porr, MA, Founder and President*

## Foundations

169 **Borderline Personality Disorder Society of B.C.**
info@bpdbc.ca
www.bpdbc.ca

Offers help to individuals with Borderline Personality Disorder (BPD), and their family and friends. Provides peer support groups in Victoria, Nanaimo, Vancouver and New Westminster.

*Baylie McKnight, BSW, MSW, RSW, President/Co-Founder*
*Deborah McKnight, Secretary/Treasurer*

170 **Brain & Behavior Research Foundation**
747 Third Avenue 646-681-4888
New York, NY 10017 800-829-8289
info@bbrfoundation.org
www.bbrfoundation.org
The Brain and Behavior Research Foundation awards grants aimed at advancing scientific understandings of mental health treatments and mental disorders such as depression and schizophrenia. The Brain and Behavior Research Foundation's mission is to eliminate the suffering caused by mental illness.
*Geoffrey A. Simon, Chairman*
*Miriam E. Katowitz, CPA, Vice President*

171 **TLC Foundation for Body-Focused Repetitive Behaviors**
716 Soquel Avenue 831-457-1004
Santa Cruz, CA 95062 info@bfrb.org
www.bfrb.org
The TLC Foundation, formerly The Trichotillomania Learning Center, serves to raise awareness on trichotillomania and related body-focused repetitive disorders; support research; disseminate scientifically-based information about trichotillomania; and offer support services for individuals and families affected by the disorders. The TLC Foundation aims to eliminate the suffering caused by trichotillomania and body-focused repetitive behaviors.
*Jen Monteleone, Interim Executive Director*
*Alice Kelly, Director, Business Services*

## Libraries & Resource Centers

172 **National Mental Health Consumers' Self-Help Clearinghouse**
selfhelpclearinghouse@gmail.com
mhselfhelp.org
The Clearinghouse is a peer-run national technical assistance center focused on achieving respect and equality of opportunity for those with mental illnesses. The Clearinghouse helps with the growth of the mental health consumer movement by evaluating mental health services, advocating for mental health reform, and providing consumers with news, information, publications, and consultation services.
*Joseph Rogers, Founder & Executive Director*
*Susan Rogers, Director*

## Research Centers

173 **Centre for Addiction and Mental Health (CAMH)**
1001 Queen Street West 416-535-8501
Toronto, ON, M6J-1H4 800-463-2338
info@camh.ca
camh.ca
The Centre for Addiction and Mental Health is a mental health, addiction teaching hospital and research centre based in Canada. CAMH seeks to support people affected by mental health and addiction issues through research, education, policy development, clinical care, and the promotion of health.
*Sarah Downey, President & CEO*

174 **Child & Family Center**
Menninger Clinic
21545 Centre Pointe Parkway 661-259-9439
Santa Clarita, CA 91350 800-351-9058
webmaster@menninger.edu
www.childfamilycenter.org/
The Center's goals: to further develop emerging understanding of the impact of childhood maltreatment and abuse; to chart primary prevention strategies that will foster healthy patterns of caregiving and attachment and reduce the prevalence of maltreatment and abuse; and to develop secondary prevention strategies that will promote early detection of attachment-related problems and effective interventions to avert the development of chronic and severe disorders.
*Steven Zimmer, Board Chair*
*Darrell Paulk, CEO*

175 **Impulse Control Disorders Clinic**
University of Minnesota
231 Pillsbury Drive,South East. 612-625-2008
Minneapolis, MN 55455 800-752-1000
TTY: 612-625-9051
A group of doctors and trainees engaged in research in Impulse-Control Disorders (ICD) and Obsessive-Compulsive Disorder (OCD) and treating patients in a specialty clinic. Conducts research to elucidate pathophysiological links to the ICD and OCD and conducts clinical trials to come up with better and improved treatments for patients.

## Support Groups & Hotlines

176 **Gam-Anon Family Groups International Service Office, Inc.**
P.O. Box 307 718-352-1671
Massapequa Park, NY 11762 gamanonoffice@gam-anon.org
gam-anon.org
A 12-step self-help fellowship of men and women who have been affected by the gambling problems of a loved one. Their program works through literature and meetings. At meetings, individuals learn how other members applied the Gam-Anon program to find serenity and a more normal way of thinking and living.

177 **Gamblers Anonymous**
P.O. Box 17173 626-960-3500
Los Angeles, CA 90017 isomain@gamblersanonymous.org
gamblersanonymous.org
Fellowship of men and women who share their experience, strength and hope with each other so that they may solve their common problem and help others recover from a gambling problem.

178 **Kleptomaniacs Anonymous**
The Shulman Center for Compulsive Theft, Spending
P.O. Box 250008 248-358-8508
Franklin, MI 48025 kleptomaniacsanonymous.com
Kleptomaniacs Anonymous is a unique, independent and secular weekly self-help group.
*Terrence Shulman, JD, LMSW, Founder/Director*

179 **Out of the FOG**
www.outofthefog.net
Providing information and support to the family members and loved-ones of individuals who suffer from a personality disorder. A supportive, close-knit community encouraging one another through the many challenges that come with having a family member or significant other who has a personality disorder. FOG stands for Fear, Obligation, and Guilt, feelings which often result from being in a relationship with a person who suffers from a Personality Disorder.

180 **Paranoid Personality Disorder Forum**
Mental Health Matters
www.psychforums.com/paranoid-personality
A helpful user to user forum for support and information about Paranoid Personality Disorders.

181 **S.A.F.E. Alternatives**
7115 W North Avenue 708-366-9066
Oak Park, IL 60302 800-366-8288
info@selfinjury.com
selfinjury.com
A world-renowned treatment program that in it's more than twenty years of operation has helped thousands of people successfully end self-injurious behavior. A treatment team of experts uses therapy, education, and support to empower clients to identify healthier ways to cope with emotional distress. The S.A.F.E. Alternatives philosophy and model of treatment focus on shifting control to the client, empowering them to make healthy choices, including the choice to not self-injure.
*Karen Conterio, CEO & Founder*
*Wendy Lader, PhD, M.Ed, Clinical Director*

182 **TLC Foundation for Body-Focused Repetitive Behaviors**
716 Soquel Avenue 831-457-1004
Santa Cruz, CA 95062 info@bfrb.org
www.bfrb.org
The TLC Foundation, formerly The Trichotillomania Learning Center, serves to raise awareness on trichotillomania and related body-focused repetitive disorders; support research; disseminate scientifically-based information about trichotillomania; and offer

support services for individuals and families affected by the disorders. The TLC Foundation aims to eliminate the suffering caused by trichotillomania and body-focused repetitive behaviors.
*Jen Monteleone, Interim Executive Director*
*Alice Kelly, Director, Business Services*

## Print Resources

183 **American Journal of Psychiatry**
American Psychiatric Association Publishing
800 Maine Avenue, S.W. 202-459-9722
Washington, DC 20024 800-368-5777
Fax: 202-403-3094
appi@psych.org
ajp.psychiatryonline.org
The American Journal of Psychiatry - "the most widely read psychiatric journal in the world" - publishes the latest research in the field of psychiatry.
*Monthly*
*Ned H. Kalin, M.D., Editor-in-Chief*

184 **Psychiatric Services**
American Psychiatric Association Publishing
800 Maine Avenue, S.W. 202-459-9722
Washington, DC 20024 800-368-5777
Fax: 202-403-3094
ps.psychiatryonline.org
This peer-reviewed journal publishes research on mental health services.
*Monthly*
*Lisa Dixon, M.D., M.P.H., Editor*

## Digital Resources

185 **PsychiatryOnline.org**
American Psychiatric Association Publishing
800 Maine Avenue, S.W. 202-459-9722
Washington, DC 20024 800-368-5777
Fax: 202-403-3094
appi@psych.org
psychiatryonline.org
Hosts numerous psychiatry and mental health publications, including the journals The American Journal of Psychiatry, FOCUS, The Journal of Neuropsychiatry and Clinical Neurosciences, Psychiatric Services, Psychiatric Research and Clinical Practice, and The American Journal of Psychotherapy.

## Web Sites

186 **Center for Family Support (CFS)**
www.cfsny.org
Devoted to providing support and assistance to individuals with developmental and related disabilities, and to the family members who care for them.

187 **MentalHealth.com**
www.mentalhealth.com
Offers online psychiatric diagnosis in the hope of reaching the two-thirds of individuals with mental illness who do not seek treatment.

188 **National Association for the Dually Diagnosed (NADD)**
www.thenadd.org
An association for persons with developmental disabilities and mental health needs.

189 **National Mental Health Consumers' Self-Help Clearinghouse**
www.mhselfhelp.org
A national consumer technical assistance center.

190 **Out of the Fog**
www.outofthefog.net
Information and support for those with a family member or loved one who suffers from a personality disorder.

191 **Psych Central**
www.psychcentral.com
The Internet's largest and oldest independent mental health social network created and run by mental health professionals to guarantee reliable, trusted information and support communities to you.

192 **Substance Abuse and Mental Health Services Administration (SAMHSA)**
www.store.samhsa.gov
Resources on mental disorders as well as treatment and recovery.

# SUBSTANCE-RELATED & ADDICTIVE DISORDERS

*Addiction differs from substance abuse in that it is a chronic disease that is incredibly difficult to control according to the National Institute on Drug Abuse. Substance use disorder combines the categories of substance abuse and substance dependence on a scale from mild to severe, according to the Diagnostic and Statistical Manual of Mental Disorders (DSM-5) of the American Psychiatry Association. Substance use disorders are defined as primary, progressive, chronic, relapsing and treatable diseases. Addictions remold the brain to assign more value to compulsions than health, work family and even life.*

Individuals often link substance dependence with addiction, when in fact, dependance can be a normal body response to a substance. Addictive disorders, in addition to substance related disorder, include behavioral disorders such as gambling disorder and internet gaming disorder. For example, gambling disorder is similar to substance use disorder in clinical expression, comorbidity, physiology, brain origin and treatment. Additional behavioral disorders, including general use of the internet and social media use, are being researched to determine if these activities can rise to the level of behavioral disorders. Regardless of formal diagnoses, any behavior that interferes with activities of daily life to the detriment of self and others should be monitored.

Risk factors for substance related and addictive disorders include:

- A family history of addiction that likely includes a genetic component
- Mental health disorders
- Lack of family support and involvement
- Peer pressure
- Abusing substances at an early age
- Taking a highly addictive drug

Alcohol use disorder remains the most common substance use disorder encouraged by both the social aspects of alcohol consumption and the perceived health benefits of a daily glass of wine. In adults reporting alcohol dependence, over half also experienced anxiety and one-third experienced a personality disorder. Tobacco use disorder causes almost half a million deaths each year and may do damage to nearly every organ in the human body.

Opioids, even when used correctly for pain control, may be addictive if continued for too long, and are used for the euphoria created by the drug after the pain subsides. Opioid abuse may lead to the use of other chemicals. Marijuana is the most-used drug in the United States after alcohol and tobacco, and over 4 million people 12 and up met the criteria for substance use disorder based on the drug.

Cannabis use disorder disrupts function in perception, thinking and problem solving as well as creating poor motor coordination. Stimulant use disorder may be created by drugs commonly used to treat obesity, attention deficit hyperactivity disorder and depression, but may also include cocaine, methamphetamines and amphetamines.

Hallucinogen use disorder produces visual and auditory hallucinations and feelings of detachment from one's environment.

Addiction is not a homogenous disease, with individuals experiencing differing reactions to substances or behaviors. For example, there are two sub-types of gambling addiction. The primary sub-type of gambling addiction is when the person is addicted to the activity itself, while the secondary sub-type is when the person uses the behavior to escape or de-stress.

Substance use disorder and addiction are complicated diseases that are highly personalized to the individual. The physiological and emotional makeup of the person may result in some people being able to resist substance abuse and behavioral abuse while others experience crippling addiction. Addiction is said to exist when the activity becomes the most important activity in the individual's life. When the individual seeks mood modification from an agent or activity, requires increasing amounts of agents or interactions, e.g., internet gaming time, or experiences withdrawal when the person is unable to engage in the desired activity, addiction is said to exist. Addiction creates conflict in all settings and even when moderated, relapse my occur.

## Agencies & Associations

193 **AMERSA**
P.O. Box 952 | 401-230-2165
Charlestown, RI 02813 | doreen@amersa.org
amersa.org
The Association for Multidisciplinary Education and Research in Substance use and Addiction (AMERSA) is a nonprofit organization of healthcare professionals dedicated to improving education and clinical care in the management of problems related to substance abuse.
*Rebecca Northup, Executive Director*

194 **Adult Children of Alcoholics World Service Organization, Inc.**
P.O. Box 811 | 310-534-1815
Lakewood, CA 90714 | adultchildren.org
Adult Children of Alcoholics is a 12 Step, 12 Tradition program for adult women and men who grew up in alcoholic or otherwise dysfunctional homes, and for adults who have experienced abuse or neglect in the past. The program involves ACA members meeting with each other in a mutually respectful, safe environment and sharing their experiences, as well as applying the program's 12 Steps for recovery to their own lives.

195 **African American Family Services (AAFS)**
410 North 21st Street | 719-636-1100
Colorado Springs, CO 80904 | Fax: 719-636-1993
dgrogan@aafs.org
www.aafs.net
African American Family Services works with individuals, families and communities affected by addiction and mental illness. Provides culturally-specific mental health services.
*Donna M. Grogan, Executive Director*
*Kimberly Wrasse, Assistant Director*

196 **Al-Anon Family Group Headquarters**
1600 Corporate Landing Parkway | 757-563-1600
Virginia Beach, VA 23454-5617 | 888-425-2666
Fax: 757-563-1656
wso@al-anon.org
www.al-anon.org
At Al-Anon Family Group meetings, family members and friends of problem drinkers share their experiences and learn how to apply the principles of the Al-Anon program to their individual situations.

197 **Alcoholics Anonymous**
475 Riverside Drive at W. 120th St. | 212-870-3400
New York, NY 10115 | www.aa.org
Alcoholics Anonymous is an international alliance of supportive individuals who have had a drinking problem. Membership is available to anyone wanting to improve their situation.

198 **American Academy of Addiction Psychiatry (AAAP)**
400 Massasoit Avenue | 401-524-3076
East Providence, RI 02914 | Fax: 401-272-0922
aaap.org
An organization of healthcare professionals dedicated to helping those with mental health disorders. Promotes the use of evidence-based research in the assessment and treatment of substance abuse and mental disorders, as well as in public policy and clinical practice. Provides education to healthcare professionals and the public on patient care, recovery, and the safe treatment of those suffering from substance abuse disorders.
*Larissa Mooney, MD, President*
*Kathryn Cates-Wessel, CEO*

199 **American Chronic Pain Association**
11936 W. 119th Street | ACPA@theacpa.org
Overland Park, KS 66213-2216 | www.theacpa.org
The ACPA facilitates peer support and education for individuals with chronic pain in its many forms, in order to increase quality of life. Also raises awareness in the healthcare community.
*Trupti Gokani, MD, President*
*Kathy Sapp, Chief Executive Officer*

200 **American Public Human Services Association**
1300 17th St. N | 202-682-0100
Arlington, VA 22209 | Fax: 202-289-6555
memberservice@aphsa.org
aphsa.org
APHSA is a nonprofit organization dedicated to improving health and human services by supporting state and local agencies, and working with partners and policymakers to drive effective policies.
*Tracy Wareing Evans, President & CEO*
*Ray Davidson, Chief Operating Officer*

201 **American Society of Addiction Medicine**
11400 Rockville Pike | 301-656-3920
Rockville, MD 20852 | Fax: 301-656-3815
email@asam.org
asam.org
ASAM's mission is to support the practice of Addiction Medicine and to improve the quality of care and treatment for people struggling with addiction.
*William F. Haning, III, MD, President*
*Brian Hurley, MD, MBA, President-Elect*

202 **Center for Family Support (CFS)**
333 Seventh Avenue | 888-813-5014
New York, NY 10001 | svernikoff@cfsny.org
www.cfsny.org
The Center for Family Support offers assistance to individuals with developmental and related disabilities, as well as their families, and provides support services and programs that are designed to accommodate individual needs. Offers services throughout New York City, Westchester County, Long Island, and New Jersey.
*Steven Vernikoff, Executive Director*
*Barbara Greenwald, Chief Operating Officer*

203 **Center for Mental Health Services (CMHS)**
Substance Abuse and Mental Health Services Admin.
5600 Fishers Lane | 240-276-1310
Rockville, MD 20857 | samhsa.gov
Promotes the treatment of mental illness and emotional disorders by increasing accessibility to mental health programs; supporting outreach, treatment, rehabilitation, and support programs and networks; and encouraging the use of scientifically-based information when treating mental disorders. CMHS provides information about mental health via a toll-free number and numerous publications.
*Anita Everett, M.D., DFAPA, Director*

204 **Center for Substance Abuse Prevention: Substance Abuse & Mental Health Services**
5600 Fishers Lane | 240-276-2420
Rockville, MD 20857 | 877-726-4727
TTY: 800-487-4889
www.samhsa.gov
Connects people and resources with strategies and programs designed to encourage efforts aimed at reducing and eliminating alcohol, tobacco and other drug problems in society. Works with federal, state, public and private organizations to develop prevention programs.
*Jennifer Fan, Pharm.D., J.D., Acting Director*

205 **Cocaine Anonymous World Services**
21720 S. Wilmington Ave | 310-559-5833
Long Beach, CA 90810-1641 | Fax: 310-559-2554
cawso@ca.org
www.ca.org
Members are recovering from addiction, and offer support and maintain their sobriety by working together.

206 **Community Anti-Drug Coalitions of America (CADCA)**
500 Montgomery Street | 703-706-0560
Alexandria, VA 22314 | Fax: 703-706-0565
international@cadca.org
cadca.org
Community Anti-Drug Coalition of America is a national organization representing the interests of over 5,000 anti-drug coalitions across the United States. CADCA participates in public policy advocacy and provides community coalitions with marketing pro-

grams, technical assistance and training, and special events with the purpose of making communities safe and drug-free.
*Mary Bono, Chairman*
*Larry P. Cote, Vice Chairman*

207 **Drug Abuse Resistance Education of America**
P.O. Box 512090
Los Angeles, CA 90051
310-215-0575
800-223-3273
Fax: 310-215-0180
dare.org
Provides information, resources, tips, warning signs and other information for parents and kids to help keep children off drugs.
*Francisco X. Pegueros, President & CEO*
*Thomas Hazelton, President, Development*

208 **FASD United**
P.O. Box 251
McLean, VA 22101
202-785-4585
fasdunited.org
Educates the public about the risks associated with alcohol use during pregnancy, including Fetal Alcohol Spectrum Disorders, which causes birth defects and developmental disabilities in children. Dedicated to preventing alcohol consumption during pregnancy and reducing the number of birth defects. Provides support for individuals and families concerned with Fetal Alcohol Spectrum Disorders.
*Tom Donaldson, President & CEO*
*Kathleen Tavenner Mitchell, MHS, Vice President & National Spokesperson*

209 **Families Anonymous, Inc.**
701 Lee Street
Des Plaines, IL 60016
800-736-9805
847-294-5877
Fax: 847-294-5837
info@familiesanonymous.org
www.familiesanonymous.org
Addresses the needs of families who are concerned about a relative with a drug problem and with related behavioral problems. Offers informational packets, meetings and support networks for these families.

210 **Goodwill Industries-Suncoast, Inc.**
727-523-1512
888-279-1988
TTY: 727-579-1068
goodwill-suncoast.org
A nonprofit, community-based organization whose mission is to help people achieve self-sufficiency through the dignity and power of work, serving people who are disadvantaged, disabled or elderly. The mission is accomplished through providing independent living skills, affordable housing, and training and placement in community employment.
*Sandra Young, Chair*
*Deborah A. Passerini, President & CEO*

211 **Grief Recovery After a Substance Passing (GRASP)**
11819 N. Deerfield Dr.
Dunlap, IL 61614
302-492-7717
administrator@grasphelp.org
grasphelp.org
GRASP provides information resources, offers support, and organizes meetings and events for families or individuals who have experienced the death of a loved one as a result of substance abuse or addiction.
*Tamara Olt, Executive Director*
*Darleen Berg, Chair*

212 **Indian Health Service**
5600 Fishers Lane
Rockville, MD 20857
605-226-7456
800-225-0241
www.ihs.gov
Provides a comprehensive program of alcoholism and substance abuse prevention and treatment for Native Americans and Alaskan natives.

213 **Lawyers Concerned for Lawyers**
2550 University Avenue W.
Saint Paul, MN 55114
651-646-5590
866-525-6466
help@mnlcl.org
www.mnlcl.org
A non-profit organization of recovering lawyers, judges, law students, and concerned others. Educates and arranges interventions and offers lawyer-only AA meetings.
*Joan Bibelhausen, Executive Director*
*Judith Rush, Outreach Manager*

214 **Marijuana Anonymous World Services**
5551 Hollywood Blvd.
Hollywood, CA 90028-6814
800-766-6779
support@marijuana-anonymous.org
www.marijuana-anonymous.org
Non-profit fellowship of individuals with marijuana addiction, seeking sobriety and support.

215 **Mental Health America**
500 Montgomery Street
Alexandria, VA 22314
703-684-7722
800-969-6642
Fax: 703-684-5968
mhanational.org
Mental Health America is a community-based nonprofit organization committed to enabling the mental wellness of all Americans. MHA advocates for greater access to quality health services and seeks to educate individuals on identifying symptoms, as well as intervention and prevention.
*Schroeder Stribling, President & CEO*

216 **MindWise Innovations**
270 Bridge Street
Dedham, MA 02026
781-239-0071
SOS@mindwise.org
www.mindwise.org
Formerly known as Screening For Mental Health, MindWise Innovations provides resources to schools, workplaces, and communities to address mental health issues, substance abuse, and suicide.

217 **Mothers Against Drunk Driving (MADD)**
511 E. John Carpenter Freeway
Irving, TX 75062
877-275-6233
www.madd.org
Founded by a small group of mothers and currently one of the largest crime victims organizations in the world. Resources available online.
*Ellen Willmott, Interim CEO*
*Andrew Robinson, Chair*

218 **NCADD**
28 East Ostend Street
Baltimore, MD 21230
adminl@ncadd.us
www.ncadd.org
The National Council on Alcoholism and Drug Dependence, Inc. (NCADD) is a national leading organization dedicated to fighting the addiction epidemic, providing awareness, support, and resources.

219 **Narcotics Anonymous World Services**
P.O. Box 9999
Van Nuys, CA 91409
818-773-9999
Fax: 818-700-0700
fsmail@na.org
www.na.org
A fellowship of individuals who meet to help one another with their drug dependency. Support and resources are available.

220 **National Alliance on Mental Illness (NAMI)**
4301 Wilson Boulevard
Arlington, VA 22203
703-524-7600
800-950-6264
nami.org
NAMI is an organization dedicated to raising awareness on mental health and providing support and education for Americans affected by mental illness. NAMI advocates for access to services and treatment and fosters an environment of awareness and understanding for those concerned with mental health.
*Joyce A. Campbell, President*
*Daniel H. Gillison, Jr., CEO*

221 **National Association for Children of Alcoholics (NACOA)**
10920 Connecticut Avenue
Kensington, MD 20895
301-468-0985
888-554-2627
nacoa@nacoa.org
www.nacoa.org
Advocates for all children and families affected by alcohol and other drug dependencies. Programs, training, and other resources are available.
*Denise Bertin Epp, MS, RN, CEO*

222 **National Association of Addiction Treatment Providers (NAATP)**
P.O. Box 271686 888-574-1008
Denver, CO 80203 info@naatp.org
naatp.org

NAATP ensures the availability and accessibility of high quality addiction treatment across the country through leadership, advocacy, training, and other member support services.
*Marvin Ventrell, JD, CEO*

223 **National Association of Alcoholism and Drug Abuse Counselors (NAADAC)**
44 Canal Center Plaza 703-741-7686
Alexandria, VA 22314 Fax: 703-741-7698
naadac@naadac.org
www.naadac.org

Largest membership organization serving addiction counselors, educators and other addiction-focused health care professionals who specialize in addiction prevention, treatment and education.
*Cynthia Moreno Tuohy, BSW, SAP, Executive Director*
*Jessica Gleason, JD, Deputy Director*

224 **National Association of State Alcohol/Drug Abuse Directors**
1919 Pennsylvania Avenue NW 202-293-0090
Washington, DC 20006 Fax: 202-293-1250
dcoffice@nasadad.org
nasadad.org

The National Association of State Alcohol and Drug Abuse Directors is a private, not-for-profit organization focused on the promotion of educational and scientific materials on alcohol, drug abuse, and related fields. NASADAD seeks to support and further the development of effective alcohol and other drug abuse treatment programs in the United States.
*Sara Goldsby, President*
*Robert Morrison, Executive Director*

225 **National Association on Drug Abuse Problems**
355 Lexington Avenue 212-986-1170
New York, NY 10017 info@nadap.org
www.nadap.org

Private non-profit corporation providing skills, evaluation, job training and job placement to recovering drug addicts in the metropolitan New York area.
*John A. Darin, President & CEO*
*Gary Stankowski, EVP, COO & CCO*

226 **National Coalition for the Homeless**
2201 P Street Northwest 202-462-4822
Washington, DC 20037 info@nationalhomeless.org
nationalhomeless.org

The National Coalition for the Homeless is an organization serving to protect the needs of those experiencing homelessness, while striving to prevent and end homelessness. NCH promotes effective treatment, services, and programs for those struggling with homelessness as well as substance abuse problems.
*Barbara Anderson, Treasurer*
*Donald Whitehead, Executive Director*

227 **National Council for Behavioral Health**
1400 K Street NW 202-684-7457
Washington, DC 20005 communications@thenationalcouncil.org
www.thenationalcouncil.org

The National Council for Behavioral Health serves to unify America's behavioral health organizations. The council is dedicated to ensuring that quality mental health and addictions care is readily accessible to all Americans.
*Linda Rosenberg, MSW, President*
*Jeannie Campbell, Executive Vice President & COO*

228 **National Crime Prevention Council**
1100 15th Street, NW
Washington, DC 20005 www.ncpc.org

Organization working to prevent crime and drug use by developing materials for parents and children, teaching strategies to communities, and raising awareness by coodinating with local agencies.
*Paul DelPonte, Executive Director*

229 **National Families in Action (NFIA)**
P.O. Box 133136 nfia@nationalfamilies.org
Atlanta, GA 30333 www.nationalfamilies.org

Non-profit organization that obtained the nation's first state laws banning the sale of drug paraphernalia. Leads a national effort to help parents replicate Georgia's laws in other states to prevent the marketing of drugs and drug use to children.
*Bill Carter, Board Chairman*
*Sue Rusche, President & CEO*

230 **National Institute on Alcohol Abuse and Alcoholism (NIAAA)**
National Institute on Health
9000 Rockville Pike 301-443-3860
Rockville, MD 20892 niaaaweb-r@exchange.nih.gov
www.niaaa.nih.gov

NIAAA seeks to reduce alcohol-related problems by conducting scientific research in a range of areas, including neuroscience, treatment, prevention, and epidemiology; working with other research institutes, federal programs, and organizations focused on the issues surrounding alcohol abuse; and disseminating information to healthcare providers, researchers, policymakers, and the public.
*George F. Koob, PhD, Director*
*Patricia A. Powell, Deputy Director*

231 **National Institute on Drug Abuse (NIDA)**
251 Bayview Blvd. 443-740-2463
Baltimore, MD 21224 800-535-8254
www.irp.drugabuse.gov

NIDA's mission is to lead the Nation in bringing the power of science to bear on drug abuse and addiction.
*Amy H. Newman, Ph.D., Scientific Director*
*Lorenzo Leggio, M.D., Ph.D., Deputy Scientific Director*

232 **Office of Women's Services: Substance Abuse & Mental Health Services**
5600 Fishers Lane 877-726-4727
Rockville, MD 20857 www.samhsa.gov

Provides leadership and guidance in creating and maintaining an agency-wide focus for addressing the substance abuse and mental health needs of women.

233 **Office on Smoking and Health: Centers for Disease Control & Prevention**
1600 Clifton Road 800-232-4636
Atlanta, GA 30329 TTY: 888-232-6348
tobaccoinfo@cdc.gov
www.cdc.gov/tobacco

Offers reference services to researchers through the Technical Information Center. Publishes and distributes a number of titles in the field of smoking and health.

234 **Partnership to End Addiction**
633 Third Avenue 212-922-1560
New York, NY 10011 855-378-4373
www.drugfree.org

Dedicated to transforming how addiction is addressed by the nation, from prevention to recovery.
*Creighton Drury, CEO*
*Emily Feinstein, J.D., COO*

235 **Recovered**
99 Wall Street info@recovered.org
New York, NY 10005 recovered.org

An organization of writers and editors dedicated to raising awareness on susbtance abuse.

236 **Remove Intoxicated Drivers (RID-USA)**
P.O. Box 520 518-372-0034
Schenectady, NY 12301 ridusa@verizon.net
rid-usa.org

Volunteers working to deter impaired driving, to help its victims obtain justice, restitution and peace of mind while navigating the criminal justice systems, and to curb the alcohol abuse which leads to drunk driving.
*Doris Aiken, Founder*

237 **Research Society on Alcoholism**
7801 North Lamar Blvd. 512-454-0022
Austin, TX 78752-1038 debbyrsa@sbcglobal.net
researchsocietyonalcohol.org

The Research Society on Alcoholism, founded in 1976, serves as a forum for scientists and researchers focused on the fields of alcoholism and alcohol-related problems. The Society promotes re-

search with the purpose of advancing treatment of alcoholism and finding potential cures.
*Lara Ray, PhD, President*
*Howard Becker, PhD, Vice President*

238 **Section for Psychiatric and Substance Abuse Services (SPSPAS)**
155 North Wacker Drive 312-422-3000
Chicago, IL 60606 800-424-4301
www.aha.org
A membership section that represents over 1,660 behavioral health providers and professionals who are members of the American Hospital Association (AHA). The Section applies AHA policy, advocacy, and service efforts to advance understandings of behavioral health care and to emphasize its importance.
*Richard J. Pollack, President & CEO*
*Michelle Hood, EVP & COO*

239 **Students Against Destructive Decisions**
655 15th Street NW 508-481-3568
Washington, DC 20005 www.sadd.org
Provides students with prevention tools to deal with the issues of underage drinking, drug use, risky and impaired driving, and other destructive decisions.
*Rick Birt, President & CEO*
*Elizabeth Vermette, VP, Public Affairs*

240 **Substance Abuse and Mental Health Services Administration (SAMHSA)**
5600 Fishers Lane 877-726-4727
Rockville, MD 20857 TTY: 800-487-4889
www.samhsa.gov
Part of the U.S. Department of Health and Human Services, SAMHSA promotes, monitors, evaluates and coordinates programs for the prevention and treatment of alcoholism and alcohol abuse.
*Miriam E. Delphin-Rittmon, Ph.D., Asstistant Secretary, Mental Health*

## *Alabama*

241 **Alabama Department of Mental Health: Div. of Mental Health & Substance Abuse**
100 North Union Street 334-242-3642
Montgomery, AL 36130 Alabama.DMH@mh.alabama.gov
www.mh.alabama.gov

## *Alaska*

242 **Alaska Department of Health: Office of Substance Abuse and Addiction Prevention**
3601 C Street 907-269-7800
Anchorage, AK 99503 osmap@alaska.gov
health.alaska.gov/Pages/default.aspx
*Heidi Hedberg, Commissioner*

## *Delaware*

243 **Delaware Division of Substance Abuse and Mental Health (DSAMH)**
Alcohol And Drug Services
1901 N. Du Pont Highway 302-255-9399
New Castle, DE 19720 DHSSInfor@state.de.us
dhss.delaware.gov/dsamh/
*Renata J. Henry, Director*

## *Florida*

244 **Alcohol and Drug Abuse Program**
Department of Children and Families
P.O. Box 1770 850-300-4323
Ocala, FL 34478-1770 Fax: 866-886-4342
myflfamilies.com/service-programs/samh/
The Substance Abuse and Mental Health (SAMH) Program, within the Florida Department of Children and Families, is the single state authority on substance abuse and mental health as designated by the federal Substance Abuse and Mental Health Services Administration (SAMHSA). The Department's SAMH Program oversees a statewide system of care for the prevention, treatment, and recovery of children and adults with serious mental illnesses and/or substance abuse disorders.

## *Georgia*

245 **Alcohol and Drug Services**
Addictive Diseases Program
Two Peachtree Street NW 404-657-2331
Atlanta, GA 30303 dbhdd.georgia.gov/be-supported/help-subs
DBHDD contracts with providers in all 6 regions to provide outpatient and residential substance abuse treatment to men and women who are struggling with the disease of addiction

## *Hawaii*

246 **Alcohol and Drug Abuse Division**
Department of Health
601 Kamokila Blvd. 808-692-7506
Kapoleiu, HI 96707 health.hawaii.gov/substance-abuse/
The mission of the Department of Health is to protect and improve the health and environment for all people in Hawai'i.
*Loretta J. Fuddy, Director*
*Keith Yamamoto, Asst. Director*

## *Illinois*

247 **Illinois Department of Alcoholism and Susbstance Abuse**
Department of Human Services
2605 Woodlawn Rd 815-632-4045
Sterling, IL 61081 www.dhs.state.il.us

## *Indiana*

248 **Indiana Division of Addiction Services**
800-901-1133
www.in.gov/fssa/dmha/home/

## *Iowa*

249 **Department of Public Health: Division of Substance Abuse**
Lucas State Office Bldg. 515-281-7689
Des Moines, IA 50319 866-227-9878
Fax: 515-281-4535
www.idph.state.ia.us
The Iowa Department of Public Health (IDPH) partners with local public health, policymakers, health care providers, business and many others to fulfill their mission of promoting and protecting the health of Iowans.
*DeAnn Decker, Bureau Chief*

## *Louisiana*

250 **Alcohol and Drug Abuse Council of South Louisiana**
1155 St. Charles Street 985-879-2273
Houma, LA 70360 Fax: 985-879-3766
ftoups@adacsl.org
www.dhh.louisiana.gov

## *Massachusetts*

251 **Bureau of Substance Addiction Services**
250 Washington Street 617-624-5111
Boston, MA 02108 800-327-5050
Fax: 617-624-5185
TTY: 888-448-8321
mass.gov/orgs/bureau-of-substance-addict

## *Nebraska*

252 **Department of Public Instruction: Division of Alcoholism and Drug Abuse**
301 Centennial Mall South 402-471-3121
Lincoln, NE 68509 866-866-8660
TTY: 800-833-7352
dhhs.ne.gov/Pages/Addiction-Treatment-an

## *New Jersey*

253 **New Jersey Division of Mental Health and Addiction Services**
5 Commerce Way 800-382-6717
Hamilton, NJ 08691 www.state.nj.us/humanservices/dmhas/home
*Valerie L. Mielke, MSW, Assistant Commissioner*

### New York

254 **New York Office of Addiction Services and Supports**
Substance Abuse Services
1450 Western Avenue 518-473-3460
Albany, NY 12203 877-846-7369
Fax: 518-457-5474
communications@oasas.ny.gov
www.oasas.ny.gov
*Chinazo Cunningham, Commissioner*
*Sean Byrne, Executive Deputy Commissioner*

### North Carolina

255 **North Carolina Mental Health and Substance Abuse**
NC Department of Health and Human Services
2001 Mail Service Center 800-662-7030
Raleigh, NC 27699-2000 www.dhhs.state.nc.us

### Oklahoma

256 **Oklahoma Department of Mental Health and Substance Abuse Services**
Substance Abuse Program
2000 N. Classen Blvd. 405-248-9200
Oklahoma City, OK 73106 oklahoma.gov/odmhsas.html

### Rhode Island

257 **Rhode Island Department of Behavioral Healthcare: Substance Use/Addiction**
14 Harrington Rd. 401-462-2339
02920ton, RI 02920 Fax: 401-462-3204
bhddh.ri.gov/substance-useaddiction
*Richard Charest, Director*

### South Carolina

258 **South Carolina Department of Alcohol and Drug Abuse Services**
1801 Main Street 803-896-5555
Columbia, SC 29201 www.daodas.org

### Tennessee

259 **Tennessee Department of Mental Health and Substance Abuse Services**
500 Deaderick Street 800-560-5767
Nashville, TN 37243 www.tn.gov/behavioral-health.html
*Marie Williams, Commissioner*

### Texas

260 **Texas Health And Human Service: Mental Health & Substance Use**
www.hhs.texas.gov
*Cecile Erwin Young, Executive Commissioner*

### Utah

261 **Utah Department of Health & Human Services : Substance Abuse & Mental Health**
195 North 1950 West dsamh@utah.gov
Salt Lake City, UT 84116 sumh.utah.gov

### Vermont

262 **Vermont Department of Health: Division of Substance Use Programs (DSU)**
108 Cherry Street 802-651-1550
Burlington, VT 05402 AHS.VDHADAP@vermont.gov
www.healthvermont.gov

### Virginia

263 **Virginia Department of Behavioral Health & Developmental Services**
Substance Use Disorder Services
1220 Bank Street 804-786-3921
Richmond, VA 23219 Fax: 804-371-6638
TTY: 804-371-8977
dbhds.virginia.gov
*Nelson Smith, Commissioner*

### Wyoming

264 **Wyoming Department of Health: Substance Use and Tobacco Prevention Program**
122 West 25th St. 307-777-6541
Cheyenne, WY 82002 wdh.prevention@wyo.gov
health.wyo.gov
*Mica Moeller, Program Manager*

## Foundations

265 **AAA Foundation for Traffic Safety**
607 14th Street NW 202-638-5944
Washington, DC 20005 info@aaafoundation.org
www.aaafoundation.org
A non-profit foundation that conducts research with the goal of preventing traffic deaths. Raises awareness on road safety measures and driver education.
*C. Y. David Yang, President & Executive Director*
*William J. Horrey, Technical Director*

266 **ABMRF/The Foundation for Alcohol Research**
1200-C Agora Dr. 800-688-7152
Bel Air, MD 21401 grantinfo@abmrf.org
www.abmrf.org
Founded in 1982 to promote research on testing systems that could diagnose the metabolic aspects of alcoholism. Seeks to educate the public on the validity of the disease concept of alcoholism.

267 **Brain & Behavior Research Foundation**
747 Third Avenue 646-681-4888
New York, NY 10017 800-829-8289
info@bbrfoundation.org
www.bbrfoundation.org
The Brain and Behavior Research Foundation awards grants aimed at advancing scientific understandings of mental health treatments and mental disorders such as depression and schizophrenia. The Brain and Behavior Research Foundation's mission is to eliminate the suffering caused by mental illness.
*Geoffrey A. Simon, Chairman*
*Miriam E. Katowitz, CPA, Vice President*

268 **Hazelden Betty Ford Foundation**
P.O. Box 11 844-598-4521
Center City, MN 55012 800-257-7810
info@hazeldenbettyford.org
www.hazelden.org
Helps individuals, families, and communities struggling with alcohol abuse, substance abuse, and drug addiction by offering prevention and recovery solutions nationwide.
*James A. Blaha, Vice President, CFO & CAO*
*Alta DeRoo, MD, Chief Medical Officer*

## Libraries & Resource Centers

269 **National Mental Health Consumers' Self-Help Clearinghouse**
selfhelpclearinghouse@gmail.com
mhselfhelp.org
The Clearinghouse is a peer-run national technical assistance center focused on achieving respect and equality of opportunity for those with mental illnesses. The Clearinghouse helps with the growth of the mental health consumer movement by evaluating mental health services, advocating for mental health reform, and providing consumers with news, information, publications, and consultation services.
*Joseph Rogers, Founder & Executive Director*
*Susan Rogers, Director*

270 **Parents Resource Institute for Drug Education**
160 Vanderbilt Court
Bowling Green, KY 42103
800-279-6361
Fax: 270-746-9598
info@pridesurveys.com
www.pridesurveys.com
Offers national information and educational materials pertaining to alcohol and drug dependency.
*Thomas J. Gleaton, EdD, President*
*Janie Pitcock, President*

## Research Centers

271 **Alcohol Research Group Public Health Institute**
Public Health Institute
6475 Christie Avenue
Emeryville, CA 94608
510-597-3440
Fax: 510-985-6459
info@arg.org
www.arg.org
The Alcohol Research Group (ARG) of the Public Health Institute was established in 1959 to conduct and disseminate high-quality research in epidemiology of alcohol consumption and problems including alcohol use disorders, alcohol-related health services research, and analyses of alcohol policy and its impacts.
*Thomas K. Greenfield, Scientific Director*

272 **Boston University Laboratory of Neuropsychology**
Dept of Behavioral Neuroscience
80 E Concord Street M9
Boston, MA 02118
617-638-4803
Fax: 617-638-4806
www.bu.edu
Offers research and studies into the effects of Alcoholism pertaining to aphasia, apraxia, dementia, memory disorders and various other neurological malfunctions.

273 **Center for Alcohol & Addiction Studies Brown University**
Brown University
121 South Main Street
Providence, RI 02903
401-863-6600
Fax: 401-863-6697
caas@brown.edu
www.caas.brown.edu
The Center for Alcohol and Addiction Studies, through its affiliation with the Brown Medical School, occupies a unique position within the University. The Center brings together more that 90 faculty and professional staff members, from 11 University departments and eight affiliated hospitals, to promote the identification, prevention, and effective treatment of alcohol and other substance abuse.
*Peter M. Monti, PhD, Center Director*
*Suzanne Colby, PhD, Associate Director*

274 **Centre for Addiction and Mental Health**
1001 Queen Street West
Toronto, ON, M6J-1H4
416-535-8501
800-463-2338
info@camh.ca
camh.ca
The Centre for Addiction and Mental Health is a mental health and addiction teaching hospital and research centre based in Canada. CAMH seeks to support people affected by mental health and addiction issues through research, education, policy development, clinical care, and the promotion of health.
*Sarah Downey, President & CEO*

275 **Cornerstone Treatment Facilities Network**
Medical Arts Center Hospital
159-05 Union Turnpike
Fresh Meadows, NY 11366
718-906-6700
800-233-9999
Fax: 718-906-6840
admin@cornerstoneny.com
www.cornerstoneny.com
Offers a complete integrated program for alcohol assessment alcohol and drug rehabilitation continuing care community education and comprehensive family recovery.
*Norine Hurtado, Senior Vice President, Human Resources*

276 **Dorothea Dix Hospital Clinical Research Unit**
809 Ruggles Drive
Raleigh, NC 27603
919-733-5227
866-349-5627
Fax: 919-733-5351
www.med.unc.edu
Researches the biological risk factors of alcoholism using young adults without the disease but with history of familial alcoholism.
*Terry Spell, Director*
*William L. Roper, CEO*

277 **Ernest Gallo Clinic and Research Center**
5858 Horton Street
Emeryville, CA 94608
510-985-3100
Fax: 510-985-3101
www.galloresearch.org
Alcoholism studies with a special emphasis on genetics.
*John A. De Luca, PhD, Chairman of the Board/President*
*Joseph E. Gallo, President/Chief Executive Officer*

278 **Families in Action**
National Drug Abuse Center
P.O. Box 3553
Wilson, NC 27895
252-237-1242
Fax: 252-237-6544
phil@familiesinaction.org
www.familiesinaction.org
Publish prevention materials and serves as an information clearinghouse for families with a member suffering from a drug or alcohol addiction.
*Phillip A. Mooring, Executive Director*
*Anna Godwin, Coordinator*

279 **Friends Medical Science Research Center**
1229 West Mount Royal Avenue
Baltimore, MD 21217
410-752-4218
Fax: 310-477-9601
www.wellness.com
Studies narcotic addictions.
*John Valenty, President*
*Rob Greenstein, President*

280 **Hahnemann University Laboratory of Human Pharmacology**
Department of Pharmacology
Broad and Vine
Philadelphia, PA 19102
215-762-7000
Fax: 215-762-8109
www.hahnemannhospital.com
Hahnemann University hospital is committed to providing quality patient care in an academic setting.

281 **Harvard Cocaine Recovery Project**
1493 Cambridge Street
Cambridge, MA 02139
617-498-1000
Fax: 617-642-58
Six-year study of relapse and recovery in cocaine addicts.

282 **Interdisciplinary Program in Cell and Molecular Pharmacology**
Medical University of South Carolina
173 Ashley Avenue BSB 358
Charleston, SC 29425
843-792-8975
Fax: 843-792-0481
www.musc.edu/pharm
Research into pharmacology and toxicology.
*Kenneth D. Tew, Ph.D., D.Sc., Professor and Chairman*
*Michelle Shorter, Administrative Coordinator*

283 **Johns Hopkins University: Behavioral Pharmacology Research Unit**
John Hopkins Bay View Campus
5510 Nathan Shock Drive
Baltimore, MD 21224
410-955-5000
Fax: 410-550-0030
bigelow@jhmi.edu
www.hopkinsmedicine.org
An internationally recognized center of excellence in research on psychoactive drugs. As the name implies BPRU's orientation is behavioral and pharmacological, emphasizing a behavioral analysis of drug action.
*George E. Bigelow, PhD, Scientific Director*
*Eric C. Strain, MD, Medical Director*

284 **Kettering-Scott Magnetic Resonance Laboratory**
Wright State University, School of Medicine
P.O. Box 927
Dayton, OH 45435
937-775-2934
www.med.wright.edu
No information found on the website.
*Marjorie Bowman, MD, Dean*
*Betty Kangas, Assistant to the dean*

285 **Marin Institute**
24 Belvedere Street
San Rafael, CA 94901
415-456-5692
Fax: 415-456-0491
www.marinInstitute.org

The mission of this Institute is to reduce the toll of alcohol and other drug problems on Marin County and society in general. The Institute fulfills this mission by developing, implementing, evaluating and disseminating innovative approaches to prevention locally, nationally and internationally.
*Bruce Lee Livingston, MPP, Executive Director*

286 **Narcotic and Drug Research**
11 Beach Street 212-966-8700
New York, NY 10013 Fax: 212-334-8058
Nonprofit organization that is devoted to drug abuse education treatment and prevention.
*Douglas S. Lipton, PhD, Director*

287 **National Center on Addiction and Substance Abuse**
Columbia University
633 3rd Avenue 212-841-5200
New York, NY 10017 800-622-4357
Fax: 212-956-8020
www.casacolumbia.org
The only nation-wide organization that brings together under one roof all the professional disciplines needed to study and combat abuse of all substances - alcohol nicotine as well as illegal prescription and performance enhancing drugs - in all sectors of society.
*Lee C. Bollinger, President*
*Ursula M. Burns, Chairman & CEO*

288 **National Prevention Resource Center CSAP Division of Communications Programs**
CSAP Division of Communications Programs
5600 Fishers Lane 301-443-9936
Rockville, MD 20857
Supports an array of prevention program evaluation approaches including individual grantee evaluations program evaluations and a National Evaluation Project. Also offers a National Data Base to provide information on programs for prevention of substance abuse.

289 **National Volunteer Training Center for Substance Abuse Prevention**
CSAP Division of Communications Programs
5600 Fishers Lane 301-443-9936
Rockville, MD 20857
Volunteers are always on hand to provide answers, information, referrals and resources pertaining to alcohol, drugs and substance abuse.

290 **Ohio State University Clinical Pharmacology Division**
College of Medicine
370 Western 9th Avenue 614-292-2220
Columbus, OH 43210 800-252-3636
Fax: 614-292-4293
www.medicine.osu.edu
Substance abuse and alcohol related research.
*Robert Bornstein, PhD, Vice Dean, Academic Affairs*
*Glen Apsloss, Director*

291 **Research Institute on Alcoholism**
State University of New York at Buffalo
1021 Main Street 716-887-2566
Buffalo, NY 14203 Fax: 716-872-52
connors@ria.buffalo.edu
www.ria.buffalo.edu
Integral part of the New York State Division of Alcoholism and Alcohol Abuse.
*Kenneth E. Leonard, PhD, Director*
*Kimberly S. Walitzer, PhD, Deputy Director*

292 **Rockefeller University Laboratory of Biology**
1230 York Avenue 212-327-8000
New York, NY 10065 Fax: 212-327-7974
www.rockefeller.edu

293 **Rutgers University Center of Alcohol Studies**
Busch Campus
607 Allison Road 732-445-2190
Piscataway, NJ 08854 Fax: 732-445-3500
alclib@rci.rutgers.edu
alcoholstudies.rutgers.edu
Causes and treatment of alcoholism.

294 **Ruth E. Golding Clinical Pharmacokinetics Laboratory**
College of Pharmacy
1703 E Mabel 520-626-1938
Tucson, AZ 85721 www.pharmacy.arizona.edu
Conducts studies of drugs in humans and animals.

295 **Southern California Research Institute**
7065 Hayvenhurst Avenue 310-390-8481
Van Nuys, CA 90066 Fax: 310-390-8482
www.scri.org
Effects of alcohol and drugs on behavior studies.
*Dary Fiorent, PhD, Executive Director*

296 **Stanford Center for Research in Disease Prevention**
Stanford University School of Medicine
1070 Arastradero Road 650-723-6254
Palo Alto, CA 94304 Fax: 650-723-6254
prevention.stanford.edu
Prevention and control of alcohol and drug abuse related disorders.
*John P.A Loannidis, MD, DSc, Director*

297 **State University of New York at Buffalo Toxicology Research Center**
3435 Main Street 716-831-2125
Buffalo, NY 14214 Fax: 716-829-2806
www.smbs.buffalo.edu
Toxicology-related research and services, including the development of tests to evaluate toxins, chemicals and drugs.
*Michale E. Cain, Director*
*Dr. James R. Olson, Assistant Director*

298 **UAMS Psychiatric Research Institute**
4224 Shuffield Drive 501-526-8100
Little Rock, AR 72205 kramerteresal@uams.edu
www.psychiatry.uams.edu
Combining research, education and clinical services into one facility, PRI offers inpatiend and outpatient services, with 40 psychiatric beds, therapy options, and specialized treatment for specific disorders, including: addictive eating, anxiety, deppressive and post-traumatic stress disorders. Research focuses on evidence-based care takes into consideration the education of future medical personnel while relying on research scientists to provide innovative forms of treatment.

299 **University of California: Los Angeles Alcohol Research Center**
405 Hilgard Ave 310-825-4321
Los Angeles, CA 90095 Fax: 310-206-7309
www.ucla.edu
Causes of alcoholism, including genetics.
*Dr. Ernest Noble, Director*

300 **University of Michigan: Alcohol Research Center**
400 E Eisenhower Parkway 734-764-1817
Ann Arbor, MI 48108 Fax: 734-998-7994
www.umich.edu
Alcohol abuse studies among the elderly, including the relationship between alcohol and aged disorders.
*Robert A. Zucker, PhD, Contact*

301 **University of Michigan: Psychiatric Center**
4250 Plymouth road 734-936-5900
Ann Arbor, MI 48109 Fax: 734-936-9761
www.umich.edu
Psychiatric disease research pertaining to the effects of alcoholism and drug abuse.

302 **University of Minnesota: Program on Alcohol/Drug Control**
Stadium Gate 27 612-624-6861
Minneapolis, MN 55455
Alcohol, tobacco and drug research.
*Dr. James Schaefer, Director*

303 **University of Missouri: Kansas City Drug Information Service**
2464 Charlotte 816-235-5490
Kansas City, MO 64108 Fax: 816-235-5491
umkcdruginformation@umkc.edu
dic.umkc.edu

Literature research and evaluation of clinical drug problems and questions.
*Pat Bryant, PhD, Director*
*Heather A. Pace, PhD, Assistant Director*

**304 University of Tennessee Drug Information Center**
875 Monroe Avenue 901-528-5555
Memphis, TN 38163 Fax: 901-448-5419
dop.utmem.edu/dic
*Katie Suda, Director*
*Camille Thornton, Assistant Professor*

**305 University of Texas Health Science Center Neurophysiology Research Center**
Speech & Hearing Institute
7000 Fannin 713-500-4472
Houston, TX 77030 Fax: 713-792-4513
Conducts clinical and animal studies aimed at combating alcohol, drug and tobacco dependence.
*Giuseppe N. Colasurdo, Director*

**306 University of Texas at Austin: Drug Synamics Institute**
1 University Station 512-475-9746
Austin, TX 78712 Fax: 512-471-2746
www.utexas.edu
Pharmaceutical and drug research.
*Janet C. Walkow, PhD, Director*
*Carla Van Den Berg, PhD, Associate Professor*

**307 University of Utah: Center for Human Toxicology**
30 South 2000 East 801-581-6731
Salt Lake City, UT 84112 Fax: 801-581-3716
dwilkins@alanine.pharm.utah.edu
www.pharmacy.utah.edu
Clinical, forensic and toxicology research.
*Chris M. Ireland, PhD, Dean*
*Dennis Crouch, Director*

**308 University of Wisconsin Milwaukee Medicinal Chemistry Group**
University of Wisconsin
P.O. Box 413 414-229-1122
Milwaukee, WI 53201 www4.uwm.edu
Research on drugs, including studies of valium receptors.
*Michael R. Lovell, Chancellor*

## Support Groups & Hotlines

**309 Adult Children of Alcoholics**
P.O. Box 811 310-534-1815
Lakewood, CA 90714 adultchildren.org
An anonymous twelve-step, twelve-tradition program of women and men who grew up in an alcoholic or otherwise dysfunctional homes.

**310 Al-Anon Alateen Family Group Hotline**
1600 Corporate Landing Parkway 757-563-1600
Virginia Beach, VA 23454 888-425-2666
Fax: 757-563-1655
wso@alanon.org
www.al-anon.alateen.org
A mutual peer-to-peer support program with groups meeting worldwide to provide hope and help to the families of alcoholics. Although a seperate entity from Alcoholics Anonymous, this program is based upon the Twelve Steps.
*Ric Buchanan, Executive Director*

**311 Al-Anon Family Group National Referral Hotline**
1600 Corporate Landing Parkway 757-563-1600
Virginia Beach, VA 23454 wso@al-anon.org
al-anon.alateen.org
Al-Anon is a mutual support group of peers who share their experience in applying the Al-Anon principles to problems related to the effects of a problem drinker in their lives. It is not group therapy and is not led by a counselor or therapist; This support network complements and supports professional treatment.

**312 Alateen and Al-Anon Family Groups**
1600 Corporate Landing Parkway 757-563-1600
Virginia Beach, VA 23454 888-425-2666
wso@al-anon.org
A fellowship of men, women, children and adult children affected by another persons drinking.
*Mary Ann Keller, Director, Members Services*

**313 Alcohol Drug Treatment Referral**
1316 South Coast Highway 800-454-8966
Laguna Beach, CA 92651 Fax: 949-281-1933
National Help and Referral Network, a nonprofit organization available 24 hours a day to assist people troubled by drug or alcohol abuse. Here to provide information on addiction treatment and support services and to help save lives and mend broken dreams.
*Mike Cohan, Director*

**314 Alcoholics Anonymous (AA): World Services**
475 Riverside Drive at W. 120th St. 212-870-3400
New York, NY 10115 www.aa.org
For men and women who share the common problems of alcoholism.

**315 Chemically Dependent Anonymous**
P.O. Box 423 888-232-4673
Severna Park, MD 21146 www.cdaweb.org
A 12-step fellowship for anyone seeking freedom from drug and alcohol addiction. The basis of the program is abstinence from all mood-changing and mind-altering chemicals, including street-type drugs, alcohol and unnecessary medication.

**316 Cocaine Anonymous**
21720 S. Wilmington Ave 310-559-5833
Long Beach, CA 90810-1641 cawso@ca.org
ca.org
Fellowship of men and women who share their experience, stength and hope with each other in hope that they may solve their common problem and help others recover from their addiction.

**317 Drug Free Workplace Hotline**
Division of Workplace Programs
Samhsa Diagonal CSAP 1 Choke Cherry 240-276-2612
Rockville, MD 20857 877-726-4727
Fax: 240-276-1210
TDD: 800-457-4889
webmaster@samhsa.hhs.gov
www.drugfreeworkplace.gov
A hotline for businesses to obtain information on a wide range of drug abuse related problems, issues and services.
*Robert Stephenson II, Director*

**318 Friday Night Live**
California Dept of Drug & Alcohol Programs
1700 K Street 916-445-7456
Sacramento, CA 95814 Fax: 916-230-59
www.communitycounseling.org/fnl
These groups, located in California, are all run by students with a faculty adviser. They arrange local alcohol and drug free events, from dances and movies to visiting hospitalized children. Students not only have fun but they learn to have fun sober.
*Jim Kooler, Administrator*
*Laura Purcellabuzo, Project Coordinator*

**319 Images Within: A Child's View of Parental Alcoholism**
Children of Alcoholics Foundation
P.O. Box 4185 212-595-5810
New York, NY 10163 800-359-2623
www.coaf.org
An innovative program designed to teach all children about family alcoholism. Middle-school-aged children learn how to get help for themselves or give help to their friends.

**320 Infoline**
United Way of Connecticut
1344 Silas Deane Highway 860-571-7500
Rocky Hill, CT 06067 800-203-1234
TTY: 800-671-0737
ctunitedway.org
Infoline is a free, confidential, help-by-telephone service for information, referral, and crisis intervention. Trained professionals help callers find information, discover options or deal with a crisis

by locating hundreds of services in their area on many different issues, from substance abuse to elder needs to suicide to volunteering in your community. Infoline is certified by the American Association of Suicidology. Operates 24 hours a day, everyday. Multilingual caseworkers are available.
*Richard Porth, CEO*

321 **MADD-Mothers Against Drunk Drivers**
511 E. John Carpenter Freeway 877-275-6233
Irving, TX 75062 www.madd.org
Mission is to stop drunk driving, support the victims of this violent crime and prevent underage drinking. MADD's work has saved nearly 300,000 lives and counting.
*Ellen Willmott, Interim CEO*
*Andrew Robinson, Chair*

322 **Marijuana Anonymous**
5551 Hollywood Blvd. 800-766-6779
Hollywood, CA 90028-6814 support@marijuana-anonymous.org
marijuana-anonymous.org
A fellowship of men and women who share experience, strength and hope with each other to solve common problem and help others to recover from marijuana addiction.

323 **Nar-Anon Family Groups**
22527 Crenshaw Blvd 310-534-8188
Torrance, CA 90505 800-477-6291
nar-anon.org
Twelve-step program for families and friends of addicts.
*Cathy Khaledi, Executive Director*

324 **Narcotics Anonymous**
P.O. Box 9999 818-773-9999
Van Nuys, CA 91409 na.org
Peer support for recovered addicts.

325 **National Health Information Center**
Office of Disease Prevention & Health Promotion
1101 Wootton Pkwy Fax: 240-453-8281
Rockville, MD 20852 odphpinfo@hhs.gov
www.health.gov/nhic
Supports public health education by maintaining a calendar of National Health Observances; helps connect consumers and health professionals to organizations that can best answer questions and provide up-to-date contact information from reliable sources; updates on a yearly basis toll-free numbers for health information, Federal health clearinghouses and info centers.
*Don Wright, MD, MPH, Director*

326 **Pathways to Promise**
5400 Arsenal Street
Saint Louis, MO 63139 pathways2promise.org
An interfaith cooperative of many faith groups, providing assistance and a resource center which offers liturgical and educational materials, program models, caring ministry with people experiencing a mental illness and their families.

327 **Rational Recovery**
P.O. Box 800 530-621-2667
Lotus, CA 95651 rational.org
Exclusive, worldwide source of counseling, guidance and direct instruction on self-recovery from addiction to alcohol and other drugs through planned, permanent abstinence.
*Jack Trimpey, President*

328 **SMART Recovery**
7304 Mentor Avenue 440-951-5357
Mentor, OH 44060 866-951-5357
info@smartrecovery.org
smartrecovery.org
The leading self-empowering addiction recovery support group. Participants learn tools for addiction recovery based on the latest scientific research and participate in a world-wide community which includes free, self-empowering, science-based mutual help groups.
*Shari Allwood, Executive Director*

329 **Students Against Destructive Decisions (SADD)**
655 15th Street NW 508-481-3568
Washington, DC 20005 www.sadd.org
SADD's mission is to provide students with the best prevention tools possible to deal with the issues of underage drinking, other drug use, risky and impaired driving, and other destructive decisions.
*Rick Birt, President & CEO*
*Elizabeth Vermette, VP, Public Affairs*

330 **ToughLove International**
P.O. Box 1069 215-348-7090
Doylestown, PA 18901 800-333-1069
www.toughlove.org
This national self-help group for parents, children and communities emphasizes cooperation, personal initiative and action. Publishes books, brochures and promotional information and holds workshops and seminars across the country.

331 **WFS' New Life Program**
Women for Sobriety
P.O. Box 618 215-536-8026
Quakertown, PA 18951 Fax: 215-538-9026
newlife@nni.com
www.womenforsobriety.org
A self-help program for women that can be used independent from AA or with AA. Groups are in many states in the United States. Donations suggested.
*Rebecca M. Fenner, Director*

## Print Resources

332 **ACAP Recap**
American Council on Alcohol Problems
3426 Bridgeland Drive 314-739-5944
Bridgeton, MO 63044 Fax: 314-739-0848
www.lifemanagement.com
Offers information on organization activities and events, updates on resources and publications and legislative information for affiliate executives.
*Dr. Curt Scarborough, Executive Director*

333 **Alcohol Research: Current Reviews (ARCR)**
National Institute on Alcohol Abuse and Alcoholism
9000 Rockville Pike 301-443-3860
Bethesda, MD 20892 arcr.niaaa.nih.gov
An open-access, peer-reviewed journal available online with no subscription or pay-per-view fees. Publishes reviews on the field of alcohol research.
*Pamela Wernett, PhD, PMP, Editor-in-Chief*
*Sheri Grabus, PhD, Managing Editor*

334 **American Issue**
American Council on Alcohol Problems
3426 Bridgeland Drive 314-739-5944
Bridgeton, MO 63044 Fax: 314-739-0848
www.lifemanagement.com
Offered to contributors of the organization.
*Dr. Curt Scarborough, Executive Director*

335 **Drug Abuse Update**
2296 Henderson Mill Road 770-934-6364
Atlanta, GA 30345
A journal of news and information for persons interested in drug prevention.

336 **Forum Magazine**
Al-Anon Alateen Family Group Headquarters
1600 Corp Landing Pkwy. 757-563-1600
Virginia Beach, VA 23454-5617 888-425-2666
Fax: 757-563-1655
wso@al-anon.org
www.al-anon.alateen.org
Contains many personal stories of inspiration, some of which are maade available each month on the Internet by authorization of Al-Anon Family Group Headquarters, Inc.

337 **Lead Line**
Grapevine
P.O. Box 1980 212-870-3400
New York, NY 10163 Fax: 212-870-3301

AA members all over the world communicate with each other through the pages of this magazine. It contains: insight into how AAs stay sober; readers' views; old-timers corner, beginners meeting, youth enjoying sobriety, and spotlight on service.

338 **Substance Abuse: Research and Treatment**
Sage Publishing
katy.shanahan@sagepub.co.uk
journals.sagepub.com/home/sata
An international, peer-reviewed journal that publishes content on human substance abuse research and treatment.
*Gregory L. Stuart, Editor-in-Chief*
*Susan Ramsey, Deputy Editor-in-Chief*

## Web Sites

339 **AA-Alcoholics Anonymous**
www.aa.org
Group sharing their experience, strength and hope with each other to recover from alcoholism.

340 **AAA Foundation for Traffic Safety**
www.aaafoundation.org
The AAA Foundation for Traffic Safety was founded in 1947 by AAA to conduct research to address growing highway safety issues. The organization's mission is to identify traffic safety problems, foster research that seeks solutions and disseminate information and educational materials.

341 **Addiction Resource Guide**
www.addictionresourceguide.com
A comprehensive directory of addiction treatment facilities online.

342 **Adult Children of Alcoholics & Dysfunctional Families World Srvc. Org.**
www.adultchildren.org
A 12-step and 12-tradition program for adults raised in an environment including alcohol or other dysfunctions.

343 **Al-Anon**
www.al-anon.alateen.org
The single purpose of this organization is to help families and friends of alcoholics, whether the alcoholic is still drinking or not.

344 **Alateen**
www.al-anon.org/for-alateen
A part of the Al-Anon program, Alateen is for teenagers who have been affected by someone else's drinking, whether it be a family member or a friend.

345 **American Council for Drug Education**
www.acde.org
This organization provides information on drug use, publishes books and offers films and curriculum materials for prevention.

346 **Association for Addiction Professionals (NAADAC)**
www.naadac.org
NAADAC is the premier global organization of addiction focused professionals who enhance the health and recovery of individuals, families and communities. NAADAC's mission is to lead, unify and empower addiction focused professionals to achieve excellence through education, advocacy, knowledge, standards of practice, ethics, professional development and research.

347 **Center for Family Support (CFS)**
www.cfsny.org
Devoted to providing support and assistance to individuals with developmental and related disabilities, and to the family members who care for them.

348 **Cocaine Anonymous**
www.ca.org
A support group based on the twelve steps of Alcoholics Anonymous that focuses specifically on problems of cocaine addiction.

349 **FASD United**
fasdunited.org
Develops and implements innovative prevention and education strategies assessing fetal alcohol syndrome.

350 **Families Anonymous**
www.familiesanonymous.org
Addresses the needs of families who are concerned about a relative with a drug problem and with related behavioral problems.

351 **Hazelden**
www.hazelden.com
Organization dedicated to providing quality rehabilitation, education and professional services for chemical dependency and related addictive behaviors.

352 **Healing Well**
www.healingwell.com
A social network and support community for patients, caregivers, and families coping with the daily struggles of diseases, disorders and chronic illness.

353 **Healthlink USA**
www.healthlinkusa.com
Health information concerning treatment, cures, prevention, diagnosis, risk factors, research, support groups, email lists, personal stories and much more. Updated regularly.

354 **Higher ED Center**
www.higheredcenter.org
One-stop resource for information about abuse prevention and addiction treatment.

355 **Indian Health Service**
www.ihs.gov
Charged with providing a comprehensive program of alcoholism and substance abuse prevention and treatment for Native Americans and Alaskan natives.

356 **Jewish Alcoholics, Chemically Dependent Persons and Significant Others (JACS)**
www.jacsweb.org
Ten articles dealing with denial and ignorance.

357 **Lawyers Concerned for Lawyers**
www.mnlcl.org
Lawyers Concerned for Lawyers provides free, confidential peer and professional assistance to Minnesota lawyers, judges, law students, and their immediate family members on any issue that causes stress or distress.

358 **LifeRing Secular Recovery**
www.lifering.org
Offers nonreligious approach with links to groups.

359 **MedicineNet**
www.medicinenet.com
An online resource for consumers providing easy-to-read, authoritative medical and health information.

360 **Medscape**
www.medscape.com
Medscape offers specialists, primary care physicians, and other health professionals the Web's most robust and integrated medical information and educational tools.

361 **MentalHealth.com**
www.mentalhealth.com
Online information and a virtual encyclopedia related to mental disorders, possible causes and treatments. News, articles, on-line diagnostic programs and related links. Designed to improve understanding, diagnosis and treatment of mental illness throughout the world. Awarded the Top Site Award and the NetPsych Cutting Edge Site Award.

362 **Mothers Against Drunk Driving**
www.madd.org
A crusade to stop alcohol consumption and underage drinking.

363 **MyHealthfinder**
www.healthfinder.gov
Searchable, carefully developed web site offering information on over 1000 topics. Developed by the US Department of Health and Human Services, the site can be used in both English and Spanish.

364 **National Clearinghouse for Alcohol and Drug Information**
www.health.org

365 **National Council for Mental Wellbeing**
www.thenationalcouncil.org
A network for sharing information and provding assistance among those working in the healthcare management field.

366 **National Council on Alcoholism and Drug Dependence**
www.ncadd.org
Provides education, information, help and hope in the fight against addictions. Nationwide network of affiliates, advocates prevention, intervention and treatment, and is committed to ridding the disease of its stigma and its sufferers of their denial and shame.

367 **National Crime Prevention Council**
www.ncpc.org
This organization works to prevent crime and drug use in many ways, including developing materials for parents and children.

368 **National Institute on Alcohol Abuse & Alcoholism**
www.niaaa.nih.gov
Supports research nationwide on alcohol abuse and alcoholism.

369 **National Institute on Drug Abuse (NIDA)**
www.drugabuse.gov
NIDA's mission is to lead the Nation in bringing the power of science to bear on drug abuse and addiction.

370 **National Mental Health Consumers' Self-Help Clearinghouse**
www.mhselfhelp.org
Encourages the development and growth of consumer self-help groups.

371 **Office on Smoking and Health**
www.cdc.gov/tobacco/
Offers reference services to researchers through the Technical Information Center. Publishes and distributes a number of titles in the field of smoking and health.

372 **Psych Central**
www.psychcentral.com
Personalized one-stop index for psychology, support, and mental health issues, resources, and people on the Internet.

373 **SMART Recovery**
www.smartrecovery.org
Four-Point program includes maintaining motivation, coping with urges, managing feelings and behavior, balancing momentary/enduring satisfactions.

374 **Safe Homes**
www.yescap.org/safehomes/safehomes.htm
This national organization encourages parents to sign a contract stipulating that when parties are held in one another's homes they will adhere to a strict no-alcohol/no-drug-use rule.

375 **Souls Self Help**
www.soulselfhelp.on.ca/coda.html
Discusses self-help, mental health, issues of co-dependency.

376 **Students Against Destructive Decisions (SADD)**
www.sadd.org
Peer leadership organization dedicated to preventing destructive decisions.

377 **Substance Abuse and Mental Health Services Administration (SAMHSA)**
www.samhsa.gov
Provides links to government resources related to substance abuse and mental health.

378 **The Alcoholism Home Page**
www.alcoholism.about.com
Information about addictive drug use, behaviors, and alcoholism.

379 **WebMD**
www.webmd.com
Provides credible information, supportive communities, and in-depth reference material about health subjects. A source for original and timely health information, as well as material from well-known content providers.

# SECTION THREE:
# HEALTH COMPLICATIONS OF ADDICTION

# AIDS/HIV

*Human immunodeficiency virus, commonly called HIV, is a virus that attacks the immune system. If HIV is not treated, it can lead to acquired immunodeficiency syndrome, or AIDS. There is no cure for HIV, and carrying the virus lasts for life. With appropriate medical care, HIV can be controlled and individuals with the virus can live a long, healthy life and protect their partners. The only way to detect HIV is through testing. Early symptoms mimic flu, making it difficult to know of exposure and infection with testing. The stages of HIV are acute HIV infection, chronic HIV infection and lastly, AIDS, the most severe stage of HIV infection, which badly damages the immune system and leads to infections and other serious illnesses. If HIV transitions to AIDS, life expectancy is approximately three years.*

HIV is spread by contact with bodily fluids of an infected person—most commonly during unprotected sex, or sex without a condom or HIV medicine to prevent or treat HIV; or through sharing of injection drug equipment such as needles. Body fluids that may carry the virus include blood, pre-seminal fluid and semen, vaginal fluids, rectal fluids and breast milk. Risky health behaviors such as having unprotected sex or sharing needles are often seen when individuals have a substance use disorder. In an attempt to get a euphoric high, individuals may turn to prostitution to get money or drugs, resulting in exposure to HIV-positive individuals or, if infected, may expose others. Sharing needles as seen in drug abuse situations is a source of viral transmission. Having oral sex rarely transmits the HIV virus, but is possible if ejaculation in the mouth occurs or there are sores or bleeding gums in the mouth. Receiving blood transfusion, blood products or organ or tissue transplants rarely transmit the virus because of testing of both blood and organs prior to use. A very small number of cases of transmission have occurred as the result of a bite from an infected person.

Viral load is the amount of HIV in the blood stream. The higher the load, the greater the chance of transmission from the infected person to the non-infected person. Taking HIV medicine as prescribed can usually allow the individual to achieve an undetectable viral load with six months. With continual medication and healthy behaviors, the infected individual will not transmit the virus to the HIV-negative partner through sex. The problem with substance use disorder is that it may cloud focus and make it difficult to stick to a daily HIV medication regime.

HIV and substance use disorders are an integrated problem when patterns of alcohol abuse or abuse of other substances such as crack cocaine, methamphetamine (meth), prescription opioids, and heroin lead to risky behaviors. Because substance abuse often lowers the ability to make rational decisions, impaired judgement often leads to unprotected sexual encounters, sharing of drug paraphernalia, having multiple partners and other behaviors designed to help the individual obtain their substance of abuse. Drug interactions between HIV medications and recreational drugs can increase the risk of dangerous side effects.

Seeking help for substance use disorder is vitally important, but not all individuals will follow this guidance. If you do not seek help, get tested if there is any chance you may be HIV-positive. Substance use in the person with HIV who abuses drugs and alcohol may create a weakened immune system. A damaged liver from drugs and alcohol must work harder to remove toxins from the body. If the individual cannot control alcohol and drug use, they should not have sex if high. Condom use is vital but there is no guarantee that using a condom will protect the individual or partner. Using only new, sterile needles each time you inject will decrease HIV transmission risk. And never have sex with a non-infected person, as you are creating a problem for another individual based on poor personal choices.

Substance use disorder creates an opportunity for risky behaviors. HIV/AIDS is just one example of the dangers that may occur.

## Agencies & Associations

380 **AIDS Coalition of Nova Scotia**
5516 Spring Garden Road 902-425-4882
Sydney, Nova Scotia, B3J-1G6 800-566-2437
Fax: 902-422-6200
acns.ns.ca
Provides support and advocacy services for PLW HIV/AIDS (people living with HIV/AIDS). Services provided deal with social, legal, ethical and spiritual issues.
*Chris Aucoin, Executive Director*
*Ned Macinnis, Program Support*

381 **AIDS Committee of Durham Region**
115 Simcoe Street South 905-576-1445
Oshawa, Ontario, L1H-4G7 877-361-8750
Fax: 905-576-4610
info@aidsdurham.com
www.aidsdurham.com
To provide HIV/AIDS related services to the infected or affected and the general community in the region of Durham.
*Dr. Warren Keyes, President*
*Miriam Philips, Vice President*

382 **AIDS Committee of North Bay & Area**
102-147 McIntyre St. W. 705-497-3560
North Bay, Ontario, P1B-2Y5 800-387-3701
Fax: 705-497-7850
oaacnba@gmail.com
aidsnorthbay.ca
To assist and support all persons infected or affected by HIV/AIDS and to limit the spread of the virus through education and outreach strategies.
*Stacey Mayhall, Executive Director*
*Steve Lamb, Support Services Coordinator*

383 **AIDS Committee of Ottawa**
19 Main Street 613-238-5014
Ottawa, Ontario, K1S-1A9 Fax: 613-238-3425
info@aco-cso.ca
www.aco-cso.ca
Works to empower people living with HIV/AIDS and the PLWHA (persons living with HIV/AID) community in Ottawa through promoting the well being and quality of life of those living with, or close affected by HIV/AIDS.
*Khaled Salam, Executive Director*
*Cory Wong, Manager, Support Services*

384 **AIDS Committee of Toronto**
543 Yonge Street 416-340-2437
Toronto, Ontario, M4Y-1Y5 Fax: 416-340-8224
ask@actoronto.org
www.actoronto.org
Delivers responsive, effective, and valued community-based HIV support services and education, prevention, outreach and fundraising programs that promote health, well-being, worth and rights of individuals and communities living with, affected by and at risk for HIV/AIDS, and increase awareness of HIV/AIDS.
*John Maxwell, Executive Director*
*Katie Wilson, Communications Coordinator*

385 **AIDS Network: Halton, Haldimand, Norfolk and Brant**
140 King Street East 905-528-0854
Hamilton, ON, L8N 866-563-0563
Fax: 905-528-6311
www.aidsnetwork.ca
The AIDS Network provides supportive services to individuals affected by or living with HIV/AIDS in Hamilton, Halton, Haldimand, Norfolk and Brant.

386 **AIDS New Brunswick**
440 Wilsey Road 833-561-4009
Fredericton, NB, E3B-6E9 Fax: 506-455-2625
info@aidsnb.com
www.aidsnb.com
A provincial organization committed to facilitating community-based responses to the issues of HIV/AIDS. The aim is to promote and support the health and well-being of persons living with and affected by HIV/AIDS and to reduce the spread of HIV/AIDS in New Brunswick.
*Linda Thompson-Brown, Executive Director*
*Meaghan Coughlan, Education Managers Manager*

387 **AIDS Outreach Center (AOC)**
400 North Beach Street 817-335-1994
Fort Worth, TX 76111 info@aoc.org
www.aoc.org
The staff and volunteers of the AIDS Outreach Center (AOC) provide a wide range of social services, outreach activities, testing and counseling, prevention education programs and public policy advocacy for men, women and children living with HIV, and their loved ones.
*Kelly Allen Gray, Executive Director*
*Johnnie Wellborne, Associate Executive Director*

388 **AIDS United**
1634 Eye St. NW 202-408-4848
Washington, DC 20006 Fax: 202-408-1818
www.aidsunited.org
Dedicated to ending the HIV epidemic in the U.S. through their public policy work.
*Jesse Milan, Jr., President & CEO*
*Carl Baloney, Jr., Vice President & Chief Advocacy Officer*

389 **ANKORS: Kootenay & Boundary HIV/AIDS and Hepatitis C Support Services**
101 Baker Street 250-505-5506
Nelson, BC, V1L-4H1 Fax: 250-505-5507
information@ankors.bc.ca
www.ankors.bc.ca
ANKORS' mission is to respond to the evolving needs of those living with and affected by HIV/AIDS and Hepatitis C.
*Cheryl Dowden, Executive Director*

390 **American Autoimmune Related Diseases Association**
19176 Hall Road 586-776-3900
Clinton Township, MI 48038 hello@autoimmune.org
www.autoimmune.org
Provides awareness, education, and referrals for patients with any type of autoimmune disease.
*Jason Gamel, President/CEO*
*Rob Dunn, RRP, Chief Financial Officer*

391 **Black Coalition for AIDS Prevention**
20 Victoria Street 416-977-9955
Toronto, M5C Fax: 416-977-7664
info@black-cap.com
www.blackcap.ca
A volunteer-driven, charitable, not-for-profit, community-based organization.
*Luka Amona, Chair*
*Rose-Ann Bailey, Vice Chair*

392 **CAYR Community Connections**
17665 Leslie Street 905-884-0613
Newmarket, Ontario, L3Y-3E3 800-243-7717
Fax: 905-884-7215
info@cayrcc.org
cayrcc.org
CAYR Community Connections was originally founded as the AIDS Committee of York Region in 1993. CAYR's mission is to create safe, confidential, and inclusive spaces and services in York Region where people can access dignified support and meaningfully engagement. Offers specialized services to people living with HIV/AIDS, people affected by or are at risk of HIV and Hep C, people who use drugs, people who identify as LGBTQ+, people of marginalized communities.
*Marie Morton, Executive Director*
*Monica Meza-Opazo, Manager, HIV & HCV Support*

393 **Children's AIDS Fund International**
P.O. Box 16433 703-433-1560
Washington, DC 20041 Fax: 703-433-1561
info@childrensaidsfund.org
www.childrensaidsfund.org
The Children's AIDS Fund aims to limit the suffering of children and their families caused by HIV, by providing care, services, re-

sources, referrals, and education. The fund operates in the U.S. and abroad.

394 **Elevate NWO**
102-106 Cumberland Street N. 807-345-1516
Thunder Bay, Ontario, P7A-4M2 Fax: 807-345-2505
info@elevatenwo.org
www.elevatenwo.org
Provides support, education and advocacy around HIV and AIDS, and Hepatitis C for communities in Thunder Bay and Northwestern Ontario.

395 **HIV West Yellowhead**
102 Government Road 780-740-0066
Hinton, Alberta, T7V-2A6 877-291-8811
director@hivoptions.ca
www.hivoptions.ca
Services include harm reduction, needle exchange, overdose prevention, free safe sex supplies, care and support, prevention, and education.
*Lori Phillips, Executive Director*
*Stacey Dickerson, Prevention & Engagement Coordinator*

396 **Housing Works**
57 Willoughby St. 347-473-7400
Brooklyn, New York, NY 11201 info@housingworks.org
www.housingworks.org
Housing Works provides advocacy services for those living with HIV/AIDS, as well as housing, healthcare, nutrition, counseling, mental health and substance abuse treatment, job training, and legal assistance. Also runs thrift shops and bookstores that raise money for the organization's services.
*Charles King, Chief Executive Officer*
*Matthew Bernardo, Executive Director*

397 **International Council of AIDS Service Organization**
120 Carlton Street 416-921-0018
Toronto, Ontario, M5A-4K2 icaso@icaso.org
www.icaso.org
A global network of non-governmental and community-based organizations.
*Mary Ann Torres, Executive Director*
*Galina Godovanny, Financial Manager*

398 **Keep A Child Alive**
17 State Street 646-975-5559
New York, NY 10004 info@keepachildalive.org
www.keepachildalive.org
Mission is to make a positive difference in the lives of children infected with HIV and affected by AIDS.
*Antonio Ruiz-Giminez, Jr., Executive Chair & CEO*
*Alicia Keys, Co-Founder*

399 **Legal Council for Health Justice**
17 N. State St. 312-427-8990
Chicago, IL 60602 Fax: 312-427-8419
legalcouncil.org
Provides legal advice and services for persons who are HIV positive or have AIDS, as well as their families. Also serves individuals with disabilities and chronic illnesses, senior citizens, and the homeless.
*Tom Yates, Executive Director*
*Ruth Edwards, Senior Director, Program Services*

400 **Medical Library Association**
225 West Wacker Drive 312-419-9094
Chicago, IL 60606 Fax: 312-419-8950
websupport@mail.mlahq.org
www.mlanet.org
Non-profit, educational organization comprised of more than 400 institutions and 3,000 individual members in the health sciences information field, committed to educating health information professionals, supporting health information research and promoting access to information.
*Kate E. Corcoran, Chief Operating Officer*
*Kevin Baliozian, Executive Director*

401 **MidAtlantic AIDS Education and Training Center (MAAETC)**
www.maaetc.org
Provides educational programs about HIV infection for healthcare providers to Delaware, District of Columbia, Maryland, Pennsylvania, Virginia, and West Virgina.

402 **Moyo Health & Community Services**
7700 Hurontario Street 905-361-0523
Brampton, Ontario, L6Y 866-896-8700
Fax: 905-595-1443
moyohcs.ca
Committed to serving people living with and affected by HIV/AIDS and to limit the spread of the virus through support, education, advocacy, and volunteerism. Serves communities in Mississauga, Brampton and Caledon.

403 **National Hospice & Palliative Care Organization (NHPCO)**
1731 King Street 703-837-1500
Alexandria, VA 22314 Fax: 703-837-1233
www.nhpco.org
This organization seeks to improve end-of-life care, widen access to hospice care, and improve quality of life for the dying and their loved ones.
*Cathy L. Gibney, CPA, Chief Financial Officer*
*Ben Marcantonio, MS, MEd, COO & Interim CEO*

404 **National Native American AIDS Prevention Center**
todd@nnaapc.org
www.nnaapc.net
Aims to eliminate HIV/AIDS, HCV, and other STI's in Native communities, including American Indian, Alaska Native, Native Hawaiian, and other Indigenous peoples.
*Todd Theringer, Executive Director*
*Bernadette Wolfe, Vice Chair*

405 **Ontario HIV Treatment Network**
1300 Yonge Street 416-642-6486
Toronto, Ontario, M4T-1X3 877-743-6486
Fax: 416-640-4245
info@ohtn.on.ca
www.ohtn.on.ca
Mission is to optimize the quality of life of people living with HIV in Ontario and to promote excellence and innovation in treatment, research, education and prevention through a collaborative network of excellence representing consumers, providers, researchers and other stakeholders.
*Hazelle Palmer, President*
*Jean Bacon, Executive Director*

406 **PEERS Alliance**
250 B Queen Street 902-566-2437
Charlottetown, PE, C1A-4B8 info@peersalliance.ca
www.peersalliance.ca
Previously known as AIDS PEI, the organization aims to create a supportive environment for Persons Living with AIDS/HIV, to increase public understanding of the impact of HIV/AIDS, and to reduce the incidence of HIV/AIDS in Prince Edward Island.
*Josie Baker, Executive Director*
*Angeles DesRoches, Program Director*

407 **Positive Living Niagara**
120 Queenston Street 905-984-8684
St. Catharines, Ontario, L2R info@positivelivingniagara.com
positivelivingniagara.com
AIDS Niagara is dedicated to improving the quality of life for those infected and/or affected by HIV/AIDS.
*Glen Walker, BA, BSW, RSW, Executive Director*

408 **Positive Women's Network - USA**
436 14th Street 510-698-3811
Oakland, CA 94612 info@pwn-usa.org
www.pwn-usa.org
Aims to empower women living with HIV through social justice and human rights.
*Venita Ray, Co-Executive Director*
*Naina Khanna, Co-Executive Director*

409 **Regional HIV/AIDS Connection**
201-602 Queens Avenue 519-434-1601
London, Ontario, N6B-1Y8 866-920-1601
Fax: 519-434-1843
info@hivaidsconnection.ca
www.hivaidsconnection.ca

A community-based, charitable organization providing HIV-related services to people living with and concerned about HIV/AIDS in Perth, Huron, Lambton, Elgin, Middlesex and Oxford Counties.
*Chris Moss, Chair*
*Nancy Griffiths, Vice Chair*

410 **Reseau ACCESS Network**
111 Larch Street 705-688-0500
Sudbury, Ontario, P3E-4T5 800-465-2437
www.reseauaccessnetwork.com
A non-profit, community-based charitable organization, promoting wellness, education, harm and risk reduction.

411 **South Central AIDS Education and Training Center (SCAETC)**
1650 University Blvd. NE 550-750-3246
Albuquerque, NM 87102 scaetcECHO@salud.unm.edu
hsc.unm.edu/scaetc/
Provides educational programs about HIV infection for healthcare providers to Arkansas, Louisiana, New Mexico, Oklahoma, and Texas.

412 **Southeast AIDS Education and Training Center (SEAETC)**
Vanderbilt Health
719 Thompson Lane 615-875-7873
Nashville, TN 37204 Fax: 615-936-1583
www.seaetc.com
Provides educational programs about HIV infection for healthcare providers to Alabama, Florida, Georgia, Kentucky, Mississippi, North Carolina, South Carolina, and Tennessee.
*Cody Chastain, MD, Co-Principal Investigator*
*Stephen P. Raffanti, MD, MPH, Co-Principal Investigator*

413 **Test Positive Aware Network (TPAN)**
5537 N Broadway Street 773-989-9400
Chicago, IL 60640 Fax: 773-989-9494
tpan@tpan.com
www.tpan.com
Empowers people living with HIV through peer-led programming support services, information dissemination, and advocacy. Provides services to the broader community to increase HIV knowledge and sensitivity and to reduce the risk of infection.
*Kara Eastman, Chief Executive Officer*
*Lorraine Hayes, MA, Chief Development Officer*

414 **Turning Point Society of Central Alberta**
4611-50th Avenue 403-346-8858
Red Deer, Alberta, T4N-3Z9 877-346-8858
Fax: 403-346-2352
administration@turningpoint-ca.org
www.turningpoint-ca.org
Turning Point (formerly Central Alberta AIDS Network Society) is a local charity and agency offering support to individuals who are infected or affected by HIV/AIDS, and also provides prevention and education throughout Central Alberta.
*Stacey Carmichael, Executive Director*

415 **UNICEF USA**
125 Maiden Lane 800-367-5437
New York, NY 10038 www.unicefusa.org
Supports child survival, protection and development worldwide through education, advocacy, and fundraising for AIDS and other conditions.
*Michael J. Nyenhuis, President & CEO*
*V. Renee Cutting, Chief Philanthropy Officer*

416 **Well Project**
www.thewellproject.org
The Well Project is a not for profit corporation and an initiative conceived, developed, and administered by HIV+ women and those who are affected by the disease.
*Kelly Bower, Operations Manager*
*Grissel Granados, Deputy Director*

### *Alabama*

417 **Alabama Department of Public Health**
201 Monroe Street 334-206-5364
Montgomery, AL 36104 800-228-0469
Fax: 334-206-2092
www.alabamapublichealth.gov/hiv/
Offers health education and risk education activities, including a mobile app called Know Your Status, Manage Your Health, and Live Your Best Life (KML AL), intended to inform, prevent HIV/AIDS transmission, and assist those who have the disease.
*Scott Harris, State Health Officer*
*Karen Landers, Chief Medical Officer*

### *Alaska*

418 **Alaska Department of Health and Social Services: HIV/STD Program**
Section of Epidemiology
3601 C Street 907-269-8000
Anchorage, AK 99503 Fax: 907-561-4239
hiv-std@alaska.gov
health.alaska.gov/dph/Epi/hivstd
The HIV/STD Program addresses public health issues and activities with the goal of preventing sexually transmitted diseases (STDs) and HIV infection in Alaska as well as their impact on health. AIDS program offers education to providers and organizations.

### *Arizona*

419 **Arizona Department of Health Services: HIV Prevention Program**
150 N 18th Avenue 602-542-1025
Phoenix, AZ 85007 Fax: 602-542-0883
www.azdhs.gov
Provides HIV and AIDS seropositive surveillance, case investigation, and analysis, as well as AIDS health education and training for the public.

420 **Southwest Center For HIV/AIDS**
1101 North Central Avenue 602-307-5330
Phoenix, AZ 85004 Fax: 602-307-5021
www.swcenter.org
Formerly The Phoenix Body Positive, the organization is a non-profit created by and for people infected and affected by HIV/AIDS, that provides the community with the knowledge, resources and collective strength necessary for individuals to live long and well with HIV and to prevent the spread of the disease.
*Jessica Jessyca, Executive Director*
*Andrew Rascon, Outreach & Community Engagement Manager*

421 **Tucson Interfaith HIV/AIDS Network (TIHAN)**
2660 North 1st Avenue 520-299-6647
Tucson, AZ 85719 www.tihan.org
Serving interfaith communities of Tucson through compassionate care, education, training and spiritual support to make more individuals aware of the health crisis which affects all of us. Also provides non-medical in-home help.
*Scott Blades, Executive Director*
*Deidre Demers, Program Manager*

### *Arkansas*

422 **Arkansas Department of Health: HIV Prevention Program**
AIDS Prevention Program
4815 W. Markham St. 501-661-2408
Little Rock, AR 72205 800-232-4636
Fax: 501-661-2082
TTY: 888-232-6348
www.healthyarkansas.com
Engages in policy development, grants, training, and collaboration with community organizations and state agencies to prevent and control the spread of HIV, as well as monitoring cases across the state.

### *California*

423 **California Collaborative Treatment Group**
UC San Diego School Of Medicine

9500 Gilman Drive
La Jolla, CA 92093 avrc.ucsd.edu/programs/cctg
The CCTG is a multi-center clinical trials organization whose primary mission is to improve the scientific basis for HIV patient care and HIV prevention. CCTG develops treatment protocols and drug therapies.

424 **California Department of Public Health: Office of AIDS**
Office of AIDS
P.O. Box 997426 916-558-1784
Sacramento, CA 95899-7426 www.cdph.ca.gov
Works to develop strategies and implement programs for education and prevention, testing and counseling, supportive care and treatment and research to control the spread of HIV infection.
*Tomas J. Aragon, M.D., Ph.D., Director & State Public Health Officer*

425 **County of Los Angeles Public Health: Division of HIV and STD Programs**
AIDS Programs
600 S Commonwealth Avenue 213-351-8000
Los Angeles, CA 90005 Fax: 213-387-0912
dhsp@ph.lacounty.org
publichealth.lacounty.gov/dhsp
Responsible for planning, coordinating, and implementing county wide HIV/AIDS and STD efforts.
*Mario J. Perez, Director, Division of HIV & STD Programs*

426 **Pacific AIDS Education and Training Center (PAETC)**
University Of California San Francisco
550 16th Street, 3rd Floor 415-476-6153
San Francisco, CA 94158 paetcmail@ucsf.edu
paetc.org
Provides educational programs about HIV infection for healthcare providers to Arizona, California, Hawaii, Nevada, and the 6 U.S.-affiliated Pacific Jurisdictions.
*Prescott Chow, MUP, Co-Principal Investigator*
*Monica Hahn, MD, MPH, Co-Principal Investigator*

427 **San Francisco Community Health Center: HHOME/GTZ-ICM**
730 Polk Street 415-292-3400
San Francisco, CA 94109 Fax: 415-292-3404
sfcommunityhealth.org
HIV Homeless Outreach and Mobile Engagement (HHOME) is a mobile program operating throughout San Francisco, serving homeless people living with HIV/AIDS. Getting to Zero Intensive Case Management (GTZ-ICM) aims to end new HIV infections across the city by 2020.
*Lance Toma, LSCW, Chief Executive Officer*
*Ming Ming Kwan, MSW, Chief Operating Officer*

## *Connecticut*

428 **Connecticut Department of Health Services AIDS Programs**
800-232-4636
TTY: 888-232-6348
cdcinfo@cdc.gov
portal.ct.gov/dph/AIDS—Chronic-Diseases
Operates a speakers bureau, provides training, workshops, seminars, and counseling services, and conducts meetings and offers information and referral services.

## *Delaware*

429 **Delaware Department of Health and Social Services: HIV Prevention Program**
Division of Public Health
540 S. Dupont Highway 302-744-1000
Dover, DE 19901 www.dhss.delaware.gov/dhss/dph/index.htm
Provides HIV counseling and testing, prevention education and AIDS surveillance and studies.

## *Florida*

430 **Florida Department of Health: HIV/AIDS Section**
4052 Bald Cypress Way 850-245-4422
Tallahassee, FL 32399 DiseaseControl@flhealth.gov
www.floridahealth.gov
Seeks to eliminate HIV transmission by making voluntary HIV testing a routine part of medical care, implementing new models for diagnosing HIV infections outside medical settings, and preventing new infections by working with persons diagnosed with HIV and their partners.
*Kenneth A. Scheppke, MD, FAEMS, Deputy Secretary, Health*
*Michele Tallent, Deputy Secretary, Operations*

431 **Pridelines**
6360 NE 4th Court 305-571-9601
Miami, FL 33138 info@pridelines.org
pridelines.org
This organization seeks to support, educate, and empower LGBTQ youth and the community as a whole in South Florida, including providing HIV/AIDS-related health services and support.
*Victor Diaz Herman, Chief Executive Officer*
*Williamson Bellot, HIV Prevention Manager*

## *Georgia*

432 **Georgia Department of Public Health: Office of HIV/AIDS**
AIDS Section
2 Peachtree Street NW 404-657-3100
Atlanta, GA 30303 dph.georgia.gov
Partners with local health districts, hospitals, colleges/universities, community-based organizations, and other stakeholders to provide prevention and care services.

## *Hawaii*

433 **Hawaii Department of Health: Harm Reduction Services Branch**
728 Sunset Avenue 808-733-8443
Honolulu, HI 96816 health.hawaii.gov/harmreduction/
Offers research, education, surveillance and testing components. AIDS information and guidelines about the placement of infants, children and adolescents who test positive for HIV in nursery or school settings are also available.
*Timothy McCormick, Branch Chief*

## *Idaho*

434 **Idaho Department of Health and Welfare: The STD/AIDS Program**
208-334-5612
Fax: 208-332-7346
IDPreventHIV@dhw.idaho.gov
www.healthandwelfare.idaho.gov
Program receives federal funding to support testing treatment and prevention services for Idaho's reportable sexually transmitted infections.

## *Illinois*

435 **Chicago Department of Public Health**
333 S State Street 312-747-9884
Chicago, IL 60604 www.chicago.gov/city/en/depts/cdph.html
Offers core medical and support services via funding from the federal Ryan White HIV/AIDS Program.

436 **Illinois Department of Public Health: Division of Infectious Diseases**
525-535 W Jefferson Street 217-782-4977
Springfield, IL 62761 800-243-2437
TTY: 800-547-0466
www.dph.illinois.gov
Provides HIV/AIDS initiatives, surveillance, training, and care services.

## *Kansas*

437 **Kansas Department of Health & Environment: STI/HIV Section**
1000 SW Jackson 785-296-5651
Topeka, KS 66612 Fax: 785-559-4228
Kristen.Row@ks.gov
www.kdheks.gov
Conducts surveillance of HIV/AIDS in Kansas. Conducts Prevention Program with training for counselors and educators, partial funding of counseling test sites and distribution of educational materials. Provides medications and primary care.
*Kristen Row, STI/HIV Surveillance Program Manager*

## Louisiana

438 **Louisiana Department of Health: STD/HIV Program**
1450 Poydras Street 504-568-7474
Baton Rouge, LA 70802 Fax: 504-568-7044
ldh.la.gov/page/928
The SHP runs statewide programs intended to prevent the transmission of STDs and HIV, track current cases, and provide medical services to those who have STDs and HIV.
*Sam Burgess, STD/HIV Program Director*
*Anthony James, STD/HIV Program Deputy Director*

## Maine

439 **Maine Dept. of Health & Human Services: HIV, STD, & Viral Hepatitis Program**
Division of Disease Surveillance
286 Water St. 207-287-3747
Augusta, ME 04330 www.maine.gov/dhhs/mecdc
The program seeks to stop the spread of STDs, viral hepatitis, and HIV, and by doing so reduce the prevalence of illness and death. The proigram also promotes the health and well-being of individuals who have, or are at risk of contracting, these diseases.

## Massachusetts

440 **Massachusetts Department of Public Health: Office of HIV/AIDS**
250 Washington Street 617-624-6000
Boston, MA 02108 Fax: 617-624-6001
TTY: 617-624-5206
www.mass.gov/hiv
The Massachusetts Department of Public Health coordinates HIV/AIDS response with the Bureau of Infectious Disease and Laboratory Services. Resources are provided for the public and healthcare professionals, including treatment guidelines, epidemiologic profiles, educational materials, and other resources.

441 **New England AIDS Education and Training Center**
Center for Health Policy and Research
333 South Street 617-262-5657
Shrewsbury, MA 01545 Fax: 617-502-1701
aidsed@neaetc.org
www.neaetc.org
NEAETC serves health care professionals in New England with consultation, technical assistance, and resource materials.
*Philip Bolduc, MD, Clinical Director*
*Jennifer Daly, MD, Co-Clinical Director*

## Michigan

442 **Michigan Department of Health & Human Services: Division of HIV & STD Programs**
www.michigan.gov/mdch
The divison focuses on prevention, care, and treatment of HIV and STDs. It also administers the Ryan White HIV/Aids Program in the state.

## Minnesota

443 **Minnesota Department of Health**
P.O. Box 64975 651-201-5810
St. Paul, MN 55164-0975 www.health.state.mn.us
The Infectious Disease Epidemiology, Prevention and Control Division oversees HIV/AIDS response in the state. The focus is on prevention and care, with resources offered to the public and to healthcare professionals.
*Jan Malcolm, Commissioner*

## Mississippi

444 **Mississippi State Department of Health: STD/HIV Office**
P.O. Box 1700 866-458-4948
Jackson, MS 39215-1700 800-826-2961
msdh.ms.gov
The STD/HIV Program aims to reduce incidents of death as a result of STDs and HIV through services for disease prevention and control.
*Dr. Daniel Edney, State Health Officer*
*Melody M. Winston, Communicable Diseases*

## Missouri

445 **Missouri Department of Health & Senior Services: Bureau of HIV, STD & Hepatitis**
P.O. Box 570 573-751-6439
Jefferson City, MO 65102 Fax: 573-751-6447
STD@health.mo.gov
health.mo.gov
The department offers a range of programs and services for individuals and communities affected by HIV/AIDS, with a focus on prevention, counseling and testing, and healthcare for those living with the disease.
*Paula F. Nickelson, Acting Director*

## Montana

446 **Montana Deptartment of Public Health & Human Services: HIV/STD/HepC Program**
1400 Broadway 406-444-3565
Helena, MT 59620 dfejes@mt.gov
dphhs.mt.gov/publichealth/hivstd
Provides services and resources for the prevention and treatment of HIV, STDs, and Hepatitis C.
*Kristi Aklestad, STD/HIV/HCV Section Supervisor*

## Nevada

447 **Nevada Department of Health & Human Services: Office of HIV Prevention**
Division of Public & Behavioral Health
1840 East Sahara Ave. 702-486-8105
Las Vegas, NV 89104 Fax: 702-486-8101
dhhs.nv.gov
Works to promote health and reduce the impact of HIV/AIDS, through the lens of public health and social justice.
*Lisa Sherych, Administrator*

## New Hampshire

448 **New Hampshire Department of Health and Human Services**
29 Hazen Drive 603-271-9000
Concord, NH 03301 800-852-3345
TTY: 800-735-2964
nhbidc@dhhs.nh.gov
www.dhhs.nh.gov/dphs/bchs/std
The Infectious Disease Prevention, Investigation and Care Services Section focuses on HIV and STD prevention, including Ryan White Care for the state, as well as viral hepatitis, tuberculosis prevention and control, and more.

## New Jersey

449 **New Jersey AIDS Services**
800-353-3232
www.njas-inc.org
Provides support services, housing, prevention techniques, and community education to counter the HIV/AIDS crisis in New Jersey.
*Laurie Litt, Chief Executive Officer*
*Joann McEniry, Chief Operating Officer*

450 **New Jersey Department of Health: Division of HIV, STD and TB Services**
P.O. Box 360 800-624-2377
Trenton, NJ 08625 www.nj.gov/health/hivstdtb
Focuses on pevention and care for those affected by HIV, STDs, and tuberculosis.
*Judith M. Persichilli, RN, BSN, MA, Commissioner of Health*

### New Mexico

451 **New Mexico Department of Health: HIV Services Program**
1190 S. St. Francis Drive 505-476-3628
Santa Fe, NM 87505 nmhealth.org/about/phd/idb/hats
Provides a range of resources for those living with HIV/AIDS, as well as promoting professional development for healthcare providers, and coordinating with community-based organizations.
*Laine Snow, Program Manager*

### New York

452 **New York Department of Health: AIDS Institute**
New York State Department of Health
Empire State Plaza 800-541-2437
Albany, NY 12237 www.health.ny.gov/diseases/aids/
Awards grants and maintains relationships with regional AIDS service groups, crisis intervention, psychosocial counseling and legal, financial and housing assistance. The Institute also offers preventive education, risk reduction education, HIV counseling and testing and patient care.
*Mary T. Bassett, M.D., M.P.H., Commissioner*

453 **Northeast/Caribbean AIDS Education and Training Center (NECAAETC)**
Columbia University, HIV Center
601 West 168th Street 646-774-6978
New York, NY 10032 Fax: 212-568-3060
necaaetc@columbia.edu
necaaetc.org
Provides educational programs about HIV infection for healthcare providers to New Jersey, New York, Puerto Rico and the U.S. Virgin Islands.
*Daria Boccher-Lattimore, Director & Principal Investigator*
*Francine Cournos, Co-Principal Investigator*

### North Carolina

454 **North Carolina Department of Health and Human Services**
1905 Mail Service Center 919-733-3419
Raleigh, NC 27699 Fax: 919-733-0490
epi.dph.ncdhhs.gov/cd/stds/program.html
Oversees the AIDS surveillance program, HIV counseling, testing, partner notification, health education, risk reduction, and public information efforts in North Carolina.

### Ohio

455 **Ohio Department of Health: HIV/AIDS Surveillance Program**
246 N High Street 614-995-5599
Columbus, OH 43215 Fax: 614-728-0876
odh.ohio.gov
Consists of AIDS surveillance, seroprevalence programs, health care worker education, health education and risk reduction projects.

### Oklahoma

456 **Oklahoma Department of Health: HIV/STD Service**
123 Robert S. Kerr Ave. 405-372-8200
Oklahoma City, OK 73102-6406 www.ok.gov/health
Services include prevention and intervention, care delivery, and surveillance and analysis.
*Keith Reed, RN, MPH, CPH, Commissioner of Health*

### Oregon

457 **Oregon Health Authority: HIV Prevention Program**
500 Summer Street, NE, E-20 503-947-2340
Salem, OR 97301-1097 Fax: 503-947-5461
TTY: 711
OHA.DirectorsOffice@odhsoha.oregon.gov
www.oregon.gov/DHS/ph
The program focuses on prevention, training, and resources for the public and healthcare providers.

### Pennsylvania

458 **Pennsylvania Department of Health: Division of HIV Disease**
Bureau of Communicable Diseases
625 Forster Street 717-783-0572
Harrisburg, PA 17120 Fax: 717-772-6975
www.health.pa.gov
The division seeks to develop and implement a multi-dimensional, coordinated strategy to prevent disease and change high-risk behaviors, as well as provide resources and direction for sustaining preventive behavior and avoiding infection. HIV/AIDS Surveillance and Epidemiology is also run by the Bureau of Epidemiology.
*Dr. Denise A. Johnson, Acting Secretary, Health & Physical Gen.*

459 **Philadelphia Department of Public Health: STD Control Program**
AIDS Activities Coordinating Office (AACO)
1101 Market Street 215-685-5600
Philadelphia, PA 19107 www.phila.gov/health
Works to stop the spread of STDs, including HIV, in Philadelphia. Other city programs include: Club 1509, providing resources for men and transpeople of color; Take Control Philly, offering free condoms; and Do You, Philly, providing sexual information and resources to young men.

### Rhode Island

460 **Rhode Island Department of Health**
3 Capitol Hill 401-222-5960
Providence, RI 02908 www.health.ri.gov/diseases/hivaids
The Division of Preparedness, Response, Infectious Disease and Emergency Medical Services oversees a number of programs related to controlling the spread of STDs, including HIV.

### South Carolina

461 **South Carolina Department of Health & Environmental Control**
Bureau of Preventive Health Services
2600 Bull Street 803-898-3301
Columbia, SC 29201 info@dhec.sc.gov
www.scdhec.gov
Provides services to prevent the spread of sexually transmitted diseases (STD's) and HIV infection, to reduce associated illness and death, and to provide care and support resources for persons with HIV.
*Rick Toomey, Director*

### Tennessee

462 **Tennessee Department of Health: HIV Prevention Services**
710 James Robertson Parkway 615-741-7500
Nashville, TN 37243 tn.health@tn.gov
www.tn.gov
Provides HIV/STD education and information, as well as collecting monitoring and distributing data. Provides assistance to individuals, and intervention and treatment services.
*Morgan McDonald, MD, FACP, FAAP, Interim Executive Director*

### Texas

463 **Houston Health Department: HIV-STD Viral Hepatitis Prevention**
Houston HIV Prevention Community Planning Group
190 Heights Blvd. 832-393-5010
Houston, TX 77007 www.houstontx.gov/health/HIV-STD
Plans and implements public health strategies to reduce the spread of HIV and other STDs in Houston.

464 **Texas Department of State Health Services: HIV-STD Program**
P.O. Box 149347 737-255-4300
Austin, TX 78714-9347 800-255-1090
Fax: 512-989-4011
hivstd@dshs.texas.gov
www.dshs.texas.gov/hiv-std-program
Mission is to prevent, treat, and/or control the spread of HIV, STD, and other communicable diseases to protect the health of the citizens of Texas.

### *Utah*

465 **Utah Department of Health: HIV/Aids Program**
Bureau of Epidemiology
288 North 1460 West 801-538-6191
Salt Lake City, UT 84114-2104 Fax: 801-538-9913
epi@utah.gov
epi.health.utah.gov/hiv-aids/
Secures and distributes funds for HIV/AIDS prevention services, provides educational programs and counseling to the general public, HIV/AIDS service organizations, health workers and groups at risk.

### *Vermont*

466 **Vermont Department of Health: Health Surveillance Division**
P.O. Box 70 802-863-7240
Burlington, VT 05402 Fax: 802-865-7701
healthvermont.gov/disease-control/hiv
Focuses on HIV prevention, care, and surveillance, as well as providing resources for healthcare providers and the public.

### *Virginia*

467 **Virginia Department of Health: Division of Disease Prevention**
P.O. Box 2448 800-533-4148
Richmond, VA 23218-2448 hiv-stdhotline@vdh.virginia.gov
www.vdh.virginia.gov
Supports local health departments and community-based organizations in the prevention, surveillance and treatment of HIV and other STDs, including their complications, through provision of education, information, and health care services.

### *Washington*

468 **Mountain West AIDS Education and Training Center (MWAETC)**
325 9th Avenue 206-543-2704
Seattle, WA 98104 aetcinfo@uw.edu
mwaetc.org
Provides educational programs about HIV infection for healthcare providers to Alaska, Colorado, Idaho, Montana, Oregon, North and South Dakota, Utah, Washington, and Wyoming.
*David Spach, MD, Principal Investigator/Clinical Director*
*Laurie Sylla, MHSA, Director*

469 **Washington DC Department of Health: HIV/AIDS, Hepatitis, STD and TB Admin.**
899 North Capitol Street NE 202-442-5955
Washington, DC 20002 Fax: 202-442-4795
TTY: 711
doh@dc.gov
dchealth.dc.gov/service/hivaids
Mission is to reduce the incidence of HIV/AIDS and number of deaths related to HIV/AIDS in the District of Columbia by the application of sound public health practices and initiatives through HIV disease surveillance, tracking, monitoring, and intervention.
*Sharon Lewis, Interim Director, DC Health*

470 **Washington Department of Health: HIV Program**
P.O. Box 47841 360-236-3426
Olympia, WA 98504-7841 877-376-9316
Fax: 360-664-2216
ask.EIP@doh.wa.gov
www.doh.wa.gov
Provides information and referrals to local, state and national resources relating to HIV/AIDS, provides informational and educational materials to individuals, agencies and organizations and actively works with print and broadcast media to promote HIV/AIDS awareness.

### *West Virginia*

471 **West Virginia Department of Health & Human Resources: Division of STD and HIV**
350 Capitol Street 800-642-8244
Charleston, WV 25301 oeps.wv.gov
A division of the West Virginia Office of Epidemiology and Prevention Services, it seeks to prevent and control the spread of disease through surveillance, intervention, testing, education, and care.

### *Wisconsin*

472 **AIDS Resource Center of Wisconsin**
600 Williamson Street 608-316-8603
Madison, WI 53703 Jenny.Kreisler@arcw.org
www.arcw.org
Provides critical AIDS care and prevention services. Sustained in these efforts by the resources, expertise and passion of hundreds of volunteers and donors.
*Jenny Kriesler, Associate Director, Prevention Services*

473 **Wisconsin Department of Health Services: Wisconsin HIV Program**
1 West Wilson Street 608-266-1865
Madison, WI 53703 800-947-3529
dhswebmaster@dhs.wisconsin.gov
www.dhs.wisconsin.gov/hiv/index.htm
Coordinates counseling and testing sites activities and services to HIV-infected persons, produces a report that contains information and recommendations for health care workers, emergency medical technicians and food service workers.
*Jacob Dougherty, Co-Supervisor, HIV Prevention Unit*
*Syd Robinson, Co-Supervisor, HIV Prevention Unit*

### *Wyoming*

474 **Wyoming Department of Health: Communicable Disease Unit**
401 Hathaway Building 307-777-7529
Cheyenne, WY 82002 866-571-0944
Fax: 307-777-7439
debi.anderson@wyo.gov
health.wyo.gov/publichealth
Provides services for individuals living with HIV and their loved ones, plus healthcare providers and case managers.
*Debi Anderson, CDU Unit Manager*

## Foundations

475 **AIDS Healthcare Foundation**
6255 Sunset Blvd. 323-860-5200
Los Angeles, CA 90028 www.aidshealth.org
The AHF is a non-profit organization that provides state-of-the-art medicine and advocacy services. Funding is derived from a network of organization-run pharmacies, thrift stores, healthcare agreements, and other partnerships.
*Michael Weinstein, President*
*Peter Reis, Senior Vice President*

476 **American Foundation for AIDS Research**
120 Wall Street 212-806-1600
New York, NY 10005 Fax: 212-806-1601
info@amfar.org
www.amfar.org
Supports research in basic, clinical, prevention and public policy. Publishes the HIV/AIDS Treatment Directory.
*Kevin Robert Frost, Chief Executive Officer*
*Kyle Clifford, Chief Development Officer*

477 **American Foundation for Children with AIDS**
1520 Greening Lane 888-683-8323
Harrisburg, PA 17110 info@afcaids.org
www.afcaids.org
A nonprofit organization founded to improve the quality of life for drug-effected and HIV-infected children and their families in Africa. The foundation raises funds for family and community-based services for children and their families affected by HIV.
*Tanya Weaver, Executive Director*
*Michelle Miller, Finance Director/Executive Assistant*

478 **Canadian Foundation for AIDS Research**
2200 Yonge Street 416-361-6281
Toronto, Ontario, M4S 844-422-6327
admin@canfar.com
canfar.ca

CANFAR is a national charitable foundation whose goal is to raise awareness in order to generate funds for research into all aspects of HIV infection and AIDS.
*Alex Filiatrault, Chief Executive Officer*
*Logan Thayalan, Dir., Development & Stewardship*

479 **Elizabeth Glaser Pediatric AIDS Foundation**
1350 Eye St NW 888-499-4673
Washington, DC 20005 info@pedaids.org
www.pedaids.org
Creates a future of hope for children and families worldwide by eradicating pediatric AIDS, providing care and treatment to people with HIV/AIDS, and accelerating the discovery of new treatments for other serious and life-threatening pediatric illnesses.
*Charles Lyons, President & CEO*
*Craig Molyneaux, Chief Operating Officer*

480 **Immune Deficiency Foundation**
7550 Teague Road 800-296-4433
Hanover, MD 21076 Fax: 410-321-9165
www.primaryimmune.org
A national charitable organization aimed at fighting the primary immune deficiency diseases. The founders included parents of children with primary immune deficiency, immunologists who treat immune deficient patients, and other individuals with an immune deficiency.
*Jorey Berry, President & CEO*

481 **National Hemophilia Foundation**
7 Penn Plaza 212-328-3700
New York, NY 10001 888-463-6643
info@hemophilia.org
www.hemophilia.org
The National Hemophilia Foundation is dedicated to finding better treatments and cures for bleeding and clotting disorders and to preventing the complications of these disorders through education, advocacy and research.
*Leonard Valentino, MD, President & CEO*

482 **Quebec Aids Foundation**
1 Sherbrooke Street East 514-642-4004
Montreal, QC, H2X-3V8 fqsida.org
The Quebec AIDS Foundation seeks to support the fight against HIV/AIDS in Quebec.

483 **San Francisco AIDS Foundation (SFAF)**
1035 Market Street 415-487-3000
San Francisco, CA 94103 info@sfaf.org
www.sfaf.org
SFAF provides confidential array of services-including financial benefits counseling, client advocacy, housing assistance, HIV prevention efforts, and needle exchange.
*Tyler Termeer, PhD, Chief Executive Officer*
*LB Brooks, Chief Program Officer*

484 **Toronto People with AIDS Foundation**
200 Gerrard Street E 416-506-1400
Toronto, Ontario, M5A-2E6 Fax: 416-506-1404
info@pwatoronto.org
www.pwatoronto.org
Promotes the health and well-being of all people living with HIV/AIDS by providing accessible, direct, and practical support services.
*Suzanne Paddock, Executive Director*
*Ian McKnight, Director, Programs & Services*

## Libraries & Resource Centers

485 **AIDS Library of Philadelphia**
1233 Locust Street 215-985-4851
Philadelphia, PA 19107 Fax: 215-985-4492
library@aidslibrary.org
www.aidslibrary.org
Improving access to health and support services, preventing HIV transmission, and raising the public awareness of HIV/AIDS related issues.
*Allie Frase, Collection Management Librarian*
*Ben Remsen, Public Services*

486 **AIDSinfo**
5601 Fishers Lane 800-448-0440
Rockville, MD 20892 hivinfo@nih.gov
hivinfo.nih.gov
AIDSinfo is a U.S. Department of Health and Human Services (DHHS) project that offers the latest federally approved information on HIV/AIDS clinical research, treatment and prevention, and medical practice guidelines for people living with HIV/AIDS, their families and friends, health care providers, scientists, and researchers.

487 **CDC National Prevention Information Network**
1600 Clifton Road NPIN-Info@cdc.gov
Atlanta, GA 30329 npin.cdc.gov
The CDC National Prevention Information Network (NPIN) is the U.S. reference, referral, and distribution service for information on HIV/AIDS, sexually transmitted diseases (STDs), and tuberculosis (TB). NPIN produces, collects, catalogs, processes, stocks, and disseminates materials and information on HIV/AIDS, STD's, and TB to organizations and people working in those disease fields in international, national, state, and local settings.

488 **Educational Materials Database**
Centers for Disease Control
1600 Clifton Road 404-639-3534
Atlanta, GA 30333 800-232-4636
TTY: 888-232-6348
cdcinfo@cdc.gov
www.cdc.gov
An information awareness resource produced by the Division of Adolescent and School Health. The database offers descriptions of various educational resources for professionals relevant to the education of children and youth about HIV infection and AIDS.
*Thomas R. Frieden, Director*
*Ileana Arias, Principal Deputy Director*

489 **Health Information Network**
206-784-5655
information@healthinfonetwork.org
healthinfonetwork.org
Offers information, public awareness and support for women with HIV/AIDS and the public in general.

490 **National AIDS Treatment Advocacy Project**
212-219-0106
Fax: 212-219-8473
info@natap.org
www.natap.org
Seeks to educate by sending out literature, e-mail lists, and host forums on how to prevent HIV, or how to live with it.
*Jules Levin, Executive Director*
*Jessica Gibson Schilling, Chief Operating Officer*

491 **National Library of Medicine**
8600 Rockville Pike 301-594-5983
Bethesda, MD 20894 888-346-3656
Fax: 301-402-1384
TDD: 800-735-2258
custserv@nlm.nih.gov
www.nlm.nih.gov/
The National Library of Medicine (NLM), on the campus of the National Institutes of Health in Bethesda, Maryland, is the world's largest medical library. The Library collects materials in all areas of biomedicine and health care, as well as works on biomedical aspects of technology, the humanities, and the physical, life, and social sciences.
*Dr. Donald Lindberg, Director*
*Betsy L. Humphreys, Deputy Director*

## Research Centers

492 **AIDS Clinical Trials Unit CARES Clinic**
CARES Clinic
2315 Stocktown blvd. 916-734-2011
Sacramento, CA 95817 800-2 U- DAV
Fax: 916-325-1955
actu@ucdavis.edu
www.ucdmc.ucdavis.edu/actu

The ACTU at Davis Medical Center is dedicated to offering the latest in research clinical trials to HIV/AIDS patients throughout Northern Central California.
*Thomas S. Nesbitt, Vice Chancellor*
*David A. Acosta, Associate, Vice Chancellor*

493 **AIDS School Health Education Database Centers for Disease Control**
Centers for Disease Control
1600 Clifton Road 404-639-3534
Atlanta, GA 30333 800-232-4636
TTY: 888-232-6348
cdcinfo@cdc.gov
www.cdc.gov
An information awareness resource produced by the Division of Adolescent and School Health. The database offers descriptions of various educational resources for professionals relevant to the education of children and youth about HIV infection and AIDS.
*Thomas R. Frieden, Director*
*Ileana Arias, Principal Deputy Director*

494 **Aaron Diamond AIDS Research Center**
455 First Avenue 212-448-5000
New York, NY 10016 Fax: 212-725-1126
www.adarc.org
Committed to finding solutions to end the AIDS epidemic. In the decade and a half since HIV was identified researchers have learned more about this virus than about any other in history.
*David Ho, Director & CEO*
*Gerald Friedland, MD, Chairman*

495 **Adult Research Opportunities**
220 Dickinson Street 619-543-8080
San Diego, CA 92103 Fax: 619-543-5066
www.avrctrials.org
A university-based nonprofit clinical trials unit. Conduct's patient-oriented research and educational programs on HIV and other chronic infections. Studies have pioneered the development of treatments that continue to change the course of the HIV epidemic.
*Constance Benson, Director*
*Richard Garfein, Professor & Chairman*

496 **CDC National Prevention Information Network**
1600 Clifton Road NPIN-info@cdc.gov
Atlanta, GA 30329 npin.cdc.gov
The CDC National Prevention Information Network (NPIN) is the U.S. reference, referral, and distribution service for information on HIV/AIDS, sexually transmitted diseases (STDs), and tuberculosis (TB). NPIN produces, collects, catalogs, processes, stocks, and disseminates materials and information on HIV/AIDS, STD's, and TB to organizations and people working in those disease fields in international, national, state, and local settings.

497 **Center for AIDS Prevention Studies**
AIDS Research Institute, University of California
50 Beale Street 415-597-9100
San Francisco, CA 94105 Fax: 415-597-9213
CAPS.Web@ucsf.edu
www.caps.ucsf.edu
The mission of the Center for AIDS Prevention Studies is to conduct domestic and international research to prevent the acquisition of HIV and to optimize health outcomes among HIV-infected individuals.
*Stephen F. Morin, Director*
*Susan Kegeles, Co-Director*

498 **Center for AIDS Research: Emory University Rollins School of Public Health**
1518 Clifton Road NE 404-727-2924
Atlanta, GA 30322 Fax: 404-727-9853
cfar@emory.edu
www.cfar.emory.edu
*James Curran, Director*
*Carlos del Rio, Co-Director for Clinical Science*

499 **Center for AIDS Research: Johns Hopkins University School of Medicine**
733 N. Broadway 410-955-3182
Baltimore, MD 21205 www.hopkinsmedicine.org/aidsresearch
*Ronald Peterson, President, JHH/HS*
*Edward Miller, MD, Dean/CEO*

500 **Center for Blood Research**
Harvard Medical School/CBR
200 Longwood Avenue 617-278-3140
Boston, MA 02115 Fax: 617-278-3131
kirchhausen@crystal.harvard.edu
www.idi.harvard.edu
Offers research into blood disorders including multidisciplinary studies on AIDS and hemophilia, cancer, and diabetes research as well.
*Fredrick Alt, President/Director*
*Stephen Carriuolo, Financial Manager*

501 **Center for Interdisciplinary Research in Immunology and Diseases at UCLA**
UCLA School of Medicine
924 Westwood Blvd. #545 310-825-6373
Los Angeles, CA 90095 dgsom.healthsciences.ucla.edu
Research into immunology and blood disorders with special focus on AIDS and HIV infections.
*Albert Glover, Director, Academic Affairs*

502 **Centers for AIDS Research: Albert Einstein College of Medicine**
Albert Einstein College of Medicine
Jack and Pearl Resnick Campus 718-430-2000
Bronx, NY 10461 Fax: 718-430-2374
www.aecom.yu.edu/cfar
Provides consultation and support to the medical and research community in the scientific evaluation of CAM therapies.
*Allen Spiegel, Dean*
*Matthew Scharff, CFAR Investigator*

503 **Centers for AIDS Research: Baylor College of Medicine**
Department of Molecular Virology & Microbiology
One Baylor Plaza 713-798-3006
Houston, TX 77030 Fax: 713-798-5019
jbutel@bcm.edu
www.bcm.edu/cfar
A research center that is a branch of the Centers for AIDS Research.
*Janet S. Butel, Director*
*William T. Shearer, Co-Director*

504 **Centers for AIDS Research: Brown University**
The Miriam Hospital
CFAR/RISE Building 401-793-4068
Providence, RI 02906 Fax: 401-793-4704
vgodleski@lifespan.org
www.lifespan.org/cfar
*Charles Carpenter, Director*
*Susan Cu-Uvin, HIV & Women Core Co-Director*

505 **Centers for AIDS Research: Case Western University**
Department of Medicine
Division of Infectious Diseases 216-368-0271
Cleveland, OH 44106 Fax: 216-368-3055
mxl6@case.edu
www.clevelandactu.org
*Michael Lederman, Co-Director*
*Jonathan Karn, Associate Director*

506 **Centers for AIDS Research: Columbia University College of Physicians**
Center for AIDS Research
630 W 168th Street 212-305-1296
New York, NY 10032 jka8@columbia.edu
www.cumc.columbia.edu
Provides a comprehensive framework for training, educational programs and research which addresses health promotion, disease prevention, symptom management and quality of life for individuals with HIV. The goal of the Center is to create innovative research and service approaches for the prevention and management of

HIV. This objective is fulfilled through research, program development and program evaluations.
*Lee Goldman MD, Executive Vice President*
*Lee Bollinger, JD, President of the University*

507 **Centers for AIDS Research: NYU School of Medicine**
522 First Avenue 212-263-8527
New York, NY 10016 www.hivinfosource.org/hivis/cfar
*Derya Unutmanz, MD, Director*
*David Levy, Associate Dean*

508 **Centers for AIDS Research: North-Central California**
UC Davis, Division of Infectious Diseases
4150 V Street 916-734-8033
Sacramento, CA 95817 Fax: 916-734-7766
nccfar@ucdavis.edu
www.ucdmc.ucdavis.edu/nccfar
*Richard Pollard, Division Chief*
*Krystin Cheung, Director*

509 **Centers for AIDS Research: USCD Center for AIDS Research**
Center for AIDS Research
9500 Gilman Drive 858-534-5545
La Jolla, CA 92093 Fax: 858-822-5840
cfar@ucsd.edu
cfar.ucsd.edu
*Douglas Richman, Director*
*Kim Schafer, Administrative Director*

510 **Centers for AIDS Research: Univeristy of North Carolina at Chapel Hill**
UNC Center For AIDS Research
Lineberger Cancer Center 919-966-8645
Chapel Hill, NC 27599 cfar@med.unc.edu
cfar.med.unc.edu
Administrative and shared research support to synergistically enhance and coordinate high quality AIDS research projects.
*Ronald Swanstrom, Director*
*Myron Cohen, Associate Director*

511 **Centers for AIDS Research: University of Washington, Harborview Medical Center**
Center For AIDS & STDs
325 Ninth Avenue 206-744-4239
Seattle, WA 98104 Fax: 206-744-3693
worthy@u.washington.edu
www.depts.washington.edu/cfas
Provides administrative and shared research support to synergistically enhance and coordinate high quality AIDS research projects. CFARs accomplish this through core facilities that provide expertise, resource, and services not otherwise readily obtained through more traditional funding mechanisms.
*King K. Holmes, Director*
*Mary Fielder, Assistant to the Director*

512 **Centers for AIDS Research: Vanderbilt University Medical Center**
Division of Infectious Disease
1161 21st Avenue S 615-322-8972
Nashville, TN 37232 richard.daquila@vanderbilt.edu
www.mc.vanderbilt.edu/cfar
*Richard D'Aquila, Director*
*G. Fatima Lima, PhD, Associate Director*

513 **City of Hope National Medical Center Drug Discover/AIDS Group**
City of Hope
1500 E Duarte Road 626-256-4673
Duarte, CA 91010 www.cityofhope.org
*Michael A. Friedma, MD, CEO*
*Robert Stone, President*

514 **Clinical Research Center - Northwestern Center for Clinical Research**
Northwestern Center for Clinical Research
633 Clark Street, 312-503-8649
Chicago, IL 60611 nucats@northwestern.edu
www.nucats.northwestern.edu
*Colleen De Luca, Associate Director, Administration*
*Philip Greenland, Director*

515 **Dana Farber Cancer Institute National Drug Discovery Group for AIDS Treatment**
Dana-Farber Cancer Institute
450 Brookline Avenue 617-632-3000
Boston, MA 02215 800-408-3324
TTY: 617-632-5330
TDD: 617-632-5330
dana-farbercontactus@dfci.harvard.edu
www.dana-farber.org
*Edward Benz, President & CEO*
*Dorthy E. Puhy, Executive Vice President & COO*

516 **Department of Epidemiology and Health Policy Research: University of Florida**
1329 SW 16th Street 352-265-8035
Gainesville, FL 32608 Fax: 352-265-8047
www.ehpr.ufl.edu
Studies into child and adolescent health, financing and organization of health care delivery systems, community health, chronic conditions, transition from pediatric to adult health care, access to health care for vulnerable populations, quality of life, and outcomes research.
*Clifford J. Crook, Chair*
*John C. Bierly, Program Assistant*

517 **Developmental Medicine Center Children's Hospital Boston**
Children's Hospital Boston
300 Longwood Avenue 617-355-6000
Boston, MA 02115 Fax: 617-730-0633
TTY: 617-730-0152
www.childrenshospital.org
Studies developmental effects of infants at risk and development effects of congenital HIV infection.
*James Mandell, CEO*
*Sandra Fenwick, President/COO*

518 **Emory University: National Cooperative Drug Discovery for AIDS Treatment**
Emory Healthcare Pediatrics Department
201 Dowman Drive 404-727-6123
Atlanta, GA 30322 Fax: 404-727-5737
www.pediatrics.emory.edu
*Barbara J. Stoll, MD, Professor, Chair*
*James W. Wagner, President*

519 **General Clinical Research Center**
Mount Sinai School of Medicine
One Gustave L Levy Place 212-241-6500
New York, NY 10029 Fax: 212-348-5811
hugh.sampson@mssm.edu
www.mssm.edu/gcrc
*Dennis S. Charney, Executive Vice President*
*Kennith Davis, President*

520 **George Washington National Cooperative: Drug Discovery/AIDS Treatment**
Department of Pharmacology & Physiology
2300 Eye Street NW 202-994-3541
Washington, DC 20037 Fax: 202-994-2870
www.gwumc.edu/pharm
Studies and researches natural products and synthetic anti-AIDS agents.
*Susan Ceryak, Associate Research Professor*
*Jian-Zhong Guo, Associate Research Professor*

521 **HIV Center for Clinical and Behavioral Studies**
1051 Riverside Drive 212-543-5969
New York, NY 10032 Fax: 212-543-6003
www.hivcenternyc.org
Interdisciplinary research center that investigates the behavioral causes and consequences of HIV/AIDS. Focusing on the intersections of HIV infection, gender, and sexuality; treatment strategies for infected populations; and innovative dissemination of scientific findings.
*Anke A. Ehrhardt, Director*
*Heino F. L. Meyer-Bahlbur, Associate Director*

522 **HIV Prevention Trials Unit**
University of Washington/Seattle HPTU Site

Cabrini Medical Tower 901 Boren Av
Seattle, WA 98104
206-520-3800
Fax: 206-520-3801
www.depts.washington.edu

A worldwide collaborative clinical trials network established by the National Institutes of Health (NIH) to evaluate the safety and efficacy of non-vaccine prevention interventions, alone or in combination, using HIV incidence as the primary endpoint.
*Connie Celum, Principal Investigator*

523 **HIV/AIDS Prevention Program**
Centers for Disease Control and Prevention
1600 Clifton Road
Atlanta, GA 30333
404-639-3534
800-232-4636
TTY: 888-232-6348
cdcinfo@cdc.gov
www.cdc.gov

An information awareness resource produced by the Division of Adolescent and School Health. The database offers descriptions of various educational resources for professionals relevant to the education of children and youth about HIV infection and AIDS.
*Thomas R. Frieden, Director*
*Ileana Arias, Principal Deputy Director*

524 **Institute for Clinical Research**
Weill Cornell Medical College
1300 York Avenue
New York, NY 10065
212-746-5454
Fax: 212-746-8970
cto@med.cornell.edu
www.med.cornell.edu

The mission of the ICR is.to support, advance and promote clinical and translational research enterprises at WCMC. As part of Research and Sponsored Programs (RASP), the ICR streamlines the clinical research process and offers a wide range of services, resources and training.
*David J. Skorton, MD, President of the University*
*Michelle A. Lewis, MS, Director, Research & Sponsored Programs*

525 **Johns Hopkins University: Center for Communication Programs**
Johns Hopkins Bloomberg School of Public Health
111 Market Place
Baltimore, MD 21202
410-659-6300
Fax: 410-659-6266
info@jhuccp.org
www.jhuccp.org

Health communications, family planning and AIDS prevention research.
*Susan Krenn, Director*

526 **Kaiser Foundation Research Institute**
2000 Broadway
Oakland, CA 94612
510-891-3400
www.dor.kaiser.org
*Tracy A. Lieu, Director*
*Alyce Adams, Health Care Delivery & Policy*

527 **Medical University of South Carolina Health Services Administration**
Medical University of South Carolina
171 Ashley Avenue
Charleston, SC 29425
843-792-1414
800-424-6872
Fax: 843-792-2601
www.musc.edu

Devoted to public health policy and health care management including AIDS research.
*Raymond S. Greenburg, President*
*Dr. Mark Sothman, Vice President*

528 **MidAtlantic AIDS Education and Training Center (MAAETC)**
www.maaetc.org

Provides educational programs about HIV infection for healthcare providers to Delaware, District of Columbia, Maryland, Pennsylvania, Virginia, and West Virgina.

529 **Midwest AIDS Education and Training Center (MATEC)**
1919 West Taylor
Chicago, IL 60612
312-996-1373
312-413-4184
matec@uic.edu
www.matec.info

*Ricardo A. Rivero, MD, MPH, Executive Director*
*Renslow Sherer, MD, Regional Clinical Director*

530 **Mountain West AIDS Education and Training Center (MWAETC)**
325 9th Avenue
Seattle, WA 98104
206-543-2704
aetcinfo@uw.edu
mwaetc.org

Provides educational programs about HIV infection for healthcare providers to Alaska, Colorado, Idaho, Montana, Oregon, North and South Dakota, Utah, Washington, and Wyoming.
*David Spach, MD, Principal Investigator/Clinical Director*
*Laurie Sylla, MHSA, Director*

531 **New England AIDS Education and Training Center**
Center for Health Policy and Research
333 South Street
Shrewsbury, MA 01545
617-262-5657
Fax: 617-502-1701
aidsed@neaetc.org
www.neaetc.org

NEAETC serves health care professionals in New England with consultation, technical assistance, and resource materials.
*Philip Bolduc, MD, Clinical Director*
*Jennifer Daly, MD, Co-Clinical Director*

532 **Northeast/Caribbean AIDS Education and Training Center (NECAAETC)**
Columbia University, HIV Center
601 West 168th Street
New York, NY 10032
646-774-6978
Fax: 212-568-3060
necaaetc.org

Provides educational programs about HIV infection for healthcare providers to New Jersey, New York, Puerto Rico and the U.S. Virgin Islands.
*Daria Boccher-Lattimore, Director & Principal Investigator*
*Francine Cournos, Co-Principal Investigator*

533 **Pacific AIDS Education and Training Center (PAETC)**
University Of California San Francisco
550 16th Street, 3rd Floor
San Francisco, CA 94158
415-476-6153
paetcmail@ucsf.edu
paetc.org

Provides educational programs about HIV infection for healthcare providers to Arizona, California, Hawaii, Nevada, and the 6 U.S.-affiliated Pacific Jurisdictions.
*Prescott Chow, MUP, Co-Principal Investigator*
*Monica Hahn, MD, MPH, Co-Principal Investigator*

534 **Purdue University Center for AIDS Research**
School of Pharmacy and Pharmaceutical Sciences
575 Stadium Mall Drive
W Lafayette, IN 47907
765-494-1361
Fax: 765-494-7880
oss@pharmacy.purdue.edu
www.pharmacy.purdue.edu

*Steve Byrn, Department Head*
*Stanley L. Hem, Associate Department Head*

535 **SUNY at Buffalo National Cooperative Drug Discovery Group for AIDS Treatment**
Department of Biochemistry
140 Farber Hall
Buffalo, NY 14214
716-829-2727
Fax: 716-829-2725
jluck@buffalo.edu
www.buffalo.edu

*Kenneth M. Blumenthal, Professor & Chairman*
*Elizabeth O'Brocta, Assistant to the Chairman*

536 **South Central AIDS Education and Training Center (SCAETC)**
1650 University Blvd. NE
Albuquerque, NM 87102
550-750-3246
scaetcECHO@salud.unm.edu
hsc.unm.edu/scaetc/

Provides educational programs about HIV infection for healthcare providers to Arkansas, Louisiana, New Mexico, Oklahoma, and Texas.

537 **Southeast AIDS Education and Training Center (SEAETC)**
Vanderbilt Health
719 Thompson Lane
Nashville, TN 37204
615-875-7873
Fax: 615-936-1583
www.seaetc.com

Provides educational programs about HIV infection for healthcare providers to Alabama, Florida, Georgia, Kentucky, Mississippi, North Carolina, South Carolina, and Tennessee.
*Cody Chastain, MD, Co-Principal Investigator*
*Stephen P. Raffanti, MD, MPH, Co-Principal Investigator*

538 **Spellman Center for HIV Related Disease**
The Spellman Center
415 W Fifty-First Street 212-459-8130
New York, NY 10019 www.stclaresny.org
*David Kaufman, Director*

539 **Stanford University General Clinical Research Center**
GCRC Administration
300 Pasteur Drive 650-723-4000
Stanford, CA 94305 Fax: 650-725-6698
gcrcstanford@stanford.edu
www.med.stanford.edu/gcrc
The Stanford General Clinical Research Center (GCRC) is the major clinical research facility for Stanford University School of Medicine. With patient care units in Stanford University Hospital and Lucile Packard Children's Hospital, the center plays a crucial role in the school's bench-to-bedside research mission.

540 **Stanford University National Cooperative Drug Discovery/AIDS Group**
School of Medicine
300 Pasteur Drive 650-723-4000
Stanford, CA 94305 Fax: 650-725-6698
www.med.stanford.edu
*Ellen Jo Baron, Director*
*Branimir I. Sikic, Program Director*

541 **State University of New York: SUNY Stony HIV Treatment Development Center**
Center for Infectious Diseases
101 Nicolls Road 631-444-4000
Stony Brook, NY 11794 Fax: 631-444-2493
rsteigbigel@notes.cc.sunysb.edu
www.stonybrookmedicalcenter.org
Human immunodeficiency virus research.
*Joyce Klien, Director*
*Laura Coppola, Assistant Director*

542 **Tampa Bay Research Institute**
10900 Roosevelt Boulevard N 727-576-6675
Saint Petersburg, FL 33716 Fax: 727-577-9862
development@tampabayresearch.org
www.tampabayresearch.org
TBRI is the first independent biomedical research organization of its kind in Florida.
*Clifford J. Crook, Chair*
*John C. Bierly, Program Assistant*

543 **Temple University Clinical Research Center Office of Clinical Research**
Office of Clinical Research
Medical Education and Research Buil 215-707-7000
Philadelphia, PA 19140 Fax: 215-201-2684
www.temple.edu/medicine
CRC Unit provides space to perform clinical research on 4 West of Temple University Hospital. The CRC Unit has the potential for three rooms for inpatient/outpatient studies and an additional room for outpatient studies.
*Antonio Giorgio, MD, President*

544 **Thomas Jefferson University: Center for Research in Medical Education**
Jefferson Medical College
1020 Walnut Street 215-955-6000
Philadelphia, PA 19107 Fax: 215-923-7583
Joseph.Gonnella@jefferson.edu
www.jefferson.edu/jmc
*Robert L. Barchi, MD, President*

545 **UCLA AIDS Clinical Research Center**
1399 S Roxbury Drive 310-557-2273
Los Angeles, CA 90035 Fax: 310-557-3450
www.uclacarecenter.org
*Dr. A. Eugene, Chancellor*
*David T. Feinberg, President*

546 **UCSD Antiviral Research Center**
220 Dickinson Street 619-543-8080
San Diego, CA 92103 Fax: 619-543-5066
www.avrctrials.org
Develops treatment protocols and drug therapies and recruits research volunteers for AIDS studies and HIV related disorders.
*Jill Kunkel, Director*
*Michael Giancola, Screening Co-ordinator*

547 **USC Internal Medicine**
1520 San Pablo Street 800-872-2273
Los Angeles, CA 90033 Fax: 213-224-6687
www.usc.edu/health/internal
Research into internal medicine with specialties in cardiovascular, endocrinology and diabetes, gastrointestinal and liver disease, geriatric medicine, hematology, infectious diseases, nephrology, oncology, pulmonary and critical care, and rheumatology and immunology.
*Alexandra Levine, Head*

548 **University of Alabama at Birmingham: National Cooperative Drug/AIDS**
UAB Center for AIDS Research
BBRB 256 205-934-4011
Birmingham, AL 35294 http://www.uab.edu
*Robert P. Kimberly, Director*
*Cheryl A. Perry, Deputy Director*

549 **University of California San Francisco Center for AIDS Prevention**
Center for AIDS Prevention Studies (CAPS)
50 Beale Street 415-597-9100
San Francisco, CA 94105 Fax: 415-597-9213
CAPS.web@ucsf.edu
www.caps.ucsf.edu
The mission of the Center for AIDS Prevention Studies is to conduct domestic and international research to prevent the acquisition of HIV and to optimize health outcomes among HIV- infected individuals.
*Stephen F Morin, Director*
*Susan Kegeles, Co-Director*

550 **University of California: Institute of Health Policy Studies**
513 Parnassus Avenue 415-476-9000
San Francisco, CA 94143 Fax: 415-476-0705
claire.brindis@ucsf.edu
www.ihps.medschool.ucsf.edu
Health policy and AIDS research.
*Susan Desmond-Hellman, Chancellor*
*Phillip R. Lee, Director*

551 **University of Maryland Center for Research, Grants & Contracts**
Family Studies Depatrment
1142 School of Public Health 301-405-3672
College Park, MD 20742 Fax: 301-314-9161
fmst@umd.edu
www.hhp.umd.edu/FMST
*Erin McClure, Coordinator*
*Doris Richardson, Business Manager*

552 **University of Maryland Center for Studies Family Studies Depatrment**
1142 School of Public Health 301-405-3672
College Park, MD 20742 Fax: 301-314-9161
fmsc@umd.edu
www.sph.umd.edu/fmsc
*Erin McClure, Coordinator*
*Doris Richardson, Business Manager*

553 **University of Maryland: Medical Biotechnology Center**
701 E. PRATT ST, 410-706-8802
Baltimore, MD 21202 Fax: 410-706-8184
hill@UMCES.edu
www.umbi.umd.edu
Offers research into AIDS and HIV infection including vaccine development.
*W. Jonathan Lederer, Director*
*Kadir Aslan, Assistant Professor*

554 **University of Michigan: National Cooperative Drug/AIDS Group**
School of Dentistry

1011 N University Avenue 734-763-6933
Ann Arbor, MI 48109 Fax: 734-763-3453
www.dent.umich.edu
Focuses on the design of new drugs to fight AIDS.
*John C. Drach, PhD, Director*
*Paul H. Krebsbach, Department Chair*

555 **University of South Florida Center for HIV Education and Research**
13301 Bruce B Downs Boulevard 813-974-4430
Tampa, FL 33612 866-352-2382
Fax: 813-974-8451
www.usfcenter.org
Serves health care professionals throughout Florida by providing education and information on the transmission control treatment and prevention of HIV and AIDS and by conducting related research and community outreach.
*Jeffery Beal, Director*
*Debbie Cestaro, Project Coordinator*

556 **University of Vermont: Office of Health Promotion Research**
1 S Prospect Street 802-656-4187
Burlington, VT 05401 Fax: 802-656-8826
ohpr@uvm.edu
www.uvm.edu/~ohpr
Research done into public policy and human health including AIDS information and evaluation.
*Anne L. Dorwaldt, Assistant Director*
*Rachael Chicoine, AAS, Research Project Assistant*

557 **Wayne State University Center for Health Research**
College of Nursing
Center for Health Research 313-577-4082
Detroit, MI 48202 888-837- 08
Fax: 313-577-6949
nursinginfo@wayne.edu
www.nursing.wayne.edu/CHR
Facilitates interdisciplinary health research across diverse settings where nursing is practiced and healthcare is provided.
*Nancy T. Artinian, Director*
*Barbara K. Redman, Dean*

558 **Whitman Walker Clinic AIDS/Medical Services Programs**
1701 14th Street NW 202-745-7000
Washington, DC 20009 Fax: 202-745-0238
info@wwc.org
www.wwc.org
A non-profit community-based health organization serving the Washington, D.C. metropolitan region. Especially committed to ending the suffering of all those infected and affected by HIV/AIDS.
*Adam Falcone, Chair*
*June Crenshaw, Vice Chair*

## Support Groups & Hotlines

559 **AEGIS AIDS Education Global Information System**
P.O. Box 184 949-495-1952
San Juan Capistrano, CA 92693 Fax: 949-443-1755
www.aegis.org
A not-for-profit, tax-exempt, educational corporation that adds more than 3000 documents each month. Reach more than 10 million users annually, including: the US Federal Government, US Educational Institutions, and Nonprofit organizations both here and abroad.
*Vanessa Robison, President*
*Sister Mary Elizabeth, Assistant Operations Director*

560 **AIDS Alabama**
3521 7th Avenue S 205-324-9822
Birmingham, AL 35222 800-592-2437
Fax: 205-324-9311
maryanne@aidsalabama.org
www.aidsalabama.org
Devotes its energy and resources statewide to helping people with HIV/AIDS live healthy, independent lives and works to prevent the spread of HIV. Goal is to provide housing for those with HIV in the Birmingham area, secure and administer grants for care of persons with HIV statewide, and specialize in targeted prevention education programs.
*Elaine Cottle, Executive Director*

561 **AIDS Hotline of Central New York**
AIDS Community Resources
627 W Genesee Street 315-475-2430
Syracuse, NY 13204 800-475-2430
Fax: 315-472-6515
information@aidscommunityresources.com
www.aidscommunityresources.com
A not-for-profit, community-based organization providing prevention, education and support services to those infected with and affected by HIV/AIDS Serves Cayuga, Herkimer, Jefferson, Lewis, Madison, Oneida, Onondaga, Oswego and St. Lawrences counties in New York State.
*Michael Crinnin, Executive Director*

562 **AIDS Support Group of Cape Cod**
428 S Street 508-778-1957
Hyannis, MA 02610 866-990-2437
Fax: 508-778-4501
info@asgcc.org
www.asgcc.org
Mission is to provide services that maintain and enhance the quality of life for persons living with HIV and AIDS on Cape Cod and Martha's Vineyard and to provide health education, prevention and harm reduction outreach via timely and accurate information about HIV/AIDS, STIs and viral hepatitis.
*Krystin St. Onge, Interim Director*

563 **AIDSinfo**
US Department of Health and Human Services
P.O. Box 6303 301-315-2816
Rockville, MD 20849 800-448-0440
Fax: 301-315-2818
TTY: 888-480-3739
contactus@aidsinfo.nih.gov
www.aidsinfo.nih.gov
Offers the latest federally approved information on HIV/AIDS clinical research, treatment and prevention, and medical practice guidelines for people living with HIV/AIDS, their families and friends, health care providers, scientists, and researchers.

564 **Alaskan Statewide AIDS Helpline**
1057 W Fireweed 907-263-2050
Anchorage, AK 99503 800-478-AIDS
Fax: 907-263-2051
www.alaskanaids.org
A key collaborator within the state of Alaska in the provision of supportive services to persons living with HIV/AIDS and their families and in the elimination of the transmission of HIV infection and its stigma.
*Heather Davis, Executive Director*
*Maureen Suttman, Client Resource Services*

565 **BABES Network-YWCA**
1118 Fifth Ave 206-720-5566
Seattle, WA 98101 888-292-1912
Fax: 206-720-5901
the_staff@babesnetwork.org
www.babesnetwork.org
A peer-based program, a sisterhood of women facing HIV together. Reduces isolation, promotes self-empowerment, enhances quality of life and serves the needs of women facing HIV and their families through peer support, advocacy, education and outreach.
*Rhonda Kimm, Advocacy Coordinator*
*Amelia Vader, Program Manager*

566 **COMPASS Program**
c/o Institute for Urban Family Health
16 East 16th Street 212-924-7744
New York, NY 10003 Fax: 212-691-4610
info@institute2000.org
www.institute2000.org/health/rwp.htm
Medical services include HIV testing and specialized HIV medical care for adults in addition to women's health services including gynecology, PAP tests, family planning and birth control methods.

Mental health services includes individual, couples, and family counseling and psychiatric evaluations and monitoring.
*Neil Calman MD/ABFP/FAAFP, President/Chief Executive Officer*
*Weston Willett, Chief Information Officer*

567 **Cascade AIDS Project Hotline**
200 SW Fifth Avenue 503-223-5907
Portland, OR 97204 Fax: 503-223-6437
info@cascadeaids.org
www.cascadeaids.org
Provides HIV prevention and services information by phone and internet to youth and adults across Orgeon and the Northwest.
*Charles Washington, President*
*warren Jimanez, Vice President*

568 **Committee of Ten Thousand**
71 Winfield Street 202-681-2351
Needham, MA 02492 info@cott1.org
www.cott1.org
Represents people with hemophilia who contracted HIV/AIDS and Hepatitis C from tainted factory concentrates in the 1970s and 1980s. The only national advocacy, and support agency for this seriously disabled community.
*Chad Blair, President*
*Chris Templin, Treasurer*

569 **Dunshee House**
303-17th Avenue East 206-322-2437
Seattle, WA 98112 Fax: 206-322-1779
www.dunsheehouse.org
A non-profit organization, builds community and cultivates powerful, healthy lives by providing emotional support and personal development services to those affected by HIV/AIDS, the Queer communities, and those who love them.
*Michael Kann, President*
*Adrienne Miller, Vice President*

570 **HEAL**
Sidney Hillman Family Pracitce
16 E 16th Street 212-924-7744
New York, NY 10003 www.thorup.com/HEAL
The Health Education AIDS Liaison provides alternative and holistic support groups and resources for people with HIV.

571 **King County Crisis Clinic**
9725 3rdAvenue NE 206-461-3210
Seattle, WA 98115 866-427-4747
Fax: 206-461-8368
TDD: 206-461-3219
info@crisisclinic.org
www.crisisclinic.org
A non-profit organization, we offer an array of support services available to everyone in King County, Washington.
*Kathleen Southwick, Executive Director*
*Susan Gemmel, Director*

572 **Minnesota AIDS Project AIDSLine**
1400 Park Avenue 612-341-2060
Minneapolis, MN 55404 800-248-7321
Fax: 612-341-4057
TTY: 888-820-2437
mapaidsline@mnaidsproject.org
www.mnaidsproject.org
A statewide, toll-free information and referral service that can answer your questions about HIV and connect you to resources that can help.
*Bill Tiedmann, Executive Director*

## Print Resources

573 **AIDS Alert**
American Health Consultants
3525 Piedmont Road 404-262-5476
Atlanta, GA 30355 800-688-2421
Fax: 404-262-5560
www.ahcmedia.com
Covers up-to-the-minute developments and guidance on the entire spectrum of AIDS challenges, including treatment, education, precautions, screening, diagnosis and policy.

574 **AIDS Clinical Care**
New England Journal of Medicine
860 Winter Street 781-893-4610
Waltham, MA 02451 800-322-2303
Fax: 781-893-3800
www.massmed.org
Up to date information specifically targeted at physicians with AIDS patients.

575 **AIDS Journal**
Lippincott Williams & Wilkins
Two Commerce Square 215-521-8300
Philadelphia, PA 19103 customerservice@lww.com
journals.lww.com/aidsonline/
Publishes original scientific, clinical, epidemiological, and social research on HIV and AIDS.
*J.A. Levy, Editor-in-Chief*

576 **AIDS: The Disease State Management Resource**
American Health Consultants
P.O. Box 550669 404-262-5476
Atlanta, GA 30355 800-688-2421
Fax: 800-284-3291
www.ahcmedia.com
Covers up-to-the-minute developments and guidance on the entire spectrum of AIDS challenges, including treatment, education, precautions, screening, diagnosis and policy.

577 **Aids & Behavior**
Springer
www.springer.com/journal/10461
Publishes scholarly work and original research articles on the consequences and social impact of HIV/AIDS.
*Seth Kalichman, Editor*
*Renee El-Krab, Managing Editor*

578 **Critical Path AIDS Project**
2062 Lombard Street 215-545-2212
Philadelphia, PA 19146 www.critpath.org
Articles and reprints on experimental treatments and alternative therapies, and a listing of Philadelphia-area resources.

579 **Institute on Health Care for the Poor and Underserved at Meharry Medical College**
Sage Publications
1005 DB Todd Boulevard 615-327-6819
Nashville, TN 37208 800-669-1269
Fax: 615-327-6362
vbrennan@mmc.edu
Offers health care and public health policy research focusing on poor and underserved populations.
*100pages*
*Dr. Amy Cato, Director*
*Dr. Virginia Brennan, Editor*

580 **Journal of Acquired Immune Deficiency Syndrome**
Lippincott Williams & Wilkins
Two Commerce Square 215-521-8300
Philadelphia, PA 19103 customerservice@lww.com
www.lww.com
An interdisciplinary journal providing a synthesis of AIDS-related information from all relevant clinical and basic sciences.
*ISBN: 0-894925-5 -*
*Paul A. Volberding, MD, Editor-in-Chief*
*William A. Blattner, MD, Co-Editor-in-Chief*

581 **Journal of the International Aids Society (JIAS)**
Wiley Online Library
onlinelibrary.wiley.com/journal/17582652
Covers HIV research from a wide range of disciplines, including: basic and biomedical sciences; behavioural sciences; epidemiology; clinical sciences; health economics and health policy; operations research and implementation sciences; and social sciences and humanities.
*Kenneth H. Mayer, Editor-in-Chief*
*Annette Sohn, Co-Editor-in-Chief*

582 **Journal of the Medical Library Association**
Pitt Open Library Publishing
jmla.mlanet.org/ojs/jmla/

An international, peer-reviewed journal that aims to advance the practice and research knowledgebase of health science librarianship.
*Jill T. Boruff, AHIP, Editor-in-Chief*
*Michelle Kraft, AHIP, FMLA, Co-Editor-in-Chief*

583 **POZ Magazine**
POZ Publishing
157 Columbus Avenue 212-242-2163
New York, NY 10023-6082 Fax: 212-675-8505
www.poz.com
A magazine for people living with, and affected by, HIV/AIDS.
*Oriol R. Gutierrez, Jr., Editor-in-Chief*
*Jennifer Morton, Managing Editor*

584 **Risky Business**
San Francisco AIDS Foundation Materials Dept.
333 Valencia Street 415-861-3397
San Francisco, CA 94103
A comic book style magazine providing accurate information about AIDS using humor and real-life situations. Contains stories that stress the importance of knowing how AIDS is transmitted and prevented.

585 **Straight Talk: A Magazine for Teens About AIDS**
Custom Publishing Division of Rodale Press
33 E Minor Street 610-967-5171
Emmaus, PA 18098
A lively magazine that includes articles about teens with AIDS, teens involved in peer education and teens at risk for getting infected. Good information is presented in an interesting format for young adults.

## Web Sites

586 **AIDS Education and Training Center National Multicultural Center**
www.aetcnmc.org
Located at Howard University College of Medicine, AETC-NMC acted as an HIV/AIDS training and technical resource for providers of minority HIV-infected patients throughout the country. It functioned as the training arm of the Ryan White HIV/AIDS Program. Funding ceased in 2014, but the Center maintains its website as an archive of information.

587 **AIDS United**
www.aidsunited.org
Dedicated to ending the HIV epidemic in the U.S. through their public policy work.

588 **AIDS.ORG**
www.aids.org
The mission of AIDS.ORG is to help prevent HIV infections and to improve the lives of those affected by HIV and AIDS by providing education and facilitating the free and open exchange of knowledge at any easy-to-find centralized website.

589 **AIDSVu**
aidsvu.org
Interactive maps of the AIDS epidemic across the states, including downloadable data sets and a services directory.

590 **Act Against AIDS**
www.cdc.gov/actagainstaids
A program of the Centers for Disease Control and Prevention and the White House, aimed at raising awareness about HIV/AIDS among all Americans, and particularly among hardest-hit groups, such as gay and bisexual men, African Americans, Latinos, and other at-risk communities.

591 **Committee of Ten Thousand**
www.cott1.org
Represents people with hemophilia who contracted HIV/AIDS and Hepatitis C from tainted factory concentrates in the 1970s and 1980s. The only national advocacy, and support agency for this seriously disabled community. Website includes a digital archive of photos, gatherings, and events.

592 **HIV.gov**
www.hiv.gov
Online portal for HIV/AIDS-related resources, managed by the U.S. Department of Health & Human Services and supported by the Secretary's Minority AIDS Initiative Fund (SMAIF).

593 **Immune Deficiency Foundation**
www.primaryimmune.org
The national patient organization dedicated to improving the diagnosis, treatment and quality of life of persons with primary immunodeficiency diseases through advocacy, education and research.

594 **Keep A Child Alive**
www.keepachildalive.org
Mission is to make a positive difference in the lives of children infected with HIV and affected by AIDS.

595 **National AIDS Information Clearinghouse**
www.cdc.gov
Provides information and materials for employers on national, state and local resources related to HIV/AIDS in the workplace.

596 **National Hospice & Palliative Care Organization (NHPCO)**
www.nhpco.org
This organization seeks to improve end-of-life care, widen access to hospice care, and improve quality of life for the dying and their loved ones. NHPCO's website offers information on regulations, advocacy, quality and performance, education, and a variety of other resources.

597 **People with AIDS Health Group**
www.Aidsinfonyc.org
PWA is a non-profit buyers club organized to assist people with AIDS in obtaining medications — as well as provide support groups committed to the self-empowerment of people living with AIDS. They offer three programs: Treatment Education and Support, Advocacy and Public Policy, and Early Treatment Access.

598 **Smart & Strong**
www.smartstrong.com
A healthcare education company that supports providers and empowers HIV positive patients through publications, seminars and innovative educational programs.

599 **TheBodyPro**
www.thebodypro.com
A digital health platform that publishes relevant news on HIV/AIDS and related fields, and serves as a platform for members the HIV workforce to share their stories and perspectives.

# ALZHEIMER'S DISEASE/DEMENTIAS

*Substance use disorder involving alcohol, tobacco and some legal and illegal substances can negatively impact mental state and cognition. Dementia is a clinical diagnosis or syndrome involving cognitive impairment, including memory loss and loss of focus, and is generally associated with old age. Alzheimer's is the most common cause of dementia and accounts for 60-80% of cases. Alzheimer's disease is a type of dementia with symptoms of memory, thinking and behavior impairment, and symptoms may become severe to the point of interfering with activities of daily living. The disease worsens over time and may result in a shortened life span. Substance use disorder may develop as individuals with a dementia or Alzheimer's diagnosis have difficulty following a medication plan due to forgetfulness, or attempt to deal with the stress of the disease through the use of alcohol and mood-altering substances.*

Up to a quarter of older adults in the United States abuse alcohol, tobacco and drugs in some form. Prescription medicine abuse is often a precursor to substance abuse and may explain the higher rates of Alzheimer diagnoses in the older population. Metabolizing drugs and alcohol are difficult in the older population. Additionally, cognitive impairment may lead an older person to take too much medication, as they forget easily. Often, older adults are not comfortable talking about memory problems, and do not recognize problem behaviors and neglect talking with their physician.

The brains of individuals who abuse drugs resemble the brains of people with early Alzheimer's disease. There is a documented link between alcohol abuse and dementia. The brains of young drug abusers often reveal brain damage similar to much older people, including damage to nerve cells found in areas of the brain dealing with learning, memory and emotional wellbeing, similar to damage found in the early stages of Alzheimer's disease. Chronic substance use may increase the risk of cognitive impairment and perhaps increase the risk of dementia later in life. Mild to moderate alcohol consumption does not correlate with developing dementia, and may even have a protective effect.

There are common classes of legal drugs that may also lead to an increased risk of Alzheimer's Disease. Multiple drugs used for allergies, colds, hypertension, trigeminal neuralgia and urinary incontinence may create an increased risk for cognitive decline, especially in older adults at risk for Alzheimer's Disease. Drugs classified as anticholinergics and commonly used are linked to dementia risk may include:

- Amitriptyline (Elavil)
- Aripiprazole (Abilify)
- Carbamazepine (Tegretol)
- Chlorpheniramine (ChlorTrimetron)
- Chlorpromazine (Thorazine)

Benzodiazepines, a class of drugs that includes medications for anxiety and sleep, create a risk of dementia when used for longer than a few months. The effect increases with the dose of the drug and the length of use. Individuals with long term use of opioid pain medications can become addicted to the point of overdose and death.

People with long-term use of opioid medications are at a slightly higher risk of getting dementia.

Seeking help for a substance abuse disorder in a timely fashion may prevent or slow cognitive impairment which in term may limit the development of dementia and Alzheimer's disease. Ensuring that older individuals take drugs as prescribed is important. The use of pill boxes set up by time and day are helpful to limit overdosing due to memory loss. Observing individuals for signs of substance abuse disorder and for potential dementias is important. Talking with the individual and the physician about changes in behavior is important before substance use disorder emerges.

## Agencies & Associations

600 **Alzheimer Society of Alberta and Northwest Territories**
10430 - 61 Avenue 780-488-2266
Edmonton, Alberta, T6H-2J3 866-950-5465
Fax: 780-488-3055
reception@alzheimer.ab.ca
www.alzheimer.ca/en/ab
Provides support, education, and advocacy for all those affected by Alzheimer's disease in Alberta and the Northwest Territories, including patients, caregivers, patients' families, and the community.
*George Andrews, President & CEO*
*Christene Gordon, VP, Programs & Partnerships*

601 **Alzheimer Society of British Columbia**
828 W 8th Avenue Street 604-681-6530
Vancouver, BC, V5C-1E2 800-667-3742
Fax: 604-669-6907
info@alzheimerbc.org
www.alzheimer.ca/en/bc
Provides support, education, and advocacy for all those affected by Alzheimer's disease in British Columbia, including patients, caregivers, patients' families, and the community.
*Jen Lyle, CEO*
*Paul Brill, Director, Marketing & Communications*

602 **Alzheimer Society of Canada**
20 Eglinton Avenue W 416-488-8772
Toronto, Ontario, M4R-1K8 800-618-8816
Fax: 416-488-3778
info@alzheimer.ca
www.alzheimer.ca
Identifies, develops and facilitates national priorities that enable its members to effectively alleviate the personal and social consequences of Alzheimer's disease and related disorders; promotes research and leads the search for a cure.
*Kevin Noel, Interim CEO*
*Gail Black-Elliot, Chief Development Officer*

603 **Alzheimer Society of Manitoba**
10 - 120 Donald Street 204-943-6622
Winnipeg, Manitoba, R3C-4G2 800-378-6699
Fax: 833-638-0760
alzmb@alzheimer.mb.ca
alzheimer.mb.ca
Provides support, education, and advocacy for all those affected by Alzheimer's disease in Manitoba, including patients, caregivers, patients' families, and the community.
*Wendy Schettler, Chief Executive Officer*
*Rebecca Krowelski, Marketing & Communications Director*

604 **Alzheimer Society of New Brunswick**
320 Maple Street 506-459-4280
Fredericton, NB, E3A-3R4 800-664-8411
Fax: 506-452-0313
info@alzheimernb.ca
alzheimer.ca/en/nb
Provides support, education, and advocacy for all those affected by Alzheimer's disease in New Brunswick, including patients, caregivers, patients' families, and the community.

605 **Alzheimer Society of Newfoundland & Labrador**
835 Topsail Road 709-576-0608
Mount Pearl, NL, A1N-3J6 877-776-0608
Fax: 709-576-0798
info@alzheimernl.ca
alzheimer.ca/en/nl
Provides support, education, and advocacy for all those affected by Alzheimer's disease in Newfoundland and Labrador, including patients, caregivers, patients' families, and the community.

606 **Alzheimer Society of Nova Scotia**
112-2719 Gladstone Street 902-422-7961
Halifax, Nova Scotia, B3K-4W6 800-611-6345
Fax: 902-422-7971
alzheimer@asns.ca
alzheimer.ca/en/ns
Provides support, education, and advocacy for all those affected by Alzheimer's disease in Nova Scotia, including patients, caregivers, patients' families, and the community.

607 **Alzheimer Society of Ontario**
20 Eglinton Avenue W 416-967-5900
Toronto, Ontario, M4R-1K8 800-879-4226
Fax: 416-967-3826
staff@alzon.ca
alzheimer.ca/en/on
Provides support, education, and advocacy for all those affected by Alzheimer's disease in Ontario, including patients, caregivers, patients' families, and the community.

608 **Alzheimer Society of Prince Edward Island**
166 Fitzroy Street 902-628-2257
Charlottetown, PE, C1A-1S1 society@alzpei.ca
alzheimer.ca/en/pei
Provides support, education, and advocacy for all those affected by Alzheimer's disease in Prince Edward Island, including patients, caregivers, patients' families, and the community.
*Nelson Hagerman, President*
*Val Maclean, Treasurer*

609 **Alzheimer Society of Saskatchewan**
2550 - 12th Avenue 306-949-4141
Regina, Saskatchewan, S4P-3X1 800-263-3367
Fax: 306-949-3069
info@alzheimer.sk.ca
www.alzheimer.ca/en/sk
Provides support, education, and advocacy for all those affected by Alzheimer's disease in Saskatchewan, including patients, caregivers, patients' families, and the community.
*Joanne Bracken, CEO*
*Leslie Quennell, Dir., Public Awareness & Comms.*

610 **Alzheimer's Association**
225 N. Michigan Avenue
Chicago, IL 60601 www.alz.org
Dedicated to research for the prevention, cure, and treatment of Alzheimer's disease and related disorders, and to providing support and assistance to patients and their families.
*Sarah Lorance, Chair*
*Harry Johns, Chief Executive Officer*

611 **Federation of Quebec Alzheimer Societies**
507-460 Rue Sainte-Catherine Ouest 514-369-7891
Montreal, Quebec, H4A-1A7 888-636-6473
info@alzheimerquebec.ca
alzheimer.ca/en/federationquebecoise
Provides support, education, and advocacy for all those affected by Alzheimer's disease in Quebec, including patients, caregivers, patients' families, and the community.
*Luc Pinard, President*
*Charles Cyr-Gill, Vice President*

612 **National Institute on Aging**
P.O. Box 8057 800-222-2225
Gaithersburg, MD 20898 niaic@nia.nih.gov
www.nia.nih.gov
Seeks to understand the nature of aging, and to extend healthy, active years of life. Free resources are available on topics such as Alzheimer's & dimentia, caregiving, cognitive heath, end of life care, and more.
*Richard J. Hodes, M.D., Director*
*Amy Kelley, M.D., M.S.H.S., Deputy Director*

### *Alabama*

613 **Alzheimer's Association: Alabama**
1 Metroplex Drive 205-379-8065
Birmingham, AL 35209 800-272-3900
jcmiller@alz.org
www.alz.org/al
*Jessica Miller, Executive Director*
*Billy Curtis, Director, Programs*

*Alaska*

614 **Alzheimer's Association: Alaska**
206-245-6431
800-272-3900
jwilgus@alz.org
www.alz.org/alaska

*Jim Wilgus, Regional Leader*
*Elizabeth Bolling, Public Policy Manager*

*Arizona*

615 **Alzheimer's Association: Desert Southwest**
340 E Palm Lane
Phoenix, AZ 85004
602-528-0545
800-272-3900
tgspitz@alz.org
www.alz.org/dsw
Serving the state of Arizona and Southern Nevada offices in Phoenix, Tucson, Sun City, Prescott and Las Vegas.
*Terri Spitz, Executive Director*
*Sarah Boerner, Development Director*

616 **Alzheimer's Association: Northern Arizona**
3111 Clearwater Drive
Prescott, AZ 86305
928-771-9257
800-272-3900
alramirez@alz.org
www.alz.org/dsw
*Alexis Ramirez, Community Engagement Coordinator*
*Susie James, Helpline Manager*

617 **Alzheimer's Association: Southern Arizona**
2990 N Swan Road
Tucson, AZ 85712
520-322-6601
800-272-3900
rbuenobarron@alz.org
www.alz.org/dsw
*Raul Bueno, Community Engagement Coordinator*
*Nallelhy Ballesteros, Program Manager*

*Arkansas*

618 **Alzheimer's Association: Arkansas**
11300 N. Rodney Parham Road
Little Rock, AR 72212
501-265-0027
800-272-3900
kedickins@alz.org
www.alz.org/arkansas
*Kirsten Dickens, Executive Director*
*Taco Price, Director, Programs*

*California*

619 **Alzheimer's Association: Cali. - Southland**
1401 Commericial Way
Baskersfield, CA 93309
661-912-3053
800-272-3900
mbarron@alz.org
www.alz.org/socal
*Meg Barron, Regional Leader & Executive Director*

620 **Alzheimer's Association: California - Central Coast**
1528 Chapala Street
Santa Barbara, CA 93101
805-892-4259
800-272-3900
Fax: 805-892-4250
lmleonard@alz.org
www.alz.org/cacentralcoast
*Lindsey Leonard, Executive Director*
*Karen Ortiz, Director, Development*

621 **Alzheimer's Association: Northern California**
2290 North First Street
San Jose, CA 95131
408-372-9900
800-272-3900
www.alz.org/norcal
*Elizabeth Edgerly, PhD, Executive Director*
*Shelley Dombroski, Senior Regional Director*

622 **Alzheimer's Association: Orange County**
38 Executive Park
Irvine, CA 92614
949-426-8544
800-272-3900
dblevy@alz.org
www.alz.org/oc
*Deborah Levy, Executive Director*
*Gregory Mathes, Director, Programs*

623 **Alzheimer's Association: San Diego**
5075 Shoreham Place
San Diego, CA 92122
619-678-8322
800-272-3900
klcroskrey@alz.org
www.alz.org/sandiego
*Janet Hamada Kelley, Executive Director*
*Ana Gonzalez Seda, MPH, Director, Programs*

*Colorado*

624 **Alzheimer's Association: Boulder and Mountain Region**
5353 Manhattan Circle
Boulder, CO 80303
303-813-1669
800-272-3900
Fax: 720-974-1583
rpatrick@alz.org
www.alz.org/co
Serving residents in Boulder, Broomfield, Chaffee, Clear Creek, Eagle, Gilpin, Lake, Park, Pitkin, and Summit counties.
*Ralph Patrick, Regional Director*
*Jeff Bird, Executive Director*

625 **Alzheimer's Association: Great Denver Region**
455 N. Sherman Street
Denver, CO 80203
303-813-1669
800-272-3900
Fax: 303-813-1670
toclark@alz.org
www.alz.org/co
Serving residents in Adams, Arapahoe, Denver, Douglas, and Jefferson Counties.
*Tom Clark, Community Engagement Manager*

626 **Alzheimer's Association: Northeastern Colorado Region**
P.O. Box 336672
Greeley, CO 80633
303-795-5465
Fax: 970-346-9025
www.alz.org/c
Serving residents in Cheyenne, Elbert, Kit Carson, Lincoln, Logan, Morgan, Phillips, Sedgwick, Washington, Weld, and Yuma Counties.
*Sarah Gostenik, Regional Director*

627 **Alzheimer's Association: Northern Colorado Region**
5010 Aspen Drive
Littleton, CO 80123
303-795-5465
800-272-3900
Fax: 303-794-0487
alhoffman@alz.org
www.alz.org/co
Serving residents in Grand, Jackson, Larimer, Moffat, Rio Blanco, and Routt Counties.
*Angel Hoffman, Regional Director*

628 **Alzheimer's Association: Southern and Central Colorado Region**
1520 N Union Blvd.
Colorado Springs, CO 80909
303-795-5465
Fax: 719-266-8798
rmjaramillo@alz.org
www.alz.org/co
Serving residents in Alamosa, Baca, Bent, Conejos, Costilla, Crowley, Custer, El Paso, Fremont, Hu,rfano, Kiowa, Las Animas, Mineral, Otero, Prowers, Pueblo, Rio Grande, Saguache, and Teller counties.
*RoseMary Jaramillo, Regional Director*

629 **Alzheimer's Association: Western Colorado Region**
2232 N. 7th Ave.
Grand Junction, CO 81501
303-795-5465
Fax: 970-243-6924
wlbandel@alz.org
www.alz.org/co
Serving residents in Archuleta, Delta, Dolores, Gunnison, Hinsdale, La Plata, Montezuma, Mesa, Montrose, Ouray, San Juan, and San Miguel counties.
*Woo Bandel, Community Engagement Manager*

*Connecticut*

630 **Alzheimer's Association: Connecticut**
200 Executive Blvd
Southington, CT 06489
860-406-3040
Fax: 860-571-8613
ckovel@alz.org
www.alz.org/ct
*Ginny Hanbridge, Executive Director*

### Delaware

631 **Alzheimer's Association: Delaware**
399 Market St.
Philadelphia, PA 19106
800-272-3900
klfransel@alz.org
www.alz.org/delval

*Kristina Fransel, Executive Director*
*Abbey Hunton, Sr. Dir., Marketing & Communications*

### District of Columbia

632 **Alzheimer's Association: National Capital Area**
8180 Greensboro Drive
McLean, VA 22102
703-359-4440
Fax: 703-359-4441
kgrooper@alz.org
www.alz.org/nca

*Kate Rooper, Chapter President & CEO*
*Ana Nelson, VP, Programs & Services*

### Florida

633 **Alzheimer's Association: Central and North Florida**
2170 W State Rd 434
Longwood, FL 32779
407-951-7992
800-272-3900
Fax: 407-951-7993
jhmarshall@alz.org
www.alz.org/cnfl

*Jessica Marshall, Executive Director*
*Deann Marasco, Regional Director, Health Systems*

634 **Alzheimer's Association: Florida Gulf Coast**
14010 Roosevelt Blvd.
Clearwater, FL 33762
727-578-2558
800-272-3900
Fax: 727-578-2286
admcauley@alz.org
www.alz.org/flgulfcoast

*Angela McAuley, Regional Leader*

635 **Alzheimer's Association: Southeast Florida**
100 W. Cypress Creek Rd.
Ft. Lauderdale, FL 33309
954-786-1533
800-272-3900
Fax: 954-497-4049
twpaige@alz.org
www.alz.org/seflorida

*Tracey Wekar-Paige, Executive Director*

### Georgia

636 **Alzheimer's Association: Georgia**
41 Perimeter Center East
Atlanta, GA 30345
404-728-1181
800-272-3900
Fax: 404-636-9768
lidavidson@alz.org
www.alz.org/georgia

*Linda Davidson, Executive Director*

### Hawaii

637 **Alzheimer's Association: Hawaii**
677 Ala Moana Boulevard
Honolulu, HI 96813
808-591-2771
800-272-3900
Fax: 808-591-9071
alohainfo@alz.org
www.alz.org/hawaii

*LJ R. Duenas, Executive Director*

### Idaho

638 **Alzheimer's Association: Greater Idaho**
P.O. Box 4746
Boise, ID 83711
208-206-0041
800-272-3900
Fax: 866-201-5957
www.alz.org/idaho

### Illinois

639 **Alzheimer's Association: Illinois**
8430 W. Bryn Mawr
Chicago, IL 60631
847-933-2413
800-272-3900
djervier@alz.org
www.alz.org/illinois

*Delia Jervier, Chapter Executive*

### Indiana

640 **Alzheimer's Association: Greater Indiana**
50 E 91st St.
Indianapolis, IN 46240
317-575-9620
800-272-3900
Fax: 317-575-9624
nmsutton@alz.org
www.alz.org/indiana

*Natalie Sutton, Chapter Executive*

### Iowa

641 **Alzheimer's Association: Iowa**
1415 28th St.
West Des Moines, IA 50266
515-440-2722
800-272-3900
Fax: 515-440-6385
dabickford@alz.org
www.alz.org/iowa

Serves the following counties: Adair, Clarke, Dallas, Decatur, Guthrie, Jasper, Lucas, Madison, Marion, Polk, Ringgold, Union, Warren and Wayne.
*Doug Bickford, Executive Director*

### Kansas

642 **Alzheimer's Association: Central and Western Kansas**
1820 East Douglas
Wichita, KS 67214
316-267-7333
800-272-3900
Fax: 316-267-6369
lbelton@alz.org
www.alz.org/cwkansas

*Juliette B. Bradley, Kansas State Director of Communications*

643 **Alzheimer's Association: Heart of America**
3846 W. 75th Street
Prairie Village, KS 66208
913-831-3888
800-272-3900
kjjackson@alz.org
www.alz.org/kansascity

*Ken Jackson, Executive Director*

### Kentucky

644 **Alzheimer's Association: Greater Kentucky and Soutern Indiana**
2808 Palumbo Dr.
Lexington, KY 40509
859-266-5283
800-272-3900
Fax: 859-268-4764
ShWhite@alz.org
www.alz.org/kyin

*Shannon White, Chapter Executive*

### Maine

645 **Alzheimer's Association: Maine**
383 Us Route One
Scarborough, ME 04074
207-772-0115
800-272-3900
dwyman@alz.org
www.alz.org/maine

*Drew Wyman, Executive Director*
*Amy Angelo, Program Manager*

### Maryland

646 **Alzheimer's Association: Greater Maryland**
502 Washington Avenue
Towson, MD 21204
410-561-9099
800-272-3900
djmcshea@alz.org
www.alz.org/maryland

*David McShea, Executive Director*

### *Massachusetts*

647 **Alzheimer's Association: Massachusetts and New Hampshire**
309 Waverley Oaks Road
Waltham, MA 02452
617-868-6718
800-272-3900
Fax: 617-868-6720
www.alz.org/manh

### *Michigan*

648 **Alzheimer's Association: Greater Michigan**
25200 Telegraph Rd.
Southfield, MI 48033
248-351-0280
800-272-3900
jlepard@alz.org
www.alz.org/gmc

*Jennifer Lepard, President & CEO*
*Kathryn Ribant Payne, Communications Director*

### *Minnesota*

649 **Alzheimer's Association: Minnesota and North Dakota**
7900 West 78th Street
Minneapolis, MN 55439
952-830-0512
800-272-3900
Fax: 952-830-0513
sjparriott@alz.org
www.alz.org/mnnd

*Susan Parriott, CEO*

### *Mississippi*

650 **Alzheimer's Association: Mississippi**
601-331-6115
800-272-3900
capolk@alz.org
www.alz.org/ms

*Chad Polk, Executive Director*
*Kristen White, LMSW, Program Coordinator*

### *Missouri*

651 **Alzheimer's Association: Greater Missouri**
9370 Olive Blvd.
St. Louis, MO 63132
800-272-3900
www.alz.org/greatermissouri

### *Montana*

652 **Alzheimer's Association: Montana**
3010 11th Ave N
Billings, MT 59101
406-252-3053
800-272-3900
jfunyak@alz.org
www.alz.org/montana

*Jami Funyak, Executive Director*
*Melanie Williams, Program Director, Programs & Edu.*

### *Nebraska*

653 **Alzheimer's Association: Nebraska**
402-260-7912
800-272-3900
sstephens@alz.org
www.alz.org/nebraska

*Sharon Stephens, Executive Director*
*Julie Chytil, Director, Programs*

### *Nevada*

654 **Alzheimer's Association: Northern Nevada**
639 Isbell Road
Reno, NV 89509
775-786-8061
800-272-3900
www.alz.org/norcal

*Elizabeth Edgerly, PhD, Executive Director*
*Shelley Dombroski, Senior Regional Director*

655 **Alzheimer's Association: Southern Nevada**
5190 S Valley View Boulevard
Las Vegas, NV 89118
702-248-2770
800-272-3900
Fax: 702-248-2771
cbaumis@alz.org
www.alz.org/dsw

*Johna Meints, Community Engagement Coordinator*
*Caroline Baumis, Program Manager*

### *New Jersey*

656 **Alzheimer's Association: Greater New Jersey**
23 Vreeland Road
Florham Park, NJ 07932
732-504-2347
800-272-3900
criccifrancione@alz.org
www.alz.org/nj

*Cheryl Ricci-Francione, Executive Director*
*Robyn Kohn, Director, Programs & Services*

### *New Mexico*

657 **Alzheimer's Association: New Mexico**
6731 Academy Rd NE
Albuquerque, NM 87109
505-266-4473
800-272-3900
Fax: 505-266-0108
tisheahan@alz.org
www.alz.org/newmexico

*Tim Sheahan, Executive Director*
*Ron D. Eppes, Program Director*

### *New York*

658 **Alzheimer's Association: Hudson Valley**
2649 South Road
Poughkeepsie, NY 12601
845-471-2655
800-272-3900
Fax: 845-471-8960
dsobel@alz.org
www.alz.org/hudsonvalley

*David Sobel, Executive Director*
*Meg Boyce, Director, Programs & Services*

659 **Alzheimer's Association: Central New York**
P.O. Box 12226
Syracuse, NY 13218
315-472-4201
800-272-3900
Fax: 315-472-4202
cny-info@alz.org
www.alz.org/centralnewyork

*Catherine James, CEO*
*Kristen Campbell, LMSW, Director, Programs & Services*

660 **Alzheimer's Association: Long Island**
300 Broadhollow Road
Melville, NY 11747
631-629-6950
800-272-3900
ddavidson@alz.org
www.alz.org/longisland

*Doug Davidson, Executive Director*
*Kate Anastasia, Program Director*

661 **Alzheimer's Association: New York City**
60 East 42nd Street
New York, NY 10165
646-418-4466
800-272-3900
NYCinfo@alz.org
www.alz.org/nyc

*Christopher Smith, Executive Director*
*Gwen Bolden, Program Operations Specialist*

662 **Alzheimer's Association: Northeastern New York**
1003 New Loudon Road
Cohoes, NY 12047
518-867-4999
800-272-3900
Fax: 518-867-4997
www.alz.org/northeasternny

*Elizabeth Smith-Boivin, Executive Director & CEO*
*Shannon Lawler, Director, Programs & Services*

663 **Alzheimer's Association: Rochester and Finger Lakes Region**
200 Meridian Centre Blvd.
Rochester, NY 14618
800-272-3900
inforochny@alz.org
www.alz.org/rochesterny

*Teresa Galbier, Chapter Executive*
*Amanda Drobnica, Senior Director, Programs & Services*

664 **Alzheimer's Association: Western New York**
6400 Sheridan Drive
Amherst, NY 14421
716-626-0600
800-272-3900
program.wny@alz.org
www.alz.org/wny

*Jill Horner, Executive Director*
*Lauren Ashburn, Associate Director, Advocacy*

## North Carolina

665 **Alzheimer's Association: Eastern North Carolina**
5171 Glenwood Avenue
Raleigh, NC 27612
919-803-8285
800-272-3900
Fax: 866-586-6307
encinfo@alz.org
www.alz.org/nc

*Madison Buchanan, Program Manager*

## Ohio

666 **Alzheimer's Association: Greater Cincinnati**
800-272-3900
anbarnett@alz.org
www.alz.org/cincinnati

667 **Alzheimer's Association: Central Ohio**
1379 Dublin Road
Columbus, OH 43215
614-457-6003
800-272-3900
vmcgrail@alz.org
www.alz.org/centralohio

*Vince McGrail, Executive Director*
*Katie Kirby, Director, Public Relations & Comms.*

668 **Alzheimer's Association: Cleveland Area**
23215 Commerce Park Drive
Beachwood, OH 44122
216-721-8457
800-272-3900
Fax: 216-831-8585
www.alz.org/cleveland

*Cheryl Kanetsky, Interim Executive Director*

669 **Alzheimer's Association: Greater East Ohio**
408 Ninth St. SW
Canton, OH 44707
330-966-7343
800-272-3900
Fax: 330-966-7757
ckanetsky@alz.org
www.alz.org/eastohio

*Cheryl Kanetsky, Interim Executive Director*
*Mary Ertle, Program Director*

670 **Alzheimer's Association: Miami Valley**
6077 Far Hills Ave.
Dayton, OH 45459
937-291-3332
800-272-3900
Fax: 937-291-0463
mvprograms@alz.org
www.alz.org/dayton

671 **Alzheimer's Association: Northwest Ohio**
480 Dussel Dr.
Maumee, OH 43537
419-537-1999
800-272-3900
Fax: 419-536-5591
jpechlivanos@alz.org
www.alz.org/nwohio

*Julia Faulkner Pechlivanos, Executive Director*

## Oklahoma

672 **Alzheimer's Association: Oklahoma**
6601 N. Broadway Ext.
Oklahoma City, OK 73116
405-319-0780
800-272-3900
www.alz.org/oklahoma

## Oregon

673 **Alzheimer's Association: Oregon and SW Washington**
5285 Meadows Road
Lake Oswego, OR 97035
503-416-0201
800-272-3900
www.alz.org/orswwa

## Pennsylvania

674 **Alzheimer's Association: Delaware Valley**
399 Market St.
Philadelphia, PA 19106
800-272-3900
klfransel@alz.org
www.alz.org/delval

*Kristina Fransel, Executive Director*
*Abbey Hunton, Senior Director, Marketing & Comms.*

675 **Alzheimer's Association: Greater Pennsylvania**
2595 Interstate Drive
Harrisburg, PA 17110
717-651-5020
800-272-3900
cjacobs@alz.org
www.alz.org/pa

*Clay Jacobs, Executive Director*
*Sara Murphy, VP, Programs & Services*

## Rhode Island

676 **Alzheimer's Association: Rhode Island**
245 Waterman Street
Providence, RI 02906
800-272-3900
Donna.McGowan@alz.org
www.alz.org/ri

*Jacqueline Waldon, CPA, President*
*Thomas Enright, Esq., Vice President*

## South Carolina

677 **Alzheimer's Association: South Carolina**
123 W. Antrim Drive
Greenville, SC 29607
800-272-3900
calewine@alz.org
www.alz.org/sc

*Cindy Alewine, President & CEO*
*Sam Wiley, VP, Programs*

## South Dakota

678 **Alzheimer's Association: South Dakota**
5915 S. Remington Place
Sioux Falls, SD 57108
605-339-4543
800-272-3900
www.alz.org/sd

## Tennessee

679 **Alzheimer's Association: East Tennessee**
9050 Executive Park Drive
Knoxville, TN 37923
800-272-3900
skthompson@alz.org
www.alz.org/tn

*Sara Dickson, Development Manager*

680 **Alzheimer's Association: Middle Tennessee**
1801 West End Ave., Suite 200
Nashville, TN 37203
800-272-3900
dcbunn@alz.org
www.alz.org/tn

*Dawne Bunn, Executive Director*
*Misa Acox, Director, Communications*

681 **Alzheimer's Association: Northeast Tennessee**
P.O. Box 41428
Nashville, TN 37204
800-272-3900
www.alz.org/tn
*George Jensen, Chair*
*Sarah Wood, Local Contact*

682 **Alzheimer's Association: Southeast Tennessee**
7625 Hamilton Park Dr.
Chattanooga, TN 37421
800-272-3900
afrench@alz.org
www.alz.org/tn

*Amy French, Programs Manager*

## Texas

683 **Alzheimer's Alliance: Dallas and Northeast Texas**
5000 Quorum Drive
Dallas, TX 75254
800-272-3900
madenzin@alz.org
www.alztexark.org/dallasnetexas

*Mark Denzin, Executive Director*
*Kathy Shockley, MA, LNHA, Program Director*

684 **Alzheimer's Association: Capital of Texas**
5508 Highway 290 West — 512-592-0990
Austin, TX 78735 — 800-272-3900
Fax: 512-692-3813
ataurins@alz.org
www.alz.org/texascapital

*Andrea Taurins, Executive Director*
*Christine Casebeer, Development Director*

685 **Alzheimer's Association: Houston and Southeast Texas**
6055 South Loop East — 713-314-1313
Houston, TX 77087-1005 — 800-272-3900
Fax: 713-314-1316
relbein@alz.org
www.alz.org/texas

*Richard Elbein, CEO*
*Alexis Eaton, Chief Development Officer*

686 **Alzheimer's Association: North Central Texas**
2630 West Freeway — 817-336-4949
Fort Worth, TX 76102 — 800-272-3900
www.alz.org

*Brenda Shuttlesworth, Executive Director*
*Jenna Perales, LMSW, Director, Program Services*

687 **Alzheimer's Association: San Antonio and South Texas**
1100 Northwest Loop 410 — 800-272-3900
San Antonio, TX 78213 — gsciuto@alz.org
www.alz.org

*Gregory Sciuto, Executive Director*
*Ginny Funk, Director, Programs*

688 **Alzheimer's Association: West Texas**
110 Mesa Park Dr. — 915-544-1799
El Paso, TX 79912 — 800-272-3900
westtexas@alz.org
www.alz.org/westtexas

*Dave Hernandez, Chapter Executive*
*Maria Llamas, Director, Programs*

### *Utah*

689 **Alzheimer's Association: Utah**
12894 S. Pony Express Road — 801-265-1944
Draper, UT 84020 — 800-272-3900
stkulp@alz.org
www.alz.org/utah

*Stacie Kulp, Executive Director*
*Raven Albertson, Program Director*

### *Vermont*

690 **Alzheimer's Association: Vermont**
75 Talcott Road — 802-316-3839
Williston, VT 05495 — 800-272-3900
www.alz.org/vermont

*Howard Goodrow, Executive Director*
*Jordan Cotto, Program Manager*

### *Virginia*

691 **Alzheimer's Association: Central and Western Virginia**
355 Rio Road West — 434-973-6122
Charlottesville, VA 22901 — 800-272-3900
alzcwva@alz.org
www.alz.org/cwva

*Lissa Greenlee, Executive Director*
*Jeanne Snyder, Community Executive*

692 **Alzheimer's Association: Greater Richmond**
4600 Cox Road — 804-967-2580
Glen Allen, VA 23060 — 800-272-3900
Fax: 804-967-2588
lagreenlee@alz.org
www.alz.org/grva

*Lissa Greenlee, Executive Director*
*Tabitha Cox, Regional Office Operations Manager*

693 **Alzheimer's Association: Southeastern Virginia**
6350 Center Drive — 757-459-2405
Norfolk, VA 23502 — 800-272-3900
Fax: 757-461-7902
kmcdonough@alz.org
www.alz.org/seva

*Katie McDonough, LCSW, Executive Director*
*Douglas Panto, Community Programs Manager*

694 **Alzheimer's Association: West Virginia**
1601 2nd Avenue — 304-343-2717
Charleston, WV 25387 — 800-272-3900
Fax: 304-343-2723
wvinfo@alz.org
www.alz.org/wv

*Sharon M. Covert, Executive Director*
*Teresa Morris, Program Director*

### *Washington*

695 **Alzheimer's Association: Washington State**
19031 33rd Ave West — 206-363-5500
Lynnwood, WA 98036 — 800-272-3900
Fax: 206-363-5700
jwilgus@alz.org
www.alz.org/alzwa

*Jim Wilgus, Executive Director*
*Brad Forbes, Director, Public Policy*

### *West Virginia*

696 **Alzheimer's Association: West Virginia**
1601 2nd Avenue — 304-343-2717
Charleston, WV 25387 — 800-272-3900
Fax: 304-343-2723
wvinfo@alz.org
www.alz.org/wv

*Sharon M. Covert, Executive Director*
*Teresa Morris, Program Director*

### *Wisconsin*

697 **Alzheimer's Association: Wisconsin**
2700 Vernon Ave. — 920-469-2110
Green Bay, WI 54304 — 800-272-3900
Fax: 920-469-2131
dgrams@alz.org
www.alz.org/wi

*Dave Grams, Executive Director*
*Wendy Betley, Senior Program Director*

### *Wyoming*

698 **Alzheimer's Association: Wyoming**
2232 Dell Range Blvd. — 307-316-2892
Cheyenne, WY 82009 — 800-272-3900
debianchi@alz.org
www.alz.org/wyoming

*Debra Antista-Bianchi, MPH, MS, Executive Director*
*Robin McIntyre, Development Manager*

## Foundations

699 **Alzheimer Society of Toronto**
20 Eglinton Ave. West — 416-322-6560
Toronto, ON, M4R-1K8 — write@alz.to
alz.to

Provides information, programs, and educational resources to individuals living with dementia, and their families and caregivers. Serves the Greater Toronto Area.
*Kari Quinn-Humphrey, Interim CEO*
*Kristy McKay, Dir., Community Support Services*

700 **Alzheimer's Foundation of America**
322 Eighth Avenue — 866-232-8484
New York, NY 10001 — info@alzfdn.org
alzfdn.org

Offers support and resources to individuals, families, and caregivers affected by Alzheimer's disease, and funds research for advanced treatment and a cure.
*Bert E. Brodsky, Founder & Chair*
*Charles J. Fuschillo Jr., President & CEO*

701 **John Douglas French Alzheimer's Foundation**
1191 Brookmere Road 213-219-3575
Pasadena, CA 91105 cheryl@jdfaf.org
www.jdfaf.org
Provides seed money for promising research including the cause cure and prevention of Alzheimer's disease. Also gives funding to scientists who might not otherwise be funded.
*B.J. Kirwan Hanna, Chair*
*Cheryl Mae Craft, Ph.D., President & CEO*

## Libraries & Resource Centers

702 **Alzheimer's Disease & Related Dementias**
National Institute on Aging
P.O. Box 8057 800-438-4380
Gaithersburg, MD 20898 adear@nia.nih.gov
www.nia.nih.gov/health/alzheimers
A service of the National Institute on Aging, the center distributes information on Alzheimer's disease, on current research activities and on services available to patients and family members. Offers a free list of publications available upon request.
*Nina Silverberg, Program Director, Alzheimer's*

703 **Green-Field Library-Alzheimer's Association**
225 N. Michigan Avenue 847-324-0356
Chicago, IL 60601 800-272-3900
Fax: 866-699-1238
TTY: 312-335-5886
TDD: 312-335-8700
greenfield@alz.org
www.alz.org
Located at the national Alzheimer's Association in Chicago this library offers a sizable collection of videos on a variety of subjects that may interest the Alzheimer's patient family members and caregivers.
*Richard Hovland, COO*

## Research Centers

704 **Aging and Alzheimer's Disease Center Oregon Health Sciences University**
Oregon Health Sciences University
3181 SW Sam Jackson Park Road 503-494-8311
Portland, OR 97239 Fax: 503-494-6695
kaye@ohsu.edu
www.ohsu.edu/research/alzheimers
Researches causes and consequences of Alzheimer's disease and ways of clinical services. Publishes a newsletter twice a year.
*Jeffrey Kaye, Director*
*Joan Benedict, Administrative Coordinator*

705 **Alzheimer's Disease & Memory Disorders Center**
ADMDC
One Baylor Plaza 713-798-5971
Houston, TX 77030 Fax: 713-798-7434
neurons@bcm.edu
www.bcm.edu/neurology/admdc
Researchers work to translate advances into improved care and diagnosis for Alzheimer's Disease and other memory disorders.
*Eli M. Mizrahi, Chair, Department of Neurology*
*Keith Davis, Department Administrator*

706 **Alzheimer's Disease Center Emory University/VA Medical Center**
201 Dowman Drive 404-727-6069
Atlanta, GA 30322 Fax: 404-286-55
emoryadrc@emory.edu
www.med.emory.edu/ADRC
Researchers work to translate advances into improved care and diagnosis for Alzheimer's patients.
*Allan Levey, Director*
*Stuart Zola, Co-Director*

707 **Alzheimer's Disease Center Kentucky University**
Sanders-Brown Center on Aging
1030 South Broadway 859-257-1412
Lexington, KY 40504 Fax: 859-323-2866
rdavi3@email.uky.edu
/www.mc.uky.edu/coa
Researchers work to translate advances into improved care and diagnosis for Alzheimer's patients.
*Linda J. Van Eldik, Ph.D., Director*
*Vince J Kellen, Chief Information Officer*

708 **Alzheimer's Disease Center Mayo Clinic Mayo Medical School**
Mayo Medical School
200 First Street SW 507-284-2511
Rochester, MN 55905 Fax: 507-538-0161
TDD: 507-2849786
mayoADC@mayo.edu
www.mayoclinic.com
Researchers work to translate advances into improved care and diagnosis for Alzheimer's patients.
*John H. Noseworhty, M.D., President*
*William C. Rupp, M.D., Vice President, CEO*

709 **Alzheimer's Disease Center Pennsylvania University School of Medicine**
Ralston House
3615 Chestnut Street 215-662-7810
Philadelphia, PA 19104 Fax: 215-662-7812
jason.karlawish@uphs.upenn.edu
www.pennadc.org
Researchers work to translate advances into improved care and diagnosis for Alzheimer's patients.
*John Q. Trojanowski, Director*

710 **Alzheimer's Disease Center: Boston University**
Boston University School of Medicine
72 E Concord Street 617-638-5426
Boston, MA 02118 888-458-2823
Fax: 617-414-1197
buad@bu.edu
www.bu.edu/alzresearch
Researchers work to translate advances into improved care and diagnosis for Alzheimer's patients.
*Neil W. Kowall, Director*
*Richard Fine, Associate Director*

711 **Alzheimer's Disease Center: Johns Hopkins University School of Medicine**
Johns Hopkins University Department of Pathology
720 Rutland Avenue 410-502-5164
Baltimore, MD 21205 Fax: 410-955-9777
edelman1@jhmi.edu
www.alzresearch.org
Researchers work to translate advances into improved care and diagnosis for Alzheimer's patients.
*Marilyn Albert, Director*
*Philip Wong, Associate Director*

712 **Alzheimer's Disease Center: University of California, Davis**
4860 Y Street 916-734-5496
Sacramento, CA 95817 wjjagust@lbl.gov
alzheimer.ucdavis.edu/
Researchers work to translate advances into improved care and diagnosis for Alzheimer's patients.
*Charles DeCarli, M.D., Clinical Core Director*

713 **Alzheimer's Disease Center: University of Alabama at Birmingham**
1720 7th Avenue S 205-934-3847
Birmingham, AL 35294 Fax: 205-975-7365
adbrain@uab.edu
www.main.uab.edu/adc
Researchers work to translate advances into improved care and diagnosis for Alzheimer's patients.
*Daniel Marson, Director*
*J. Michael Wyss, Associate Director*

714 **Alzheimer's Disease Center: Washington University**
1660 S Columbian Way 206-764-2069
Seattle, WA 98108 800-317-5382
Fax: 206-768-5456
wamble@u.washington.edu
www.depts.washington.edu/adrcweb
Researchers work to translate advances into improved care and diagnosis for Alzheimer's patients.
*Sydney Lewis, Education & Outreach Coordinator*
*Nancy Brown, Lead Psychometrist*

715 **Alzheimer's Disease Research Center Washington University School of Medicine**
Washington University School of Medicine
4488 Forest Park Avenue 314-286-2683
St Louis, MO 63108 Fax: 314-286-2763
morrisj@abraxas.wustl.edu
www.adrc.wustl.edu
Researchers work to translate advances into improved care diagnosis and treatment for Alzheimer's patients.
*John Morris, Director*
*Virginia D. Buckles, Executive Director*

716 **Alzheimer's Disease Research Center Duke University**
Bryan ADRC
2200 W Main Street Suite A200 919-668-0820
Durham, NC 27705 866-444-2372
kwe@duke.edu
adrc.mc.duke.edu
Researchers work to translate advances into improved care and diagnosis for Alzheimer's patients.
*Kathleen A. Welsh-Bohmer, Director*
*James Robert Burke, Associate Director*

717 **Cognitive Neurology and Alzheimer's Disease Center**
CNADC
320 E Superior Street 312-908-9339
Chicago, IL 60611 Fax: 312-908-8789
CNADC-Admin@northwestern.edu
www.brain.northwestern.edu
Researchers work to translate advances into improved care and diagnosis for Alzheimer's patients.
*Megan Atchu, Research Administrator*
*Kevin Connolly, Business Administrator*

718 **Cornell University: Winifred Masterson Burke Medical Research-Dementia**
1300 York Avenue 212-746-5454
New York, NY 10065 Fax: 212-821-0576
publicaffairs@med.cornell.edu
www.med.cornell.edu
Clinical and basic studies in metabolic aspects of the nervous system especially Alzheimer's disease.
*David J. Skorton, MD, President*
*Thomas H. Blair, III, Senior Director Administrator*

719 **Duke University Center for the Study of Aging and Human Development**
Duke University
Box 3003 919-660-7500
Durham, NC 27710 Fax: 919-668-0453
webmaster@geri.duke.edu
www.geri.duke.edu
Basic and clinical research into geriatrics and gerontology focusing on a number of chronic diseases in the elderly including osteoporosis, cancer, heart disease, infectious diseases, Alzheimer's disease and other disorders leading to dysmobility.
*Harvey Jay Cohen, MD, Director*
*Linda K. George, Associate Director*

720 **Duke University Clinical Research Institute**
Headquarters
2400 Pratt Street 919-668-8700
Durham, NC 27705 www.dcri.duke.edu
Multidisciplinary clinical research into the cause and prevention of human diseases such as Alzheimer's.
*Robert Harrington, Director*

721 **Indiana University Center for Aging Research**
The Center for Aging Research
1050 Wishard Blvd 317-630-6083
Indianapolis, IN 46202 Fax: 317-423-5695
www.medicine.iupui.edu/iucar/?
Researchers work to translate advances into improved care and diagnosis for Alzheimer's patients.
*Christopher Callahan, Director*
*Douglas Miller, Associate Director*

722 **Indiana University: Human Genetics Center of Medical & Molecular Genetics**
School of Medicine
340 West 10th Street 317-274-8157
Indianapolis, IN 46202 kcornett@iupui.edu
www.medicine.iu.edu
Comprised of a core group of scientists with primary appointments in the Department and a group of molecular biologists from other departments who hold joint appointments in Medical and Molecular Genetics.
*Craig Brater, Dean*
*John F. Fitzgerald, MD, MBA, Executive Associate Dean*

723 **Institute for Basic Research in Developmental Disabilities**
1050 Forest Hill Road 718-494-0600
Staten Island, NY 10314 866- 94- 973
TTY: 866- 933-488
ibr@opwdd.ny.gov
www.opwdd.ny.gov/institute-for-basic-res
*James Moran, Acting Commissioner*

724 **Long Island Alzheimers Foundation**
5 Channel Drive 516-767-6856
Port Washington, NY 11050 Fax: 516-767-6856
info@liaf.org
www.liaf.org
Researchers work to translate advances into improved care and diagnosis for Alzheimer's patients.
*Fred Jenny, Executive Director*
*Anna Maria Warmuz, Executive Assistant*

725 **Massachusetts Alzheimers Disease Research Center**
Massachusetts ADRC
16th Street 617-726-3987
Charlestown, MA 02129 Fax: 617-724-1480
www.madrc.org
Multi-institutional consortium of Harvard affiliated facilities that encompasses five Core units: an Administrative Core, a Clinical Core, a Database Management and Statistics Core, a Neuropathology Core, and an Education and Information Transfer Core. The ADRC also supports four specific research projects funded for 3-5 years, and annually designates three or four pilot research projects that are funded for 1 year.
*John Growdon, Clinic Director*
*Bradley Hyman, Center Director*

726 **Medical College of Georgia Alzheimers Research Center**
1120 15th Street 706-721-0211
Augusta, GA 30912 Fax: 706-721-7063
www.mcg.edu/centers/alz
Clinical and basic research of Alzheimer's disease.

727 **Michigan Alzheimer's Disease Research Center**
University of Michigan
2101 Commonwealth Blvd., 734-936-4000
Ann Arbor, MI 48105 www.med.umich.edu/alzheimers
Researchers work to translate advances into improved care and diagnosis for Alzheimer's patients.
*Sid Gilman, M.D., Director*
*Bruno Giordani Ph.D., Core Director*

728 **Mount Sinai School of Medicine: Alzheimers Disease Research Center**
Alzheimer's Disease Research Center
One Gustave L Levy Place 212-241-6696
New York, NY 10029 Fax: 212-369-2344
mary.sano@mssm.edu
www.mssm.edu
Focuses on Alzheimer's disease research.
*Mary Sano, Director*
*Samuel Gandy, Associate Director*

729 **Neurosciences Institute of the Neurosciences Research Program**
The Neurosciences Institute
10640 John Jay Hopkins Drive 858-626-2000
San Diego, CA 92121 Fax: 858-626-2099
info@nsi.edu
www.nsi.edu
Nonprofit organization focusing on Alzheimer's and related disorders.
*Gerald M. Edelman, President*

730 **Ohio State University Neuroscience Program**
1835 Neil Avenue 614-292-8185
Columbus, OH 43210 Fax: 614-921-44
www.psy.ohio-state.edu
Specializes in brain disorders such as Alzheimer's disease.
*Richard Petty, Chair*
*Scott Burch, Behavioral Neurosciences Area Assistant*

731 **Taub Institute for Research on Alzheimers Disease and the Aging Brain**
630 West 168th Street 212-305-1818
New York, NY 10032 Fax: 212-342-2849
taubinstitute@columbia.edu
www.alzheimercenter.org
Researchers work to translate advances into improved care and diagnosis for Alzheimer's patients.
*Michael L. Shelanski, Co-Director*
*Richard Mayeux, Co-Director*

732 **UC San Diego Center for Healthy Aging**
University of California San Diego
9500 Gilman Drive 858-534-6299
La Jolla, CA 92093 Fax: 858-534-5475
steininstitute@ucsd.edu
www.sira.ucsd.edu
Research on aging and Alzheimer's disease.
*Debra Kaine, Director*
*Maureen Halp, Executive Director*

733 **University Alzheimer Center University of Alabama at Birmingham**
University of Alabama at Birmingham
1530 3rd Avenue S 205-934-4011
Birmingham, AL 35294 800-333-6543
Fax: 205-975-7365
TTY: 205-934-4642
adbrain@uab.edu
main.uab.edu
Researchers work to translate advances into improved care and diagnosis for Alzheimer's patients.
*Dr. Carol Garrison, President*
*Kristen Burdick, Director of Executive Affairs*

734 **University Alzheimer Center UHC: Case Western Reserve University**
12200 Fairhill Road 216-844-6400
Cleveland, OH 44120 Fax: 216-844-6446
Kathy.Shaw@Case.Edu
www.ohioalzcenter.org
Researchers work to translate advances into improved care and diagnosis for Alzheimer's patients.
*Alan Lerner, Co-Director*
*Kathleen Smyth, Administrator*

735 **University of Chicago Dept of Neurology University of Chicago Hospital**
University of Chicago Hospital
5841 S Maryland Avenue 773-702-6390
Chicago, IL 60637 Fax: 773-702-9076
cgomez@neurology.bsd.uchicago.edu
neurology.uchicago.edu
Covers Translational Neuroscience Research and research programs in neuroimmunology neuromuscular disease and neurovirology provided the initial foundation and brought national recognition.
*Kenneth Goodell, Senior Executive Administrator*
*Judith Maratea, Administrative Assistant*

736 **University of Illinois Health Services Research**
University of Illinois College of Medicine
1601 Parkview Avenue 815-395-0600
Rockford, IL 61107 Fax: 815-395-5887
prrockford@uic.edu
www.uirockford.com
A unit of the University of Illinois College of Medicine at Rockford serves faculty students health care providers human services agencies and other community organizations throughout Illinois with demographic health social and economic data. The skills data and resources available to faculty and students at the college are also available to individuals and organizations needing assistance.
*Joann Glacken, Research Support Services*

737 **University of Maryland: Division of Infectious Diseases**
UM Baltimore Department of Medicine
655 West Baltimore Street 410-706-7410
Baltimore, MD 21201 Fax: 410-706-0235
rredfield@ihv.umaryland.edu
www.medschool.umaryland.edu
Focuses research on elderly studies including drug use treatments and infectious diseases of the aged.
*E. Albert Reece, Vice President*
*Richard Pierson, III, M.D., Senior Associate Dean for Academic Affai*

738 **University of Miami: Center on Aging Center on Aging**
Center on Aging
1695 NW 9th Avenue 305-355-9080
Miami, FL 33136 Fax: 305-355-9076
centeronaging.med.miami.edu
Focuses on aged disorders such as Alzheimer's research.
*Sara Czaja, Co-Director*
*Charles B. Nemeroff, M.D., Ph.D, Director*

739 **Yeshiva University: Resnick Gerontology Center**
Albert Einstein College of Medicine
Jack and Pearl Resnick Campus 718-920-6722
Bronx, NY 10467 866-633-8255
Fax: 718-655-9672
www.aecom.yu.edu
Alzheimer's disease and other dementia studies.
*Allen Spiegel, Dean*
*Amy Ehrlich, Geriatrics Fellowship Program Director*

## Support Groups & Hotlines

740 **Alzheimer's Association Autopsy Assistance Network**
Alzheimer s Association
Western/Central Washington Chapter 206-363-5500
Seattle, WA 98125 800-848-7097
Fax: 206-363-5700
rowena.rye@alz.org
http://alzwa.org/resources6.htm
The primary purposes of the Autopsy Assistance Network are: to provide families with information regarding autopsy; to assist in obtaining a confirmed diagnosis; provide tissue for Alzheimer's disease research; and establish diagnosis for purpose of clinical and epidemiological studies.
*Nancy Dapper, Executive Director*
*Rowena Rye, Community Resources*

741 **Alzheimer's Support Group**
Columbus Health Rehabilitation Center
2100 Midway Street 812-372-8447
Columbus, IN 47201 Fax: 812-375-5117
www.columbushrc.com/
The skilled Nursing Center includes a separate unit dedicated to the care of residents with Alzheimer's disease and other forms of dementia. The Alzheimer's program is designed to celebrate the spirit of their residents, striving to offer a comfortable and compassionate environment that emphasizes positive life experiences and active involvement in a daily routine.
*Mike Spencer, Executive Director*

742 **National Health Information Center**
Office of Disease Prevention & Health Promotion
1101 Wootton Pkwy Fax: 240-453-8281
Rockville, MD 20852 odphpinfo@hhs.gov
www.health.gov/nhic

Supports public health education by maintaining a calendar of National Health Observances; helps connect consumers and health professionals to organizations that can best answer questions and provide up-to-date contact information from reliable sources; updates on a yearly basis toll-free numbers for health information, Federal health clearinghouses and info centers.
*Don Wright, MD, MPH, Director*

## Print Resources

743 **Alzheimer Disease and Associated Disorders: An International Journal**
Raven Press
1185 Ave of the Americas 212-930-9500
New York, NY 10036 800-777-2295
journals.lww.com
A leading international forum for reports of new research findings and new approaches to diagnosis and treatments. Contributions are offered from all scientific and medical fields.
*Dr. Jose Luchsinger-Stuart, Editor-in-Chief*

744 **Alzheimer's & Dementia: The Journal of the Alzheimer's Association**
Alzheimer's Association
225 North Michigan Avenue 314-447-8871
Chicago, IL 60601 800-654-2452
www.alz.org
A peer-reviewed journal that publishes reviews, clinical trials, and investigations on dementia research.
*Donna M. Wilcock, PhD, Editor-in-Chief*

745 **Journal of Alzheimer's Disease (JAD)**
IO Press
george.perry@j-alz.com
www.j-alz.com
An international multidisciplinary journal that publishes research reports, reviews, and hypotheses on Alzheimer's disease.
*George Perry, PhD, Editor-in-Chief*
*Beth Kumar, Managing Editor*

746 **The Journal of Neuropsychiatry and Clinical Neurosciences**
American Neuropsychiatric Association
P.O. Box 97 anpaoffice@gmail.com
Abilene, KS 67410-1707 neuro.psychiatryonline.org
Publishes peer-reviewed articles on neuroscience and behavioral disrders, and addresses subjects like Alzheimer's disease, traumatic brain injury, Parkinson's disease, epilepsy, and seizure disorders.
*David B. Arciniegas, M.D., Editor*
*C. Alan Anderson, M.D., Deputy Editor*

## Web Sites

747 **Alzheimer Research Forum**
www.alzforum.org
The web's most dynamic scientific community dedicated to understanding alzheimer's disease and related disorders.

748 **Alzheimer Support**
www.alzheimersupport.com
Serves Alzheimer's sufferers and their loved ones by reporting the latest news in research and treatment, making hard-to-find, recommended nutritional supplements available at manufacturer-direct low prices, and, most importantly, donating profits from each purchase to fund Alzheimer's medical research.

749 **Alzheimer's Association**
www.alz.org
The leading, global voluntary health organization in Alzheimer care and support, and the largest private, nonprofit funder of Alzheimer research.

750 **Alzheimer's Disease International**
www.alz.co.uk/adi
The international federation of 73 Alzheimer associations around the world, in relations with the World Health Organization.

751 **Healing Well**
www.healingwell.com
A social network and support community for patients, caregivers, and families coping with the daily struggles of diseases, disorders and chronic illness.

752 **Healthlink USA**
www.healthlinkusa.com
Health information concerning treatment, cures, prevention, diagnosis, risk factors, research, support groups, email lists, personal stories and much more. Updated regularly.

753 **MEDLINEplus Health Information**
www.nlm.nih.gov/medlineplus
MedlinePlus is the National Institutes of Health's Web site for patients and their families and friends.

754 **MedicineNet**
www.medicinenet.com
An online resource for consumers providing easy-to-read, authoritative medical and health information.

755 **Medscape**
www.medscape.com
Medscape offers specialists, primary care physicians, and other health professionals the Web's most robust and integrated medical information and educational tools.

756 **MyHealthfinder**
www.healthfinder.gov
Searchable, carefully developed web site offering information on over 1000 topics. Developed by the US Department of Health and Human Services, the site can be used in both English and Spanish.

757 **Neurology Channel**
www.healthcommunities.com
Find clearly explained, medically accurate information regarding conditions, including an overview, symptoms, causes, diagnostic procedures and treatment options. On this site it is possible to ask questions and get information from a neurologist and connect to people who have similar health interests.

758 **WebMD**
www.webmd.com
Provides credible information, supportive communities, and in-depth reference material about health subjects. A source for original and timely health information, as well as material from well-known content providers.

# AUTOIMMUNE DISEASES

*Autoimmune disease is said to occur when the body's immune system attacks and destroys healthy tissue by mistake. There are more than 80 types of autoimmune diseases. Blood cells in the immune system protect against bacteria, viruses, cancer cells, and toxins such as chemical agents (antigens). Antibodies created by the immune system protect the body from these antigens by destroying harmful substances. When an autoimmune disease is present, the immune system does not distinguish between harmful antigens and healthy tissue, leading to a reaction that destroys normal tissue.*

Exact causes of autoimmune disorders are unknown. Triggers such as a bacteria or virus may confuse the immune system, perhaps occurring when an individual has a gene or genes that make them more prone to immune disease.

One or more organs or tissue types may be affected when an autoimmune disease is present, including:

- Endocrine glands
- Joints and muscles
- Blood vessels and red blood cells
- Connective tissue
- Skin

Drugs, both prescription and illegal, can cause drug-induced autoimmune syndromes. A classic example is drug-induced systemic lupus erythematosus. Some autoimmune syndromes have life-threatening complications, so identifying drug-induced disease is critical. Substance abuse can directly harm the immune system, making it difficult to function and resist disease. Substance use disorders may lead to infections from shared needles and unprotected sex, for example, and a weakened immune system is unable to mount a strong immune response. Snorting drugs can interrupt the mucous membranes of the nose and make the individual more prone to respiratory diseases when the immune system is compromised.

### Types of Autoimmune Disorders

While there are more than 80 types of autoimmune disorders, some of the more common disorders and a brief definition include:

- Rheumatoid arthritis-antibodies attach to joint linings, with the immune system creating swelling, pain and inflammation.
- Inflammatory bowel disease including Crohn's disease and ulcerative colitis-the immune system attacks the lining of the intestines, leading to diarrhea, rectal bleeding, loss of bowel control and abdominal pain, often accompanied by weight loss and fever.
- Diabetes mellitus-in Type I diabetes mellitus, the immune system destroys insulin-producing cells in the pancreas. Diagnosis is often at an early age and individuals need insulin to live a more normal life.

- Multiple sclerosis-a disease that may include muscle weakness and poor coordination, pain, blindness, weakness and muscle spasms caused when the immune system attacks nerve cells throughout the body.
- Systemic lupus erythematosus-a severe autoimmune disease where antibodies attack tissues throughout the body, including tissues in joints, lungs, blood cells, nerves and kidneys.

With an autoimmune disorder, a weakened immune system creates an even greater risk to the individual. A compromised immune system at a time with new viruses, such as COVID-19, and the evolution of existing viruses, as seen in flu and avian variations, pose a real threat of death. An inability to fight infection increases with substance use disorder.

### Substance Use and the Immune System

Side effects of substance use and abuse include addiction, overdose and death, but also a weakening of the immune system. The body attempts to attack a foreign substance when the immune system is activated, but in the case of a foreign drug substance, repeated use "wears out" or weakens the immune system. A compromised immune system is dangerous if the individual is exposed to germs, viruses and bacteria and the body's response is too weak to control the resulting disease. COVID-19 and its variants, flu and other infectious disease processes such as hepatitis, are significantly more aggressive in the individual with a weakened immune system. While drugs are perceived as potentially fatal, complicating factors such as infections are often just as dangerous.

The use of both legal and illegal drugs can alter the immune system. While there is often an understanding of illegal drug use, the misuse of prescription drugs is often less-well understood. Misuse can be taking a medication or dose other than as prescribed by the physician; for example, taking too much opioid pain medication after pain has lessened. Using someone else's prescription, even if for a legitimate reason, or taking a medication to feel euphoric (high) is prescription drug abuse. Teens and adults with diabetes mellitus requiring insulin may increase their dose of insulin to lose weight. The most commonly misused prescription drugs are opioids prescribed for pain control; tranquilizers, sedatives and hypnotics (central nervous system depressants); and stimulants often prescribed for attention-deficit hyperactivity disorder (ADHD). Abuse of prescription drugs can both alter the immune system and lead to eventual addiction.

Using illegal drugs with injection, smoking, snorting or in other manners, introduces a chemically harmful, foreign substance to the body and activates the immune system. Because illegal drug use often escalates into a substance use disorder, repeated use over activates the immune system, leaving it incapable of fighting off real threats. Illegal drug use often escalates risky behaviors that can expose the individual to infections, which with a weakened immune system, may be life threatening.

Excessive use of alcohol can limit the body's ability to fight infection. Lung infections like pneumonia are more likely with marijuana use, as the lung's defenses become weakened over time. Methamphetamines leave the body exhausted, dehydrated and deprived of essential nutrients needed to fight infection. All mind-altering drugs negatively impact the body's immune system in some manner.

### A Chronic Illness

Autoimmune diseases are generally considered chronic illnesses that can be managed with appropriate health care. Treatment protocols are often quite regimented, and variations are not helpful to the disease management. Introducing substances, whether legal or illegal, without consulting the physician managing the autoimmune disease is dangerous.

## Agencies & Associations

759 **American Association of Diabetes Care & Education Specialists**
125 S. Wacker Dr. 800-338-3633
Chicago, IL 60606 www.diabeteseducator.org
An independent, multidisciplinary organization of health professionals involved in teaching persons with diabetes. The mission is to enhance the competence of health professionals who teach persons with diabetes and advance the specialty practice of diabetes.
*Matthew Hornberger, Chief Executive Officer*
*Leslie Kolb, Chief Science, Practice & Learning Off.*

760 **American Autoimmune Related Diseases Association**
19176 Hall Road 586-776-3900
Clinton Township, MI 48038 hello@autoimmune.org
www.autoimmune.org
Provides awareness, education, and referrals for patients with any type of autoimmune disease.
*Jason Gamel, President/CEO*
*Rob Dunn, RRP, Chief Financial Officer*

761 **American Chronic Pain Association**
11936 W. 119th Street ACPA@theacpa.org
Overland Park, KS 66213-2216 www.theacpa.org
The ACPA facilitates peer support and education for individuals with chronic pain in its many forms, in order to increase quality of life. Also raises awareness among the healthcare community, and with policy makers.
*Trupti Gokani, MD, President*
*Kathy Sapp, Chief Executive Officer*

762 **American Diabetes Association**
2451 Crystal Drive 888-342-2383
Arlington, VA 22202 askada@diabetes.org
www.diabetes.org
Voluntary organization concerned with diabetes and its complications. The mission of the organization is to prevent and cure diabetes and to improve the lives of persons with diabetes. Offers a network of offices nationwide.
*Charles Henderson, Chief Executive Officer*
*Robert A. Gabbay, MD, PhD, Chief Science & Medical Officer*

763 **American Gastroenterological Association**
4930 Del Ray Avenue 301-654-2055
Bethesda, MD 20814 Fax: 301-654-5920
member@gastro.org
www.gastro.org
AGA fosters the development and application of the science of gastroenterology by providing leadership and aid including patient care, research, teaching, continuing education, scientific communication, and matters of national health policy.
*Tom Serena, CEO*
*Jessica Duncan, VP, Communications*

764 **Arthritis Foundation**
1355 Peachtree St NE 800-283-7800
Atlanta, GA 30309 www.arthritis.org
A council of the Arthritis Foundation devoted to serving the special needs of children, teens and young adults with childhood rheumatic diseases (including systemic lupus erythematosus) and their families. Provides support groups, information, advocacy, research updates, and conferences.
*Steven Taylor, President & CEO*
*Vickie Fung, MPH, Senior Vice President, Mission Delivery*

765 **Arthritis Society Canada**
393 University Avenue 416-979-7228
Toronto, Ontario, M5G-1E6 800-321-1433
Fax: 416-979-8366
info@arthritis.ca
www.arthritis.ca
Promotes, evaluates, and funds research in the areas of causes, prevention, treatment, and cures of arthritis.
*Trish Barbato, President & CEO*
*Sian Bevan, PhD, Chief Science Officer*

766 **Diabetes Action Network for the Blind**
200 East Wells Street 410-659-9314
Baltimore, MD 21230 Fax: 410-685-5653
nfb@nfb.org
www.nfb.org
DAN is a division of the National Federation of the Blind. It is a support and information organization of persons losing vision due to diabetes. Provides personal contact and resource information with other blind diabetics about non-visual techniques of independently managing diabetes and monitoring glucose levels.
*Mark A. Riccobono, President*
*Pam Allen, First Vice President*

767 **Multiple Sclerosis Association of America**
375 Kings Highway North 800-532-7667
Cherry Hill, NJ 08034 Fax: 856-661-9797
MSquestions@mymsaa.org
www.mymsaa.org
A national non-profit organization dedicated to enriching the quality of life for everyone affected by multiple sclerosis.
*Jennifer L. Schwartz, Chair*
*Eric K. Bossard, Vice Chair*

768 **Myositis Association of America**
6950 Columbia Gateway Drive 800-821-7356
Columbia, MD 21046 tma@myositis.org
www.myositis.org
The MMA seeks to improve the lives of individuals affected by myositis, an inflammation of the muscles, through funding research and increasing public awareness.
*Chrissy Thornton, Executive Director*
*Aisha Morrow, Senior Manager, Operations*

769 **National Institute of Arthritis & Musculoskeletal & Skin Diseases**
National Institutes of Health
9000 Rockville Pike 301-495-4484
Bethesda, MD 20892 877-226-4267
Fax: 301-718-6366
TTY: 301-565-2966
NIAMSinfo@mail.nih.gov
www.niams.nih.gov
Supports research into the causes, treatment, and prevention of arthritis and musculoskeletal and skin diseases, the training of basic and clinical scientists to carry out this research, and the dissemination of information on research programs.
*Lindsey A. Criswell, MD, MPH, DSc, Director*

770 **National Institute of Diabetes & Digestive & Kidney Diseases**
31 Center Drive 800-860-8747
Bethesda, MD 20892 TTY: 866-569-1162
healthinfo@niddk.nih.gov
www.niddk.nih.gov
Research areas include diabetes, digestive diseases, endocrine and metabolic diseases, hematologic diseases, kidney disease, liver disease, urologic diseases, as well as matters relating to nutrition and obesity.
*Griffin P. Rodgers, Director*
*Gregory Germino, Deputy Director*

771 **National Institute of Neurological Disorders and Stroke**
P.O. Box 5801 800-352-9424
Bethesda, MD 20824 www.ninds.nih.gov
Seeks to reduce the burden of neurological disease affecting individuals from all walks of life.
*Walter Koroshetz, MD, Director*
*Amy Bany Adams, PhD, Acting Principal Deputy Director*

772 **National Multiple Sclerosis Society**
800-344-4867
www.nationalmssociety.org
The Society helps people affected by MS by funding cutting-edge research, driving change through advocacy, facilitating professional education, and providing programs and services that help people with MS and their families move their lives forward.
*Sylvia Lawry, Founder*
*Cynthia Zagieboylo, President & CEO*

773 **United Ostomy Associations of America, Inc.**
P.O. Box 525 800-826-0826
Kennebunk, ME 04043-0525 www.ostomy.org

A national network for bowel and urinary diversion support groups in the United States. Its goal is to provide a non-profit association that will serve to unify and strengthen its member support groups, which are organized for the benefit of people who have, or will have intestinal or urinary diversions and their caregivers.
*James Murray, President*
*Christine Ryan, Executive Director*

774 **Wound Ostomy and Continence Nurses Society (WOCN)**
1120 Rt. 73 888-224-9626
Mt Laurel, NJ 08054 Fax: 856-439-0525
info@wocn.org
www.wocn.org
Membership comprises nurses that specialize in enterostomal therapy.
*Nicolette Zuecca, MPA, CAE, Chief Staff Officer*
*Anna Shnayder, Chief Operations Officer*

## Alabama

775 **American Diabetes Association: Georgia & Alabama**
P.O. Box 7023 404-320-7100
Merrifield, VA 22116 ADAGA@diabetes.org
www.diabetes.org

776 **National Multiple Sclerosis Society: Alabama-Louisiana-Mississippi**
2200 Woodcrest Place 800-344-4867
Birmingham, AL 35209 www.nationalmssociety.org/Chapters/ALC
*John Bentley, Chair*
*Andy Tunnell, Vice Chair*

## Alaska

777 **American Diabetes Association: Alaska & Washington**
P.O. Box 7023 907-272-1424
Merrifield, VA 22116 ADAAlaska@diabetes.org
www.diabetes.org
*Michelle Cassano, Executive Director*
*Phoebe O'Connell, Manager*

## Arizona

778 **American Diabetes Association: Arizona & New Mexico**
P.O. Box 7023 602-861-4731
Merrifield, VA 22116 adunn@diabetes.org
www.diabetes.org
*Aaron Dunn, Executive Director*
*Nichole Brown, Associate Director, Development*

## Arkansas

779 **American Diabetes Association: Arkansas**
P.O. Box 7023 479-464-4121
Merrifield, VA 22116 ADAAR@diabetes.org
www.diabetes.org

## California

780 **American Diabetes Association: Northern California**
P.O. Box 7023 510-654-4499
Merrifield, VA 22116 ADANoCA@diabetes.org
www.diabetes.org

781 **American Diabetes Association: Southern California & Nevada**
P.O. Box 7023 323-966-2890
Merrifield, VA 22116 ADASOCAL@diabetes.org
www.diabetes.org

782 **National Multiple Sclerosis Society: Southern California**
5150 W. Goldleaf Circle 800-344-4867
Los Angeles, CA 90056 jennifer.wise@nmss.org
www.nationalmssociety.org/Chapters/CAL
*Jennifer Wise, Chapter President*

783 **National Multiple Sclerosis Society: Northern California**
4153 Northgate Blvd. 800-344-4867
Sacramento, CA 95834 can_info@nmss.org
www.nationalmssociety.org/Chapters/CAN
*Linda Glassel, Chapter President*

## Colorado

784 **American Diabetes Association: Rocky Mountain Area**
P.O. Box 7023 720-855-1102
Merrifield, VA 22116 ADARockyMtn@diabetes.org
www.diabetes.org
Serves Colorado, Montana, Utah, and Wyoming.
*Beth Muehlethaler, Executive Director*
*Anna Berry, Development Director*

785 **National Multiple Sclerosis Society: Colorado-Wyoming**
900 S. Broadway 800-344-4867
Denver, CO 80209 robyn.moore@nmss.org
www.nationalmssociety.org/Chapters/COC
*Robyn Moore, Chapter President*

## Connecticut

786 **American Diabetes Association: New England**
P.O. Box 7023 617-482-4580
Merrifield, VA 22116 ADANewEngland@diabetes.org
www.diabetes.org
Serves Massachusetts, New England, Connecticut, Rhode Island, Maine, and Vermont.

787 **National Multiple Sclerosis Society: Connecticut-Rhode Island**
1111 Cromwell Ave. 800-344-4867
Rocky Hill, CT 06067 www.nationalmssociety.org/Chapters/CTN
*Marcia Maslo, Chapter President*

## Delaware

788 **American Diabetes Association: Eastern Pennsylvania & Delaware**
P.O. Box 7023 610-828-5003
Merrifield, VA 22116 ADAEastPA@diabetes.org
www.diabetes.org

789 **National Multiple Sclerosis Society: Greater Delaware Valley**
30 South 17th Street 800-344-4867
Philadelphia, PA 19103 www.nationalmssociety.org/chapters/DED/i
*Kevin Moffitt, Chapter President*

## District of Columbia

790 **American Diabetes Association: DC National Capital Area**
P.O. Box 7023 202-331-8303
Merrifield, VA 22116 ADAWashDC@diabetes.org
www.diabetes.org

791 **National Multiple Sclerosis Society: Greater DC-Maryland**
One M Street S.E. 202-375-5616
Washington, DC 20003 800-344-4867
Chartese.Berry@nmss.org
www.nationalmssociety.org/Chapters/MDM
*Chartese Berry, Chapter President*

## Florida

792 **American Diabetes Association: Florida**
P.O. Box 7023 407-660-1926
Merrifield, VA 22116 ADAFL@diabetes.org
www.diabetes.org

793 **National Multiple Sclerosis Society: Mid-South Florida**
3250 W. Commercial Blvd. 800-344-4867
Fort Lauderdale, FL 33309 Robin.Nunley@nmss.org
www.nationalmssociety.org/Chapters/FLS
*Robin Nunley, Chapter President*

## Georgia

794 **National Multiple Sclerosis Society: Georgia**
950 East Paces Ferry Road 800-344-4867
Atlanta, GA 30326 gaa.mailbox@nmss.org
www.nationalmssociety.org/Chapters/GAA
*Curtis W. Winston, Chapter President*

### Hawaii

795 **American Diabetes Association: Hawaii**
P.O. Box 7023
Merrifield, VA 22116
808-947-5979
ADAHawaii@diabetes.org
www.diabetes.org

796 **National Multiple Sclerosis Society: Pacific South Coast**
10089 Willow Creek Road
San Diego, CA 92131
760-448-8406
800-344-4867
Janet.Hamada@nmss.org
www.nationalmssociety.org/Chapters/CAS
*Janet Hamada-Kelley, Chapter President*

### Idaho

797 **National Multiple Sclerosis Society: Idaho-Nevada-Utah**
P.O. Box 54879
Los Angeles, CA 90054
801-523-4251
800-344-4867
www.nationalmssociety.org/Chapters/UTU
*Melisa Matthews, Chapter President*

### Illinois

798 **American Diabetes Association: Illinois**
P.O. Box 7023
Merrifield, VA 22116
312-346-1805
ADAIL@diabetes.org
www.diabetes.org

799 **National Multiple Sclerosis Society: Greater Illinois**
525 West Monroe Street
Chicago, IL 60661
312-423-1147
800-344-4867
nancy.mcinroy@nmss.org
www.nationalmssociety.org/Chapters/ILD
*Nancy McInroy, Chapter President*

### Indiana

800 **American Diabetes Association: Indiana**
P.O. Box 7023
Merrifield, VA 22116
317-352-9226
ADAIN@diabetes.org
www.diabetes.org

801 **National Multiple Sclerosis Society: Indiana-Kentucky-Tennessee**
214 Overlook Circle
Brentwood, TN 37027
615-690-5355
800-344-4867
david.haddock@nmss.org
www.nationalmssociety.org/Chapters/TNS
*David Haddock, Chapter President*

### Iowa

802 **American Diabetes Association: Iowa, Nebraska & South Dakota**
P.O. Box 7023
Merrifield, VA 22116
317-352-9226
ADAIN@diabetes.org
www.diabetes.org

803 **National Multiple Sclerosis Society: Upper Midwest**
2829 University Avenue SE
Minneapolis, MN 55414
800-344-4867
www.nationalmssociety.org/Chapters/MNM
*Kathleen O'Donnell, Chapter President*

### Kansas

804 **American Diabetes Association: Kansas - Wichita**
P.O. Box 7023
Merrifield, VA 22116
316-684-6091
ADAKS@diabetes.org
www.diabetes.org

805 **National Multiple Sclerosis Society: Mid America**
2020 W 89th Street
Leawood, KS 66206
800-344-4867
Carolyn.Fischer@nmss.org
www.nationalmssociety.org/chapters/KSG
*Carolyn Fischer, Chapter President*

### Louisiana

806 **American Diabetes Association: Louisiana**
P.O. Box 7023
Merrifield, VA 22116
504-889-0278
ADALA_MS@diabetes.org
www.diabetes.org

### Maryland

807 **American Diabetes Association: Maryland**
P.O. Box 7023
Merrifield, VA 22116
410-265-0075
ADAMD@diabetes.org
www.diabetes.org

### Massachusetts

808 **National Multiple Sclerosis Society: Greater New England**
465 Waverly Oaks Rd.
Waltham, MA 02452
800-344-4867
lori.espino@nmss.org
www.nationalmssociety.org
*Lori Espino, Chapter President*

### Michigan

809 **American Diabetes Association: Michigan**
P.O. Box 7023
Merrifield, VA 22116
248-433-3830
ADAMI@diabetes.org
www.diabetes.org

810 **National Multiple Sclerosis Society: Michigan**
29777 Telegraph Road
Southfield, MI 48034
800-344-4867
Tammy.Willis@nmss.org
www.nationalmssociety.org/Chapters/MIG
*Tammy Willis, Chapter President*

### Minnesota

811 **American Diabetes Association: Minnesota & North Dakota**
P.O. Box 7023
Merrifield, VA 22116
763-593-5333
ADAMN_WI_ND@diabetes.org
www.diabetes.org

### Missouri

812 **American Diabetes Association: Missouri**
P.O. Box 7023
Merrifield, VA 22116
317-352-9226
ADAIN@diabetes.org
www.diabetes.org

813 **National Multiple Sclerosis Society: Gateway Area**
10420 Old Olive Street Road
Creve Coeur, MO 63141
800-344-4867
www.nationalmssociety.org/chapters/MOS
*Christie Derbin, Chapter President*

### New Jersey

814 **National Multiple Sclerosis Society: New Jersey Metro Chapter**
1480 U.S. Highway 9 North
Woodbridge, NJ 07095
201-977-6055
800-344-4867
Yasmin.Nielsen@nmss.org
www.nationalmssociety.org/Chapters/NJM
*Yasmin Nielsen, Chapter President*

### New York

815 **American Diabetes Association: New York (Greater NYC and New Jersey)**
P.O. Box 7023
Merrifield, VA 22116
703-549-1500
Kmagnifico-riggio@diabetes.org
www.diabetes.org
*Kristine Riggio, Executive Director*
*Joseph Abrams, Director, Development*

816 **Lupus Alliance of Upstate New York**
732 West Delavan Avenue
Buffalo, NY 14222
800-300-4198
judy@lupusupstateny.org
www.lupusupstateny.org
*Judith Burnett Christian, President & CEO*

817 **National Multiple Sclerosis Society: Greater N.Y. City-Long Island Chapter**
733 Third Avenue
New York, NY 10017
800-344-4867
dana.miele@nmss.org
www.nationalmssociety.org/Chapters/NYN
*Dana Miele, Chapter President*

*North Carolina*

818 **National Multiple Sclerosis Society: Greater Carolinas**
2610 Wycliff Road 714-791-8587
Raleigh, NC 27607 800-344-4867
jennifer.wise@nmss.org
www.nationalmssociety.org/Chapters/NCT
*Jennifer Wise, Chapter President*

*Ohio*

819 **American Diabetes Association: Northeast Ohio**
P.O. Box 7023 216-328-9989
Merrifield, VA 22116 ADAOH@diabetes.org
www.diabetes.org

820 **American Diabetes Association: Southwest Ohio**
P.O. Box 7023 317-352-9226
Merrifield, VA 22116 ADAIN@diabetes.org
www.diabetes.org

821 **National Multiple Sclerosis Society: Ohio**
6133 Rockside Rd. 800-344-4867
Independence, OH 44131 julie.leggett@nmss.org
www.nationalmssociety.org/Chapters/OHA
*Julie Leggett, Chapter President*

*Oklahoma*

822 **American Diabetes Association: Oklahoma**
P.O. Box 7023 918-492-3839
Merrifield, VA 22116 ADAOK@diabetes.org
www.diabetes.org

823 **National Multiple Sclerosis Society: Oklahoma**
1050 N. Post Oak Road 713-394-2976
Houston, TX 77055 800-344-4867
Linda.Bates@nmss.org
www.nationalmssociety.org/chapters/OKE/i
*Linda Bates, Chapter President*

*Oregon*

824 **American Diabetes Association: Oregon & SW Washington**
P.O. Box 7023 503-736-2770
Merrifield, VA 22116 ADAOR_WA@diabetes.org
www.diabetes.org

825 **National Multiple Sclerosis Society: Oregon**
5331 Sw Macadam Ave. 503-445-8342
Portland, OR 97239 800-344-4867
Tracy.leeper@nmss.org
www.nationalmssociety.org/chapters/ORC
*Tracy Leeper, Chapter President*

*Pennsylvania*

826 **American Diabetes Association: Eastern Pennsylvania & Delaware**
P.O. Box 7023 610-828-5003
Merrifield, VA 22116 ADAEastPA@diabetes.org
www.diabetes.org

827 **American Diabetes Association: Western Pennsylvania**
P.O. Box 7023 412-824-1181
Merrifield, VA 22116 ADAWestPA@diabetes.org
www.diabetes.org

828 **National Multiple Sclerosis Society: Pennsylvania**
1501 Reedsdale Street 412-261-6347
Pittsburgh, PA 15233 800-344-4867
anne.mageras@nmss.org
www.nationalmssociety.org/Chapters/PAX
*Anne Mageras, Chapter President*

*South Carolina*

829 **American Diabetes Association: Southern Carolina & Nevada**
P.O. Box 7023 323-966-2890
Merrifield, VA 22116 ADASOCAL@diabetes.org
www.diabetes.org

*Tennessee*

830 **American Diabetes Association: Tennessee**
P.O. Box 7023 317-352-9226
Merrifield, VA 22116 ADAIN@diabetes.org
www.diabetes.org
*Glenda Berry, Executive Director*
*Harlyn Hardin, Director of Programs*

*Texas*

831 **American Diabetes Association: Central South Texas**
P.O. Box 7023 713-977-7706
Merrifield, VA 22116 ADACSTX@diabetes.org
www.diabetes.org

832 **American Diabetes Association: North Texas**
P.O. Box 7023 972-392-1181
Merrifield, VA 22116 ADANTX@diabetes.org
www.diabetes.org

833 **American Diabetes Association: West Texas**
P.O. Box 7023 806-794-0691
Merrifield, VA 22116 ADAWestTX@diabetes.org
www.diabetes.org

834 **National Multiple Sclerosis Society: Texas**
1050 N. Post Oak Road 800-344-4867
Houston, TX 77055 linda.bates@nmss.org
www.nationalmssociety.org/Chapters/TXH
*Linda Bates, Chapter President*

*Virginia*

835 **American Diabetes Association: Virginia/West Virginia**
P.O. Box 7023 757-424-6662
Merrifield, VA 22116 ADAVA_WV_NC@diabetes.org
www.diabetes.org

836 **National Multiple Sclerosis Society: Virginia/West Virginia**
4200 Innslake Drive 804-591-3030
Glen Allen, VA 23060 800-344-4867
sherri.ellis@nmss.org
www.nationalmssociety.org/chapters/VAR
*Sherri Ellis, Chapter President*

*Washington*

837 **National Multiple Sclerosis Society: Greater Northwest**
180 Nickerson St. 206-515-4568
Seattle, WA 98109 800-344-4867
laurie.johnson@nmss.org
www.nationalmssociety.org/Chapters/WAS
*Laurie Johnson, Chapter President*

*Wisconsin*

838 **American Diabetes Association: Wisconsin**
P.O. Box 7023 414-778-5500
Merrifield, VA 22116 ADAWI@diabetes.org
www.diabetes.org

839 **National Multiple Sclerosis Society: Wisconsin**
1120 James Drive 262-369-4428
Hartland, WI 53029 800-344-4867
robert.multerer@nmss.org
www.nationalmssociety.org/Chapters/WIG
*Rob Multerer, Chapter President*

## Foundations

840 **Arthritis Foundation**
1355 Peachtree Street NE 800-283-7800
Atlanta, GA 30309 www.arthritis.org
A non-profit organization that depends on volunteers to provide services to help people with arthritis. Supports research to find ways to cure and prevent arthritis and provides services to improve the quality of life for those affected by arthritis. Provides help through information, referrals, speakers bureaus, forums,

self-help courses, and various support groups and programs nationwide.
*Steven Taylor, President & CEO*
*Vickie Fung, MPH, Senior Vice President, Mission Delivery*

841 **Crohn's & Colitis Foundation**
733 Third Avenue 800-932-2423
New York, NY 10017 info@crohnscolitisfoundation.org
www.crohnscolitisfoundation.org
CCF's mission is to cure and prevent Crohn's disease and ulcerative colitis through research, and to improve the quality of life of children and adults affected by the disease through education and support. The foundation offers patient and professional support.
*Michael Osso, President & CEO*
*Allison Coffrey, Chief Development Officer*

842 **International Foundation for Functional Gastrointestinal Disorders (IFFGD)**
537 Long Point Rd. 414-964-1799
Mount Pleasant, SC 29464 www.iffgd.org
Non-profit education, support, and research organization devoted to increasing awareness and understanding of functional gastrointestinal disorders, including irritable bowel syndrome (IBS), constipation, diarrhea, pain, and incontinence. Mission is to inform, assist, and support people affected by these disorders.
*Nancy J. Norton, Founder*
*Ceciel T. Rooker, President*

843 **Juvenile Diabetes Research Foundation**
International Office
200 Vesey Street 800-533-2873
New York, NY 10281 Fax: 212-785-9595
info@jdrf.org
www.jdrf.org
Focuses energies on fund-raising, referrals, educational materials and information pertaining to juvenile diabetes.
*Aaron J. Kowalski, PhD, Chief Executive Officer*
*Bala Balasubramanian, Chief Information Officer*

844 **Juvenile Diabetes Research Foundation - Canada**
235 Yorkland Blvd. 877-287-3533
Toronto, Ontario, M2J-4Y8 Fax: 416-491-2111
general@jdrf.ca
www.jdrf.ca
*Dave Prowten, President & CEO*
*Sarah Linklater, Chief Scientific Officer*

845 **Lupus Foundation of America**
2121 K Street NW 202-349-1155
Washington, DC 20037 Fax: 202-349-1156
info@lupus.org
www.lupus.org
The nation's leading non-profit voluntary health organization dedicated to finding the causes and cure for lupus.
*Andrew T. Brophy, Board Chair*
*Stevan W. Gibson, President & CEO*

846 **Multiple Sclerosis Foundation**
6520 N Andrews Avenue 954-776-6805
Fort Lauderdale, FL 33309-2132 800-225-6495
Fax: 954-938-8708
admin@msfocus.org
www.msfocus.org
The foundation offers free services including educational programs, homecare, support groups, assistive technology for individuals with MS.
*Natalie Blake, Executive Director*
*Kasey Minnis, Co-Executive Director*

### *Alabama*

847 **Crohn's & Colitis Foundation: Alabama/Northwest Florida Chapter**
P.O. Box 59486 646-387-2149
Birmingham, AL 35259 alabama@crohnscolitisfoundation.org
www.crohnscolitisfoundation.org

### *Arizona*

848 **Crohn's & Colitis Foundation: Arizona Chapter**
P.O. Box 6317 602-734-1392
Mesa, AZ 85216 arizona@crohnscolitisfoundation.org
www.crohnscolitisfoundation.org

849 **JDRF: Desert West Chapter**
4343 E. Camelback Road 602-224-1800
Phoenix, AZ 85018 Fax: 602-224-1801
desertwest@jdrf.org
www.jdrf.org/desertwest/
*Lorry Bottrill, President/Executive Committee*
*Steve Zanella, Co-President/Executive Committee*

850 **Lupus Foundation of America: Arizona Chapter**
2121 K Street NW 202-349-1155
Washington, DC 20037 Fax: 800-558-0121
info@lupus.org
www.lupus.org/az/home-arizona

### *California*

851 **Crohn's & Colitis Foundation: Greater Los Angeles/Orange County Chapter**
10350 Santa Monica Blvd 310-478-4500
Los Angeles, CA 90025 866-831-9157
greaterla-oc@crohnscolitisfoundation.org
www.crohnscolitisfoundation.org

852 **Crohn's & Colitis Foundation: Northern California Chapter**
4104 24th Street 415-356-2232
San Francisco, CA 94114 ncal@crohnscolitisfoundation.org
www.crohnscolitisfoundation.org

853 **JDRF: Northern California Chapter**
1215 4th Avenue 415-977-0360
Seattle, WA 98161 Fax: 415-977-0355
norcal@jdrf.org
www.jdrf.org/norcal/

854 **JDRF: Southern California Chapter**
1391 Warner Avenue 949-553-0363
Tustin, CA 92780 Fax: 949-553-8813
southernca@jdrf.org
www.jdrf.org/southernca/

### *Colorado*

855 **Crohn's & Colitis Foundation: Rocky Mountain Chapter**
1805 S Bellaire St 303-639-9163
Denver, CO 80222 rockymountain@crohnscolitisfoundation.or
www.crohnscolitisfoundation.org
Serves Colorado, Utah and Wyoming.

### *Connecticut*

856 **Crohn's & Colitis Foundation: Connecticut - Westchester Chapter**
3010 Westchester Ave 914-328-2874
Purchase, NY 10577 connecticutwestchester@crohnscolitisfoun
www.crohnscolitisfoundation.org

857 **JDRF: Greater Connecticut and Western Massachusetts Chapter**
20 Batterson Park Road 860-470-0020
Farmington, CT 06032 Fax: 860-674-0880
connecticutwestma@jdrf.org
www.jdrf.org/ctma/

858 **Lupus Foundation of America: Northeast Chapter**
65 High Ridge Road 866-225-0348
Stamford, CT 06905 infone@lupus.org
www.lupus-arkansas.com
*Jamesetta Smith, President*

### *District of Columbia*

859 **Crohn's & Colitis Foundation: DC - Maryland - Virginia Chapter**
2202 18th St NW 646-799-8132
Washington, DC 20009 dmv@crohnscolitisfoundation.org
www.crohnscolitisfoundation.org

860 **JDRF: Mid Atlantic Chapter**
1400 K Street NW 202-371-0044
Washington, DC 20005 Fax: 833-749-0382
midatlantic@jdrf.org
www.jdrf.org/midatlantic/

*Jaclyn Toll Basse, Executive Director*
*Danielle Cohen, Associate Executive Director*

861 **Lupus Foundation of America: DC - Maryland - Virginia Chapter**
2121 K Street NW 202-349-1155
Washington, DC 20037 800-558-0121
info@lupus.org
www.lupus.org/dmv/home-dc-maryland-virgi

## *Florida*

862 **Crohn's & Colitis Foundation: Central & Northeastern Florida Chapter**
P.O. Box 701130 646-203-1214
St Cloud, FL 34770 centralandnorthernfl@crohnscolitisfounda
www.crohnscolitisfoundation.org

863 **Crohn's & Colitis Foundation: Southern Florida Chapter**
21301 Powerline Road 561-218-2929
Boca Raton, FL 33433 florida@crohnscolitisfoundation.org
www.crohnscolitisfoundation.org

864 **JDRF: Northern Florida Chapter**
1850 Lee Road 407-774-2166
Winter Park, FL 32789 Fax: 407-774-2168
northernflorida@jdrf.org
www.jdrf.org/northernflorida/

*Diane Meiller Cook, Executive Council President*
*Tom Warsop, Board President*

865 **JDRF: Southern Florida Chapter**
3369 Pine Ridge Road 239-591-2825
Naples, FL 34109 Fax: 239-591-2833
southernflorida@jdrf.org
www.jdrf.org/southernflorida/

866 **Lupus Foundation of America: Southeast Chapter**
2300 High Ridge Road 561-279-8606
Boynton Beach, FL 33426 infose@lupus.org
www.lupus.org/southeast/

*Judy Barlin, Director, Florida*
*Lynn Blandford, Director, Texas*

## *Georgia*

867 **Crohn's & Colitis Foundation: Georgia Chapter**
2751 Buford Hwy NE 404-982-0616
Atlanta, GA 30324 georgia@crohnscolitisfoundation.org
www.crohnscolitisfoundation.org

868 **JDRF: Georgia and South Carolina Chapter**
3525 Piedmont Road N.E. 404-420-5990
Atlanta, GA 30305 Fax: 404-420-5995
georgiasouthcarolina@jdrf.org
www.jdrf.org/georgiasouthcarolina/

*Sara Orrell, Executive Director, Georgia*
*Kevin Simmons, Market Director, South Carolina*

869 **Lupus Foundation of America: Georgia Chapter**
1850 Lake Park Drive 770-333-5930
Smyrna, GA 30080 Fax: 770-333-5932
info@lfaga.org
www.lupus.org/georgia/

*Teri Emond, President & CEO*
*Consuelo Farley, Operations Manager*

## *Illinois*

870 **Crohn's & Colitis Foundation: Illinois Chapter**
2200 E Devon Ave 847-827-0404
Des Plaines, IL 60018 illinois@crohnscolitisfoundation.org
www.crohnscolitisfoundation.org

871 **JDRF: Illinois Chapter**
1 East Wacker Dr. 312-670-0313
Chicago, IL 60601 Fax: 312-670-0250
illinois@jdrf.org
www.jdrf.org/illinois/

*Laura Dunne, Board President*
*Michael Mayberry, Executive Director*

## *Indiana*

872 **Crohn's & Colitis Foundation: Indiana Chapter**
5325 East 82nd Street 317-259-8071
Indianapolis, IN 46250 800-332-6029
indiana@crohnscolitisfoundation.org
www.crohnscolitisfoundation.org

873 **Diabetes Youth Foundation of Indiana**
5050 East 211th St 317-750-9310
Noblesville, IN 46060-9212 Fax: 317-877-1846
dyfjenna@gmail.com
www.dyfi.org

The Diabetes Youth Foundation of Indiana (DYFI) is a non-profit organization that aims to empower and support children living with Type 1 diabetes, and their families.
*Jenna White, Executive Director*
*Emily Butera, Development Director*

874 **JDRF: Indiana and Kentucky Chapter**
225 S. East St. 317-469-9604
Indianapolis, IN 46202 Fax: 317-469-9607
indianakentucky@jdrf.org
www.jdrf.org/inky/

875 **Lupus Foundation of America: Indiana Chapter**
9302 N. Meridian Street 317-225-4400
Indianapolis, IN 46260 800-948-8806
brian@lupusindiana.org
www.lupus.org/indiana/

*Brian Rothenberg, Chief Executive Officer*
*Chanel Barrett, Director, Operations & Programs*

## *Kansas*

876 **JDRF: Kansas and Missouri Chapter**
215 West Pershing Road 816-472-7997
Kansas City, MO 64108 Fax: 816-472-7617
kansasmissouri@jdrf.org
www.jdrf.org/kansasmissouri/

*Sherri Lozano, MPA, Executive Director*
*Tori Freeman, Development Director*

## *Louisiana*

877 **Louisiana Lupus Foundation**
P.O. Box 1003 225-774-7999
Baker, LA 70741 800-355-7473
www.louisianalupusfoundation.org

A non-profit dedicated to providing information, education and referrals to individuals with Lupus in Louisiana and southwest Mississippi.
*Linda B. Perkins, President*

## *Massachusetts*

878 **Crohn's & Colitis Foundation: New England Chapter**
72 River Park St 781-449-0324
Needham Heights,, MA 02494 ne@crohnscolitisfoundation.org
www.crohnscolitisfoundation.org

Serves Maine, Massachusetts, New Hampshire, Rhode Island, and Vermont

879 **JDRF: Greater New England Chapter**
62 Walnut Street 781-431-0700
Wellesley, MA 02481 833-910-1166
greaternewengland@jdrf.org
www.jdrf.org/greaternewengland/

*Craig Comins, Executive Director*
*Lauren Shields, Associate Executive Director*

### Michigan

880 **Crohn's & Colitis Foundation: Michigan Chapter**
25882 Orchard Lake Rd. 248-737-0900
Farmington Hills, MI 48336 michigan@crohnscolitisfoundation.org
www.crohnscolitisfoundation.org

881 **JDRF: Michigan and Northern Ohio Chapter**
24359 Northwestern Highway 248-355-1133
Southfield, MI 48075 Fax: 248-355-1188
michigannorthernoh@jdrf.org
www.jdrf.org/michigannoh/
*Nikki Borges, Executive Director*
*Krystal Dunlap, Sr. Development Director*

882 **MI Lupus Foundation**
30200 Telegraph Rd. 248-901-7299
Bingham Farms, MI 48025 info@milupus.org
www.milupus.org

### Minnesota

883 **Crohn's & Colitis Foundation: Minnesota - Dakotas Chapter**
2277 Hwy 36 W 651-917-2424
Roseville, MN 55113 minnesota@crohnscolitisfoundation.org
www.crohnscolitisfoundation.org

884 **JDRF: Minnesota and Dakotas Chapter**
3001 Metro Drive 952-851-0770
Bloomington, MN 55425 Fax: 952-851-0766
minnesotadakotas@jdrf.org
www.jdrf.org/minnesotadakotas/
*Erica Rooney, Executive Director*
*Elizabeth Anderson, Associate Executive Director*

885 **JDRF: Mountain West Chapter**
3001 Metro Drive 303-770-2873
Bloomington, MN 55425 Fax: 303-955-1282
mountainwest@jdrf.org
www.jdrf.org/mountainwest/
*Ellen Penrod, Executive Director*
*Mike Somers, Market Director*

### Mississippi

886 **JDRF: Southern States Chapter**
2630 Southerland Street 601-981-1184
Jackson, MS 39216 Fax: 601-981-1280
southernstates@jdrf.org
www.jdrf.org/southernstates/

### Missouri

887 **Crohn's & Colitis Foundation: Mid-America Chapter**
1034 South Brentwood Blvd 314-863-4747
Richmond Heights, MO 63117 800-783-8006
midamerica@crohnscolitisfoundation.org
www.crohnscolitisfoundation.org
Serves Missouri, Kansas, and Arkansas.

888 **Lupus Foundation of America: Heartland Chapter**
8050 Watson, Road 314-644-2222
St. Louis, MO 63119 800-958-7876
info@lfaheartland.org
www.lupus.org
*Amy Ondr, President & CEO*
*Beka Rich, Chief Operating Officer*

### Nebraska

889 **Crohn's & Colitis Foundation: Nebraska - Iowa Chapter**
268 N 115th Street 402-505-9901
Omaha, NE 68154 888-422-3266
ne-ia@crohnscolitisfoundation.org
www.crohnscolitisfoundation.org

890 **JDRF: Nebraska and Iowa Chapter**
9202 West Dodge Road 402-397-2873
Omaha, NE 68114 Fax: 402-397-6509
nebraskaiowa@jdrf.org
www.jdrf.org/nebraskaiowa/
*AnnElise Walsh, Executive Director*
*Chris Dunn, Associate Executive Director*

### New Jersey

891 **Crohn's & Colitis Foundation: New Jersey Chapter**
766 Shrewsbury Avenue 732-786-9960
Tinton Falls, NJ 07724 newjersey@crohnscolitisfoundation.org
www.crohnscolitisfoundation.org

892 **JDRF: New Jersey Metro and Rockland County**
1480 Us Highway 9 North 732-219-6654
Woodbridge, NJ 07095 Fax: 732-219-8722
newjerseymetro@jdrf.org
www.jdrf.org/newjerseymetro/

893 **Lupus Foundation of America: New Jersey Chapter**
65 E. Northfield Road 973-379-3226
Livingston, NJ 07039 800-322-5816
Fax: 973-992-5840
info@lupusnj.org
www.lupus.org/newjersey/node/179

### New York

894 **Crohn's & Colitis Foundation: Greater New York Chapter**
120 Broadway 212-679-1570
New York, NY 10271 newyork@crohnscolitisfoundation.org
www.crohnscolitisfoundation.org

895 **Crohn's & Colitis Foundation: Long Island Chapter**
585 Stewart Avenue 516-222-5530
Garden City, NY 11530 longisland@crohnscolitisfoundation.org
www.crohnscolitisfoundation.org

896 **Crohn's & Colitis Foundation: Upstate Northeastern New York Chapter**
103 Patroon Dr 518-608-5069
Guilderland, NY 12084 upstateny@crohnscolitisfoundation.org
www.crohnscolitisfoundation.org

897 **Crohn's & Colitis Foundation: Western - Cental New York Chapter**
733 Third Ave 585-967-0266
New York, NY 10017 pgeller@crohnscolitisfoundation.org
www.ccfa.org/chapters/rochester

898 **JDRF: Greater New York City Chapter**
200 Vesey Street 212-689-2860
New York, NY 10281 Fax: 212-253-4171
greaternyc@jdrf.org
www.jdrf.org/greaternyc/

899 **JDRF: Upstate New York Chapter**
1757 Central Ave. 518-477-2873
Albany, NY 12205 Fax: 518-477-7004
upstateny@jdrf.org
www.jdrf.org/upstateny/
*Thomas Guagliardo, Executive Director*
*Denise Nicastro, Market Director*

900 **Lupus Foundation of America: Northeast Regional Office**
500 Fashion Avenue 866-225-0348
New York, NY 10018 infone@lupus.org
www.lupus.org/northeast/home-ne
Serves New York, Connecticut, and New England.
*Susan J. Gloor, Senior Region Director*
*Jessica Orr, Development Manager*

### North Carolina

901 **Crohn's & Colitis Foundation: Carolinas Chapter**
8508 Park Road 704-264-0587
Charlotte, NC 28210 carolinas@crohnscolitisfoundation.org
www.crohnscolitisfoundation.org

902 **JDRF: North Carolina Chapter**
205 Regency Executive Park Dr.
Charlotte, NC 28217
704-561-0828
Fax: 704-561-9920
northcarolina@jdrf.org
www.jdrf.org/northcarolina/
*Jamie R. Hayes, CFRE, Executive Director*
*Sally Langan, Associate Executive Director*

903 **Lupus Foundation of America: North Carolina Chapter**
2820 Selwyn Avenue
Charlotte, NC 28209
704-716-5640
info@lupusnc.org
www.lupus.org/northcarolina/node/264

## *Ohio*

904 **Crohn's & Colitis Foundation: North Ohio Chapter**
4700 Rockside Rd
Independence, OH 44131
216-524-7700
northeastohio@crohnscolitisfoundation.or
www.crohnscolitisfoundation.org

905 **Crohn's & Colitis Foundation: South Ohio Chapter**
6797 N. High St.
Worthington, OH 43085
614-889-6060
centralohio@crohnscolitisfoundation.org
www.crohnscolitisfoundation.org

906 **JDRF: Southern and Central Ohio Chapter**
8035 Hosbrook Rd.
Cincinnati, OH 45236
513-793-3223
Fax: 513-936-5333
socentralohio@jdrf.org
www.jdrf.org/socentralohio/
*Cathy Chisholm, Interim Executive Director*
*Kristy Emch-Roby, Market Director*

907 **Lupus Foundation of America: Greater Ohio Chapter**
12930 Chippewa Road
Brecksville, OH 44141
440-717-0183
Fax: 440-717-0186
info@lupusgreaterohio.org
lupusgreaterohio.org
*Suzanne Tierney, CEO & President*
*Leslie Vizcarra, VP, Operations & Lead Patient Navigator*

## *Pennsylvania*

908 **Crohn's & Colitis Foundation: Philadelphia - Delaware Chapter**
2 Bala Plaza
Bala Cynwyd, PA 19004
215-396-9100
philadelphia@crohnscolitisfoundation.org
www.crohnscolitisfoundation.org

909 **Crohn's & Colitis Foundation: Western Pennsylvania/West Virginia Chapter**
6425 Living Place
Pittsburgh, PA 15206
412-823-8272
wpawv@crohnscolitisfoundation.org
www.crohnscolitisfoundation.org
*10-12 pages*

910 **JDRF: Greater Delaware Valley Chapter**
555 Croton Road
King of Prussia, PA 19406
610-664-9255
Fax: 215-559-5684
greaterdelawarevalley@jdrf.org
www.jdrf.org/greaterdelawarevalley/

911 **JDRF: Western and Central Pennsylvania Chapter**
501 Martindale Street
Pittsburgh, PA 15212
412-471-1414
Fax: 412-471-1417
westcentralpa@jdrf.org
www.jdrf.org/westcentralpa/
*Becky Withrow, Executive Director*
*Carling Nolan, Development Director*

912 **Lupus Foundation of America: Philadelphia Tri-State Chapter**
101 Greenwood Avenue
Jenkintown, PA 19046
215-517-5070
866-517-5070
Fax: 215-517-8483
info@lupustristate.org
www.lupus.org/tristate
Serves Delaware, New Jersey and Pennsylvania.
*Cindy Messerle, Chief Executive Officer*
*Adrienne Randall, Program & Communications Manager*

## *Tennessee*

913 **Crohn's & Colitis Foundation: Tennessee Chapter**
P.O. Box 2145
Brentwood, TN 37024
615-356-0444
tennessee@crohnscolitisfoundation.org
www.crohnscolitisfoundation.org

914 **JDRF: Tennessee Chapter**
105 Westpark Drive
Nashville, TN 37027
615-383-6781
Fax: 833-914-0694
tennessee@jdrf.org
www.jdrf.org/tennessee/
*Andi Holbrook, Executive Director*
*Savannah Lee, Development Manager*

## *Texas*

915 **Crohn's & Colitis Foundation: North Texas - Oklahoma Chapter**
12801 N Central Expy
Dallas, TX 75243
972-386-0607
ntexas@crohnscolitisfoundation.org
www.crohnscolitisfoundation.org

916 **JDRF: Northern Texas and Oklahoma Chapter**
8140 Walnut Hill Lane
Dallas, TX 75231
214-373-9808
Fax: 214-373-6337
northtexasoklahoma@jdrf.org
www.jdrf.org/northtexasoklahoma/
*Amy Camp, Executive Director*
*Cati Freeman, Development Manager*

917 **JDRF: Southern Texas Chapter**
1776 Yorktown
Houston, TX 77056
713-334-4400
Fax: 713-334-4040
southerntexas@jdrf.org
ww.jdrf.org/southerntexas/
*Rick Byrd, Executive Director*
*Deandrea Dillard, Associate Executive Director*

918 **Lupus Foundation of America: Lone Star Chapter**
13155 Noel Road
Dallas, TX 75240
972-919-6191
info@lupuslonestar.org
www.lupus.org/lonestar/
*Liz Roth, President & CEO*
*Shawana Black, Programs & Communications Director*

919 **Lupus Foundation of America: Texas Gulf Coast Chapter**
405 Main Street
Houston, TX 77002
713-529-0126
Fax: 713-529-0780
info@LupusTexas.org
www.lupus.org/texasgulfcoast/
*Anne Marie Blacketer, CFRE, CEO*
*Jacinda Bishop, Program Manager*

## *Washington*

920 **Crohn's & Colitis Foundation: Northwest Chapter**
7683 Se 27th St.
Mercer Island, WA 98040
425-451-8455
877-703-6900
northwest@crohnscolitisfoundation.org
www.crohnscolitisfoundation.org
Serves Washington, Oregon, Idaho, Montana, and Alaska.

921 **JDRF: Pacific Northwest Chapter and Seattle Guild**
1215 4th Avenue
Seattle, WA 98161
206-838-5153
Fax: 206-838-5158
pacificnw-sguild@jdrf.org
www.jdrf.org/pacificnwandseattleguild/

922 **Lupus Foundation of America: Pacific Northwest Chapter**
1417 Nw 54th Street
Seattle, WA 98101
425-336-2309
877-774-2992
InfoPNW@lupus.org
www.lupus.org/pacificnorthwest/
*Matt Degooyer, Senior Regional Director, PNW Region*

## *Wisconsin*

923 **Crohn's & Colitis Foundation: Wisconsin**
17100 W Bluemound Rd
Brookfield, WI 53005
414-475-5520
wisconsin@crohnscolitisfoundation.org
www.crohnscolitisfoundation.org

924 **JDRF: Wisconsin Chapter**
1800 Appleton Road
Menasha, WI 54952
920-997-0038
Fax: 833-914-0698
wisconsin@jdrf.org
www.jdrf.org/wisconsin/

925 **Lupus Foundation of America: Wisconsin Chapter**
2600 N Mayfair Road
Milwaukee, WI 53226
414-443-6400
866-587-8794
lupuswi@lupuswi.org
www.lupus.org/wisconsin/
*Dawn T. Thomas-Semanko, President & CEO*
*Angie L. Eakley, Administrative & Content Coordinator*

## Libraries & Resource Centers

926 **Diabetes Control Program**
California Department of Health Services
P.O. Box 997413
Sacramento, CA 95899
916-552-9888
Fax: 916-552-9988
http://www.caldiabetes.org/
Mission is to prevent diabetes and its complications in California's diverse communities.
*Susan Lopez-Payan, Interim Chief*

927 **Division of Diabetes Translation**
National Center for Chronic Disease Prevention
1600 Clifton Rd
Atlantia, GA 30333
800-232-4636
Fax: 770-488-5966
TTY: 888-232-6348
cdcinfo@cdc.gov
www.cdc.gov/diabetes
The Division of Diabetes Translation's (DDT) goal is to reduce the burden of diabetes in the United States. The division works to achieve this goal by combining support for public health-oriented diabetes prevention and control programs (DPCPs) and translating diabetes research findings into widespread clinical and public health practice.

928 **Health Science Library**
Marshall University
1600 Medical Center Drive
Huntington, WV 25701
304-691-1700
www.musom.marshall.edu/library
The Health Sciences Library's primary mission is serving the informational needs of the students, faculty, and staff at Marshall University and the Cabell-Huntington Hospital. The Library also plays an important role in providing information services to hospitals and healthcare professionals in the Huntington and the Tri-State area.
*Edward Dzierzak, Director*

929 **Inflammatory Bowel Disease Program**
www.nm.org
A fully integrated clinical GI program that is part of the Northwestern Medicine Digestive Health Center.

930 **Joslin Center at University of Maryland Medicine**
22 S Greene Street
Baltimore, MD 21201
800-492-5538
TDD: 800735225800
www.umm.edu/joslindiabetes
The Joslin Center at University of Maryland Medicine meets the highest standards of care for people with diabetes. Its programs reflect a philosophy which have been the hallmark of Joslin's care - a comprehensive team approach to diabetes treatment with programs designed to help children and adults with diabetes take charge of their own health and well-being.
*Thomas W Donner, MD, Director*

931 **Naomi Berrie Diabetes Center at Columbia University Medical Center**
Russ Berrie Medical Science Pavillion
1150 St. Nicholas Avenue
New York, NY 10032
212-851-5494
Fax: 212-851-5459
diabetes@columbia.edu
nbdiabetes.org
The special focus of the Naomi Berrie Diabetes Center is on families — a concept that differentiates it from almost every other diabetes treatment facility in America. People with diabetes are strongly encouraged to involve their entire families in the treatment process.
*Robin Goland, MD, Co-Director*
*Rudolph Liebel, Co-Director*

932 **Schulze Diabetes Institute**
University of Minnesota
420 Delaware Street SE
Minneapolis, MN 55455
612-626-3016
diitinfo@umn.edu
www.med.umn.edu
Formerly the Diabetes Institute for Immunology and Transplantation.
*David Sutherland MD, PhD, Director*
*Bernard Hering, Director*

933 **St. Agnes Hospital Medical: Health Science Library**
305 North Street
White Plains, NY 10605
914-681-4500
Fax: 914-328-6408
*Labe C Scheinberg MD, Director*

934 **Tallahassee Memorial Diabetes Center**
Tallahassee Memorial Health Care
1300 Miccosukee Road
Tallahassee, FL 32308
850-431-5404
800-662-4278
Fax: 850-431-6325
www.tmh.org/diabetes
TMH provides comprehensive, patient-centered services to both children and adults. The Diabetes Center uses a team approach that involves the patient, physicians, nurse educators, registered dietitians with access to a diabetes counselor and registered pharmacists and social worker.
*Richard M Bergenstal, MD, Medical Director*

## Research Centers

935 **Affiliated Children's Arthritis Centers of New England**
New England Medical Center
750 Washington Street
Boston, MA 02111
617-636-7285
Fax: 617-350-8388
Research organization comprised of a network of 15 territory pediatric centers throughout New England and based at the Floating Hospital of New England Medical Center.
*Jane G Schaller MD, Coordinator*

936 **Alliance for Lupus Research**
28 W 44th Street
New York, NY 10036
212-218-2840
800-867-1743
info@lupusresearch.org
www.lupusresearch.org
Research foundation dedicated to providing information about lupus.
*Robert Wood Johnson IV, Chairman*
*Ira Akselrad, Director*

937 **Arthritis and Musculoskeletal Center: UAB**
Shelby Interdisciplinary Biomedical Research Bldg
1825 University Boulevard
Birmingham, AL 35294
205-934-0245
Fax: 205-934-1564
rpk@uab.edu
www.main.uab.edu/amc
Arthritis and related rheumatic disorders are studied.
*Robert Kimbe MD, Director*
*Jennifer A Croker, Executive Administrator*

938 **Barbara Davis Center for Childhood Diabetes**
13001 E 17th Place
Aurora, CO 80045
303-724-2323
Fax: 303-724-6839
www.uchsc.edu/misc/diabetes
Research and educational organization.
*Marian Rewers, Clinical Director*
*George S Eisenbarth, Executive Director*

939 **Baylor College of Medicine: Children's General Clinical Research Center**
One Baylor Plaza
Houston, TX 77030
713-798-4780
Fax: 713-790-1345
pedi-webmaster@bcm.edu
www.bcm.edu/pediatrics

Offers research into juvenile aspects of immunology and infectious diseases including diabetes research activities.
*Lisa Bomgaars, Medical Director*
*Mark A Ward, Director*

940 **Benaroya Research Institute**
Virginia Mason Medical Center
1201 9th Avenue 206-583-6525
Seattle, WA 98101 Fax: 206-223-7543
info@benaroyaresearch.org
www.benaroyaresearch.org
Immunology and diabetes research.
*Robert B Lemon, Chair*
*Gerald Nepom, Director*

941 **Boston University Arthritis Center**
580 Harrison Avenue 617-638-4590
Boston, MA 02118 Fax: 617-638-5226
mikyork@bu.edu
www.bumc.bu.edu
The research efforts of the Rheumatology Section relate to basic biologic mechanisms in the pathogenesis of scleroderma vasculitis amyloidosis osteoarthritis and systemic lupus erythematosus. There are concordant research efforts in clinical investigation of these disorders including testing of novel therapies.
*Karen H Antman, Dean*
*Paul Monach, Associate Fellowship Program Director*

942 **Boston University Medical Campus General Clinical Research Center**
72 E Concord Street 617-638-4542
Boston, MA 02118 Fax: 617-638-8890
jkopp@bu.edu
www.ctsi.bu.edu
Integral unit of the University Hospital specializing in arthritis and connective tissue studies.
*Courtney Alpert, Administrative Coordinator*
*Janice Kopp, Executive Director*

943 **Brigham and Women's Hospital: Center for Neurologic Diseases**
LMRC Building
75 Francis Street 617-732-5500
Boston, MA 02115 800-294-9999
TTY: 617-732-6458
www.brighamandwomens.org
Offers research relating to Multiple Sclerosis and other autoimmune diseases.
*Dennis J. Selkoe, Co-Director*
*Howard L. Weiner, Co-Director*

944 **Brigham and Women's Orthopedica and Arthritis Center**
Brigham and Women's Hospital
75 Francis Street 617-732-5500
Boston, MA 02115 800-BWH-9999
TTY: 617-732-6458
www.brighamandwomens.org
Research studies into arthritis and rheumatic diseases.
*Matthew Lian MD, Director*

945 **Center for Neuroimmunology: University of Alabama at Birmingham**
1720 7th Ave S 205-934-0683
Birmingham, AL 35294 Fax: 205-996-4039
www.main.uab.edu/neurology
Evaluate and treat acute and chronic neurological and neuromuscular diseases which are caused by autoimmune mechanisms or linked to presumed abnormalities affecting the immune system.
*Khurram Bashir, Director*

946 **Central Missouri Regional Arthritis Center**
Stephen's College Campus
1205 University Ave 573-882-8097
Columbia, MO 65211 888-702-8818
Fax: 573-884-5509
TDD: 0
marrtc.missouri.edu
Research into arthritis and rheumatic diseases.
*Liz Raine, MPH, CHES, Health Educator*
*Beth Richards, BS, TRS, Director*

947 **Department of Pediatrics, Division of Rheumatology**
Duke University School of Medicine
T909 Children's Health Center 919-684-6575
Durham, NC 27710 Fax: 919-684-6616
rheum.pediatrics.duke.edu
Clinical and laboratory pediatric rheumatoid studies.
*Laura Schanberg MD, Cochairman*
*Egla Rabinovich MD, Co-Chairman*

948 **Diabetes Education and Research Center**
The Franklin House
P.O. Box 897 215-829-3426
Philadelphia, PA 19105 Fax: 215-829-5807
www.diabeteseducationandresearchcenter.o
Is a non-profit organization serving the needs of people living in Philadelphia PA and surrounding communities. The goal of the Foundation is to improve the health of people with diabetes.

949 **Diabetes Research and Training Center: University of Alabama at Birmingham**
Department of Medicine
1530 3rd Avenue S 205-934-4011
Birmingham, AL 35294 Fax: 205-934-4389
TTY: 205-934-4642
www.main.uab.edu
The DRTC works to develop and evaluate new models of diabetes care and to facilitate translational diabetes research.
*Dr Carol Garrison, President*
*William Ferniany, CEO*

950 **Division on Endocrinology**
Northwestern Uni. Feinberg School of Medicine
251 East Huron Street 312-926-6895
Chicago, IL 60611 Fax: 312-503-7757
help@medicine.northwestern.edu
www.medicine.northwestern.edu
Nonprofit organization focusing research activities on endocrinology metabolism nutrition and specializing in diabetes.
*Joe Bass, MD, PhD, Chief of the Division of Endocrinology*
*Grazia Aleppo, MD, Director, Endocrinology Clinical Practic*

951 **Endocrinology Research Laboratory**
Cabrini Medical Center
227 E 19th Street 212-222-7464
New York, NY 10003 www.cabrininy.org
Focuses on the effects of insulin and insulin-like growth factors on human body functions.
*Dr Leonid Poretsky, Director*

952 **Hahnemann University Hospital, Orthopedic Wellness Center**
Hahnemann University Hospital
230 N Broad St 215-762-7000
Philadelphia, PA 19102 Fax: 215-762-8109
www.hahnemannhospital.com
Research activity at Hahnemann University into the areas of arthritis.
*Dr. Arnold Berman, Director*

953 **Hahnemann University Lupus Study Center**
Hahnemann University Medical Center
Broad and Vine Street 215-762-7000
Philadelphia, PA 19102 866-884-4HUH
Fax: 215-762-8109
www.hahnemannhospital.com
*Raphael J Gotthelf, President*

954 **Hahnemann University, Krancer Center for Inflammatory Bowel Disease Research**
230 N Broad St 215-762-7000
Philadelphia, PA 19102 Fax: 215-762-8109
www.hahnemannhospital.com
Research into the causes and treatments of ulcerative colitis and Crohn's disease.
*Dr. Harris Clearfield, Director*

955 **Indiana University: Area Health Education Center**
714 N Senate Avenue 317-278-8893
Indianapolis, IN 46202 Fax: 317-278-0392
ahec@iupui.edu
www.ahec.iupui.edu

A collaborative statewide system for community-based primary health care professions education that fosters the continuing improvement of health care services for all citizens in Indiana.
*Richard D Kiovsky, MD, Director*
*Jonathan C Barclay, Associate Director*

956 **Indiana University: Center for Diabetes Research**
340 West 10th Street 317-274-8157
Indianapolis, IN 46202 Fax: 317-274-1437
rconsidi@iupui.edu
www.medicine.iu.edu
Goal is to promote the training of scientists whose research will develop new understandings of the basis of the disease and its complications and to cultivate basic science research that can speed the discovery of more effective therapies.
*Robert Considine, Associate Professor of Medicine*
*D Craig Brater MD, Dean*

957 **Indiana University: Pharmacology Research Laboratory**
Division of Clinical Pharmacology
1001 W 10th Street 317-630-8795
Indianapolis, IN 46202 Fax: 317-630-8185
www.medicine.iupui.edu/clinpharm
*David A Flockhart, Division Director*
*John T Callaghan, Associate Professor of Medicine*

958 **International Diabetes Center at Nicollet**
3800 Park Nicollet Boulevard 952-993-3393
Saint Louis Park, MN 55416 888-825-6315
Fax: 952-993-1302
idcdiabetes@parknicollet.com
www.parknicollet.com/diabetes
Research center which improves the quality of life of individuals with diabetes and those at risk of developing diabetes by undertaking clinical care, education, research, and outreach activities that stimulate and support health.
*Richard Berg MD, Executive Director*

959 **Jimmie Heuga Center**
27 Main Street 970-926-1290
Edwards, CO 81632 800-367-3101
Fax: 970-926-1295
info@mscando.org
www.mscando.org
Conducts research and studies on multiple sclerosis patients.
*Kim Lennox Sharkey, Chief Executive Officer*
*Carrie Van Beek, Office Coordinator*

960 **Joslin Diabetes Center**
One Joslin Place 617-732-2400
Boston, MA 02215 800-567-5461
Fax: 617-322-40
diabetes@joslin.harvard.edu
www.joslin.org
An internationally recognized leader in diabetes and endocrine disease treatment, research and patient and professional education affiliated with Harvard Medical School. In addition to its headquarters in Boston's Longwood Medical area, Joslin has affiliated treatment centers across the nation. Established in 1898.
*John L Brooks, Chairman of the Board*
*Martin J Abrahamson, Senior VP, Medical Director*

961 **Juvenile Diabetes Research Foundation International**
International Office
200 Vesey Street 800-533-2873
New York, NY 10281 Fax: 212-785-9595
info@jdrf.org
www.jdrf.org
Focuses energies on fund-raising, referrals, educational materials and information pertaining to juvenile diabetes.
*Aaron J. Kowalski, PhD, Chief Executive Officer*
*Bala Balasubramanian, Chief Information Officer*

962 **Medical University of South Carolina: Division of Rheumatology & Immunology**
96 Jonathan Lucas Street 843-792-1991
Charleston, SC 29403 Fax: 843-792-7121
www.musc.edu
Offers basic and clinical research on various types of arthritis.
*Richard M Silver, Division Director/Professor*
*Gary S Gilkeson, Vice Chairman Research*

963 **Metabolic Research Institute**
1515 N Flagler Drive 561-802-3060
West Palm Beach, FL 33401 Fax: 561-802-3260
www.metabolic-institute.com
The Metabolic Research Institute specializes in clinical studies involving endocrinology disorders, complications of endocrinology disorders, metabolic problems and selected renal disease.
*William A Kaye, Co-Director*
*Barry Horowitz, Co-Director*

964 **Multipurpose Arthritis and Musculoskeletal Disease Center**
School of Medicine Rheumatology Division
545 Barnhill Drive 317- 27- 843
Indianapolis, IN 46202 Fax: 317-274-1437
medicine.iupui.edu
The mission of this center is to pursue major biomedical research interests relevant to the rheumatic diseases. Current areas of emphasis include articular cartilage biology, pathogenesis and treatment of various forms of amyloidosis, the pathogenesis of dermatomyositis, and immunologic and biochemical markers of cartilage breakdown and repair.
*Bernetta Hartman, Executive Assistant to the Chairman*
*Martin Friedman, VP Medicine Specialties Division, IUHP*

965 **National Institute of Arthritis & Musculoskeletal & Skin Diseases**
National Institutes of Health
9000 Rockville Pike 301-495-4484
Bethesda, MD 20892 877-226-4267
Fax: 301-718-6366
TTY: 301-565-2966
NIAMSinfo@mail.nih.gov
www.niams.nih.gov
Supports research into the causes, treatment, and prevention of arthritis and musculoskeletal and skin diseases, the training of basic and clinical scientists to carry out this research, and the dissemination of information on research programs.
*Lindsey A. Criswell, MD, MPH, DSc, Director*

966 **Neuromuscular Treatment Center: Univ. of Texas Southwestern Medical Center**
Department of Neurology 214-648-3111
Dallas, TX 75390 www.utsouthwestern.edu
Basic and clinical studies of myasthenia gravis.
*Daniel Podolsky, MD, President*
*Diane Jeffries, Director*

967 **Oklahoma Medical Research Foundation**
825 NE 13th Street 405-271-6673
Oklahoma City, OK 73104 800-522-0211
Fax: 405-271-OMRF
contact@omrf.org
www.omrf.ouhsc.edu
Focuses on arthritis and muscoloskeletal disease research.
*Dr. Paul Kincade, Head of OMRF's Immunobiology*
*Philip M. Silverman, PhD, Member*

968 **Rehabilitation Institute of Chicago**
345 E Superior Street 312-238-1000
Chicago, IL 60611 800-354-7342
TTY: 312-238-1059
www.ric.org
Expertise in treating a range of conditions, from the most complex conditions including cerebral palsy, spinal cord injury, stroke and traumatic brain injury, to the more common, such as arthritis, chronic pain and sports injuries.
*Edward Case, Executive Vice President and Chief Finan*
*Joanne Smith, President and Chief Executive Officer*

969 **Rosalind Russell Medical Research Center for Arthritis at UCSF**
350 Parnassus Avenue 415-476-1141
San Francisco, CA 94117 Fax: 415-476-3526
rrac@medicine.ucsf.edu
www.rosalindrussellcenter.ucsf.edu
Arthritis research and its probable causes.
*Ephraim Engelman, MD, Director*
*David Wofsy, Associate Director*

970 **Rush University Multiple Sclerosis Center**
1653 W. Congress Parkway 312-942-5000
Chicago, IL 60612 888-352-RUSH
TTY: 312-942-2207
complaint@jointcommission.org
www.rush.edu
The Multiple Sclerosis Center combines comprehensive treatment with clinical and laboratory research to provide the highest quality patient care.
*Floyd Davis, Director*

971 **Sansum Diabetes Research Institute**
2219 Bath Street 805-682-7638
Santa Barbara, CA 93105 Fax: 805-682-3332
info@sansum.org
www.sansum.org
A research institute devoted to the prevention, treatment and cure of diabetes.
*Lois Jovanovich, CEO & Chief Scientific Officer*
*Wendy Bevier, Associate Investigator*

972 **Terri Gotthelf Lupus Research Institute**
3 Duke Place 800-828-87
S Norwalk, CT 06854 Fax: 203-852-9720
Founded to help millions of lupus victims in the world and to encourage, coordinate and direct future progress in the etiology, diagnosis and treatment of this disease.

973 **University of Chicago: Comprehensive Diabetes Center**
5841 S Maryland Avenue 773-702-2371
Chicago, IL 60637 800-989-6740
diabetes@uchospitals.edu
www.kovlerdiabetescenter.org
The University of Chicago Kovler Diabetes Center offers a unique. fully comprehensive approach to diagnosing and treating diabetes. Focuses on children, adolescents and adults with diabetes as well as individuals at the highest risk for serious complications.
*Louis H. Philipson, Medical Director*
*Christopher Rhodes, Kovler Diabetes Center Pediatric Program*

974 **University of Colorado: General Clinical Research Center, Pediatric**
13001 E 17th Place 720-777-2957
Aurora, CO 80045 www.uchsc.edu/pedsgcrc
Focuses on developmental studies and diabetes research.
*Ronald J. Sokol, Program Director*
*Philip S. Zeitler, Associate Program Director*

975 **University of Iowa: Diabetes Research Center**
Department of Internal Medicine
200 Hawkins Drive 319-353-7842
Iowa City, IA 52242 www.int-med.uiowa.edu
The Diabetes Research Center combines the talents of experienced clinical investigators, molecular biologists and vascular physiologists in an integrated multidisciplinary approach toward the study and treatment of abnormalities of vascular reactivity which characterize diabetes mellitus.
*Ken Kates, Chief Executive Officer*
*John Swenning, Associate Director*

976 **University of Kansas Cray Diabetes Center**
3901 Rainbow Boulevard 913-588-5000
Kansas City, KS 66160 Fax: 913-588-4023
TTY: 913-588-7963
geaks@kumc.edu
www.kumc.edu
The KU Medical Center is a complex institution whose basic functions include research, education, patient care, and community service involving multiple constituencies at state and national levels.
*Barbara Atkinson, Executive Vice Chancellor*

977 **University of Massachusetts: Diabetes and Endocrinology Research Center**
55 Lake Avenue N 508-856-8989
Worcester, MA 01655 evelyn.vignola@umassmed.edu
www.umassmed.edu
UMMS has exploded onto the national scene as a major center for research, and in the past four decades, UMMS researchers have made pivotal advances in HIV, cancer, diabetes, infectious disease and in understanding the molecular basis of disease.
*Micheal F. Collins, Md, Senior VP*
*Michael P. Czech, Professor & Chair*

978 **University of Miami: Diabetes Research Institute**
200 S Park Road 954-964-4040
Hollywood, FL 33021 800-321-3437
Fax: 954-964-7036
info@drif.org
www.diabetesresearch.org
The Diabetes Research Institute (DRI) is an innovator in many fields of diabetes research but one of its primary strengths lies in islet cell transplantation, a cellular therapy that restores insulin production to normalize blood sugar control.
*Thomas D. Stern, Chairman*
*Camillo Ricordi, DRI Scientific Director*

979 **University of Michigan: Orthopaedic Research Laboratories**
University of Michigan Mott Hospital
109 Zina Pitcher Place 734-936-7417
Ann Arbor, MI 48109 Fax: 734-647-0003
www.orl.med.umich.edu
Develops and studies the causes and treatments for arthritis including new devices and assistive aids.

980 **University of New Mexico General Clinical Research Center**
University of New Mexico Hospital
The University of New Mexico 505-277-0111
Albuquerque, NM 87131 Fax: 505-272-0266
mburge@salud.unm.edu
hsc.unm.edu/som/gcrc
Diabetes research.
*Steve McKernan, CEO*
*Richard Larson, Vice President for Research*

981 **University of Pennsylvania Diabetes and Endocrinology Research Center**
700 Clinical Research Building (CRB 215-898-4365
Philadelphia, PA 19104 Fax: 215-898-5408
www.med.upenn.edu/idom/derc
The Penn Diabetes and Endocrinology Research Center (DERC) participates in the nationwide inter-disciplinary program established over two decades ago by the NIDDK to foster research and training in the areas of diabetes and related endocrine and metabolic disorders.
*Mitchell Lazar, Director*
*Morris Birnbaum, Co Director*

982 **University of Pittsburgh: Department of Molecular Genetics and Biochemistry**
200 Lothrop Street 412-648-9570
Pittsburgh, PA 15261 Fax: 412-624-8997
info@mmg.pitt.edu
www.mgb.pitt.edu
MMG students and fellows routinely publish their research in outstanding journals, present their science at international conferences and go on to achieve positions at prestigious laboratories and institutions.
*J. Richard Chaillet, Associate Professor*
*Bruce A. McClane, Professor*

983 **University of Tennessee: General Clinical Research Center**
1265 Union Avenue 901-516-2212
Memphis, TN 38104 Fax: 901-516-7013
www.utmem.edu/crc
Congress directed the National Institutes of Health to establish clinical research centers throughout the United States to launch an all-out attack on human diseases.
*Bruce S. Alpert, MD, Program Director*

984 **University of Texas General Clinical Research Center**
7400 Merton Minter Boulevard 409-772-1950
San Antonio, TX 78229 Fax: 409-772-8097
public.affairs@utmb.edu
www.utmb.edu/gcrc
Focuses on diabetes and infectious disease research.

985 **University of Washington Diabetes: Endocrinology Research Center**
DVA Puget Sound Health Care System

1660 S Columbian Way
Seattle, WA 98108
206-616-4860
Fax: 206-764-2693
derc@u.washington.edu
www.depts.washington.edu/diabetes
The primary purpose of the DERC is to facilitate and enhance the diabetes-related research of approximately 100 Affiliate Investigators at the University of Washington
*Jerry Palmer, MD, Director*
*David Cummings, Deputy Director*

986 **Vanderbilt University Diabetes Center**
1211 Medical Center Drive
Nashville, TN 37232
615-322-5000
Fax: 615-936-1667
dc.brown@vanderbilt.edu
www.mc.vanderbilt.edu/diabetes/vdc
The Vanderbilt Diabetes Center provides complete care for children and adults with diabetes under one roof
*Joe C. Davis, Chair in Biomedical Sciences*
*Alvin C. Powers, Director Vanderbilt Diabetes Center*

987 **Veterans Affairs Medical Center: Research Service**
500 Foothill Drive
Salt Lake City, UT 84148
801-582-1565
Fax: 801-584-1289
www.va.gov
Diabetes and cancer research.
*James Floyd, Director*
*Byron Bair, Director*

988 **Warren Grant Magnuson Clinical Center**
National Institute of Health
9000 Rockville Pike
Bethesda, MD 20892
301-496-4000
800-411-1222
Fax: 301-480-9793
TTY: 866-411-1010
prpl@mail.cc.nih.gov
clinicalcenter.nih.gov
Established in 1953 as the research hospital of the National Institutes of Health. Designed so that patient care facilities are close to research laboratories so new findings of basic and clinical scientists can be quickly applied to the treatment of patients. Upon referral by physicians, patients are admitted to NIH clinical studies.
*John Gallin, Director*
*David Henderson, Deputy Director for Clinical Care*

989 **Washington University: Diabetes Research and Training Center**
School of Medicine
660 S Euclid Avenue
Saint Louis, MO 63110
314-362-0558
Fax: 314-747-2692
drtc.im.wustl.edu
DRTC investigators were involved in conducting 60 investigator-initiated diabetes-related clinical research protocols on the WU GCRC
*Jean Schaffer, MD, Professor of Medicine*
*Kristin E. Mondy, Medicine/Infectious Diseases*

## Support Groups & Hotlines

990 **Arthritis Foundation Information Helpline**
1355 Peachtree Street NE
Atlanta, GA 30309
800-283-7800
www.arthritis.org
Offers information and referrals, counseling, physicians information and more to persons living with arthritis.
*Ann M. Palmer, President & CEO*

991 **Diabetes Society**
1165 Lincoln Avenue
San Jose, CA 95125
408-287-3785
Fax: 408-287-2701
ckassouf@diabetessociety.org
www.diabetessociety.org
The Diabetes Society was organized in 1963 as the result of efforts by a group of mothers of children with diabetes. Today, the Diabetes Society offers its services to the estimated 140,000 people with diabetes in the Santa Clara Valley.
*Greg Price, Board President*
*Carol Kassouf, CEO*

992 **Kids on the Block Arthritis Programs**
Arthritis Foundation
P.O. Box 19000
Atlanta, GA 31126
404-872-7100
800-283-7800
Fax: 404-872-0457
State and local programs that use puppetry to help children understand what it is like for children and adults who have arthritis.

993 **MS Toll-Free Information Line**
National Multiple Sclerosis Society
733 3rd Avenue
New York, NY 10017
800-344-4867
Offers public and professional information, brochures and referrals to MS patients, their families and health care professionals.

994 **MSWorld**
1943 Morrill Street
Sarasota, FL 34236
415-701-1117
877-710-0302
msworld@msworld.org
www.msworld.org/
MSWorld is for people with multiple sclerosis their families and friends, offer support via chat, e-mail, message boards, magazines.
*Kathleen Wilson, Founder/President*

995 **Multiple Sclerosis Action Group**
National Multiple Sclerosis Society
733 3rd Avenue
New York, NY 10017
409-883-2282
800-344-4867
msag@erasems.com
www.nationalmssociety.org/index.aspx
*Richard J. Mengel, Treasurer*
*Fred J. Lublin, Director*

996 **National Health Information Center**
Office of Disease Prevention & Health Promotion
1101 Wootton Pkwy
Rockville, MD 20852
Fax: 240-453-8281
odphpinfo@hhs.gov
www.health.gov/nhic
Supports public health education by maintaining a calendar of National Health Observances; helps connect consumers and health professionals to organizations that can best answer questions and provide up-to-date contact information from reliable sources; updates on a yearly basis toll-free numbers for health information, Federal health clearinghouses and info centers.
*Don Wright, MD, MPH, Director*

997 **National Multiple Sclerosis Society**
800-344-4867
www.nationalmssociety.org
The Society helps people affected by MS by funding cutting-edge research, driving change through advocacy, facilitating professional education, and providing programs and services that help people with MS and their families move their lives forward.

998 **Traditional Tibetan Healing**
13 Harrison Street
Sommerville, MA 2143
617-666-8635
866-628-6504
Kelob@gte.net
www.tibetanherbalhealing.com/
To rid mankind from chronic illnesses using alternative methods.
*Keyzon Bhutti, Chief Physician*

## Print Resources

999 **Arthritis Today**
Arthritis Foundation
1355 Peachtree St NE
Atlanta, GA 30309
800-283-7800
arthritis.org/arthritis-today-magazine
The authoritative and respected source of information for persons with arthritis, their families and health professionals who manage their care. As the official magazine of the Arthritis Foundation, it is backed by the Foundation's years of experience and leadership in the fight against arthritis. This magazine gives its readers the advice, information and inspiration they need to live better with arthritis.

1000 **Clinical Diabetes**
American Diabetes Association
2451 Crystal Drive
Arlington, VA 22202
diabetesjournals.org/clinical

Provides health professionals responsible for the care of patients with diabetes with recent research, case studies, and education materials.
*Stephen A. Brunton, MD, FAAFP, Editor-in-Chief*

1001 **Diabetes**
American Diabetes Association
2451 Crystal Drive
Arlington, VA 22202
800-342-2383
Fax: 703-549-6995
diabetesjournals.org/diabetes
A peer-reviewed journal focusing on the physiology and pathophysiology of diabetes.
*David A. D'Alessio, MD, Editor-in-Chief*

1002 **Diabetes Care**
American Diabetes Association
2451 Crystal Drive
Arlington, VA 22202
800-342-2383
Fax: 703-549-6995
diabetesjournals.org/care
A peer-reviewed journal emphasizing reviews, commentaries and original research on topics of interest to clinicians.
*Steven E. Kahn, MB, CHB, Editor-in-Chief*

1003 **Diabetes Spectrum**
American Diabetes Association
2451 Crystal Drive
Arlington, VA 22202
800-342-2383
Fax: 703-549-6995
diabetesjournals.org/spectrum
A journal translating research into practice and focusing on diabetes education and counseling.
*Curtis L. Triplitt, PharmD, CDCES, Editor-in-Chief*

1004 **Multiple Sclerosis Journal**
National Multiple Sclerosis Society
733 3rd Avenue
New York, NY 10017
212-986-3240
800-344-4867
Fax: 212-986-7981
journals.sagepub.com/home/msj
A peer-reviewed international journal that publishes research on multiple sclerosis and other related autoimmune diseases.
*64 pages*
*Alan J. Thompson, Editor-in-Chief*
*Jeffrey Cohen, Co-Editor, Americas*

1005 **Phoenix Magazine**
United Ostomy Association of America
P.O. Box 15755
North Hollywood, CA 91615-5755
800-750-9311
publisher@phoenixuoaa.org
phoenixuoaa.org
America's leading ostomy patient magazine providing colostomy, ileostomy, urostomy, and continent diversion information, management techniques, new products, and much more.
*Ian Settlemire, Publisher*

1006 **Voice of the Diabetic**
National Federation of the Blind
1412 I-70 Drive SW
Columbia, MO 65203
673-875-8911
Fax: 573-875-8902
nfb@nfb.org
www.nfb.org
The leading publication in the diabetes field. Each issue addresses the problems and concerns of diabetes, with a special emphasis for those who have lost vision due to diabetes. Available in print and on cassette.
*28 pages*
*Ed Bryant, Editor*

## Web Sites

1007 **American Association of Diabetes Care & Education Specialists**
www.diabeteseducator.org
An independent, multidisciplinary organization of health professionals involved in teaching persons with diabetes. The mission is to enhance the competence of health professionals who teach persons with diabetes and advance the specialty practice of diabetes.

1008 **American Diabetes Association**
www.diabetes.org
Voluntary organization concerned with diabetes and its complications. The mission of the organization is to prevent and cure diabetes and to improve the lives of persons with diabetes. Offers a network of offices nationwide.
*Tracey D. Brown, MBA, BChE, Chief Executive Officer*
*Eloise Scavella, MA, Chief Operating & Strategy Officer*

1009 **American Juvenile Arthritis Organization**
www.arthritis.com
Serves the special needs of young people with arthritis and their families. Provides information, inspiration and advocacy.

1010 **Arthritis Foundation**
www.arthritis.org
Provides services to help through information, referrals, speakers bureaus, forums, self-help courses, and various support groups and programs nationwide.

1011 **Crohn's & Colitis Foundation**
www.crohnscolitisfoundation.org
CCF's mission is to cure and prevent Crohn's disease and ulcerative colitis through research, and to improve the quality of life of children and adults affected by the disease through education and support. The foundation offers patient and professional support.

1012 **Diabetes Exercise**
www.diabetes-exercise.org
Exists to enhance the quality of life for people with diabetes through exercise and physical fitness.

1013 **Healing Well**
www.healingwell.com
An online health resource guide to medical news, chat, information and articles, newsgroups and message boards, books, disease-related web sites, medical directories, and more for patients, friends, and family coping with disabling diseases, disorders, or chronic illnesses.

1014 **Healthlink USA**
www.healthlinkusa.com
Health information concerning treatment, cures, prevention, diagnosis, risk factors, research, support groups, email lists, personal stories and much more. Updated regularly.

1015 **Lupus Foundation of America**
www.lupus.org
The LFA mission is to assist local chapters in their efforts to provide supportive services to individuals living with lupus, educate the public about lupus, and supports research into the cause and cure of lupus.

1016 **MedicineNet**
www.medicinenet.com
An online resource for consumers providing easy-to-read, authoritative medical and health information.

1017 **Medscape**
www.medscape.com
Medscape offers specialists, primary care physicians, and other health professionals the Web's most robust and integrated medical information and educational tools.

1018 **Multiple Sclerosis Foundation**
www.msfocus.org
Dedicated to helping create a brighter tomorrow for those with MS, the foundation offers a wide array of free services including: national toll-free support, educational programs, homecare, support groups, assitive technology, publications, a comprehensive website and more to improve the quality of life for those affected by MS.

1019 **MyHealthfinder**
www.healthfinder.gov
Searchable, carefully developed web site offering information on over 1000 topics. Developed by the US Department of Health and Human Services, the site can be used in both English and Spanish.

1020 **National Arthritis & Musculoskeletal & Skin Diseases Information Clearinghouse**
www.niams.nih.gov
The mission of the National Institute of Arthritis and Musculoskeletal and Skin Diseases is to support research into the

causes, treatment, and prevention of arthritis and musculoskeletal and skin diseases; the training of basic and clinical scientists to carry out this research; and the dissemination of information on research progress in these diseases.

1021 **National Institute of Diabetes & Digestive & Kidney Diseases**

www.niddk.nih.gov

Offers various materials, resources, books, pamphlets. and more for persons and families in the area of diabetes.

1022 **Neurology Channel**

www.healthcommunities.com

Find clearly explained, medically accurate information regarding conditions, including an overview, symptoms, causes, diagnostic procedures and treatment options. On this site it is possible to ask questions and get information from a neurologist and connect to people who have similar health interests.

1023 **United Ostomy Associations of America, Inc.**

www.ostomy.org

A national network for bowel and urinary diversion support groups in the United States. Its goal is to provide a non-profit association that will serve to unify and strengthen its member support groups, which are organized for the benefit of people who have, or will have, intestinal or urinary diversions.

1024 **WebMD**

www.webmd.com

Provides credible information, supportive communities, and in-depth reference material about health subjects. A source for original and timely health information, as well as material from well-known content providers.

# CANCER

*Substance use disorder is complex when any co-morbid condition is present. A co-morbid condition is one that presents simultaneously with another disease; for example, substance use and any type of cancer. Substance use disorder may exist prior to a disease diagnosis or may occur as a result of a diagnosis. A cancer diagnosis may be both emotionally and physically devasting and many types of cancer cause significant pain. An oncology patient may present with a substance use disorder or may develop a substance use disorder during treatment. An active substance use disorder may limit the type of treatment a cancer patient may receive.*

Certain agents that may be classified within a substance use disorder may cause cancer. A substance use disorder may develop in an attempt to escape the emotional effects of the diagnosis. Rarely does a substance use disorder develop during pain treatment as a part of cancer therapy when pain is managed correctly.

Carcinogenic agents are substances capable of causing cancer. For example, smoking is known to contribute to 80 percent of lung cancer, according to the American Cancer Society. Alcohol consumption has been linked to oral, liver and colon cancer. Illicit drugs such as cocaine and heroin may be laced with cancer-causing cutting agents. Carcinogens may cause cancer due to changes in metabolism, by acting with another chemical, or as a direct acting carcinogen that causes cancer as-is.

Substance use disorder may occur as a result of a cancer diagnosis. The diagnosis of cancer is a life-altering situation leading to stress, anger, fear and a host of emotions. In an attempt to deal with the disease, individuals may self-medicate using legal or illegal means. Prescription drug abuse using drugs prescribed for other reasons or other people, or purchasing illicit drugs on the street, may occur.

Cancer pain can be caused by the cancer, tests, surgery and treatments. Pain can impact all parts of the cancer patient's life. While cancer pain can be controlled, keeping it from starting and preventing it from getting worse is the goal. If the cancer patient takes the medications as prescribed by the doctor, addiction rarely occurs. A written pain management protocol is often provided by the cancer care team. If not, the following questions should be asked of the cancer care team:

- How much medication should I take, and how often? Review the prescription with the doctor and nurse to be sure the dosage and timing is well-understood.
- If the amount prescribed is not helping my pain, should I call the doctor before taking more? The answer is yes.
- If I skip a dose or forget to take a dose of pain medication, the physician will likely tell the patient to take the dose and restart the timing. For example, if the dosing is every four hours and you go eight hours by accident, just restart the dosing and count four hours before the next dose. Contact the physician with any questions.
- Is it safe to drive or operate machinery? This should be discussed with the doctor, but if any drowsiness or clumsiness, for example, is a side effect, most likely it is not safe to drive or operate machinery.
- Are there other medicines I can take with the pain medicine, or are there medications I should stop taking? This is a decision between the physician and patient.

- How do I manage side effects?

Cancer pain management is a vital part of cancer therapy. Taking drugs for cancer pain does not cause euphoria or a high, as the body interprets the drug as needed. The pain associated with cancer often requires significant pain medications including opioids, a highly addictive medication. As the pain increases, some drug doses are significantly higher than normal, as the type of pain requires aggressive management. Conversely as, for example, a tumor shrinks and pain lessens, the dose may be adjusted downward.

The individual should be educated continually about ongoing pain management. For example, using medication to control pain and not to escape the emotions of the disease. One of the significant issues in cancer pain management is that often family want the doctor to reduce dosages to prevent the patient from becoming addicted to pain medications. There is no way to describe how severe cancer pain can be. Using a scale of 1, being no pain, to 10 being worst possible pain, most cancer patients with severe pain say its way beyond 10. Educating family to the fact that dosing is pain-dependent is important. If pain is not managed appropriately, the patient may seek additional drugs to help manage the pain without the doctor or family's knowledge, leading to a true addiction and interfering with response to cancer therapy.

With a terminal patient at end of life, pain medication doses may be well outside the normal range of prescription recommendations. An oncologist or pain management physician knowledgeable about cancer pain should decide what is in the best interest of the patient. At the end of life, addiction should not be a worry. The worry is whether the last few days of a patient's life are comfortable and of the best quality possible. Family should understand that near death, addiction is not an issue.

## Agencies & Associations

1025 **American Cancer Society**
3380 Chastain Meadows Pkwy NW 800-227-2345
Kennesaw, GA 30144 www.cancer.org
A nationwide community-based voluntary health organization dedicated to eliminating cancer as a major health problem by preventing, saving lives, and diminishing suffering through research, education, advocacy, and services. Provides free printed materials.
*Karen E. Knudsen, MBA, PhD, Chief Executive Officer*
*Andre Bokhoor, Chief People Officer*

1026 **American Childhood Cancer Organization**
P.O. Box 498 240-965-5581
Kensington, MD 20895-0498 855-858-2226
Fax: 301-962-3521
rhoffman@acco.org
www.acco.org
Founded by parents of children with cancer. The ACCO helps families of pediatric and adolescent cancer patients cope with the educational and emotional needs of the disease. The organization is the largest distributor of free childhood cancer books and other materials.
*Ken Wegner, President*
*Ruth I. Hoffman, MPH, CEO*

1027 **American Chronic Pain Association**
11936 W. 119th Street ACPA@theacpa.org
Rocklin, CA 95677 www.theacpa.org
The ACPA facilitates peer support and education for individuals with chronic pain in its many forms, in order to increase quality of life. Also raises awareness among the healthcare community, and with policy makers.
*Trupti Gokani, MD, President*
*Kathy Sapp, Chief Executive Officer*

1028 **American Institute for Cancer Research**
P.O. Box 97167 800-843-8114
Washington, DC 20090 Fax: 202-328-7226
www.aicr.org
Not-for-profit research and educational organization. Provides grants for research into the causes, development, prevention and treatment of cancer through diet and nutrition. Offers publications, research results, conferences and various public services.

1029 **American Society of Colon and Rectal Surgeons (ASCRS)**
2515 Waukegan Road 847-607-6410
Bannockburn, IL 60015 ascrs@fascrs.org
www.fascrs.org
ASCRS represents colon and rectal surgeons dedicated to advancing and promoting the science and practice of the treatment of patients with cancer, and other diseases affecting the colon and related areas.
*Elizabeth Collens Wick, MD, President*
*Larissa K. F. Temple, MD, Vice President*

1030 **Americas Association for the Care of the Children**
P.O. Box 2154 303-527-2742
Boulder, CO 80306 aacchildren.org
Carries out a variety of programs to promote the health of children. Publishes educational materials on child health of interest to parents, educators and health professionals.
*Deborah Young, Executive Director & Founder*
*Judi Jackson, President*

1031 **Breast Cancer Action (BCAction)**
548 Market Street 415-243-9301
San Francisco, CA 94104-5401 info@bcaction.org
www.bcaction.org
BCAction seeks health justice for all individuals at risk of and living with breast cancer. Focuses on systematic interventions that will produce broad public health benefits.
*Krystal Redman, Executive Director*
*Zoe Christopher, Program Officer & Operations Manager*

1032 **Canadian Breast Cancer Network (CBCN)**
185 Somerset St. West 613-230-3044
Ottawa, Ontario, K2P-0J2 800-685-8820
Fax: 613-230-4424
cbcn@cbcn.ca
www.cbcn.ca
Survivor-directed, national network of organizations and individuals concerned about breast cancer, representing the concerns of all Canadians affected by breast cancer, and those at risk.
*Jenn Gordon, Director, Operations*
*Niya Chari, Director, Public Affairs & Health Policy*

1033 **Cancer Control Society**
P.O. Box 4651 323-663-7801
Modesto, CA 95352-4651 cancercontrol@att.net
www.cancercontrolsociety.com
An informational organization offering books, films, videos, clinic tours and lists of patients with cancer.
*Lorraine Rosenthal, Co-Founder*
*Frank Cousineau, President*

1034 **CancerCare**
275 7th Avenue 212-712-8400
New York, NY 10001 800-813-4673
Fax: 212-712-8495
info@cancercare.org
www.cancercare.org
National non-profit organization that provides free, professional support services for anyone affected by a cancer diagnosis.
*Patricia J. Goldsmith, Chief Executive Officer*
*Christine Verini, RPh, Chief Operating Officer*

1035 **Center for Science in the Public Interest**
1220 L Street N.W. 866-293-2774
Washington, DC 20005 cspi@cspinet.org
www.cspinet.org
The nation's leading consumer group concerned with food and nutrition issues. Focuses on diseases that result from consuming too many calories, too much fat, sodium and sugar such as cancer and heart disease.
*Peter Lurie, MD, MPH, President & Executive Director*
*Jeff Cronin, Director of Communications*

1036 **Colorectal Cancer Canada**
1350 Sherbrooke Street West 416-785-0449
Montreal, Quebec, H3G-1J1 877-502-6566
info@colorectalcancercanada.com
www.coloncancercanada.ca
Seeks to raise public awareness of colorectal cancer, while supporting and advocating for patients. The Colorectal Cancer Association of Canada and Colon Cancer Canada amalgamated in 2017.
*Barry D. Stein, President*
*Bunnie Schwartz, Co-Founder*

1037 **International Association of Laryngectomees**
925B Peachtree Street NE 866-425-3678
Atlanta, GA 30309 office@theial.com
www.theial.com
Consists of local clubs worldwide that provide services and information to patients who have undergone laryngectomies, and their families. Members are given information on first aid, postoperative care, rehabilitation, esophageal speech and other speech alternatives. Directories of speech instructors and self-care supplies for the surgical site are distributed.
*Kyd Dieterich, President*
*Jennifer Malkiewicz, Vice President & Treasurer*

1038 **Leukemia and Lymphoma Society**
3 International Drive 888-557-7177
Rye Brook, NY 10573 www.lls.org
Dedicated to funding blood cancer research, education, and patient services.
*Louis J. DeGennaro, PhD, President & CEO*
*Troy Dunmire, EVP & Chief Operating Officer*

1039 **National Cancer Institute**
9000 Rockville Pike Drive 800-422-6237
Bethesda, MD 20892 nciinfo@nih.gov
www.cancer.gov

Offers educational information, public awareness, research grants, and more for patients, their families, and health care professionals. Information specialists answer cancer-related questions by phone, LiveHelp instant messaging, and e-mail.
*Monica Bertagnolli, M.D, Director*
*Douglas R. Lowy, M.D., Principal Deputy Director*

**1040 National Children's Cancer Society (NCCS)**
500 North Broadway 312-241-1600
St. Louis, MO 63102 800-532-6459
Fax: 314-241-1996
thenccs.org
NCSS seeks to improve the quality of life for children with cancer and their families worldwide by providing financial, emotional, educational, and medical assistance, at every stage of their illness and recovery.
*Mark Stolze, President & CEO*
*Jessica Cook, VP, Patient & Family Services*

**1041 National Coalition for Cancer Survivorship**
8455 Colesville Road 877-622-7937
Silver Spring, MD 20910 Fax: 301-565-9670
info@canceradvocacy.org
www.canceradvocacy.org
Survivor-led advocacy organization working exclusively on behalf of people with all types of cancer and their families. Dedicated to assuring quality and care for all Americans.
*Shelley Fuld Nasso, MPP, Chief Executive Officer*
*Woulita Seyoum, Senior Director, Finance & Operations*

**1042 National Health Federation**
P.O. Box 288 626-357-2181
Monrovia, CA 91017 360-325-8692
contact-us@thenhf.com
www.thenhf.com
A nonprofit, consumer-oriented organization devoted to health matters. Dedicated to preserving freedom of choice in health care issues, prevention of diseases and the promotion of wellness.
*Scott C. Tips, JD, President*
*Gregory Kunin, Vice President*

**1043 National Hospice & Palliative Care Organization (NHPCO)**
1731 King Street 703-837-1500
Alexandria, VA 22314 Fax: 703-837-1233
www.nhpco.org
This organization seeks to improve end-of-life care, widen access to hospice care, and improve quality of life for the dying and their loved ones.
*Cathy L. Gibney, CPA, Chief Financial Officer*
*Ben Marcantonio, MS, MEd, COO & Interim CEO*

**1044 National Institute on Aging**
P.O. Box 8057 800-222-2225
Gaithersburg, MD 20898 niaic@nia.nih.gov
www.nia.nih.gov
Seeks to understand the nature of aging, and to extend healthy, active years of life. Free resources are available on topics such as Alzheimer's & dimentia, caregiving, cognitive heath, end of life care, and more.
*Richard J. Hodes, M.D., Director*
*Amy Kelley, M.D., M.S.H.S., Deputy Director*

**1045 National Kidney and Urologic Diseases Information Clearinghouse**
31 Center Drive 800-860-8747
Bethesda, MD 20892 TTY: 866-569-1162
healthinfo@niddk.nih.gov
www.niddk.nih.gov
A service of the Federal Government's National Institute for Diabetes and Digestive and Kidney Diseases. Offers free information about benign prostate enlargement and other non-cancerous urinary tract problems.
*Griffin P. Rodgers, Director*
*Gregory Germino, Deputy Director*

**1046 National Marrow Donor Program**
500 N 5th Street 800-627-7692
Minneapolis, MN 55401-1206 patientinfo@nmdp.org
bethematch.org
Created to improve the effectiveness of the search for bone marrow donors so that a greater number of bone marrow transplants can be carried out. Operates the Be The Match marrow registry.
*Amy L. Ronneberg, Chief Executive Officer*
*Jeffery Auletta, MD, Senior Vice President, Patient Outcomes*

**1047 National Ovarian Cancer Coalition**
12221 Merit Drive 214-273-4200
Dallas, TX 75251 888-682-7426
nocc@ovarian.org
www.ovarian.org
Aims to raise awareness about ovarian cancer and to promote education about the disease, while dispelling myths and misunderstandings. The coalition is committed to improving the overall survival rate and quality of life for women with ovarian cancer.
*Melissa Aucoin, Chief Executive Officer*
*Sara Harris, Secretary*

**1048 People Against Cancer**
1212 Nelson Ave. 515-972-4444
Otho, IA 50569 Info@PeopleAgainstCancer.org
www.peopleagainstcancer.com
A nonprofit grassroots organization whose mission is to find the best cancer therapy for people with cancer worldwide.
*Frank D. Wiewel, Founder*

**1049 Rethink Breast Cancer**
50 Carroll Street 416-220-0700
Toronto, Ontario, M4M-3G3 hello@rethinkbreastcancer.com
www.rethinkbreastcancer.com
A charity helping young people who are concerned about and affected by breast cancer through innovative breast cancer education, research and support programs.
*M.J. DeCoteau, Founder & Executive Director*

**1050 Support for People with Oral and Head and Neck Cancer (SPOHNC)**
P.O. Box 53 800-377-0928
Locust Valley, NY 11560-0053 info@spohnc.org
www.spohnc.org
Non-profit organization addressing the broad emotional, physical, and humanistic needs of oral and head and neck cancer patients.
*James Sciubba, DMD, PhD, President*
*Mary Ann Caputo, Executive Director*

### *Alabama*

**1051 American Cancer Society: Alabama**
P.O. Box 131433 800-227-2345
Birmingham, AL 35213 www.cancer.org

### *Alaska*

**1052 American Cancer Society: Alaska**
P.O. Box 230148 800-227-2345
Anchorage, AK 99523 www.cancer.org

### *Arizona*

**1053 American Cancer Society: Arizona**
P.O. Box 81409 800-227-2345
Phoenix, AZ 85069 www.cancer.org

### *Arkansas*

**1054 American Cancer Society: Arkansas**
P.O. Box 16328 800-227-2345
Little Rock, AR 72231 www.cancer.org

### *California*

**1055 American Cancer Society: California**
P.O. Box 111417 800-227-2345
Campbell, CA 95011 www.cancer.org

### *Colorado*

**1056 American Cancer Society: Colorado**
P.O. Box 370207 800-227-2345
Denver, CO 80237 www.cancer.org

*Connecticut*

1057 **American Cancer Society: Connecticut**
P.O. Box 280285 800-227-2345
East Hartford, CT 06128 www.cancer.org

*Delaware*

1058 **American Cancer Society: Delaware**
P.O. Box 669 800-227-2345
New Castle, DE 19720 www.cancer.org

*District of Columbia*

1059 **American Cancer Society: District of Columbia**
P.O. Box 18090 800-227-2345
Middle River, MD 21220 www.cancer.org

*Florida*

1060 **American Cancer Society: Florida**
P.O. Box 17127 800-227-2345
Tampa, FL 33682 www.cancer.org

*Georgia*

1061 **American Cancer Society: Georgia**
P.O. Box 1685 800-227-2345
Atlanta, GA 30303 www.cancer.org

*Hawaii*

1062 **American Cancer Society: Hawaii**
P.O. Box 11689 800-227-2345
Honolulu, HI 96828 www.cancer.org

*Idaho*

1063 **American Cancer Society: Idaho**
P.O. Box 8449 800-227-2345
Boise, ID 83707 www.cancer.org

*Illinois*

1064 **American Cancer Society: Illinois**
P.O. Box 10393 800-227-2345
Chicago, IL 60610 www.cancer.org

*Indiana*

1065 **American Cancer Society: Indiana**
P.O. Box 681405 800-227-2345
Indianapolis, IN 46268 www.cancer.org

*Iowa*

1066 **American Cancer Society: Iowa**
P.O. Box 715 800-227-2345
Des Moines, IA 50303 www.cancer.org

*Kansas*

1067 **American Cancer Society: Kansas**
P.O. Box 171335 800-227-2345
Kansas City, KS 66117 www.cancer.org

*Kentucky*

1068 **American Cancer Society: Kentucky**
P.O. Box 2167 800-227-2345
Lexington, KY 40588 www.cancer.org

*Louisiana*

1069 **American Cancer Society: Louisiana**
P.O. Box 83930 800-227-2345
Baton Rouge, LA 70884 www.cancer.org

*Maine*

1070 **American Cancer Society: Maine**
P.O. Box 350 800-227-2345
Westbrook, ME 04092-3438 www.cancer.org

*Maryland*

1071 **American Cancer Society: Maryland**
P.O. Box 18090 800-227-2345
Baltimore, MD 21220 www.cancer.org

*Massachusetts*

1072 **American Cancer Society: Massachusetts**
P.O. Box 1120 800-227-2345
Framingham, MA 01701 www.cancer.org

*Michigan*

1073 **American Cancer Society: Michigan**
P.O. Box 10069 800-227-2345
Detroit, MI 48210 www.cancer.org

*Minnesota*

1074 **American Cancer Society: Minnesota**
P.O. Box 21600 800-227-2345
Eagan, MN 55121 www.cancer.org

*Mississippi*

1075 **American Cancer Society: Mississippi**
P.O. Box 4449 800-227-2345
Brandon, MS 39047 www.cancer.org

*Missouri*

1076 **American Cancer Society: Missouri**
P.O. Box 171335 800-227-2345
Kansas City, KS 66117 www.cancer.org

*Montana*

1077 **American Cancer Society: Montana**
P.O. Box 20893 800-227-2345
Millings, MT 59104 www.cancer.org

*Nebraska*

1078 **American Cancer Society: Nebraska**
P.O. Box 24168 800-227-2345
Omaha, NE 68124 www.cancer.org

*Nevada*

1079 **American Cancer Society: Nevada**
P.O. Box 231359 800-227-2345
Las Vegas, NV 89105 www.cancer.org

*New Hampshire*

1080 **American Cancer Society: New Hampshire**
P.O. Box 10538 800-227-2345
Bedford, NH 03110 www.cancer.org

*New Jersey*

1081 **American Cancer Society: New Jersey**
P.O. Box P. 800-227-2345
Manasquan, NJ 08736 www.cancer.org

*New Mexico*

1082 **American Cancer Society: New Mexico**
P.O. Box 36240 800-227-2345
Albuquerque, NM 87179 www.cancer.org

### New York

1083 **American Cancer Society: New York**
P.O. Box 1357 800-227-2345
New York, NY 10018 www.cancer.org

### North Carolina

1084 **American Cancer Society: North Carolina**
P.O. Box 11796 800-227-2345
Charlotte, NC 28220 www.cancer.org

### North Dakota

1085 **American Cancer Society: North Dakota**
P.O. Box 7519 800-227-2345
Fargo, ND 58106 www.cancer.org

### Ohio

1086 **American Cancer Society: Ohio**
P.O. Box 1981 800-227-2345
Cleveland, OH 44106 www.cancer.org

### Oklahoma

1087 **American Cancer Society: Oklahoma**
P.O. Box 22958 800-227-2345
Oklahoma City, OK 73123 www.cancer.org

### Oregon

1088 **American Cancer Society: Oregon**
P.O. Box 22770 800-227-2345
Portland, OR 97269 www.cancer.org

### Pennsylvania

1089 **American Cancer Society: Pennsylvania**
P.O. Box 30386 800-227-2345
Philadelphia, PA 19103 www.cancer.org

### Rhode Island

1090 **American Cancer Society: Rhode Island**
P.O. Box 7312 800-227-2345
Warwick, RI 02886 www.cancer.org

### South Carolina

1091 **American Cancer Society: South Carolina**
P.O. Box 11796 800-227-2345
Charlotte, NC 28220 www.cancer.org

### South Dakota

1092 **American Cancer Society: South Dakota**
P.O. Box 1146 800-227-2345
Sioux Falls, SD 57101 www.cancer.org

### Tennessee

1093 **American Cancer Society: Tennessee**
P.O. Box 771557 800-227-2345
Memphis, TN 38177 www.cancer.org

### Texas

1094 **American Cancer Society: Texas**
P.O. Box 632008 800-227-2345
Houston, TX 77263 www.cancer.org

### Utah

1095 **American Cancer Society: Utah**
P.O. Box 16440 800-227-2345
Salt Lake City, UT 84116 www.cancer.org

### Vermont

1096 **American Cancer Society: Vermont**
P.O. Box 1070 800-227-2345
Williston, VT 05495 www.cancer.org

### Virginia

1097 **American Cancer Society: Virginia**
P.O. Box 4110 804-613-3575
Glen Allen, VA 23058 www.cancer.org

### Washington

1098 **American Cancer Society: Washington**
P.O. Box 3682 800-227-2345
Seattle, WA 98124 www.cancer.org

### Wisconsin

1099 **American Cancer Society: Wisconsin**
P.O. Box 902 800-227-2345
Pewaukee, WI 53072 www.cancer.org

### Wyoming

1100 **American Cancer Society: Wyoming**
P.O. Box 1446 800-227-2345
Casper, WY 82602 www.cancer.org

## Foundations

1101 **Bone Marrow & Cancer Foundation**
515 Madison Avenue 212-838-3029
New York, NY 10022 800-365-1336
Fax: 212-223-0081
bmcf@bonemarrow.org
bonemarrow.org
Goal is to improve the quality of life for bone marrow and stem cell transplant patients, and their families, by providing financial aid, education, and emotional support.
*Christina Merrill, President & CEO*
*Robert Fishman, Chair*

1102 **Breast Cancer Resource Foundation of Alabama**
P.O. Box 531225 205-996-5463
Birmingham, AL 35253 BCRFA@uab.edu
www.bcrfa.org
Partners with Alabamians to fundraise for breast cancer research.
*Beth Davis, President & CEO*
*Wright Wiggins Rouse, Marketing & Communications Director*

1103 **Breast Cancer Society of Canada**
101-415 Exmouth Street 800-567-8767
Sarnia, Ontario, N7T-8A4 Fax: 519-336-5725
hello@breastcancerprogress.ca
www.breastcancerprogress.ca
Funds research into improving detection, prevention, and treatment of breast cancer, as well as to find a cure, and creates awareness through education.
*Kimberly Carson, CEO*
*Dr. Marc Webster, Chair, Scientific Advisory Committee*

1104 **Canadian Cancer Society**
55 St. Clair Avenue W. 888-939-3333
Toronto, Ontario, M4V-2Y7 TTY: 866-786-3934
info@cancer.ca
www.cancer.ca
A national community-based organization of volunteers whose mission is the eradication of cancer and the enhancement of the quality of life of people living with cancer.
*Patricia J. Goldsmith, Chief Executive Officer*
*Christine Verini, RPH, EVP/Chief Operating Officer*

1105 **Chemotherapy Foundation**
176 East 77th Street 212-213-9292
New York, NY 10075 Fax: 212-133-31
info@chemotherapyfoundation.org
www.chemotherapyfoundation.com

The Chemotherapy Foundation is dedicated to developing more effective methods of treatment for the control and cure of cancer. They provide educational materials and provide funds for innovative chemotherapy research, and sponsor professional and public educational symposia.
*Paola G. Muggia, Executive Director*

1106 **Childhood Cancer Canada**
20 Queen Street W. 416-489-6440
Toronto, Ontario, M5H-3R3 800-363-1062
Fax: 416-489-9812
info@childhoodcancer.ca
www.childhoodcancer.ca
Invests in national, collaborative research into childhood cancer, as well as supporting education and community programs.
*Sandi Hancox, Executive Director*
*Asha Lewis-Isaacs, Development Officer*

1107 **Dermatology Foundation**
1560 Sherman Avenue 847-328-2256
Evanston, IL 60201-4806 Fax: 847-328-0509
dfgen@dermatologyfoundation.org
dermatologyfoundation.org
The Foundation focuses on funding research that will advance dermatologic research, investing over $80 million in donations.
*Janet A. Fairley, MD, President*
*John E. Bournas, MA, MBA, Executive Director*

1108 **National Foundation for Cancer Research**
5515 Security Lane 800-321-2873
Rockville, MD 20852 info@nfcr.org
www.nfcr.org
Contracts with major universities for basic science cancer research in the fields of biophysics, theoretical physics, and biochemistry.
*Sujuan Ba, PhD, President & CEO*
*Brian Wachtel, Executive Director*

1109 **Prostate Cancer Foundation**
1250 Fourth Street 310-570-4700
Santa Monica, CA 90401 800-757-2873
Fax: 310-570-4701
info@pcf.org
www.pcf.org
Seeks to find better treatments and a cure for recurrent prostate cancer by reaching out to individuals, corporations, and others, to harness financial and human resources.
*Michael Milken, Founder & Chair*
*Charles J. Ryan, MD, President & CEO*

1110 **Skin Cancer Foundation**
205 Lexington Avenue 212-725-5176
New York, NY 10016 www.skincancer.org
Conducts public and medical education programs to help reduce skin cancer. Major goals are to increase public awareness of the importance of taking protective measures against the damaging rays of the sun and to teach people how to recognize the early signs.
*Deborah S. Sarnoff, MD, President*
*Dan Latore, Executive Director*

## Libraries & Resource Centers

1111 **Cancer Control Society**
P.O. Box 4651 323-663-7801
Modesto, CA 95352-4651 cancercontrol@att.net
www.cancercontrolsociety.com
An informational organization offering books, films, videos, clinic tours and lists for patients with cancer.
*Lorraine Rosenthal, Co-Founder*
*Frank Cousineau, President*

1112 **Cancer Federation**
P.O. Box 1298 951-849-4325
Banning, CA 92220 Fax: 951-849-0156
info@cancerfed.org
www.cancerfed.com
The Federation is a not-for-profit organization that provides information, counseling, educational materials and meetings for the cancer patients, their families and friends. Also, they fund research and scholarships.
*John Steinbacher, Executive Director*

1113 **International Association of Laryngectomees**
925B Peachtree Street NE 866-425-3678
Atlanta, GA 30309 office@theial.com
www.theial.com
Consists of local clubs worldwide that provide services and information to patients who have undergone laryngectomies, and their families. Members are given information on first aid, postoperative care, rehabilitation, esophageal speech and other speech alternatives. Directories of speech instructors and self-care supplies for the surgical site are distributed.
*Kyd Dieterich, President*
*Jennifer Malkiewicz, Vice President & Treasurer*

1114 **Patient Advocates for Advanced Cancer Treatments (PAACT)**
P.O. Box 141695 616-453-1477
Grand Rapids, MI 49514 Fax: 616-453-1846
paact@paactusa.org
www.paactusa.org
Provides support and advocacy for prostate cancer patients, their families, and the general public at risk. Information relative to the advancements in the detection, diagnosis, evaluation, and treatment of prostate cancer. Information, referrals, phone help, conferences, newsletter.
*Richard H. Profit, President*
*Saleem Durvesh, Executive Marketing Director*

## Research Centers

1115 **AMC Cancer Research Center**
1600 Pierce Street 303-233-6501
Denver, CO 80214 800-321-1557
Fax: 303-239-3400
www.amc.org
Offers research activities, publications, meetings, educational activities, public services, testing services, community-based cancer control programs and knowledge of cancer mortality rates.
*Alice Norton, Executive Director*
*Gail Eckhardt, Clinical Science*

1116 **Abramson Cancer Center of the University of Pennsylvania**
3535 Market Street 800-789-PENN
Philadelphia, PA 19104 Fax: 215-349-5445
www.penncancer.com
National leader in cancer research, patient care, and education.
*Douglas L. Fraker, MD, Deputy Director*
*Caryn Lerman, Interim Director*

1117 **Ackerman Institute for the Family**
149 E 78th Street 212-879-4900
New York, NY 10075 Fax: 212-744-0206
ackerman@ackerman.org
www.ackerman.org
Independent, nonprofit research organization specializing in family therapy, teaching and clinical services.
*Lois Braverman, President/CEO*

1118 **Albany Medical College Joint Center for Cancer and Blood Disorders**
43 New Scotland Avenue 518-262-3125
Albany, NY 12208 877-AMC-8008
Fax: 518-262-3165
TTY: 518-262-1180
www.amc.edu
Offers research in the fields of cancer and blood disorders, focusing on radiotherapy, pathology and surgery.
*Herbert Abbott, General Pediatric*
*Kevin Costello, Internal Medicine*

1119 **Albert Einstein Cancer Center**
Albert Einstein College of Medicine
1300 Morris Park Avenue 718-430-2302
Bronx, NY 10461 Fax: 718-430-2000
www.einstein.yu.edu/centers/cancer/

The goal of AECC is to foster basic clinical, population-based and translational research that addresses all aspects of the cancer problem.
*Allen M. Spiegel, MD, Dean*
*David Goldman, Director*

1120 **Allegheny Singer Research Institute**
West Penn Allegheny Health System
4800 Friendship Avenue 412-362-8677
Pittsburgh, PA 15224 877-284-2000
Fax: 412-359-8610
tchakurd@wpahs.org
www.wpahs.org
*Christopher Olivia, MD, President, CEO*

1121 **Association for Research of Childhood Cancer**
P.O. Box 251 716-681-4433
Buffalo, NY 14225 president@arocc.org
www.arocc.org
The Association was chartered by New York State in that year as a not-for-profit corporation whose primary purpose was to fund the major pediatric research centers in Western New York.
*Larry Lorenz, Vice President*
*Anne O'Donnel, President*

1122 **Bassett Research Institute**
One Atwell Road 607-547-3456
Cooperstown, NY 13326 800-227-7388
research.institute@bassett.org
www.bassett.org
Research institute committed to seeking new information and new strategies for preventing detecting and treating disease.
*Wiliiam F. Streck , MD, President/CEO*

1123 **Baton Rouge Regional Tumor Registry**
Mary Bird Perkins Cancer Center
4950 Essen Lane 225-767-0847
Baton Rouge, LA 70809 Fax: 225-215-1215
www.marybird.org
The Louisiana Tumor Registry is composed of a central office and regional registries that collect and process cancer incidence data from the state's eight established geographic regions. These eight geographic areas are based on Louisiana's historic health districts.
*Todd D. Stevens, President, CEO*
*J. Gerald Jolly, Chairman*

1124 **Baylor University Bone Marrow Transplantation Research Center**
Baylor Research Institute
3500 Gaston Avenue 214-820-2687
Dallas, TX 75246 800-422-9567
www.baylorhealth.com
Offers bone marrow transplantation research in leukemia studies.
*John B. McWhorter, President*
*Irving D. Prengler, VP, Medical Staff Affairs*

1125 **Birmingham VA Medical Center: Research and Development**
700 S 19th Street 205-933-8101
Birmingham, AL 35233 866-487-4243
Fax: 205-933-4484
www.birmingham.va.gov
An acute tertiary care facility with particularly strong programs in both medicine and surgery and serves as the primary referral center for the state. Provides health care services to eligible veterans in the VA Southeast Network.
*Steven L. Keller, Acting Chairman*
*Rica Lewis-Payton, Medical Center Director*

1126 **Boston University Cancer Research Center**
820 Harrison Avenue 617-638-8265
Boston, MA 02118 Fax: 617-638-6518
sfenness@bu.edu
www.bumc.bu.edu/clinicaltrials
The Office of Clinical Research (OCR) was established to serve as the central focus for clinical research support, conduct and training at Boston University Medical Center.
*Douglas V. Faller, Director*
*Salli Fennessey, Manager*

1127 **Brigham Young University Cancer Research Center**
181 Benson Science Building 801-422-3913
Provo, UT 84602 cancer_research@byu.edu
www.cancerresearch.byu.edu
Provide a rigorous research training program for students.
*Daniel L. Simmons, Director*
*Cecil O. Samuelson, President*

1128 **Brown University Division of Biology and Medicine**
BioMed Research Admin, Brown Medical School
The Warren Alpert Medical School of 401-863-3330
Providence, RI 02912 Fax: 401-863-2660
www.biomed.brown.edu
Interdisciplinary studies in biological and medical sciences including studies in health care problems and fields of research such as cancer and diabetes.
*John Perry, Senior Associate Dean*
*Edward J. Wing, Medicine/Biological Sciences*

1129 **Burnham Institute Cancer Center**
The Burnham Institute for Medical Research
10901 N Torrey Pines Road 858-646-3100
La Jolla, CA 92037 Fax: 858-646-3199
info@sanfordburnham.org
www.sanfordburnham.org
Known for world-class capabilities in stem cell research and drug discovery technologies. Dedicated to revealing the fundamental molecular causes of disease and devising the innovative therapies of tomorrow.
*Kristiina Vuori, President/CEO*
*Gary Raisl, Executive VP/CFO/Treasurer*

1130 **Cancer Center of Wake Forest University at Bowman Gray School of Medicine**
Wake Forest University School of Medicine
Medical Center Boulevard 336-716-2011
Winston-Salem, NC 27157 800-446-2255
Fax: 336-716-9593
medadmit@wfubmc.edu
www1.wfubmc.edu/cancer
Beyond the academic experiences offered at our medical school, the Center encourages the development of students as caring physicians dedicated to providing the very best care, professionally and personally, to all patients.
*William B. Applegate, MD, Dean*
*John D. McConnell, CEO*

1131 **Cancer Institute of Brooklyn**
927 49th Street 718-972-5816
Brooklyn, NY 11219 Fax: 718-972-8693
*Jo-Ann Hertz, Executive Director*

1132 **Cancer Prevention Institute**
23 Jasper St 937-227-9400
Dayton, OH 45409 877-274-4543
Fax: 937-297-6970
info@pch-dayton.org
www.premiercommunityhealth.org
Nonprofit organization focusing research activities primarily on cancer prevention, anti-cancer drugs, early diagnosis of cancer, and bone marrow toxicity. Previously known as the Hipple Cancer Research Center.
*Stephen McHugh, Treasurer*
*Diane Ewing, Chair*

1133 **Cancer Prevention Institute of California**
2201 Walnut Avenue 510-608-5000
Fremont, CA 94538 800-511-2300
Fax: 510-608-5095
www.cpic.org
The North California Cancer Center is dedicated to understanding the causes prevention and detection of cancer and to improving the quality of life for individuals living with cancer.
*Reed Goertler, Chief Operations Officer*
*Sally Glaser, PhD, CEO*

1134 **Cancer Research Center**
3501 Berrywood Drive 573-875-2255
Columbia, MO 65201 Fax: 873-443-1202
www.cancerresearchcenter.org

Not only does the Cancer Research Center offer research they also offer community outreach programs to educate church groups, civic clubs, and other organizations about their research and cancer prevention.
*Dr. Abe Eisenstark, Research Director*
*Jack Bozarth, Director*

1135 **Cancer Research Foundation of America**
1600 Duke Street 703-836-4412
Alexandria, VA 22314 800-227-2732
Fax: 703-836-4413
mmcleod@crfa.org
www.preventcancer.org
Prevention and early detection of cancer through research, education and community outreach to all populations, including children and the underserved.
*Carolyn R. Aldige, President & Founder*
*Marcia Myers Carlucci, Chairman*

1136 **Cancer Research Institute: New York**
One Exchange Plaza 55 Broadway 212-688-7515
New York, NY 10006 800-992-2623
Fax: 212-832-9376
info@cancerresearch.org
www.cancerresearch.org
The Cancer Research Institute is the world's only non-profit organization dedicated exclusively to the support and coordination of laboratory and clinical efforts that will lead to the immunological treatment control and prevention of cancer.
*Jill O'Donnel-Tormey, Executive Director*
*Leslie Anson, Assistant to the Executive Director*

1137 **Cancer Therapy and Research Center**
7979 Wurzbach Road 210-450-1000
San Antonio, TX 78229 800-340-2872
www.ctrc.net
The mission of the Cancer Therapy & Research Center is to conquer cancer through research, prevention and treatment.
*Ian M. Thompson, MD, Director*

1138 **Cancer and Leukemia Group B**
230 W Monroe 773-702-9171
Chicago, IL 60606 Fax: 312-345-0117
marciak@uchicago.edu
www.calgb.org
Integral unit of the Institute specializing in leukemia research and prevention.
*Marcia Kelly, Administrative Coordinator*
*Michael Kelly, Director, Protocol Operations*

1139 **Case Western Reserve University: Ireland Cancer Center**
University Hospitals of Cleveland
11100 Euclid Avenue 216-844-1529
Cleveland, OH 44106 888-844-8447
www.uhhospitals.org/irelandcancer
*Thomas F. Senty, CEO*

1140 **Children's Center for Cancer and Blood Disorders**
University of South Carolina School of Medicine
7 Richland Medical Park 803-434-7000
Columbia, SC 29203 www.palmettohealth.org
Joint clinical and basic research of juvenile cancer and blood disorders.
*Charles D. Beaman, Jr., CEO*

1141 **Children's Hospital Research Foundation**
700 Childrens Drive 614-722-2000
Columbus, OH 43205 800-792-8401
Fax: 61 -35 -079
www.nationwidechildrens.org
Offers research activities into Reye's Syndrome, genetics and children's cancer chemotherapy.
*Richard McClead, Medical Director*
*Richard J. Brilli, Chief Medical Officer*

1142 **City of Hope Comprehensive Cancer Research Center**
1500 E Duarte Road 626-256-4673
Duarte, CA 91010 800-256-4673
Fax: 626-930-5394
tkronitis@coh.org
www.cityofhope.org
Excellence in biomedical research patient-centered medical care and community outreach.
*Theodore G. Krontiris, MD, Director*
*Richard Jove, Deputy Director*

1143 **City of Hope National Medical Center**
Beckman Research Institute
1500 E Duarte Road 626-256-4673
Duarte, CA 91010 800-826-4673
tpogue@coh.org
www.cityofhope.org
City of Hope is an innovative biomedical research, treatment and educational institution dedicated to the prevention and cure of cancer and other life-threatening illness.
*Stephen J. Foreman, Chair*

1144 **Colorado Cancer Research Program**
2253 S Oneida Street 303-777-2663
Denver, CO 80224 888-785-6789
Fax: 303-777-2642
ccrp@co-cancerresearch.org
www.co-cancerresearch.org
A nonprofit community-based cancer program established to provide community hospitals and physicians access to a wide range of cancer research trials in order to provide their patients with greater options for the treatment control and prevention.
*Jane Hajovsky, Executive Director*
*Eduardo Pajon, Principal Investigator*

1145 **Columbia University Comprehensive Cancer Center**
630 W 168th Street 212-305-4186
New York, NY 10032 Fax: 212-305-6889
/www.cumc.columbia.edu/
*Lee Goldman, President*
*Anne L. Taylor, Vice Dean*

1146 **Dana-Farber Institute: Department of Biostatistics and Computational Biology**
450 Brookline Avenue 617-632-3000
Boston, MA 02115 Fax: 617-632-2444
biostatistics@jimmy.harvard.edu
www.dana-farber.org
Integral unit of the Institute organized into laboratories of biostatistics computing and epidemiology.
*Marvin Zelen, Researcher*
*Edward J. Benz, President, CEO*

1147 **David H. Koch Institute for Integrative Cancer Research**
MIT Center for Cancer
Koch Institute at MIT 76-158 617-253-6403
Cambridge, MA 02142 Fax: 617-324-2238
cancer@mit.edu
www.ki.mit.edu
The mission of MIT Cancer Center is to apply tools of basic science and technology to determine how cancer is caused progresses and responds to treatment. Through this effort they have developed an increasingly complete understanding of the nature of cancer cells which has led directly to improved treatments for the disease.
*Dr. Tyler Jacks, Director*
*Jaqueline Lees, Associate Director*

1148 **Duke Comprehensive Cancer Center**
2424 Erwin Road 919-684-3377
Durham, NC 27705 888-ASK-DUKE
Fax: 919-684-5653
www.cancer.duke.edu
One of only 39 centers in the country designated by the National Cancer Institute (NCI) as a 'comprehensive cancer center'. Duke combines cutting-edge research with compassionate care.
*Anthony Means, Deputy Director*

1149 **Eastern Cooperative Oncology Group**
1818 Market Street 215-789-3645
Philadelphia, PA 19103 800-4CA-NCER
Fax: 267-256-5291
www.ecog.dfci.harvard.edu
Studies into cancer, including biological response modifiers and cancer studies.

1150 **Emory University: Georgia Center for Cancer Statistics**
Rollins School of Public Health

201 Dowman Drive 404-727-6123
Atlanta, GA 30322 Fax: 404-727-7261
gccs@sph.emory.edu
www.sph.emory.edu/gccs

Serves as a cancer registry for five counties of metropolitan Atlanta and ten rural counties of central Georgia.
*James W. Wagner, President*

1151 **Emory University: Winship Cancer Institute**
1365-C Clifton Road NE 404-778-1900
Atlanta, GA 30322 888-946-7447
www.winshipcancer.emory.edu

A clinical cancer center coordinating basic and clinical cancer research.
*Walter Currans, Executive Director*
*Fadlo Khuri, MD, Deputy Directory for Basic Research*

1152 **Fox Chase Cancer Center**
333 Cottman Avenue 215-728-6900
Philadelphia, PA 19111 888-369-2427
www.fccc.edu

*Linda Fliescher, MPH, PhD, Assistant Vice President, Comms.*
*Theresa Berger, MBE, Project Manager*

1153 **Fred Hutchinson Cancer Research Center**
1100 Fairview Avenue N 206-288-7222
Seattle, WA 98109 800-804-8824
Fax: 206-288-1025
hutchdoc@fhcrc.org
www.fhcrc.org

Teams of world-renowned scientists and humanitarians work together to prevent, diagnose and treat cancer, HIV/AIDS and other diseases.
*Lee Hartwell, Director/President*
*Mark Groudine, EVP/Deputy Director*

1154 **Frederick Cancer Research Center**
P.O. Box B 301-846-1000
Frederick, MD 21702 Fax: 301-846-1108
web.ncifcrf.gov

Direct research into the causes treatment and prevention of cancer AIDS and related diseases.
*Craig W. Reynolds, Associate Director*
*Jo Anne Barb, Secretary*

1155 **Georgetown University: Vincent T Lombardi Cancer Research Center**
3800 Reservoir Road NW 202-444-4000
Washington, DC 20057 www.lombardi.georgetown.edu

Established in 1970, the Lombardi Comprehensive Cancer Center is named for the legendary Green Bay Packers and Washington Redskins coach Vince Lombardi, who was treated for cancer at Georgetown University Hospital.
*Louis M. Weiner, Director*
*Peter G. Shields, Deputy Director*

1156 **Geraldine Brush Cancer Research Institute**
California Pacific Medical Center
2333 Clay Street #201 415-600-6000
San Francisco, CA 94115 cpmcadmin@sutterhealth.org
www.cpmc.org

*Martin Brotman, President*
*Robert Tomasello, Chairman*

1157 **Gershenson Radiation Oncology Center**
Barbara Ann Karmanos Cancer Institute
4100 John Road 313-745-9191
Detroit, MI 48201 800-527-6266
Fax: 313-745-2314
info@karmanos.org
www.karmanos.org

Radiation therapy and cancer treatment and research.
*Gerold Bepler, President*

1158 **Henry Vogt Cancer Research Institute**
James Graham Brown Cancer Center
2301 S 3rd Street 502-852-5555
Louisville, KY 40208 800-334-8635
info@ulh.org
www.louisville.edu/hsc/centers

The overall goal of the scientists in the Henry Vogt Cancer Research Institute is to study mechanisms relevant to tumor cell biology at the basic and translational level in order to provide insights that will contribute to the ultimate prevention and cure of malignant diseases.
*Donald M. Miller, Director*
*John W. Eaton, Deputy Director*

1159 **Howard University Cancer Center**
2041 Georgia Avenue NW 202-806-7697
Washington, DC 20060 Fax: 202-462-8928
ladams-campbell@howard.edu
www.cancer.howard.edu

Reduce the burden of cancer through research education and service with emphasis on the unique ethnic and cultural aspects of minority and underserved populations.
*Lucile Adams-Campbel, Director*
*Wayne A. Frederick, Interim Director*

1160 **Huntsman Cancer Institute**
University of Utah School of Medicine
2000 Circle of Hope 801-585-0303
Salt Lake City, UT 84112 877-585-0303
Fax: 801-585-5886
public.affairs@hci.utah.edu
www.huntsmancancer.org

Understand cancer from its beginnings to use that knowledge in the creation and improvement of cancer treatments to relieve the suffering of cancer patients and to provide education about cancer risk prevention and care.
*Mary C. Beckerle, Executive Director*
*Wallace Akerley, Senior Director of Clinical Research*

1161 **Ida and Joseph Friend Cancer Resource Center**
1600 Divisadero St. 415-885-3693
San Francisco, CA 94143 800-444-2559
Fax: 415-885-3701
www.cancer.ucsf.edu/crc/

The Cancer Resource Center supports wellness and the healing process by providing patients and their loved ones with information, emotional support, and community resources. The CRC maintains a multimedia library, provides access to specialized health databases and offers research assistance.

1162 **Iowa Oncology Research Association**
300 E Locust 515-244-7586
Des Moines, IA 50309 888-244-6061
Fax: 515-244-3037
sherrijr@iora.org
www.iora.org

Clinical cancer studies and research.
*Sherri Rickabaugh, Administrator*
*Becky Berrett, Research Assistants*

1163 **Johns Hopkins University: Sydney Kimmel Comprehensive Cancer Center**
The Harry and Jeanette Weinberg Buidling
401 N Broadway 410-955-5222
Baltimore, MD 21231 www.hopkinskimmelcancercenter.org

Johns Hopkins Kimmel Cancer Center has active programs in clinical research, laboratory research, education, community outreach, and prevention and control.
*Ronald J. Danielles, President*
*Edward Miller, MD, Dean of Medical Faculty/CEO*

1164 **Jonsson Comprehensive Cancer Center**
University of California At Los Angeles
8-684 Factor Building 310-825-5268
Los Angeles, CA 90095 888-662-8252
Fax: 310-206-5553
jcccinfo@mednet.ucla.edu
www.cancer.ucla.edu

UCLA's Jonsson Comprehensive Cancer Center (JCCC) has established an international reputation for developing new cancer therapies, providing the best in experimental treatments, and expertly guiding and training the next generation of medical researchers.
*Judith Gasson, Director*
*James Economou, Executive Director*

1165 **Kansas State University: Terry C Johnson**
Center for Basic Cancer Research
1 Chalmers Hall 785-532-6705
Manhattan, KS 66506 Fax: 785-532-6707
marcia@k-state.edu
www.k-state.edu/cancer.center

The mission of the Terry C. Johnson Center for Basic Cancer Research is to further the understanding of cancers by funding basic cancer research, and supporting higher education, training, and public outreach.
*Rob Denell, Director*
*S. Keith Chapes, Associate Director*

1166 **Kellogg Cancer Care Center**
Evanston Hospital
2650 Ridge Avenue 847-570-2000
Evanston, IL 60201 888-364-6400
www.enh.org

Integral unit of the Evanston Hospital this center researches treatment and diagnosis of cancer, including phase 1 and phase 2 studies.
*Mark R. Neaman, President/CEO*
*Jeffery H. Hillebrand, COO*

1167 **Kentucky Cancer Program**
2365 Harrodsburg Road 859-219-0772
Lexington, KY 40504 Fax: 859-219-0548
dka@kcp.uky.edu
www.kcp.uky.edu

The KCP provides a variety of cancer programs and services to health professionals, the public, patients and survivors.
*Debra Armstong, Director*
*Diane Frasure, Administrative Associate*

1168 **Leukemia Research Foundation**
3520 Lake Avenue 847-424-0600
Wilmette, IL 60091 888-558-5385
Fax: 847-424-0606
info@lrfmail.org
www.leukemia-research.org

To conquer leukemia lymphoma and myelodysplastic syndromes by funding research into their causes and cures and to enrich the quality of life of those touched by these diseases.
*Kevin Radelet, Executive Director*
*Cindy Kane, Senior Director of Development*

1169 **Lincoln Cancer Center**
4600 Valley Road 402-483-2827
Lincoln, NE 68510 Fax: 402-483-4184
*Barb Morton, Director*

1170 **Mary Margaret Walther Program**
Walther Cancer Institute
9292 N Meridian Street 317-708-6101
Indianapolis, IN 46260 Fax: 317-708-6102
info@walther.org
www.walther.org

Focuses research on all types of cancer studies.
*Leonard J. Betley, Chairman*
*James E. Ruckle, President/CEO*

1171 **Mayo Comprehensive Cancer Center**
200 First Street SW 507-284-2511
Rochester, MN 55905 Fax: 507-284-0161
TTY: 507-284-9786
www.mayo.edu

Scientists and physician investigators conduct wide-ranging research to improve patient care, while training the next generation of medical scholars.
*Denis Cortese, President/Chief Executive Officer*
*Robert A. Rizza, Director*

1172 **Medical College of Toledo: Cancer Research Division**
Department of Pathology
3000 Arlington Avenue 419-383-4000
Toledo, OH 43614 800-321-8383
Fax: 419-383-6130
utmc.webmaster@utoledo.edu
www.utmc.utoledo.edu

Researches into all aspects of cancer.
*Jill Zyrek-Betts, Assistant Professor*

1173 **Medical Foundation of Buffalo**
Hauptman-Woodward Medical Research Institute
700 Ellicott Street 716-898-8600
Buffalo, NY 14203 Fax: 716-898-8660
www.hwi.buffalo.edu

Nonprofit organization devoted to cancer research.
*Herbert A. Hauptman, PhD, President/Nobel Laureate*
*Eaton E. Lattman, Executive Director & CEO*

1174 **Melanoma Research Foundation**
1411 K Street NW 202-347-9675
Washington, DC 20005 800-673-1290
Fax: 202-347-9678
info@melanoma.org
www.melanoma.org

Founded in October 1996 by melanoma patients and their families to support research which will lead to cure for melanoma. Strictly a volunteer organization - not one person will receive compensation for his or her efforts.
*Steve Silverstein, President & CEO*
*william G. Reilly, President/Owner*

1175 **Memorial Sloan-Kettering Cancer Center**
1275 York Avenue 212-639-2000
New York, NY 10065 888-675-7722
publicaffairs@mskcc.org
www.mskcc.org

Sloan-Kettering Institute has endeavored to lead the way in basic science research oftentimes translating those advances into clinical treatments.
*Harold Varmus, President, CEO*
*Paul A. Marks, President Emeritus*

1176 **Meyer L. Prentis Comprehensive Cancer Center**
4100 John Road 313-745-9191
Detroit, MI 48201 800-527-6266
Fax: 313-745-2314
info@karmanos.org
www.karmanos.org

*Gerald Bepler, President*

1177 **Natalie Warren Bryant Cancer Center**
St. Francis Hospital
6600 S Yale Avenue 918-488-6688
Tulsa, OK 74136 webadministrator@saintfrancis.com
www.saintfrancis.com/locations/nwbcc
*Jake Henry Jr, President/Chief Executive Officer*
*Barry Steichen, Executive Vice President/Chief Administr*

1178 **National Foundation for Cancer Research**
5515 Security Lane 800-321-2873
Rockville, MD 20852 info@nfcr.org
www.nfcr.org

Contracts with major universities for basic science cancer research in the fields of biophysics, theoretical physics, and biochemistry.
*Sujuan Ba, PhD, President & CEO*
*Brian Wachtel, Executive Director*

1179 **New York University Cancer Institute**
New York University Medical Center
530 First Avenue 212-263-7300
New York, NY 10016 888-769-8633
Fax: 212-263-0715
www.nyucancerinstitute.org

The mission of the NYU Cancer Institute is to decrease and eliminate cancer as a significant health problem throughout New York the national and the world by developing and maintaining excellent programs in patient care research education and prevention.
*William Carroll, Director*
*Lauren E. Hackett, Executive Director of Administration*

1180 **Norris Cotton Cancer Center**
Dartmouth-Hitchcock Medical Center
One Medical Center Drive 603-653-9000
Lebanon, NH 03756 800-639-6918
Fax: 603-653-9003
cancercenter@dartmouth.edu
www.cancer.dartmouth.edu

The Cancer Center provides a positive environment for treatment cure and recovery for patients with all forms of cancer.
*Mark Israel, MD, Director*
*Burton L. Eisenberg, Deputy Director*

1181 **Ohio State University Comprehensive Cancer Center**
Arthur G James Cancer Hospital
300 W 10th Avenue 614-293-7521
Columbus, OH 43210 michael.caligiuri@osumc.edu
www.osuccc.osu.edu
A national and international leader in research, which translates to high-quality patient care and educational programs for residents of Ohio and beyond.
*Michael A. Caligiuri, MD, Director*
*John C. Byrd, Associate Director*

1182 **Ohio State University General Clinical Research Center**
The Ohio State University 614-293-8750
Columbus, OH 43210 Fax: 614-293-3796
william.malarkey@osumc.edu
www.crc.osu.edu
Provides facilities and financial support for inpatient and outpatient cancer research.
*William Malaykey, Program Director*
*David Phillips, Administrative Director*

1183 **Oklahoma Medical Research Foundation Immunobiolgy & Cancer Research**
Oklahoma Medical Research Foundation
825 North East 13th Street 405-271-6673
Oklahoma City, OK 73104 800-522-0211
Fax: 405-271-7016
OMRF-President@omrf.org
www.omrf.org
*Dr. Stephen Prescott, President*

1184 **Oncology Hematology Associates of Central Illinois**
8940 N Wood Sage Road 309-243-3000
Peoria, IL 61615 866-662-6564
www.illinoiscancercare.com
Research into cancer treatments.
*Robert Cooper, Director*
*Paul A. S. Fishkin, Hematology Internal Medicine*

1185 **Pacific Health Research Institute**
3375 Koapaka Street 808-524-4411
Honolulu, HI 96819 Fax: 808-524-5559
info@phrei.org
www.phrihawaii.org
Located in Honolulu Hawaii Pacific Health Research Institute (PHRI) is the largest independent biomedical research institute in the state. Since its founding on 1960 as an independent not for profit 501(c)(3) research institute PHRI today has become a leader in biomedical research in the Pacific. Indeed its researchers are performing complex investigations aimed at conquering some of the most debilitating and lethal diseases that afflict humankind.
*Vicki L. Shambaugh, MA, MPH, Director*
*Helen Petrovitch, Executive Director*

1186 **Pediatric Cancer Research Laboratory**
Children's Hospital of Orange County
1201 W.LA Veta Ave 714-997-3000
Orange, CA 92868 Fax: 714-532-8380
www.choc.org
CHOC is the first hospital devoted exclusively to caring for children in Orange County.
*Mitchell Cairo, Director*

1187 **Purdue Cancer Center**
Purdue University
201 S University Street 765-494-9129
W Lafayette, IN 47907 Fax: 765-494-9193
cancerresearch@purdue.edu
www.cancer.purdue.edu
Provide a forum for 75 of Purdue's best and brightest scientists to collaborate across campus and nationwide to prevent cancer to ease its detection and to cure it.
*Timothy Ratliff, Director*
*Andrea Gregory-Kreps, Operations Manager*

1188 **Rambaugh-Goodwin Institute for Cancer Research**
1850 NW 69th Avenue 954-587-9020
Plantation, FL 33313 Fax: 954-587-6378
www.rgicr.org
RGI is committed to rapidly developing anti-cancer therapies in conjunction with industrial and academic partners using efficient models of cancer growth and metastasis with the aim of moving novel compounds to market in the shortest time possible.
*Claire Thuning-Robin, Director*

1189 **Rebecca and John Moores UCSD Cancer Center**
3855 Health Sciences Drive 585-534-7600
La Jolla, CA 92093 Fax: 858-534-7628
dedavis@ucsd.edu
www.cancer.ucsd.edu
One of the just 39 centers in the US to hold a National Cancer Institute designation as a Comprehensive Cancer Center. As such it ranks among the top centers in the nation conducting basic and clinical cancer research providing advanced patient care and serving the community through outreach and education programs.
*John Alksne, Professor, Surgery*
*Michael Andre, Adjunct Professor, Radiology*

1190 **Robert H Lurie Comprehensive Cancer Center of Northwestern University**
Galter Pavilion 675 N Street Clair 312-695-0990
Chicago, IL 60611 866-587-4322
Fax: 312-695-702
cancer@northwestern.edu
www.lurie.northwestern.edu
Lurie Cancer Center is a founding member of the National Comprehensive Cancer Network an exclusive alliance of 21 of the nation's leading cancer centers.
*Steven T. Rosen, Director*
*Leonidas Platanias, Deputy Director*

1191 **Roger Williams Clinical Cancer Research Center**
Roger Williams General Hospital
825 Chalkstone Avenue 401-456-2000
Providence, RI 02908 www.rwmc.com
*Kenneth Belcher, President*
*Sheri L. Smith, Ph.D., Chair*

1192 **Roswell Park Cancer Institute National Cancer Institute**
Elm & Carlton Streets 716-845-2300
Buffalo, NY 14263 877-275-7724
askrpci@roswellpark.org
www.roswellpark.org
Roswell Park Cancer Institute has made fundamental contributions to reducing the cancer burden and has successfully maintained an exemplary leadership role in setting the national standards for cancer care research and education.
*Donald L. Trump, M.D., Director*
*Ann Gioia, Director*

1193 **Salk Institute Cancer Center**
Salk Institute for Biological Studies
P.O. Box 85800 858-453-4100
San Diego, CA 92186 Fax: 858-453-8534
communications@salk.edu
www.salk.edu
The Cancer Center was established in 1970. It is one of only eight basic research cancer centers in the country designated by the National Cancer Institute. The center includes 22 faculty members 150 postdoctoral researchers 45 graduate students and 80 research assistants. It comprises about half of the research at the Salk Institute.
*Walter Eckhart, Professor & Laboratory Head*
*William R. Brody, President*

1194 **Samuel Roberts Noble Foundation: Biomedical Division**
2510 Sam Noble Parkway 580-223-5810
Ardmore, OK 73401 Fax: 580-224-6217
www.noble.org
One of the largest international offshore drilling contractors in the world.
*Michael A. Cawley, CEO/President*
*Bill Goddard, Trustee*

1195 **San Antonio Cancer Institute**
7703 Floyd Curl Drive 210-567-7000
San Antonio, TX 78229 Fax: 210-567-2709
www.uthscsa.edu/
*Tyler Curiel, Director*
*William L. Henrich, MD, President*

1196 **Santa Barbara Breast Cancer Institute**
5333 Hollister Avenue 805-964-8883
Santa Barbara, CA 93111
*Otto Sartorius, Director*

1197 **Southwest Association for Education in Biomedical Research**
P.O. Box 210101 520-621-3931
Tucson, AZ 85721 Fax: 520-621-3355
swaebr@ahsc.arizona.edu
www.swaebr.org
The mission of the Southwest Association for Education in Biomedical Research is to develop and implement a strong proactive campaign to educate school children as well as the general public in the vital role biomedical research plays in their everyday lives.
*Charles Atkinson, President*

1198 **Southwest Foundation for Biomedical Research**
P.O. Box 760549 210-258-9400
San Antonio, TX 78245 www.sfbr.org
Advancing the health of our global community through innovative biomedical research.
*John R Hurd, Chairman*
*Lewis J Moorman III, Vice-Chairman*

1199 **St. Jude Children's Research Hospital**
262 Danny Thomas Place 901-495-3300
Memphis, TN 38105 Fax: 901-495-4011
www.stjude.org
One of the world's premier pediatric cancer research centers.
*Harvey J. Cohen, Chair*

1200 **Stanford University: Beckman Center for Molecular and Genetic Medicine**
School of Medicine, Department of Biochemistry
291 Campus Drive Rm LK3C02 650-723-3622
Stanford, CA 94305 Fax: 650-724-9733
cmgm.stanford.edu
*Paul Berg, Emeritus Professor, Biochemistry*
*Philip A. Pizzo, MD, Dean*

1201 **State University of New York Health Science Center At Brooklyn**
450 Clarkson Avenue 718-270-1000
Brooklyn, NY 11203 www.downstate.edu
Downstate includes Colleges of Medicine Nursing and Health Related Professions and a School of Graduate Studies as well as its own teaching hospital an M.P.H. Program and extensive research facilities.
*John C. LaRosa, President*
*John B. Clark, Interim Chancellor*

1202 **Temple University FELS Institute for Cancer Research**
School of Medicine
3500 N Broad Street 215-707-7000
Philadelphia, PA 19140 Fax: 215-707-7000
www.temple.edu/medicine
Policies and programs are oriented toward research and training in cancer-related basic biological and biochemical sciences with progressive extension into the areas of molecular developmental and chemical biology to advance knowledge of the etiology and pathogenesis of cancer. A major goal of the Institute is to utilize the advances made in basic science programs to develop novel targeted therapies for the treatment of cancer.
*John M. Daly, MD, Dean*
*Diane Omdal, Director, Research Administration*

1203 **Tulane University Pulmonary Diseases Critical Care and Enviromental Medicine**
School of Medicine
1430 Tulane Avenue 504-988-5187
New Orleans, LA 70112 800-588-5300
medsch@tulane.edu
www.som.tulane.edu/pulmdis/facilities
Provides state-of-the-art care to patients and teaching to trainees through several areas of academic excellence that include: Interstitial Lung Diseases; Asthma; Cystic Fibrosis; Sleep Disorders; Interventional Pulmonology; Lung Cancer; Smoking Cessation; Critical Care; and Environmental Medicine.
*Lee Hamm, MD, Senior Vice President and Dean*
*Roy Weiner, Associate Dean for Clinical Research*

1204 **UM/Sylvester Comprehensive Cancer Center**
1475 NW 12th Avenue 305-243-1000
Miami, FL 33136 800-545-2292
www.sylvester.org
UMHC offers an outpatient clinic a 40-bed inpatient unit a comprehensive treatment unit the Mohs surgery center/dermatology clinic the Rosenfield GI Center a cardiology lab and clinic a radiology/imaging suite an interventional radiology clinic the Spine Institute clinics on-site laboratory and pharmacy the Courtelis Center for Psychosocial Oncology the Jill Selevan Chapel a cafeteria as well as administrative offices.
*Joan Scheiner, Chair*
*Jayne S. Malfitano, Vice Chair*

1205 **USC/Norris Comprehensive Cancer Center**
1441 Eastlake Avenue 323-865-3000
Los Angeles, CA 90033 uscnorriscancer.usc.edu
Major regional and national resource for cancer research treatment prevention and education.
*Peter A. Jones, Director*
*Nikias C.L. Max, President*

1206 **University of Alabama at Birmingham Comprehensive Cancer Center**
UAB Comprehensive Cancer Center
1802 6th Avenue S 205-934-5077
Birmingham, AL 35294 800-UAB-0933
info@ccc.uab.edu
www3.ccc.uab.edu
The Center provides advanced cancer care research and education based on stringent peer-reviewed data.
*Edward E. Partridge, Associate Director*
*Kirby I. Bland, Deputy Director*

1207 **University of Arizona Cancer Center**
1515 N Campbell Avenue 520-626-5279
Tucson, AZ 85724 800-327-2873
www.azcc.arizona.edu
Comprehensive cancer center for diagnosis treatment and prevention.
*David S. Alberts, Director*
*Paola Villar Werstler, Director, Development*

1208 **University of California Berkeley Cancer Research Laboratory**
449 Life Science Addition 510-642-4711
Berkeley, CA 94720 Fax: 510-642-5741
crl@berkeley.edu
www.crl.berkeley.edu/?q=crl
Basic research with a special emphasis on mammary cancer and tumor immunotherapy.
*Astar Winoto, Director*
*Judith Yee, Manager*

1209 **University of California: Los Angeles Bone Marrow Transplantation Program**
200 UCLA Medical Plaza 310-206-6889
Los Angeles, CA 90024 www.healthcare.ucla.edu/transplant
Treatment of leukemia and anemia.
*David W. Golde, M.D., Director*
*Gabriel Danovitch, M.D., Medical Director, Proffessor of Medicine*

1210 **University of Chicago Cancer Research Center**
5841 S Maryland Avenue 773-702-6180
Chicago, IL 60637 877-824-0600
www.cancer.uchicago.edu
The University of Chicago Cancer Research Center (UCCRC) employs a wealth of intellectual technological and financial resources to pursue a comprehensive collaborative research program involving more than 200 renowned scientists and clinicians.
*Mary Ellen Connellan, Executive Director*
*Justin Ullman, President*

1211 **University of Chicago: Clinical Nutrition Research Unit**
5841 S Maryland Avenue 773-702-6180
Chicago, IL 60637 877-824-0600
feedback@bsd.uchicago.edu
www.uchicago.edu
Provide superior healthcare in a compassionate manner ever mindful of each patient's dignity and individuality.
*Michael M. Le Beau, Ph.D., Director*
*James L. Madara, CEO*

1212 **University of Colorado Cancer Center**
13001 E 17th Place 303-724-3155
Aurora, CO 80045 800-473-2288
Fax: 303-724-3162
www.uccc.info
UCCC consortium is the hub for cancer research in Colorado. With eight programs 17 shared core resources and nearly 400 members from three universities and six institutions UCCC is responsible for the majority of cancer research in the Rocky Mountain region.
*Dan Theodorescu, M.D., Ph.D., Director*
*Laurie Gasper, M.D., Associate Director for Clinical Research*

1213 **University of Hawaii: Cancer Research Center**
1236 Lauhala Street 808-586-2985
Honolulu, HI 96813 Fax: 808-586-2982
cvogel@crch.hawaii.edu
www.crch.org
The mission of the Cancer Research Center of Hawaii is to reduce the burden of cancer through research education and service with an emphasis on the unique ethnic culture and environmental characteristics of Hawaii and the Pacific.

1214 **University of Iowa: Holden Comprehensive Cancer Center**
UI Hospitals and Clinics
University of Iowa 319-353-8620
Iowa City, IA 52242 800-777-8442
Fax: 319-353-8988
cancer-center@uiowa.edu
www.uihealthcare.com/depts/cancercenter
The Holden Cancer Center promotes interactive high-quality cancer research high-quality health care related to the prevention detection and treatment of cancer and educates cancer professionals and the citizens of Iowa about cancer.
*Jean E. Robillard, Vice President, Medical Affairs*
*Kenneth P. Kates, CEO*

1215 **University of Kentucky: Children Cancer Study Group**
Markey Cancer Center
800 Rose Street 859-257-4500
Lexington, KY 40536 800-333-8874
Fax: 859-323-2074
www.ukhealthcare.uky.edu/markey/
Kentucky Children's Hospital is the only children's hospital in the region. Patients range in age from infants through adolescents and have a variety of illness and injuries.
*Michael Karpf, EVP, Health Affairs*
*Frank Butler, VP, Medical Center Operations*

1216 **University of Kentucky: Lucille Parker Markey Cancer Center**
800 Rose Street 859-247-4500
Lexington, KY 40536 800-333-8874
Fax: 859-323-2074
www.ukhealthcare.uky.edu/markey/
The Markey Cancer Center mission is to eliminate the morbidity and mortality of cancer through a comprehensive program of research education clinical care and community outreach.
*Alfred M. Cohen, MD, FACS, Director*
*Michael Karpf, EVP, Health Affairs*

1217 **University of Michigan: Cancer Center**
Cancer Research Committee
1500 E Medical Center Drive 734-764-0039
Ann Arbor, MI 48109 800-865-1125
Fax: 734-936-9582
www.cancer.med.umich.edu
The U-M Comprehensive Cancer Center provides its patients diagnostic treatment and support services in a collaborative environment focused on excellence in patient care.
*Eric R. Fearon, Associate Director for Science*
*Max S. Wicha, Director*

1218 **University of Minnesota Masonic Cancer Center**
Division of Oncology
420 Delaware Street SE 612-624-8484
Minneapolis, MN 55455 800-226-2376
Fax: 612-626-3069
ccinfo@umn.edu
www.cancer.umn.edu
The Masonic Cancer Center fosters this mission by creating a collaborative research environment focused on the causes prevention detection and treatment of cancer; applying that knowledge to improve quality of life for patients and survivors; and sharing its discoveries with other scientists students professionals and the community.
*Brian Steeves, Deputy Director*
*Ann D. Cieslak, Executive Director*

1219 **University of Nebraska at Omaha Eppley Institute for Research in Cancer**
University of Nebraska
985950 Nebraska Medical Center 402-559-4090
Omaha, NE 68198 hmmaurer@unmc.edu
www.unmc.edu/eppley
To improve the health of Nebraska through premier educational programs innovative research the highest quality patient care and outreach to underserved populations.
*Harold M. Maurer, Chancellor*
*Thomas H. Rosenquist, Vice Chancellor*

1220 **University of New Mexico: Cancer Research and Treatment Center**
1201 Camino de Salud NE 505-272-4946
Albuquerque, NM 87131 800-432-6806
Fax: 505-925-0100
www.cancer.unm.edu
One of the nation's 60 premier National Cancer Institute (NCI)-Designated Cancer Centers and we have been named one of America's Best Cancer Hospitals by U.S. News & World Report. UNM Cancer Center provides cancer diagnosis and treatment to over 40% of the adults and virtually all of the children diagnosed with cancer each year in New Mexico.
*Cheryl Willman, Director/CEO*
*John A Trotter, Deputy EVP for Health Sciences*

1221 **University of New Mexico: Center for Non-Invasive Diagnosis**
Mind Imaging Center/University of New Mexico
1101 Yale Boulevard NE 505-277-0111
Albuquerque, NM 87131 Fax: 505-272-4056
www.hsc.unm.edu
Cardiology and cancer research.
*David Lepre, Executive Director*

1222 **University of North Carolina UNC Lineberger Comprehensive Cancer Center**
School of Medicine
450 est Dr 919-966-3036
Chapel Hill, NC 27514 866-869-1856
Fax: 919-966-3015
lccc@med.unc.edu
www.unclineberger.org
The Center provides multidisciplinary programs for most cancers giving patients the benefit of many medical specialists in one place often in one visit.
*H. Shelton Earp, Director*
*Michael O'Malley, Associate Director*

1223 **University of Pittsburgh Cancer Institute**
5150 Centre Avenue 412-647-2811
Pittsburgh, PA 15232 PCI-INFO@upmc.edu
www.upci.upmc.edu
Since 1985 the UPCI has been committed to improving the understanding of how cancer develops; to characterizing new lifesaving approaches for cancer prevention detection diagnosis and treatment; and to educating future generations of scientists and clinicians.
*Nancy E. Davidson, MD, Committee Chair*
*Adam Brufsky, MD, PhD, Associate Director*

1224 **University of Rochester: James P Wilmot Cancer Center**
601 Elmwood Avenue 585-275-5823
Rochester, NY 14642 866-494-5668
Fax: 585-276-0158
www.urmc.rochester.edu
To use education science and technology to improve health transforming the patient experience with fresh ideas and approaches steeped in disciplined science and delivered by health care professionals who innovate take intelligent risks and care about the lives they touch.
*Jonathan W. Friedberg M.D., Director*
*Gregory Connolly, M.D., Hematology Oncology*

1225 **University of Tennessee Memphis: Cancer Center**
66 N. Pauline St 901-448-5150
Memphis, TN 38163 Fax: 901-528-5033
*Alvin M. Mauer, MD, Director*

1226 **University of Texas: MD Anderson Cancer Center**
1515 Holcombe Boulevard 713-792-2121
Houston, TX 77030 800-392-1611
www.mdanderson.org
To eliminate cancer in Texas, the nation, and the world through outstanding programs that integrate patient care, research and prevention, and through education for undergraduate and graduate students, trainees, professionals employees and the public.
*John Mendelsohn, President, Executive Committee*
*Raymond DuBois, Executive Vice President*

1227 **University of Texas: Medical Branch at Galveston Cancer Center**
301 University Boulevard 409-772-1011
Galveston, TX 77555 Fax: 409-747-1938
TTY: 409-772-4200
public.affairs@utmb.edu
www.utmb.edu
The mission of The University of Texas Medical Branch at Galveston is to provide scholarly teaching, innovative scientific investigation, and state-of-the-art patient care in a learning environment to better the health of society.
*B. Mark Evers, Director*
*David L. Calender, President*

1228 **University of Vermont Cancer Center**
University of Vermont
E-213 Given Buildinge 802-656-4414
Burlington, VT 05405 877-540-4673
Fax: 802-656-8788
www.vermontcancer.org
*Richard Branda, Interim Director*
*Marianne Baggs, Assistant to the Director*

1229 **University of Wisconsin Paul P Carbone Comprehensive Cancer Center**
600 Highland Avenue 608-263-6400
Madison, WI 53792 800-622-8942
Fax: 608-263-8613
www.cancer.wisc.edu
The University of Wisconsin Paul P. Carbone Comprehensive Cancer Center is the only comprehensive cancer center in Wisconsin as designated by the National Cancer Institute. An integral part of the UW School of Medicine and public Health this cancer center unites more than 250 physicians and scientists who work together in translating discoveries from research laboratories into new treatments that benefit cancer patients.

1230 **Virginia Commonwealth University: Massey Cancer Center**
401 College Street 804-828-0450
Richmond, VA 23298 877-4MA-SSEY
Fax: 804-828-8453
massey@vcu.edu
www.massey.vcu.edu
The mission of the University of Central Arkansas is to maintain the highest academic quality and to ensure that its programs remain current and responsive to the diverse needs of those it serves.
*Gordon D. Ginder, MD, Director*
*Steven Grant, MD, Associate Director*

1231 **Warren Grant Magnuson Clinical Center**
National Institute of Health
9000 Rockville Pike 301-496-4000
Bethesda, MD 20892 800-411-1222
Fax: 301-480-9793
TTY: 866-411-1010
prpl@mail.cc.nih.gov
www.clinicalcenter.nih.gov/index.html
Established in 1953 as the research hospital of the National Institutes of Health. Designed so that patient care facilities are close to research laboratories so new findings of basic and clinical scientists can be quickly applied to the treatment of patients. Upon referral by physicians, patients are admitted to NIH clinical studies.
*John Gallin, Clinical Center Director*
*David Henderson, Deputy Director for Clinical Care*

1232 **Wayne State University Center for Molecular Medicine and Genetics**
Wayne State University School of Medicine
3127 Scott Hall 313-577-5323
Detroit, MI 48201 Fax: 313-577-5218
sshaw@wayne.edu
www.genetics.wayne.edu
Research focusing on human conditions such as cancer and neuromuscular disorders.
*Lawrence I. Grossman, Professor/Director*
*Jeffrey A. Loeb, Associate Director*

1233 **West Virginia University: Mary Babb Randolph Cancer Center**
Mary Babb Randolph Cancer Center Clinic
One Medical Center Drive 304-293-4500
Morgantown, WV 26506 877-427-2894
Fax: 304-598-4553
www.wvucancer.org/pages/
Premier cancer facility with a national reputation of excellence in cancer treatment, prevention and research.
*Augusto Ochoa, Director*
*Lori K. Acciavatti, Professional Technologists*

1234 **Yale University Comprehensive Cancer Center**
333 Cedar Street 203-785-4095
New Haven, CT 06520 866-925-3226
Fax: 203-785-4116
www.yalecancercenter.org
A National Cancer Institute designated comprehensive cancer center for over 30 years. Yale Cancer Center is one of only 40 Centers in the nation and the only comprehensive center in Southern New England.
*Thomas Lynch, Director*
*Kevin Vest, PT, MBA, FACHE, Deputy Director*

## Support Groups & Hotlines

1235 **ABCD: After Breast Cancer Diagnosis**
5775 N. Glen Park Road 800-977-4121
Glendale, WI 53209 info@abcdmentor.org
www.abcdbreastcancersupport.org
Provides free, personal support and resources to those affected by breast cancer.
*Billie Jean Smith, President*
*Ellen Friebert Schupper, Executive Director*

1236 **American Cancer Society: San Jose Prostate Cancer Support Group**
3369 Union Avenue 408-559-8553
San Jose, CA 95124 www.cancer.org

1237 **American Foundation for Urologic Disease: Us Too Line**
1128 N Charles Street 301-727-2908
Baltimore, MD 21201 800-828-7866
www.afud.org
Provides information and referrals for family members, victims and other individuals concerned with prostate cancer.

1238 **American Institute for Cancer Research**
1759 R Street NW
Washington, DC 20009
202-328-7744
800-843-8114
Fax: 202-328-7226
aicrweb@aicr.org
www.aicr.org

*Melvin Huston, Chairman*
*Lawrence Pratt, Vice-Chairman*

1239 **CanHelp**
P.O. Box 1678
Livingston, NJ 07039
800-364-2341
Fax: 888-800-0201
joan@canhelp.com
www.canhelp.com
Offers reports for cancer patients on orthodox and alternative therapies and coaching/counseling to help with treatment decision-making and coping.
*Patrick M. McGrady, Founder*

1240 **Cancer Support Community**
3276 Mc Nutt Avenue
San Francisco, CA 94597
925-933-0107
Fax: 925-933-0249
www.cancersupportcommunity.net
Offers understanding, support and guidance to people with cancer and those who care about them.
*James Bouquin, President & Executive Director*
*Margaret Stauffer, Vice President & Program Director*

1241 **CancerCare**
275 Seventh Avenue
New York, NY 10001
212-712-8400
800-813-4673
Fax: 212-712-8495
info@cancercare.org
www.cancercare.org
Provides a wide variety of support services to cancer patients, their families and friends including support groups, education classes, personal counseling and telephone helplines.
*Patricia J. Goldsmith, Chief Executive Office*
*Christine Verini, RPH, EVP/Chief Operating Officer*

1242 **Cancervive**
11636 Chayote Street
Los Angeles, CA 90049
310-203-9232
800-486-2873
Fax: 310-471-4618
cancervivr@aol.com
www.cancervive.org
Dedicated to providing support, public education and advocacy to those who have experienced this disease. The mission of Cancervive is to assist survivors to reclaim their lives after cancer.

1243 **Center for Cancer Survival**
104 W Anapamu Street
Santa Barbara, CA 93101
805-962-6221
Nonprofit, nonmedical outreach education program teaching specific emotional, mental and spiritual skills for survival on their journey of recovery from cancer.
*Richard Sheldon, Founder*

1244 **Collaborative Medicine Center**
10 Willow Street
Mill Valley, CA 94941
415-383-3197
Works with cancer patients by using a variety of supportive modalities. The emphasis at the center is on helping people learn to support and activate their own healing processes.
*Martin L. Rossman, MD*

1245 **Commonwealth Cancer Help Program**
451 Mesa Road
Bolinas, CA 94924
415-868-0970
Fax: 415-868-2230
commonweal@commonweal.org
www.commonweal.org/programs/cancer-help/
An educational program designed to help participants reduce the stress of cancer, explore health habits, be with others experiencing the same difficulties and consider information on established and complementary therapeutic options.
*Michael Lerner, President*
*Susan Braun, Executive Director*

1246 **Corporate Angel Network**
Westchester County Airport
One Loop Road
White Plains, NY 10604
914-328-1313
866-328-1313
Fax: 914-328-3938
info@corpangelnetwork.org
www.corpangelnetwork.org
To ease the emotional stress, physical discomfort and financial burden of travel for cancer patients by arranging free flights to treatment cetners, using the empty seats on corporate aircraft flying on routine business.
*Peter H. Fleiss, Executive Director*
*Randall Greene, President & CEO*

1247 **Exceptional Cancer Patients/ECaP**
532 Jackson Park Drive
Meadville, CT 16335
814-337-8192
Fax: 814-337-0699
info@ecap-online.org, info@mind-body.org
www.ecap-online.org/home.htm
The mission of EcaP/Exceptional Cancer Patients is to provide exceptional resources, comprehensive professional training programs and extraordinary interdisciplinary retreats that help people facing the challenges of cancer and other chronic illnesses discover their inner healing resources.
*Bernie Siegal MD, Founder*
*Barry Bittman MD, Chief Executive Officer*

1248 **Gilda's Club: Grand Rapids**
1806 Bridge Street NW
Grand Rapids, MI 49504
616-453-8300
Fax: 616-453-8355
info@gildasclubgr.org
www.gildasclubgr.org
A free cancer support community of children, adults, families and friends.
*Leann Arkema, President/CEO*
*Davis Sesbastian, Chair*

1249 **Gilda's Club: New York City**
502 Eigth Avenue
Brooklyn, NY 11215
718-788-1600
Fax: 718-788-0322
info@gildasclubnyc.org
www.gildasclubnyc.org
Creates welcoming communities of free support for everyone living with cancer - men, women, teens and children - along with their families and friends. The innovative program is an essential complement to medical care, providing networking and support groups, workshops, lectures and social activities, all free of charge.
*Robert Easton, Chairman of the Board*
*Lily Safani, CEO*

1250 **Gilda's Club: Quad Cities**
1234 E River Drive
Davenport, IA 52803
319-326-7504
877-926-7504
Fax: 563-323-1658
www.gildasclubqc.org
A cancer support community providing people living with cancer, and all who touch their lives, access to other people going through the same experience.
*Claudia Robinson, CEO*
*Melissa Wright, Program Director*

1251 **Gilda's Club: South Florida**
119 Rose Drive
Fort Lauderdale, FL 33316
954-763-6776
Fax: 954-763-6761
info@gildasclubsouthflorida.org
www.gildasclubsouthflorida.org
A free cancer support community for women, men, children, and teens with all types of cancer and their families and friends. Offer networking groups, lectures, workshops, specialized children's and teen programs, and social events in a nonresidential, non-medical, home-like setting.
*Shelley Goren, CEO*
*Sara Howley Callari, Chair*

1252 **I Can Cope**
American Cancer Society
1599 Clifton Road NE
Atlanta, GA 30329
404-320-3333
800-227-2345
www.cancer.org
An educational program for people facing cancer, either personally, or as a friend or family caregiver. Helps dispel cancer myths

by presenting straightforward facts and answers to your cancer-related questions

1253 **International Association of Cancer Victors and Friends**
7740 W Manchester Avenue 310-822-5032
Playa del Rey, CA 90293 Fax: 310-822-4193
Offers reports and information on alternative therapies and recent cancer studies.
*Ann Cinquina*

1254 **JamesCare For Life Support Groups & Services**
James Cancer Hospital & Solove Research Institute
300 W 10th Avenue 614-293-5066
Columbus, OH 43210 800-293-5066
Fax: 614-293-2565
jamesline@osumc.edu
www.cancer.osu.edu
JamesCare for Life Cancer Support Groups and Services provides a wide range of resources and services to assist patients and families on their journey. This group offers support for patients and families to share experiences, express concerns, and learn more about the impact of cancer and available treatments.
*Michael A. Caligiuri, CEO*
*Jeff Walker, Senior Executive Director*

1255 **Look Good... Feel Better**
American Cancer Society
1599 Clifton Road NE 404-320-3333
Atlanta, GA 30329 800-227-2345
www.lookgoodfeelbetter.org
A community-based, free, national service. Teaches female cancer patients beauty tips to look better and feel good about how they look during chemotherapy and radiation treatments

1256 **Lung Cancer Alliance Support Group**
888 16th Street NW 202-463-2080
Washington, DC 20006 800-298-2436
kay@lungcanceralliance.org
www.lungcanceralliance.org
Dedicated solely to support and advocacy for all those living with or at risk for lung cancer.
*T. Joseph Lopez, Chairman*
*Cheryl Healton, President & CEO*

1257 **National Cancer Institute**
9000 Rockville Pike Drive 800-422-6237
Bethesda, MD 20892 nciinfo@nih.gov
www.cancer.gov
Offers educational information, public awareness, research grants, and more for patients, their families, and health care professionals. Information specialists answer cancer-related questions by phone, LiveHelp instant messaging, and e-mail.
*Monica Bertagnolli, M.D, Director*
*Douglas R. Lowy, M.D., Principal Deputy Director*

1258 **National Foundation for Cancer Research Hotline**
5515 Security Lane 800-321-2873
Rockville, MD 20852 info@nfcr.org
www.nfcr.org
Contracts with major universities for basic science cancer research in the fields of biophysics, theoretical physics, and biochemistry.
*Sujuan Ba, PhD, President & CEO*
*Brian Wachtel, Executive Director*

1259 **National Health Information Center**
Office of Disease Prevention & Health Promotion
1101 Wootton Pkwy Fax: 240-453-8281
Rockville, MD 20852 odphpinfo@hhs.gov
www.health.gov/nhic
Supports public health education by maintaining a calendar of National Health Observances; helps connect consumers and health professionals to organizations that can best answer questions and provide up-to-date contact information from reliable sources; updates on a yearly basis toll-free numbers for health information, Federal health clearinghouses and info centers.
*Don Wright, MD, MPH, Director*

1260 **National Hospice Helpline**
1731 King Street 703-837-1500
Alexandria, VA 22314 Fax: 703-837-1233
www.nhpco.org
Offers information on hospice in general and offers referrals to local hospice programs.
*Cathy L. Gibney, CPA, Chief Financial Officer*
*Ben Marcantonio, MS, MEd, COO & Interim CEO*

1261 **PDQ**
National Cancer Institute
9000 Rockville Pike Drive 800-422-6237
Bethesda, MD 20892 www.cancer.gov/publications/pdq
An NCI database that contains the latest information about cancer treatment, screening, prevention, genetics, supportive care, and complementary and alternative medicine, plus clinical trials.
*Eric J. Seifter, M.D., Editor-in-Chief*

1262 **Reach to Recovery**
American Cancer Society
1599 Clifton Road NE 404-320-3333
Atlanta, GA 30329 800-227-2345
www.cancer.org
Provides support for people recentlry diagnosed with breast cancer; people facing a possible diagnosis of breast cancer; those interested in or who have undergone a lumpectomy or mastectomy; those considering breast reconstruction; those who have lymphedema; those who are undergoing or who have completed treatment such as chemotherapy and radiation therapy; people facing breast cancer recurrence or metastasis

1263 **Wainwright House Cancer Support Programs**
260 Stuyvesant Avenue 914-967-6080
Rye, NY 10580
Weeklong residential retreats offered four times a year to cancer patients. Retreats are devoted to cancer patient education, health promotion and stress management.
*Richard Grossman, Program Director*

1264 **Women's Suffrage for Prostate Cancer Awareness**
743 Caribou Court 800-776-2262
Sunnyvale, CA 94087 www.pcawomen.org
Women have banded together here to help people cope with the effects of prostate cancer on their lives and educate others about it. Members understand problems of patients and families and are here to support and educate.
*Judith P. Barnhard, CPA, Chairman*
*May Barnhard, PC, Chairman*

## Print Resources

1265 **American Journal of Clinical Oncology**
Lippincott Williams & Wilkins
Two Commerce Square 215-521-8300
Philadelphia, PA 19103 customerservice@lww.com
journals.lww.com/amjclinicaloncology/
Offers coverage of ongoing research in cancer treatment for cancer surgeons, radiation oncologists, and medical oncologists. The journal was formerly entitled Cancer Clinical Trials.
*Bimonthly*
*David E. Wazer, MD, Editor-in-Chief*

1266 **Cancer**
American Cancer Society
3380 Chastain Meadows Pkwy. N.W. 800-227-2345
Kennesaw, GA 30144 www.cancer.org
An international interdisciplinary journal that publishes original peer-reviewed research on oncology disciplines, including cancer research, risk reduction, treatment, and patient care.
*Suresh S. Ramalingam, MD, Editor-in-Chief*

1267 **Cancer Nursing: An International Journal for Cancer Care**
Lippincott Williams & Wilkins
Two Commerce Square 215-521-8300
Philadelphia, PA 19103 customerservice@lww.com
journals.lww.com/cancernursingonline/
Addresses issues within the care and support of cancer patients, such as prevention and early detection, geriatric and pediatric cancer nursing, medical and surgical oncology, ambulatory care, nu-

tritional support, psychosocial aspects of cancer, and specific nursing interventions.
*Bimonthly*
*Pamela S. Hinds, PhD, RN, FAAN, Editor-in-Chief*
*Amy Bedinger Miller, Managing Editor*

1268 **Diseases of the Colon and Rectum**
American Society of Colon and Rectal Surgeons
2515 Waukegan Road 847-607-6410
Bannockburn, IL 60015 ascrs@fascrs.org
www.fascrs.org
Diseases of the Colon and Rectum (DCR) is the official journal of the American Society of Colon and Rectal Surgeons and is mailed to all members on a mothly basis as a member benefit. Non-member subscribers have access to the online version of DCR.

1269 **Pancreas**
Lippincott Williams & Wilkins
Two Commerce Square 215-521-8300
Philadelphia, PA 19103 journals.lww.com/pancreasjournal/
Provides a central forum for communication of original works involving both basic and clinical research on the exocrine and endocrine pancreas and their consequences in the disease state.
*Vay Liang W. Go, MD, Editor-in-Chief*
*Christine Nguyen, Managing Editor*

1270 **The Melanoma Letter**
Skin Cancer Foundation
205 Lexington Avenue 212-725-5176
New York, NY 10016 www.skincancer.org
Publishes trends, topics and techniques on melanoma.
*Allan C. Halpern, MD, Co-Editor*
*Ashfaq A. Marghoob, MD, Co-Editor*

## Web Sites

1271 **American Academy of Dermatology**
www.aad.org
An organization of doctors who specialize in diagnosing and treating skin problems.

1272 **American Cancer Society**
www.cancer.org
Provides free printed materials, offers a range of services to patients and their families.

1273 **American Society of Colon and Rectal Surgeons (ASCRS)**
www.fascrs.org
ASCRS represents colon and rectal surgeons dedicated to advancing and promoting the science and practice of the treatment of patients with cancer, and other diseases affecting the colon and related areas.

1274 **Association for the Cure of Cancer of the Prostate**
www.capcure.org

1275 **Bone Marrow & Cancer Foundation**
bonemarrow.org
Goal is to improve the quality of life for bone marrow and stem cell transplant patients, and their families, by providing financial aid, education, and emotional support.
*Christina Merrill, President & CEO*
*Robert Fishman, Chair*

1276 **Healing Well**
www.healingwell.com
An online health resource guide to medical news, chat, information and articles, newsgroups and message boards, books, disease-related web sites, medical directories, and more for patients, friends, and family coping with disabling diseases, disorders, or chronic illnesses.

1277 **Healthlink USA**
www.healthlinkusa.com
Health information concerning treatment, cures, prevention, diagnosis, risk factors, research, support groups, email lists, personal stories and much more. Updated regularly.

1278 **International Association of Eating Disorders Professionals Foundation**
www.iaedp.com
Supplies printed information and sponsors meetings and other activities. Publishes a directory of speech instructors and maintains a list of sources for supplies for laryngectomee.

1279 **Leukemia and Lymphoma Society**
www.leukemia.org
A national voluntary health agency dedicated to curing leukemia, lymphoma, Hodgkin's disease and myeloma and to improving the quality of life of patients and their families.

1280 **MedicineNet**
www.medicinenet.com
An online resource for consumers providing easy-to-read, authoritative medical and health information.

1281 **Medscape**
www.medscape.com
Medscape offers specialists, primary care physicians, and other health professionals the Web's most robust and integrated medical information and educational tools.

1282 **MyHealthfinder**
www.healthfinder.gov
Searchable, carefully developed web site offering information on over 1000 topics. Developed by the US Department of Health and Human Services, the site can be used in both English and Spanish.

1283 **National Hospice & Palliative Care Organization (NHPCO)**
www.nhpco.org
This organization seeks to improve end-of-life care, widen access to hospice care, and improve quality of life for the dying and their loved ones. NHPCO's website offers information on regulations, advocacy, quality and performance, education, and a variety of other resources.

1284 **National Ovarian Cancer Coalition**
www.ovarian.org
Aims to raise awareness about ovarian cancer and to promote education about the disease, while dispelling myths and misunderstandings. The coalition is committed to improving the overall survival rate and quality of life for women with ovarian cancer.

1285 **Support for People with Oral and Head and Neck Cancer (SPOHNC)**
www.spohnc.org
Non-profit organization addressing the broad emotional, physical, and humanistic needs of oral and head and neck cancer patients.

1286 **WebMD**
www.webmd.com
Provides credible information, supportive communities, and in-depth reference material about health subjects. A source for original and timely health information, as well as material from well-known content providers.

1287 **Webhelp**
www.webhelp.com
Provides links to information, including research, treatment, prevention, support, and more.

# CARDIOVASCULAR DISEASES

*Substance use disorder is a social problem worldwide and causes physical issues that may be serious and require medical intervention. Stimulants, sedatives, sleeping pills and narcotics are often associated with abuse even when regulated by law. Agents may cause cerebrovascular and cardiovascular diseases requiring emergency medical treatment. These drugs cause a hyperadrenergic state with vasoconstriction (narrowing of blood vessels that causes high blood pressure) and tachycardia (rapid heart rate), and may cause ischemic and hemorrhagic stroke, acute coronary syndrome, aortic dissection and arrhythmias (irregular heart rate).*

Substance use disorders may also lead to cardiac enlargement (hypertrophy) and left ventricular dysfunction leading to congestive heart failure. Individuals with substance use disorder are almost three times as likely to have cardiovascular disease than individuals without substance use disorder.

Adverse cardiovascular effects such as abnormal heart rate and even heart attack may be caused by illicit drug use. Injecting illicit drugs may lead to collapsed veins and bacterial blood infections affecting blood vessels and heart valves. Cocaine, heroin and amphetamines affect the central nervous system and alter consciousness. According to the American Heart Association, addiction is always a threat, but the side effects and risks with illicit drug use also include:

- Headaches, abdominal pain and nausea
- Alterations in heart rate, blood pressure and body temperature
- Poor judgment leading to a variety of poor decisions, including unprotected sex or risky sex behaviors resulting in a greater risk of sexually transmitted diseases
- Exposure to substances used in cutting illicit drugs, such as talc, poisons and herbicides
- Heart attacks, respiratory arrest and seizures.

Cocaine is considered the perfect heart attack drug due to users having higher blood pressure, stiffer arteries (the oxygen carrying blood vessel), and thicker heart wall muscle, all increasing the risk of heart attack. Cocaine use occurs in almost 2 percent of the U.S. population over the age of 12. It is the drug most often responsible to visits to U.S. hospital emergency rooms.

Prescribed amphetamines, such as those used to treat Parkinson's disease, obesity, narcolepsy and attention deficit disorder with hyperactivity, can be addictive and prone to misuse. Heart rate and blood pressure increases are noted as the drugs stimulate the brains and nerves. Stopping drugs without a conversation with the physician is dangerous and can result in withdrawal symptoms.

Drinking, smoking and drug use are linked to premature heart disease in younger individuals. The use of tobacco, marijuana, alcohol and illegal drugs are line to premature artery disease. Misuse of drugs at an earlier age leads to worse health over the long term. Illegal drug use, including prescription drug abuse, is increasing in adults over the age of 50. As the body ages, the risk of cardiovascular disease increases especially if the individual has not maintained an adequate level of fitness. Combined with an unhealthy body, illicit and prescription drug abuse may lead to significant levels of cardiovascular disease.

Physicians should inquire about substance use disorder when an individual presents with cardiovascular disease. Most health assessments currently ask if an individual is using drugs but some do not ask about previous drug use that could have a lingering effect on the person. Active substance use disorder may predispose the individual to cardiovascular disease. There are both short- and long-term consequences of substance use disorder as it relates to cardiovascular disease.

## Agencies & Associations

1288 **American Autoimmune Related Diseases Association**
19176 Hall Road 586-776-3900
Clinton Township, MI 48038 hello@autoimmune.org
www.autoimmune.org
Provides awareness, education, and referrals for patients with any type of autoimmune disease.
*Jason Gamel, President/CEO*
*Rob Dunn, RRP, Chief Financial Officer*

1289 **American Heart Association**
7272 Greenville Avenue 214-570-5943
Dallas, TX 75231 800-242-8721
www.heart.org
The American Heart Association is the nation's oldest, largest volunteer organization devoted to fighting cardiovascular diseases and stroke. Funds research and raises public awareness of heart diseases.
*Michelle A. Albert, President*
*Nancy Brown, Chief Executive Officer*

1290 **Canadian Adult Congenital Heart Network**
222 Queen Street 877-569-3407
Ottawa, Ontario, K1P-5V9 cachnet@ccs.ca
www.cachnet.org
Organization founded to share knowledge and skills among congenital heart disease professionals in order to create a community committed to caring for individuals with congenital heart disease.
*Ariane Marelli, MD, President*
*Candice Silversides, MD, Vice President*

1291 **Canadian Cardiovascular Society**
150 Elgin Street 877-569-3407
Ottawa, ON, K2P-1L4 info@ccs.ca
ccs.ca
A non-profit organization that represents over 2,300 cardiovascular healthcare professionals.
*Dr. Michelle Graham, President*
*Dr. Sean Virani, Vice President*

1292 **National Heart, Lung & Blood Institute**
31 Center Drive nhlbiinfo@nhlbi.nih.gov
Bethesda, MD 20892 www.nhlbi.nih.gov
Trains, conducts research, and educates in order to promote the prevention and treatment of heart, lung, and blood disorders.
*Gary H. Gibbons, MD, Director*

1293 **Pulmonary Hypertension Association (PHA)**
1629 K. St. 301-565-3004
Washington, DC 20006 800-748-7274
www.PHAssociation.org
A non-profit organization for pulmonary hypertension patients, families, caregivers and PH-treating medical professionals. PHA works to provide support, education, and find a cure for pulmonary hypertension.
*Matt Granato, President & CEO*
*Elizabeth Joseloff, VP, Quality Care & Research*

## Foundations

1294 **Cardiovascular Research Foundation (CRF)**
1700 Broadway 646-434-4500
New York, NY 10019 info@crf.org
www.crf.org
CRF is an academically focused organization that supports cardiovascular research and education.
*Jack Lewin, CEO*
*Martin B. Leon, Founder*

1295 **Children's Heart Society**
12122 68 Street NW 780-454-7665
Edmonton, Alberta, T5B-1R1 childrensheart@shaw.ca
www.childrensheart.ca
Supports families of children with acquired and congenital heart disease in the Edmonton area, and funds research into pediatric heart disease.
*Cameron Kerr, President*
*Gerry Cruz, Vice President*

1296 **Heart and Stroke Foundation of Canada**
2300 Yonge St. 888-473-4636
Toronto, ON, M4P-1E4 Fax: 866-650-6167
www.heartandstroke.ca
A Canadian charity dedicated to advancing cardiovascular research through fundraising initiatives.
*Doug Roth, CEO*
*Avril Goffredo, EVP, Fundraising & Marketing*

## Research Centers

1297 **Arizona Heart Institute**
2632 N 20th Street 602-266-2200
Phoenix, AZ 85006 800-345-4278
Fax: 602-604-5047
www.azheart.com
*Edward Diethrich, Medical Director & Founder*

1298 **Baylor College of Medicine: Debakey Heart Center**
Texas Medical Center
1 Baylor Plaza 713-798-4710
Houston, TX 77030 Fax: 713-798-3692
president@bcm.edu
www.bcm.tmc.edu
Research activities have an emphasis on therapeutic intervention and prevention of heart disease.
*James T. Hackett, Chair*
*Paul Klotman, MD, President*

1299 **Bees-Stealy Research Foundation**
2001 4th Avenue 619-235-8744
San Diego, CA 92101 Fax: 619-234-8190
Basic cardiac research.

1300 **Bockus Research Institute Graduate Hospital**
Graduate Hospital
415 S 19th Street 215-893-2000
Philadelphia, PA 19146
Offers research in cardiovascular diseases with emphasis on muscle tissue studies.
*Dr. Robert Cox, Director*

1301 **Boston University, Whitaker Cardiovascular Institute**
715 Albany Street 617-638-4887
Boston, MA 02118 Fax: 617-638-4066
www.bumc.bu.edu
Offers basic and clinical care research relating to cardiovascular diseases.
*Gary J. Balady, MD, Clinical Investigator*

1302 **Cardiovascular Research and Training Center University of Alabama**
THT Room 311 205-934-3624
Birmingham, AL 35294 Fax: 205-345-96
*Robert C. Bueourge, Director*

1303 **Children's Heart Institute of Texas**
P.O. Box 3966 512-887-4505
Corpus Christi, TX 78463 Fax: 512-887-0539
Offers research and statistical information on pediatric cardiology.
*Laura Berlanga, Director*

1304 **Cleveland Clinic Lerner Research Institute**
9500 Euclid Avenue 216-444-3900
Cleveland, OH 44195 Fax: 216-444-3279
dicorlp@ccf.org
www.lerner.ccf.org
Research institute focusing on diseases of the cardiovascular system.
*Paul E. DiCorleto PhD, Institute Chairman*
*Guy M. Chisolm, III, PhD, Institute Vice-Chair*

**1305 Columbia University Irving Center for Clinical Research Adult Unit**
Presbyterian Hospital
116 Street and Broadway 212-854-1754
New York, NY 10027 Fax: 212-053-13
askcuit@columbia.edu
www.columbia.edu
Research center focusing on pulmonary diseases.
*Lee C. Bollinger, President*
*John H. Coatsworth, Provost*

**1306 Congenital Heart Disease Anomalies Support, Education & Resources CHASER**
2112 N Wilkins Road 419-825-5575
Swanton, OH 43558 Fax: 419-825-2880
www.csun.edu
An organization established to meet the emotional and educational needs of parents and professionals who deal with congenital heart disease in children. Offers resource materials and support for parent to parent networking.

**1307 Creighton University Cardiac Center**
3006 Webster Street 402-280-4566
Omaha, NE 68131 800-237-7828
Fax: 402-280-4938
thecardiaccenter.creighton.edu
Research into the clinical aspects of cardiology and heart disease.
*Tami Ward, Nurse Practitioner*
*Kimberly Harm, Nurse Practitioner*

**1308 Duke University Pediatric Cardiac Catheterization Laboratory**
T901/Children's Health Center 919-681-4080
Durham, NC 27705 Fax: 919-681-2714
john.rhodes@duke.edu
pediatrics.duke.edu
Research into pediatric cardiology.
*Joseph St. Geme, III, MD, Chair*
*Kay Marshall, Chief Administrator*

**1309 Florida Heart Research Institute**
4770 Biscayne Boulevard 305-674-3020
Miami, FL 33137 Fax: 305-535-3642
pak@floridaheart.org
www.miamiheartresearch.org
General cardiovascular research.
*Kathleen T. DuCasse, Chief Executive Officer*

**1310 Framingham Heart Study**
73 Mount Wayte Avenue 508-935-3418
Framingham, MA 01702 Fax: 508-626-1262
LLehmann1@partners.org
www.framinghamheartstudy.org
*Lisa Soleymani Lehmann, MD, Chair*

**1311 General Clinical Research Center at Beth Israel Hospital**
330 Brookline Avenue 617-667-7000
Boston, MA 02215 800-667-5356
TDD: 800-439-0183
www.bidmc.org
Studies into cardiology pulmonary disorders and heart disease.
*Stephen B. Kay, Chair*
*Kevin Tabb, MD, President & Chief Executive Officer*

**1312 General Clinical Research Center: University of California at LA**
Center for Health Sciences
10833 Le Conte Avenue 310-825-7177
Los Angeles, CA 90095 Fax: 310-206-5012
www.gcrc.medsch.ucla.edu
Cardiovascular and heart disease disorders and illness research.
*Isidro Salus, MD, Program Director*
*Gerald Levey, Principal Investigator*

**1313 Hahnemann University Likoff Cardiovascular Institute**
Broad & Vine Streets 215-854-8100
Philadelpia, PA 19102
Diseases of the heart and vessels.
*William S. Frankl, MD, Director*

**1314 Harvard Throndike Laboratory Harvard Medical Center**
Harvard Medical Center
330 Brookline Avenue 617-735-3020
Boston, MA 02215 Fax: 617-735-4833
*Dr. James Morgan, Director*

**1315 Heart Disease Research Foundation**
50 Court Street 718-649-6210
Brooklyn, NY 11201
*Robert A. Teters, Director*

**1316 Heart Research Foundation of Sacramento**
1007 39th Street 916-456-3365
Sacramento, CA 95816 www.hrfsac.org

**1317 Hope Heart Institute**
1380 112th Ave. NE 425-456-8700
Bellvue, WA 98004 Fax: 425-456-8701
info@hopeheart.org
www.hopeheart.org
Heart and blood vessel research.
*Dr. Lester R. Sauvage, MD, Founder*
*Cherie Skager, Interim Executive Director*

**1318 John L McClellan Memorial Veterans' Hospital Research Office**
4300 W 7th Street 501-257-1000
Little Rock, AR 72205 Fax: 501-671-2510
www2.va.gov
*Karl David Straub, MD, Chief Staff*

**1319 Krannert Institute of Cardiology**
1801 N Senate Boulevard 317-962-0500
Indianapolis, IN 46202 800-843-2786
Fax: 317-962-0501
medicine.iupui.edu/krannert
The cardiovascular program at the Indiana University School of Medicine is recognized throughout the world for its commitment to excellence in patient care, research, and education.
*Peng-Sheng Chen, MD, Division Director*
*Eric Williams, MD, Associate Dean*

**1320 Loyola University of Chicago Cardiac Transplant Program**
2160 S 1st Avenue 708-216-9000
Maywood, IL 60153 888-584-7888
Fax: 708-216-4918
www.loyolamedicine.org/
Loyola University Health System is committed to excellence in patient care and the education of health professionals.
*Larry M. Goldberg, President & CEO*
*Wendy S. Leutgens, Senior Vice President & COO*

**1321 Medstar Georgetown University Hospital Facility**
3800 Reservoir Road NW 202-444-2000
Washington, DC 20007 www.georgetownuniversityhospital.org
Studies of medical sciences with particular emphasis on heart disease.
*Dr. Richard Goldberg, President*

**1322 Mount Sinai Medical Center**
4300 Alton Road 305-674-2121
Miami Beach, FL 33140 Fax: 305-743-09
www.msmc.com
General cardiovascular research.
*Steven D. Sonenreich, President & Chief Executive Officer*

**1323 Oklahoma Medical Research Foundation: Cardiovascular Research Program**
825 NE 13th Street 405-271-6673
Oklahoma City, OK 73104 800-522-0211
Fax: 405-271-3980
contact@omrf.org
www.omrf.ouhsc.edu
The Cardiovascular Biology Research Program investigates fundamental mechanisms involved in blood coagulation inflammation and atherogenesis with special emphasis on the regulation of theses processes.
*Stephen M. Prescott, President*
*Mike D. Morgan, Executive Vice President & COO*

**1324 Pennsylvania State University Artificial Heart Research Project**
Milton S Hershey Medical Center

500 University Drive
Hershey, PA 17033
717-531-8407
Fax: 717-531-5011
www.psu.edu

*William S. Pierce, MD, Director*

**1325 Preventive Medicine Research Institute**
900 Bridgeway
Sausalito, CA 94965
415-332-2525
Fax: 415-325-30
Tandis@pmri.org
www.pmri.org

Nonprofit organization focusing on prevention and treatment of heart disease through modification of diet, exercise and relaxation techniques.
*Dean Ornish, MD, Founder & President*
*Anne Ornish, Director, Program Development*

**1326 Purdue University William A Hillenbrand Biomedical Engineering Center**
AA Potter Engineering Center
206 S. Martin Jischke Drive
W Lafayette, IN 47907
765-494-2995
877-598-4233
Fax: 765-494-6628
WeldonBME@purdue.edu
engineering.purdue.edu/BME

Cardiology and heart disease research.
*Brian J. Knoy, Director of Development*
*Kathryn Copper, Secretary*

**1327 Rockefeller University Laboratory of Cardiac Physiology**
1230 York Avenue
New York, NY 10065
212-327-8000
Fax: 212-327-7974
pubinfo@rockefeller.edu
www.rockefeller.edu

Causes of cardiac arrhythmias and prevention of heart disease.
*David Rockfeller, Honorary Chair*
*Russell L. Carson, Chair*

**1328 San Francisco Heart & Vascular Institute**
1900 Sullivan Avenue
Daly City, CA 94015
650-991-6712
800-82H-EART
Fax: 650-755-7315
www.sfhi.com

Committed to providing a full range of high quality services and state-of-the-art cardiovascular treatments for patients.
*Colman J. Ryan, MD, Executive Medical Director*
*Michael Girolami, MD, Chief of Cardiology*

**1329 Specialized Center of Research in Ischemic Heart Disease**
1802 6th Avenue South
Birmingham, AL 35294
205-934-4011
800-822-8816
www.health.uab.edu

Coronary artery disease.
*Will Ferniany, CEO*
*Becky Armstrong, Program Manager*

**1330 Texas Heart Institute**
St. Lukes Episcopal Hospital
6770 Bertner Avenue
Houston, TX 77030
832-355-4011
800-292-2221
Fax: 713-791-3089
www.texasheartinstitute.org

*Denton A. Cooley, MD, President Emeritus*
*James T. Willerson, MD, President, Medical Director*

**1331 University of Alabama at Birmingham: Congenital Heart Disease Center**
1720 2nd Avenue South
Birmingham, AL 35294
205-934-4011
Fax: 205-934-7514
TDD: 205-934-4642
www.uab.edu

*Ray L. Watts, MD, President*
*Linda Lucas, PhD, Provost*

**1332 University of California San Diego General Clinical Research Center**
UCSD Medical Center
200 W Arbor Drive
San Diego, CA 92103
619-543-3102
858-657-7000
Fax: 619-435-36
www.health.ucsd.edu

General clinical research.
*Paul Viviano, Chief Executive Officer*
*Margarita Baggett, Interim Chief Operating Officer*

**1333 University of California: Cardiovascular Research Laboratory**
Center for Health Sciences
UCLA Medical Center
Los Angeles, CA 90024
310-825-6824
Fax: 310-206-5777
Cellular and subcellular cardiac conditions.
*Dr. Glenn Langer, Director*

**1334 University of Cincinnati Department of Pathology & Laboratory Medicine**
234 Goodman Street
Cincinnati, OH 45219
513-584-7284
Fax: 513-584-3892
pathology@uc.edu
pathology.uc.edu

*Fred V. Lucas, MD, Chair of Pathology*
*James Hill, Business Manager*

**1335 University of Iowa: Iowa Cardiovascular Center**
College of Medicine
200 Hawkins Drive
Iowa City, IA 52242
319-335-8588
Fax: 319-335-6969
www.int-med.uiowa.edu
The purpose is to coordinate the cardiovascular programs of the College into a more cohesive unit to permit the Center to 1. utilize cardiovascular resources optimally, 2. intensify, expand and integrate basic and clinical research programs in areas related to cardiovascular research, and 3. evaluate the role of new measures for prevention diagnosis and treatment of cardiovascular disease.
*Barry London, MD, PhD, Director Cardiovascular Medicine*

**1336 University of Michigan Pulmonary and Critical Care Division**
University Hospital
1500 E Medical Center Drive
Ann Arbor, MI 48109
734-647-9342
888-287-1084
Fax: 734-763-4585
www2.med.umich.edu/healthcenters/clinic_
*Kevin Michael Chan, MD, Division Director*

**1337 University of Michigan: Cardiovascular Med Medicine**
325 Briarwood Circle
Ann Arbor, MI 48108
734-647-9000
Fax: 734-936-0133
www2.med.umich.edu/departments/cvc/servi
Focuses on the diagnosis, treatment and prevention of cardiovascular and heart diseases.
*Kim Allen Eagle, MD, Division Director*

**1338 University of Missouri Columbia Division of Cardiothoracic Surgery**
School of Medicine
Columbia, MO 65212
573-882-2121
Fax: 573-884-0437
AldenM@missouri.edu
www.missouri.edu

Cardiac surgery research.
*Mike Alden, Director*
*Brian Foster, Provost*

**1339 University of Pennsylvania Muscle Institut Institute**
School of Medicine
700A Clinical Research Building
Philadelphia, PA 19104
215-573-9758
Fax: 215-898-2653
www.med.upenn.edu/pmi/

Studies in tissue science.
*E. Michael Ostap, PhD, Director*

**1340 University of Pittsburgh: Human Energy Research Laboratory**
4200 Fifth Avenue
Pittsburgh, PA 15260
412-624-4141
www.pitt.edu
Focuses on exercise and cardiac rehabilitation.
*Mark A. Nordenberg, Chancellor*
*Patricia E. Beeson, Provost & Senior Vice Chancellor*

**1341 University of Rochester: Clinical Research Center**
601 Elmwood Avenue
Rochester, NY 14642
585-275-2907
Fax: 585-256-3805
germaine_reinhardt@urmc.rochester.edu
www.urmc.rochester.edu/crc/

Studies of normal tissue functions pertaining to heart diseases.
*Thomas A. Pearson, MD, MPH, PhD, Director, Principal Investigator*
*Giovanni Schifitto, MD, Program Director*

1342 **University of Southern California: Coronary Care Research**
1200 N State Street 213-226-7242
Los Angeles, CA 90033
*Dr. L Julian Haywood, Director*

1343 **University of Tennessee: Division of Cardiovascular Diseases**
920 Madison Avenue 901-448-5750
Memphis, TN 38163 Fax: 901-448-8084
www.utmem.edu\cardiology
Cardiovascular system disorders including heart disease prevention and treatment.
*Karl T. Weber, MD, Director*

1344 **University of Texas Southwestern Medical Center at Dallas**
University of Texas
5323 Harry Hines Boulevard 214-648-3111
Dallas, TX 75390 Fax: 214-483-11
www.utsouthwestern.edu
Cardiology department research.
*Daniel K. Podolsky, MD, President*
*J. Gregory Fitz, MD, Executive Vice President*

1345 **University of Utah: Artificial Heart Research Laboratory**
50 North Medical Drive 801-581-2121
Salt Lake City, UT 84132 Fax: 801-581-4044
healthsciences.utah.edu
Cardiac and blood vessel research.
*Allen Stephens, Associate Director*

1346 **University of Utah: Cardiovascular Genetic Research Clinic**
420 Chipeta Way 801-581-3888
Salt Lake City, UT 84132 Fax: 801-581-6862
www.medicine.utah.edu/internalmedicine/c
Cardiovascular genetics research.
*Dr. Roger Williams, Founder*

1347 **Urban Cardiology Research Center**
2300 Garrison Boulevard 410-945-8600
Baltimore, MD 21216
Causes, diagnosis and treatment of cardiovascular diseases.
*Arthur White, MD, Director*

1348 **Warren Grant Magnuson Clinical Center**
National Institute of Health
10 Center Drive MSC 1078 301-496-3311
Bethesda, MD 20892 800-411-1222
Fax: 301-496-2390
TTY: 866-411-1010
mmichael@cc.nih.gov
www.dnrc.nih.gov/reports/programs/ncc.as
Established in 1953 as the research hospital of the National Institutes of Health. Designed so that patient care facilities are close to research laboratories so new findings of basic and clinical scientists can be quickly applied to the treatment of patients. Upon referral by physicians, patients are admitted to NIH clinical studies.
*Madeline Michael, Chief, Clinical Nutrition Services*

1349 **Yeshiva University General Clinical Research Center**
500 West 185th Street 212-960-5400
New York, NY 10033 www.yu.edu
Cardiovascular research.
*Dr. Henry Kressel, Chairman*
*Richard M. Joel, President*

## Support Groups & Hotlines

1350 **Mended Hearts**
8150 N. Central Expressway 214-206-9259
Dallas, TX 75206 888-432-7899
Fax: 214-295-9552
info@mendedhearts.org
www.mendedhearts.org
Mutual support for persons who have heart disease, their families, friends, and other interested persons.
*Gordon Littlefield, President of the Board*
*Donnette Smith, Executive Vice President*

1351 **Mitral Valve Prolapse Program of Cincinnati Support Group**
10525 Montgomery Road 513-745-9911
Cincinnati, OH 45242 kscordo@wright.edu
www.nursing.wright.edu
Brings together persons frightened by their symptoms in order to learn to better cope with MVP. Fosters use of non-drug therapies. Supervised exercise sessions, diagnostic evaluations and specialized testing. Information and referrals, conferences, literature, group meetings, MVP Hot Line, and assistance in starting groups.

1352 **National Health Information Center**
Office of Disease Prevention & Health Promotion
1101 Wootton Pkwy Fax: 240-453-8281
Rockville, MD 20852 odphpinfo@hhs.gov
www.health.gov/nhic
Supports public health education by maintaining a calendar of National Health Observances; helps connect consumers and health professionals to organizations that can best answer questions and provide up-to-date contact information from reliable sources; updates on a yearly basis toll-free numbers for health information, Federal health clearinghouses and info centers.
*Don Wright, MD, MPH, Director*

1353 **National Society for MVP and Dysautonomia**
880 Montclair Road 205-595-8229
Birmingham, AL 35213 866-595-8229
Fax: 205-595-8222
nancysawyermd@bellsouth.net
Assists individuals suffering from mitral valve prolapse syndrome and dysautonomia to find support and understanding. Education on symptoms and treatment. Other areas of focus are Fibromyalgia and Sjogren's Syndrome.
*Nancy Sawyer, MD*

1354 **Society of Mitral Valve Prolapse Syndrome**
P.O. Box 431 630-250-9327
Itasca, IL 60143 Fax: 630-773-0478
bonnie0107@aol.com
www.mitralvalveprolapse.com/
Provides support and education to patients, families and friends about mitral valve prolapse syndrome.
*Jim Durante, Co-Founder*
*Bonnie Durante, Co-Founder*

## Print Resources

1355 **JRSM Cardiovascular Disease**
SAGE Publishing
albert.ferro@kcl.ac.uk
journals.sagepub.com/home/cvd
A peer-reviewd open access journal that publishes on the prevention and treatment of cardiovascular diseases.
*Albert Ferro, Editor-in-Chief*
*Orina Belton, Associate Editor*

1356 **Journal of the American Heart Association: Cardiovascular & Cerebrovascular Disease**
American Heart Association
200 5th Ave. jaha@journalaha.org
Waltham, MA 02451 www.ahajournals.org/journal/jaha
A peer-reviewed open-access journal for healthcare professionals interested in cardiovascular and cerebrovascular diseases, vascular and endovascular medicine, pediatric cardiology, and neurology.
*24/year*
*Barry London, Editor-in-Chief*
*Kathleen Sullivan, Managing Editor*

## Web Sites

1357 **American Heart Association**
www.heart.org

Supports research, education, and community service programs with the objective of reducing premature death and disability from cardiovascular diseases and stroke. Coordinates the efforts of health professionals in the fight against heart and circulatory disease.

1358 **Healing Well**

www.healingwell.com

An online health resource guide to medical news, chat, information and articles, newsgroups and message boards, books, disease-related web sites, medical directories, and more for patients, friends, and family coping with disabling diseases, disorders, or chronic illnesses.

1359 **Healthlink USA**

www.healthlinkusa.com

Health information concerning treatment, cures, prevention, diagnosis, risk factors, research, support groups, email lists, personal stories and much more. Updated regularly.

1360 **MedicineNet**

www.medicinenet.com

An online resource for consumers providing easy-to-read, authoritative medical and health information.

1361 **Medscape**

www.medscape.com

Medscape offers specialists, primary care physicians, and other health professionals the Web's most robust and integrated medical information and educational tools.

1362 **MyHealthfinder**

www.healthfinder.gov

A government web site where individuals can find information and tools to help you and those you care about stay healthy.

1363 **National Heart, Lung and Blood Institute**

www.nhlbi.nih.gov

Primary responsibility of this organization is the scientific investigation of heart, blood vessel, lung, and blood disorders. Oversees research, demonstration, prevention, education, control and training activities in these fields, and emphasizes the prevention and control of heart diseases.

1364 **WebMD**

www.webmd.com

Provides credible information, supportive communities, and in-depth reference material about health subjects. A source for original and timely health information, as well as material from well-known content providers.

# CHRONIC PAIN

*Chronic pain is defined as pain that lasts more than several months after what should be normal healing. About 25 million U.S. adults suffer from pain over a three-month period, and 40 million more adults had severe pain. Those with severe pain had poor health, engaged with the health system more often, and had more disability than those with less severe pain. Pain and responses to pain are impacted by temperament, psychological state, memory, cognition, culture, beliefs and expectations as well as age, gender, and co-occurring health conditions (comorbidities).*

Managing chronic pain in adults with substance use disorder (SUD), or in recovery from substance use disorder, pose a challenge to providers. Careful pretreatment screening and education are crucial, as are ongoing monitoring for compliance with the plan of treatment and effectiveness, especially with opioid prescriptions. It is estimated that 10 percent of chronic pain patients misuse prescription opioids. Chronic pain has physiological, social and psychological components that can harm health, functioning and well-being. While manageable, chronic pain may never be completely eliminated. Approximately one-third of patients with chronic pain may have addictive disorders. Almost two-thirds of people with opioid addiction report chronic pain. Many of the agents used in chronic pain management qualify as addictive substances, or drugs that cause a "drug seeking" behavior.

There are a variety of pain types that are defined as chronic pain. Chronic noncancer pain is not associated with a terminal condition and is unlikely to improve as a result of tissue healing. Examples are fibromyalgia, sickle cell disease and inflammatory arthritis. Chronic pain syndrome is an intractable pain lasting more than 6 months, with the individual exhibiting changes in behavior, including depression or anxiety; limitations on activities of daily living; no clear relationship to a disorder; and a history of non-productive tests, treatments or surgeries. Cancer pain must always be managed aggressively. Treatment for chronic pain may require increasing dosage of drugs as tolerance develops. Tolerance is said to occur when a drug loses full effect over time. Chronic pain, when managed correctly, rarely leads to addiction if the appropriate drugs are prescribed.

Chronic pain and substance use disorder share common components. They have similar physical, emotional, social and economic impacts on health and well-being. Chronic pain and SUD exhibit disordered central nervous system function. Genetics and environment play a role and both may have significant behavioral components. Treatments must include a variety of interventions personalized to the individual.

Substance use by an individual may be to lessen pain, but also to achieve euphoric effects, relieve stress, or overcome depression and anxiety. In some individuals, repeated exposure to substances may lead to addiction. Substances with addictive potential used in chronic pain management must be carefully managed. Only a minority of individuals will develop addiction, as pain medication used to control real pain is rarely addicting. There are other substance options that may contribute to relief from chronic pain that are not addictive. Non-steroidal anti-inflammatory drugs, tricycle antidepressants, anticonvulsants, and topical analgesics demonstrate pain-relieving capabilities in some patients. Therapeutic exercise is also effective in some individuals. Complementary and alternative medicine, while not considered conventional treatment, are effective in some individuals. Acupuncture and herbs are the most common approaches. A careful history taken initially and at each ongoing visit is important to be sure that dosing schedules and treatment protocols are carefully followed, and that providers are aware of all non-prescribed or complementary approaches people are using.

Chronic pain management and substance use disorders pose a challenge to providers, but with personalized treatment planning, successful outcomes may be achieved without the risk of addiction developing or relapse occurring. Pain treatment goals should be pain-reduction and enhanced functioning. Addiction specialists should be part of the pain management team. Educating the patient and family is important to allow them to understand how to help themselves. Treatment agreements between the patient and the pain management team are often used. Careful monitoring of the patient is the key to safe outcomes.

## Agencies & Associations

1365 **American Chronic Pain Association**
11936 W. 119th Street ACPA@theacpa.org
Overland Park, KS 66213-2216 www.theacpa.org
The ACPA facilitates peer support and education for individuals with chronic pain in its many forms, in order to increase quality of life. Also raises awareness among the healthcare community, and with policy makers.
*Trupti Gokani, MD, President*
*Kathy Sapp, Chief Executive Officer*

1366 **American Osteopathic Association**
142 E. Ontario St. 312-202-8000
Chicago, IL 60611 www.osteopathic.org
Serving as the professional family for more than 145,000 osteopathic physicians (DOs) and osteopathic medical students, the American Osteopathic Association (AOA) promotes public health and encourages scientific research.
*Ernest Gelb, President*
*Kevin M. Klauer, Chief Executive Officer*

1367 **American Physical Therapy Association**
3030 Potomac Avenue 703-684-2782
Alexandria, VA 22305 800-999-2782
Fax: 703-684-7343
www.apta.org
The American Physical Therapy Association (APTA) is an individual membership professional organization representing more than 100,000 member physical therapists (PTs), physical therapist assistants (PTAs), and students of physical therapy.
*Roger Herr, PT, MPA, President*
*Susan Appling, PT, DPT, PhD, Vice President*

1368 **Canadian Pain Society**
250 Consumers Road 416-642-6379
Toronto, Ontario, M2J office@canadianpainsociety.ca
www.canadianpainsociety.ca
Dedicated to healthcare professionals and lay persons with an interest in the field of pain.
*John Xavier Pereira, MD, CM, CCFP, President*
*Nivez Rasic, MD, Treasurer*

1369 **Chronic Pain Association of Canada**
P.O. Box 66017 780-482-6727
Edmonton, Alberta, T6J-6T4 Fax: 780-433-3128
cpac@chronicpaincanada.com
chronicpaincanada.com
Seeks to prevent and alleviate chronic pain, and to improve patients' quality of life.
*Barry Ulmer, Executive Director*
*Terry Bremner, President*

1370 **International Association for the Study of Pain**
1510 H. Street NW 202-856-7400
Washington, DC 20005-1020 Fax: 202-856-7401
iaspdesk@iasp-pain.org
www.iasp-pain.org
The International Association for the Study of Pain is the leading professional forum for science, practice, and education in the field of pain.
*Catherine Bushnell, PhD, President*
*Michael Rowbotham, MD, Treasurer*

1371 **International Pelvic Pain Society**
14305 Southcross Drive West 612-474-4140
Burnsville, MN 55306 Fax: 952-314-8212
info@pelvicpain.org
www.pelvicpain.org
Seeks to recruit, organize, and educate health care professionals actively involved with the treatment of patients who have chronic pelvic pain.
*Tessa Benitez, Executive Director*
*Bobbi Hahn, Association Manager*

1372 **National Association of Myofascial Trigger Point Therapists**
Namtpt.president@gmail.com
www.myofascialtherapy.org
The NAMTPT is a professional organization dedicated to increasing public awareness of, and access to, myofascial pain treatment.
*Mary Biancalana, President*
*Heather Brown, Vice President*

1373 **Reflex Sympathetic Dystrophy Syndrome Association (RSDSA)**
99 Cherry Street 203-877-3790
Milford, CT 06460 877-662-7737
Fax: 203-882-8362
info@rsds.org
www.rsds.org
Non-profit professional and consumer organization founded to support research into the cause, treatment, and cure of reflex sympathetic dystrophy syndrome. RSDSA also organizes support groups, promotes awareness among health professionals, and develops educational programs.
*Jim Broatch, Executive VP & Director*
*Jeri Krassner, Special Events Coordinator*

## Foundations

1374 **U.S. Pain Foundation, Inc.**
15 North Main Street 800-910-2462
West Hartford, CT 06107 contact@uspainfoundation.org
uspainfoundation.org
A nonprofit organization that supports individuals living with chronic pain, as well as their families, caregivers and care providers.
*Nicole Hemmenway, CEO*
*Pamela Lynch, CFO*

## Support Groups & Hotlines

1375 **National Health Information Center**
Office of Disease Prevention & Health Promotion
1101 Wootton Pkwy Fax: 240-453-8281
Rockville, MD 20852 odphpinfo@hhs.gov
www.health.gov/nhic
Supports public health education by maintaining a calendar of National Health Observances; helps connect consumers and health professionals to organizations that can best answer questions and provide up-to-date contact information from reliable sources; updates on a yearly basis toll-free numbers for health information, Federal health clearinghouses and info centers.
*Don Wright, MD, MPH, Director*

## Print Resources

1376 **Canadian Journal of Pain**
Country Hills Boulevard N.W. 587-896-7246
Calgary, AB T3A-5K8 office@canadianpainsociety.ca
www.canadianpainsociety.ca/page-1075355
An international, open access, multidisciplinary journal that covers all aspects of pain research.
*Joel Katz, Editor-in-Chief*
*Rebecca Lewinson, Editorial Manager*

1377 **PAIN: The Journal of the International Association for the Study of Pain**
International Association for the Study of Pain
1510 H. Street N.W. 202-856-7400
Washington, DC 20005-1020 Fax: 202-856-7401
www.iasp-pain.org/publications/pain/
Available to IASP members, this peer-reviewed journal publishes original research on the nature and treatment of pain.
*12/year*
*Francis J. Keefe, PhD, Editor-in-Chief*

## Web Sites

1378 **American Pain Society**
americanpainsociety.org
Multidisciplinary organization of basic and clinical scientists, practicing clinicians, policy analysts, and others.

1379 **Discovery Health**

www.discoverylife.com

A source of information on various health topics, including chronic pain and its symptoms and treatments.

1380 **Healing Well**

www.healingwell.com

An online health resource guide to medical news, chat, information and articles, newsgroups and message boards, books, disease-related web sites, medical directories, and more for patients, friends, and family coping with disabling diseases, disorders, or chronic illnesses.

1381 **Healthlink USA**

www.healthlinkusa.com

Health information concerning treatment, cures, prevention, diagnosis, risk factors, research, support groups, email lists, personal stories and much more. Updated regularly.

1382 **International Pelvic Pain Society**

www.pelvicpain.org

Seeks to recruit, organize, and educate health care professionals actively involved with the treatment of patients who have chronic pelvic pain.

1383 **MedicineNet**

www.medicinenet.com

An online resource for consumers providing easy-to-read, authoritative medical and health information.

1384 **Medscape**

www.medscape.com

Medscape offers specialists, primary care physicians, and other health professionals the Web's most robust and integrated medical information and educational tools.

1385 **MyHealthfinder**

www.healthfinder.gov

Searchable, carefully developed web site offering information on over 1000 topics. Developed by the US Department of Health and Human Services, the site can be used in both English and Spanish.

1386 **WebMD**

www.webmd.com

Provides credible information, supportive communities, and in-depth reference material about health subjects. A source for original and timely health information, as well as material from well-known content providers.

# DEPRESSIVE DISORDERS

*Depressive disorders, also referred to as depression or clinical depression, is a common mood disorder causing severe symptoms affecting feelings, thinking and activities of daily living. Sleeping, eating and working may all be negatively impacted by depressive disorders. Symptoms must be present for two weeks for a diagnosis of depression to be made. Feeling intermittently sad is not depression, but if not addressed, depression may eventually intrude. Individuals with depression are two times more likely to also have a substance use disorder. Individuals with bipolar disorder are seven times as likely to have a substance use disorder.*

Mood disorders and substance use disorders are often seen to potentiate the other. Mood disorders may create drug seeking behaviors or create alcohol abuse to alleviate feelings of sadness and discomfort. Individuals with substance use disorder often say they use drugs and alcohol to combat mood disorders. Individuals may seek opiates for a mellowing effect or cocaine for the exhilarating feelings it provides. Chronic substance abuse may reveal bipolar or other mood disorders. Genetic risk factors are similar in both substance abuse and mood disorders.

The most common psychiatric comorbidities in patients with substance use disorder are mood disorders, including depression and bipolar disorders. Managing substance use disorder and depressive disorders may be challenging. Treating mood disorders may reduce substance cravings and enhance overall well-being. Recognizing intoxication and withdrawal is a part of managing depressive disorders. Substance-induced mood disorders are direct physiologic consequences of substance use, and often result in persistent mood disturbances. Alcohol abuse in most people may also impact mood, as it provides a calming or depressive response when consumed to excess.

The different types of depression include:

- Major depression—lasting two weeks or more and interfering with the ability to work, sleep, study and eat
- Persistent depressive disorder—with less severe symptoms that last longer, usually for at least two years
- Seasonal affective disorder—comes and goes with changes in the season; usually starts in late fall through the winter and goes away during the spring and summer
- Perinatal depression—major depression during pregnancy or after delivery (postpartum depression)
- Depression with psychosis symptoms—a severe form of depression with psychoses including hallucinations, delusions and other.

Bipolar disorder, formerly called manic depression or manic-depressive illness, exhibits in individuals with alternating depressive episodes in which they exhibit a low energy level, sadness, indifferent or hopelessness; followed by manic episodes with unusually elevated mood, higher activity levels and feeling very happy. In between the episodes, the individual may experience periods when their mood is balanced even without medication. Alcohol is commonly abused by individuals with bipolar disorder, and they may seek out other substances to try to self-manage the depression and mania. Studies have shown that 30-50 percent of individuals diagnosed with bipolar disorders (I and II) will develop a substance use disorder sometime in their lifetime. Treatment is available and remission and recovery is possible with early intervention.

Children and adolescents may exhibit disruptive mood dysregulation disorder and premenstrual dysphoric disorder (PMDD). In the adolescent years, substance use disorder may occur as a combination of experimenting with drugs, or trying to manage mood disorders.

Individuals with both a mood disorder and a substance use disorder have a complicated and severe clinical course with worse outcomes than having just one or the other. A tragic link between substance use disorders, mood disorders and suicide has long been seen. Substance abuse disorders have a negative impact on the course and prognosis of mood disorders, resulting in frequent hospitalizations and treatment resistance. The delivery of optimal care remains difficult.

## Agencies & Associations

1387 **Anxiety and Depression Association of America**
8701 Georgia Avenue 240-485-1001
Silver Spring, MD 20910 information@adaa.org
adaa.org

An international nonprofit organization committed to the use of education and research to promote the prevention, treatment, and cure of anxiety, depressive, obssesive compulsive, and other trauma related disorders. ADAA's mission is to improve the lives of all people with anxiety and mood disorders.
*Charles B. Nemeroff, MD, President*
*Susan K. Gurley, Executive Director*

1388 **Center for Family Support (CFS)**
333 Seventh Avenue 888-813-5014
New York, NY 10001 svernikoff@cfsny.org
www.cfsny.org

The Center for Family Support offers assistance to individuals with developmental and related disabilities, as well as their families, and provides support services and programs that are designed to accommodate individual needs. Offers services throughout New York City, Westchester County, Long Island, and New Jersey.
*Steven Vernikoff, Executive Director*
*Barbara Greenwald, Chief Operating Officer*

1389 **Center for Mental Health Services (CMHS)**
Substance Abuse and Mental Health Services Admin.
5600 Fishers Lane 240-276-1310
Rockville, MD 20857 samhsa.gov

Promotes the treatment of mental illness and emotional disorders by increasing accessibility to mental health programs; supporting outreach, treatment, rehabilitation, and support programs and networks; and encouraging the use of scientifically-based information when treating mental disorders. CMHS provides information about mental health via a toll-free number and numerous publications.
*Anita Everett, M.D., DFAPA, Director*

1390 **Depression and Bipolar Support Alliance**
Depression and Bipolar Support Alliance
55 East Jackson Boulevard 800-826-3632
Chicago, IL 60604 Fax: 312-642-7243
www.dbsalliance.org

DBSA is a national organization focused on improving the lives of individuals with depression, bipolar disorder, and other mood disorders. DBSA organizes peer-led support groups; educates patients, families, professionals, and the public on mental health; and works to ensure the availability of quality care for all people.
*Michael Pollock, Chief Executive Officer*
*Maria Margaglione, Programs Director*

1391 **Freedom From Fear**
308 Seaview Avenue 718-351-1717
Staten Island, NY 10305 help@freedomfromfear.org
freedomfromfear.org

A national nonprofit organization whose mission is to aid and counsel individuals suffering from anxiety and depressive disorders through advocacy, education, research, and community support.
*Mary Guardino, Founder & Executive Director*

1392 **Mood Disorders Center**
600 North Wolfe Street 410-955-5212
Baltimore, MD 21218 877-666-3754
www.hopkinsmedicine.org

The Mood Disorders Center at Johns Hopkins Medicine provides specialized clinical services to patients with mood disorders; conducts research on the causes of mood disorders, treatment responses, and brain function and structure; and educates patients, caregivers, and the public on mood disorders through symposia, publications, community presentations, and the Adolescent Depression Awareness Program.
*J. Raymond DePaulo, MD, Co-Director*
*Kay Redfield Jamison, PhD, Co-Director*

1393 **National Alliance on Mental Illness (NAMI)**
4301 Wilson Boulevard 703-524-7600
Arlington, VA 22203 800-950-6264
nami.org

NAMI is an organization dedicated to raising awareness on mental health and providing support and education for Americans affected by mental illness. NAMI advocates for access to services and treatment and fosters an environment of awareness and understanding for those concerned with mental health.
*Joyce A. Campbell, President*
*Daniel H. Gillison, Jr., CEO*

1394 **National Association for the Dually Diagnosed (NADD)**
321 Wall Street 845-331-4336
Kingston, NY 12401 info@thenadd.org
thenadd.org

NADD is a nonprofit organization designed to increase awareness of, and provide services for, individuals with developmental disabilities and mental illness. NADD emphasizes the importance of quality mental healthcare for people with mental health needs and offers conferences, information resources, educational programs, and training materials to professionals, parents, and organizations.
*Jeanne M. Farr, MA, Chief Executive Officer*
*Robert J. Fletcher, DSW, Founder & CEO Emeritus*

1395 **National Institute of Mental Health**
6001 Executive Boulevard 866-615-6464
Bethesda, MD 20892-9663 nimhinfo@nih.gov
nimh.nih.gov

The National Institute of Mental Health conducts clinical research on mental disorders and seeks to expand knowledge on mental health treatments.
*Joshua A. Gordon, M.D., Ph. D., Director*

1396 **Postpartum Support International**
6706 Southwest 54th Avenue 503-894-9453
Portland, OR 97219 800-944-4773
Fax: 503-894-9452
postpartum.net

A nonprofit organization focused on providing support for pregnant, post-loss, and postpartum women across the world. Postpartum Support International seeks to raise awareness about the emotional and mental health issues that women face during pregnancy and postpartum.
*Wendy N. Davis, PhD, Executive Director*
*Lianne Swanson, Executive Administrator*

1397 **Sutcliffe Clinic**
851 Fremont Avenue 650-941-1698
Los Altos, CA 94024 Fax: 650-434-1953
info@sutcliffedbp.com
www.sutcliffeclinic.com

Sutcliffe Developmental & Behavioral Pediatrics is an organization that specializes in the treatment of ADHD, autism spectrum disorder, anxiety disorders, conduct disorders, learning disabilities, and more. Sutcliffe works with community services, school districs, and primary physicians, and provides family counseling.
*Trenna Sutcliffe, MD, MS, Medical Director*

1398 **Thriving Minds**
10524 E. Grand River Avenue 810-225-3417
Brighton, MI 48116 office@thrivingminds.info
www.thrivingmindsbehavioralhealth.com

Thriving Minds is an organization that offers therapy to people with anxiety, behavioral issues, and depression. With locations in Brighton and Chelsea, Thriving Minds uses a mix of research-based interventions, such as Cognitive Behavioral Therapy; parent coaching; and school interventions in order to help children, teens, and adults deal with their anxiety.
*Amiee Kotrba, PhD, Owner*
*Bryce Hella, PhD, Director, Brighton Clinic*

## Foundations

1399 **Brain & Behavior Research Foundation**
747 Third Avenue 646-681-4888
New York, NY 10017 800-829-8289
info@bbrfoundation.org
www.bbrfoundation.org

The Brain and Behavior Research Foundation awards grants aimed at advancing scientific understandings of mental health treatments and mental disorders such as depression and schizophrenia. The

Foundation's mission is to eliminate the suffering caused by mental illness.
*Geoffrey A. Simon, Chairman*
*Miriam E. Katowitz, CPA, Vice President*

1400 **Centre for Addiction and Mental Health Foundation**
1451 Queen Street West 416-979-6909
Toronto, ON, M6R-1A1 800-414-0471
foundation@camh.ca
www.camh.ca
CAMH Foundation supports people affected by mental health and addiction issues through fundraising, research, education, policy development, clinical care, and the promotion of health.
*Deborah Gillis, President & CEO*
*Gina Daya, CFO*

1401 **International Foundation for Research and Education on Depression (iFred)**
P.O. Box 17598 Fax: 443-782-0739
Baltimore, MD 21297 info@ifred.org
www.ifred.org
Mission is to alleviate mental health stigma and inspire hope through marketing campaigns, positive imagery, and celebrity engagement.
*Kathryn Goetzke, MBA, Founder*
*Tom Dean, Chair*

1402 **The Jed Foundation**
530 7th Avenue 212-647-7544
New York, NY 10018 Fax: 212-647-7542
jedfoundation.org
JED offers programs to teens and young adults to improve mental health, minimize potential harm, and prevent suicide in the U.S.
*Rebecca Benghiat, President & COO*
*John MacPhee, CEO*

## Libraries & Resource Centers

1403 **National Mental Health Consumers' Self-Help Clearinghouse**
selfhelpclearinghouse@gmail.com
mhselfhelp.org
The Clearinghouse is a peer-run national technical assistance center focused on achieving respect and equality of opportunity for those with mental illnesses. The Clearinghouse helps with the growth of the mental health consumer movement by evaluating mental health services, advocating for mental health reform, and providing consumers with news, information, publications, and consultation services.
*Joseph Rogers, Founder & Executive Director*
*Susan Rogers, Director*

## Research Centers

1404 **UAMS Psychiatric Research Institute**
University of Arkansas for Medical Sciences
4224 Shuffield Drive 501-526-8100
Little Rock, AR 72205 psychiatry.uams.edu
Combining research, education and clinical services into one facility, PRI offers inpatiend and outpatient services, with 40 psychiatric beds, therapy options, and specialized treatment for specific disorders, including: addictive eating, anxiety, deppressive and post-traumatic stress disorders. Research focuses on evidence-based care takes into consideration the education of future medical personnel while relying on research scientists to provide innovative forms of treatment.
*Donald R. Bobbitt, President*
*William Bowes, MS, Vice Chancellor, Finance*

1405 **University of Texas: Mental Health Clinical Research Center**
6363 Forest Park Road 214-648-3111
Dallas, TX 75390 utsouthwestern.edu
Research activity of major and atypical depression.

1406 **Yale Mood Disorders Research Program**
Department of Psychiatry
300 George Street 203-785-2090
New Haven, CT 06511 psychiatry.yale.edu
MDRP is dedicated to understanding the science of mood disorders, including bipolar disorder and depression. The MDRP brings together a multi-disciplinary group of scientists from across the Yale campus in a highly collaborative research effort. Goals of the MDRP include the identification of biological markers for mood disorders and discovery of new treatment strategies.
*John H. Krystal, Chair*
*Rajita Sinha, Chief, Psychology Section*

## Support Groups & Hotlines

1407 **Depressed Anonymous**
P.O. Box 17414 502-569-1989
Louisville, KY 40217 depressedanon.com
Formed to provide therapeutic resources for depressed individuals of all ages. Works with the chronically depressed and those recently discharged from health facilities who were treated for depression.

1408 **Emotions Anonymous International Service Center**
2233 University Ave W 651-647-9712
Saint Paul, MN 55114 info@emotionsanonymous.org
emotionsanonymous.org
A community-based organization to provide support managing mental health difficulties. Groups meet weekly to share experiences, strength, and hope.
*Elaine Weber Nelson, Executive Director*

1409 **Recovery International**
1415 W. 22nd Street 312-337-5661
Oak Brook, IL 60523 866-221-0302
info@recoveryinternational.org
www.recoveryinternational.org
Recovery International is an organization that uses a peer-to-peer, self-help training system developed by Abraham Low in order to help individuals with mental health issues lead more productive lives.
*Sandra K. Wilcoxon, Chief Executive Officer*
*Joanne Lampey, President*

## Digital Resources

1410 **Advocate**
National Alliance on Mental Illness (NAMI)
4301 Wilson Boulevard 703-524-7600
Arlington, VA 22203 800-950-6264
www.nami.org
NAMI's Advocate magazine is available to members at least twice a year. Digital editions can be downloaded online. Publishes a variety of mental health topics.

1411 **Insights**
Anxiety & Depression Association of America
8701 Georgia Avenue 240-485-1001
Silver Spring, MD 20910 information@adaa.org
adaa.org
ADAA's free bi-weekly e-newsletter for members and health professionals, anxiety and depression scientists, clinicians and researchers. Publishes news and research on anxiety and depression.
*Charles Nemeroff, MD, PhD, ADAA President*

1412 **NAMI Now**
National Alliance on Mental Illness (NAMI)
4301 Wilson Boulevard 703-524-7600
Arlington, VA 22203 800-950-6264
www.nami.org
NAMI's digital newsletter, available to members, features relevant news and information on mental illness.

## Web Sites

1413 **Befrienders Worldwide**
www.befrienders.org
Support, helplines, and advice.

1414 **Center for Family Support (CFS)**
www.cfsny.org

Devoted to providing support and assistance to individuals with developmental and related disabilities, and to the family members who care for them.

1415 **CyberPsych**
www.cyberpsych.org
Hosts the American Psychoanalyists Foundation, American Association of Suicideology, Society for the Exploration of Psychotherapy Intergration, and Anxiety Disorders Association of America. Also subcategories of the anxiety disorders, as well as general information, including panic disorder, phobias, obsessive compulsive disorder (OCD), social phobia, generalized anxiety disorder, post traumatic stress disorder, and phobias of childhood. Book reviews and links to web pages sharing the topics.

1416 **Depression and Bipolar Support Alliance**
www.dbsalliance.org
Mental health news updates and local support group information.

1417 **EMDR Institute**
www.emdr.com
Discusses EMDR-Eye Movement Desensitization and Reprocessing-as an innovative clinical treatment for trauma, including sexual abuse, domestic violence, combat, crime, and those suffering from a number of other disorders including depressions, addictions, phobias and a variety of self-esteem issues.

1418 **Goodwill-Suncoast**
www.goodwill-suncoast.org
A nonprofit, community-based organization that serves individuals diagnosed as developmentally disabled, with a secondary diagnosis of psychiatric difficulties as evidenced by problem behavior.

1419 **National Alliance on Mental Illness (NAMI)**
www.nami.org
From its inception in 1979, NAMI has been dedicated to improving the lives of individuals and families affected by mental illness.

1420 **National Association for the Dually Diagnosed (NADD)**
www.thenadd.org
An association for persons with developmental disabilities and mental health needs.

1421 **National Institute of Mental Health**
nimh.nih.gov/health/topics/depression
National Institute of Mental Health offers brochures organized by topic. Depression discusses symptoms, diagnosis, and treatment options.

1422 **National Mental Health Consumers' Self-Help Clearinghouse**
www.mhselfhelp.org
Encourages the development and growth of consumer self-help groups.

1423 **Psych Central**
www.psychcentral.com
Personalized one-stop index for psychology, support, and mental health issues, resources, and people on the Internet.

1424 **Psychology Information On-Line: Depression**
www.psychologyinfo.com/depression
Information on diagnosis, therapy, and medication.

1425 **Psycom**
www.psycom.net/depression
Medication-oriented site. Clearinghouse on all types of depressive disorders.

1426 **SAMHSA - Center for Mental Health Services**
www.samhsa.gov
Information about resources, technical assistance, research, training, networks, and other federal clearinghouses, fact sheets and materials.

1427 **UT Southwestern Medical Center**
www.utsouthwestern.edu
Research to find the corticosteroid effects on the human brain, dual-diagnosed patients, and depression in asthma patients.

1428 **Wing of Madness: A Depression Guide**
www.wingofmadness.com
Accurate information, advice, support, and personal experiences.

1429 **Yale School of Medicine**
www.med.yale.edu
Research center dedicated to understanding the science of mood disorders.

# GASTROINTESTINAL (GI) DISORDERS

*Digestive system damage is an increasing problem when coupled with substance use disorder. Substance abuse can contribute to cancers developing in all parts of the digestive system. The gastrointestinal tract (GI) is made up of the mouth, esophagus, stomach, small intestine, large intestine and anus; hollow tubes that move food intake through the body. The liver, pancreas and gallbladder are solid organs found in the digestive system. Digestion is the process that breaks down food into nutrients that the body uses for growth, energy and cell repair. GI disorders can be acute, chronic or long-lasting.*

The digestive process is controlled by hormones and nerves. Signals flow between the GI tract and brain. Hormones tells the body when to make digestive juices to break down food and to tell your body you are hungry or full. The pancreas makes insulin that regulates the breakdown of sugar into usable components available for energy. It also signals the liver to store blood sugar for later use. Nerves that connect the central nervous system to the digestive system control some digestive functions.

Excessive alcohol consumption is associated with colon and rectal cancer. Synthetic drugs such as ecstasy may lead to both digestive and liver (hepatic) damage and vascular complications in the stomach. Pancreatitis is also associated with heavy alcohol use and abuse. Ischemic colitis and enterocolitis may also occur as a result of substance abuse. A variety of medications can cause gastrointestinal disorders which may mimic inflammatory bowel disease (IBD) and irritable bowel syndrome (IBS). Non-steroidal anti-inflammatory drugs, antipsychotics, antidepressants and metformin should be considered as creating adverse reactions, but studies are continuing. Cocaine can impair bowel tissue and cause pain in the abdomen. Opioids tend to cause constipation, acid reflux, and abdominal pain. Hallucinogens are often associated with nausea and vomiting.

With substance use disorder, including alcohol and drugs, it is important to end dependence. Addiction affects the whole body even after cleaning the substances of abuse out of the body. Post-detoxification, treatment should focus on managing cravings and increasing resolve to stay off drugs while improving overall health and wellness. Substance abuse often results in nutritional disorders and deficiencies. Your gut health is important, as nutrients enter the body through the digestive system. For example, excessive alcohol intake causes inflammation in the gut making nutrient absorption difficult. Mood problems affect both the gut and brain, as the GI system is full of nerves. Mental health issues and addiction both can negatively impact the GI system.

Cortisol, the hormone the body produces under stress, may be activated by difficult life circumstances related to addiction. Cortisol can make the walls of the intestines overly permeable, allowing toxins and pathogens to leak into the bloodstream affecting mood and increasing sensitivity to stress. Alcohol and drugs put a strain on your GI tract and poor digestion and constipation are often seen in people with substance use disorder.

In addition to getting substance use disorder treatment, there are other things that may help:

- Take a probiotic supplement to decrease digestive symptoms and increase good bacteria. Probiotic foods can improve mood and brain function while fighting inflammation.
- Manage constipation with 400-800 mg of magnesium oxide nightly to keep bowels regular.
- Taking anti-inflammatory supplements such as vitamins C and E, curcumin and drinking green or black tea.
- A digestive enzyme supplement may help relieve symptoms of poor digestion.

Focusing on taking better care of the GI system, including with proper nutrition and stopping unneeded substances will aid in proper nutrition necessary to maintaining a healthy body.

## Agencies & Associations

1430 **Academy of Nutrition & Dietetics**
120 South Riverside Plaza 312-899-0040
Chicago, IL 60606-6995 800-877-1600
www.eatright.org
Serves the public through the promotion of optimal nutrition, health, and well-being. Formerly the American Dietetic Association.
*Ellen R. Shanley, President*

1431 **American College of Gastroenterology**
6400 Goldsboro Road 301-263-9000
Bethesda, MD 20817 www.gi.org
ACG serves clinical and scientific information needs of member physicians and surgeons, who specialize in digestive and related disorders. Emphasis is on scholarly practice, teaching, and research.
*Daniel J. Pambianco, MD, FACG, President*
*Amy S. Oxentenko, MD, FACG, Vice President*

1432 **American Gastroenterological Association**
4930 Del Ray Avenue 301-654-2055
Bethesda, MD 20814 Fax: 301-654-5920
member@gastro.org
www.gastro.org
AGA fosters the development and application of the science of gastroenterology by providing leadership and aid including patient care, research, teaching, continuing education, scientific communication, and matters of national health policy.
*Tom Serena, CEO*
*Jessica Duncan, VP, Communications*

1433 **American Motility Society**
45685 Harmony Lane 734-699-1130
Belleville, MI 48111 Fax: 734-699-1136
admin@motilitysociety.org
www.motilitysociety.org
Promotes research and sponsors professional education seminars about gastrointestinal motility topics including disorders of esophageal, gastric, small intestinal, and colonic function; and sponsors biennial meetings (even years), syposia and courses.
*John Pandolfino, MD, President*
*Lori Ennis, Executive Director*

1434 **American Pancreatic Association**
2508 West 71st Street 913-402-7102
Prairie Village, KS 66208 apa@apapancreas.org
www.american-pancreatic-association.org
Membership organization for physicians and researchers interested in diseases of the pancreas.
*Min Li, PhD, President*
*Ashok Saluja, PhD, Secretary-Treasurer*

1435 **American Society for Gastrointestinal Endoscopy**
3300 Woodcreek Drive 630-573-0600
Downers Grove, IL 60515 800-353-2743
Fax: 630-963-8332
info@asge.org
www.asge.org
ASGE provides information, training, and practice guidelines about gastrointestinal endoscopic techniques.
*Bret T. Petersen, MD, MASGE, President*
*Donald J. Palmisano, Jr., JD, CAE, CEO*

1436 **American Society for Parenteral and Enteral Nutrition (ASPEN)**
8401 Colesville Road 301-587-6315
Silver Spring, MD 20910 Fax: 301-587-2365
aspen@nutritioncare.org
www.nutritioncare.org
Offers information and continuing medical education to professionals involved in the care of parenterally and enterally fed patients. Membership includes complimentary subscriptions to peer-reviewed journals.
*Ryan T. Hurt, President*
*Wanda Johnson, CEO*

1437 **Cyclic Vomiting Syndrome Association**
P.O. Box 270341 414-342-7880
Milwaukee, WI 53227 cvsa@cvsaonline.org
www.cvsaonline.org
CVSA provides opportunities for patients, families and professionals to offer and receive support and share knowledge about cyclic vomiting syndrome. Actively promotes and facilitates medical research about nausea and vomiting.
*Blynda Killian, President*
*Kristin Koch, Secretary*

1438 **Digestive Disease National Coalition**
50 F. St. NW 202-544-7497
Washington, DC 20001 Fax: 202-546-7105
www.ddnc.org
Informs the public and the healthcare community about digestive disorders; seeks Federal funding for research, education, and training; and represents members' interests regarding Federal and State legislation that affects digestive diseases research.
*Ceciel Rooker, Chair*
*James DeGerome, MD, Director, Development*

1439 **National Kidney and Urologic Diseases Information Clearinghouse**
31 Center Drive 800-860-8747
Bethesda, MD 20892 TTY: 866-569-1162
healthinfo@niddk.nih.gov
www.niddk.nih.gov
Established to increase knowledge and understanding about digestive diseases among people with these conditions and their families, healthcare professionals, and the general public. To carry out this mission, NDDIC works closely with a coordinating panel of representatives from Federal agencies, voluntary organizations on the national level, and professional groups to identify and respond to informational needs about digestive diseases.
*Griffin P. Rodgers, Director*
*Gregory Germino, Deputy Director*

1440 **North American Society for Pediatric Gastroenterology, Hepatology & Nutrition**
714 N. Bethlehem Pike 215-641-9800
Ambler, PA 19002 Fax: 215-641-1995
naspghan@naspghan.org
www.naspghan.org
Promotes research and provides a forum for professionals in the areas of pediatric GI liver disease, gastroenterology, and nutrition. Associated with fellow organizations in Europe and Australia (ESPGAN, AUSPGAN).
*Margaret K. Stallings, Executive Director*
*Kim Rose, Associate Director*

1441 **Northwestern Medicine Digestive Health Center**
www.nm.org
Multifaceted program to meet the needs of people who suffer from gastrointestinal problems; offers literature, videotapes, and educational meetings and, if medical care is needed, appropriate referrals are made.
*Dean M. Harrison, CEO*
*Howard B. Chrisman, MD, President & COO*

1442 **Society for Surgery of the Alimentary Tract (SSAT)**
500 Cummings Center 978-927-8330
Beverly, MA 01915 Fax: 978-524-0461
www.ssat.com
SSAT provides a forum for exchange of information among physicians specializing in alimentary tract surgery.
*Jean Nicolas Vauthey, MD, Chair*
*Jennifer F. Tseng, MD, MPH, President*

1443 **Society of American Gastrointestinal Endoscopic Surgeons (SAGES)**
11300 W Olympic Boulevard 310-437-0544
Los Angeles, CA 90064 www.sages.org
SAGES encourages study and practice of gastrointestinal endoscopy, laparoscopy and minimal access surgery.
*John D. Mellinger, MD, President*
*Brent D. Matthews, MD, Secretary*

**1444 Society of Gastroenterology Nurses and Associates**
330 N. Wabash Avenue 312-321-5165
Chicago, IL 60611 Fax: 312-673-6694
info@sgna.org
www.sgna.org
SGNA provides members with continuing education opportunities, practice and training guidelines, and information about trends and development in the field of gastroenterology.
*Nancy Denton, BSN, RN, CGRN, President*
*Kim Eskew, MBA, CAE, Executive Director*

**1445 United Ostomy Associations of America**
P.O. Box 525 800-826-0826
Kennebunk, ME 04043-0525 www.ostomy.org
A national network for bowel and urinary diversion support groups in the United States. Its goal is to provide a non-profit association that will serve to unify and strengthen its member support groups, which are organized for the benefit of people who have, or will have intestinal or urinary diversions and their caregivers.
*James Murray, President*
*Christine Ryan, Executive Director*

## Foundations

**1446 American Porphyria Foundation**
3475 Valley Rd. NW 301-347-7166
Atlanta, GA 30305 866-APF-3635
general@porphyriafoundation.org
www.porphyriafoundation.com
The APF is dedicated to improving the health and well-being of individuals and families affected by porphyria. Their mission is to enhance public awareness about porphyria, develop educational programs and distributing educational material for patients and physicians and support research to improve treatment and ultimately lead to a cure.
*Warren Hudson, Chair*
*Desiree Lyon, Executive Director*

**1447 Canadian Digestive Health Foundation**
2525 Old Bronte Road 905-847-2002
Oakville, ON, L6M-4J2 cdhf.ca
CDHF is committed to providing Canadians with the latest research and information on how to manage digestive conditions.
*Tara Petch, VP, Parternships & Strategic Initiatives*
*Kelsey Cheyne, Executive Director*

**1448 Gastro-Intestinal Research Foundation**
1954 First Street 312-332-1350
Highland Park, IL 60035 info@girf.org
www.giresearchfoundation.org
Provides funds for equipment, laboratories, and the support of investigators and young physicians in the University of Chicago Gastroenterology Section - a group of full-time dedicated doctors who seek solutions to gastrointestinal illnesses affecting the esophagus, the stomach, the small intestine, the large intestine, the liver, the gallbladder, and the pancreas.
*Yekaterina Chudnovsky, President*
*Jackie Casey, Executive Director*

**1449 International Foundation for Functional Gastrointestinal Disorders (IFFGD)**
537 Long Point Rd. 414-964-1799
Mount Pleasant, SC 29464 www.iffgd.org
Non-profit education, support, and research organization devoted to increasing awareness and understanding of functional gastrointestinal disorders, including irritable bowel syndrome (IBS), constipation, diarrhea, pain, and incontinence. Mission is to inform, assist, and support people affected by these disorders.
*Nancy J. Norton, Founder*
*Ceciel T. Rooker, President*

**1450 NASPGHAN Foundation**
714 N. Bethlehem Pike 215-641-9800
Ambler, PA 19002 Fax: 215-641-1995
naspghan@naspghan.org
www.naspghan.org
The foundation's sole mission is to improve the treatment and management of gastrointestinal, hepatobiliary, pancreatic, and nutritional disorders in children.
*Menno Verhave, MD, President*
*Jeannie S. Huang, MD, MPH, Secretary-Treasurer*

**1451 Oley Foundation**
Albany Medical Center
99 Delaware Avenue 518-262-5079
Delmar, NY 12054 Fax: 518-262-5528
www.oley.org
Promotes and advocates education and research in home parenteral and enteral nutrition; provides support and networking to patients through information clearinghouse and regional volunteer networks; and sponsors meetings and conferences, including annual patient/clinician conference.
*Beth Gore, PhD, Executive Director*
*Joan Bishop, Executive Director Emeritus*

**1452 Society for Surgery of the Alimentary Foundation**
500 Cummings Center 978-927-8330
Beverly, MA 01915 Fax: 978-524-0461
ssat.com/foundation
Provides funding for surgeon-scientists.

## Libraries & Resource Centers

**1453 American Hemochromatosis Society**
www.americanhs.org
Educates the public, the medical community, and the media by distributing the most current information available on hereditary hemochromatosis (HH), including DNA screening for HH and pediatric HH. Also facilitates patient empowerment through an online network.
*Sandra Thomas, President/Founder*

**1454 Oley Foundation**
Albany Medical Center
99 Delaware Avenue 518-262-5079
Delmar, NY 12054 Fax: 518-262-5528
www.oley.org
Promotes and advocates education and research in home parenteral and enteral nutrition; provides support and networking to patients through information clearinghouse and regional volunteer networks; and sponsors meetings and conferences, including an annual patient/clinician conference.
*Beth Gore, PhD, Executive Director*
*Joan Bishop, Executive Director Emeritus*

## Research Centers

**1455 ACG Institute for Clinical Research and Education**
6400 Goldsboro Road 301-263-9000
Bethesda, MD 20817 gi.org/acg-institute
Innovation center and source of funding for clinically oriented research and education into gastroenterology.
*Neena S. Abraham, MD, MSc, MACG, Director*

**1456 Baylor College of Medicine: General Clinical Research Center for Adults**
One Baylor Plaza 713-798-4951
Houston, TX 77030 dbier@bcm.edu
www.bcm.edu/pediatrics
Endocrinology, genetics and gastroenterology research.
*Dennis M. Bier, MD, Program Director*
*Paul Klotman, President*

**1457 Digestive Disorders Associates Ridgely Oaks Professional Center**
Ridgely Oaks Professional Center
621 Ridgely Avenue 41 -22 -488
Annapolis, MD 21401 800-273-0505
Fax: 410-224-6971
TTY: 800-735-2258
www.dda.net

Specializes in the diagnosis and treatment of diseases of the entire digestive system including esophagus, stomach, small and large intestine, colon, liver, pancreas, and gall bladder.
*Michael S. Epstein, Founder*
*Charles E. King, Doctor*

1458 **Gastro-Intestinal Research Foundation**
1954 First Street 312-332-1350
Highland Park, IL 60035 info@girf.org
www.giresearchfoundation.org
Founded to help combat gastrointestinal diseases. Raises funds to support research at the Center for study of the Digestive Diseases at the University of Chicago Medical Center and to support advanced training for scientists. Sponsors educational activities for the public.
*Yekaterina Chudnovsky, President*
*Jackie Casey, Executive Director*

1459 **North American Society for Pediatric Gastroenterology, Hepatology & Nutrition**
714 N. Bethlehem Pike 215-641-9800
Ambler, PA 19002 Fax: 215-641-1995
naspghan@naspghan.org
www.naspghan.org
Promotes research and provides a forum for professionals in the areas of pediatric GI liver disease, gastroenterology, and nutrition. Provides resources and programs to encourage the advancement of pediatric gastroenterologists, hepatologists, and nutritionists.
*Margaret K. Stallings, Executive Director*
*Kim Rose, Associate Director*

1460 **University of California: Davis Gastroenterology & Nutrition Center**
Pediatric GI Medical Center
4900 Broadway 91- 73- 904
Sacramento, CA 95820 www.ucdmc.ucdavis.edu
Research into gastrointestinal mobility and electro-physiology nutrition support and references for the public and patient evaluations.
*Bonnie Hyatt, Assistant Director*
*Jenny Carrick, Sr. Dir., Communications*

1461 **University of California: Los Angeles Center for Ulcer Research**
LA Medical Center
Building 115 Room 117 310-312-9284
Los Angeles, CA 90073 Fax: 310-268-4963
cureadmn@mednet.ucla.edu
www.cure.med.ucla.edu
Offers basic and clinical research related to peptic ulcer disease, including causes, checks and balances, and stress-ulcer relationships.
*Enrique Rozengurt, Director*
*Emeran Mayer, Co-Director*

1462 **University of Michigan Michigan Gastrointestinal Peptide Research Ctr.**
U-M Health System
1500 E Medical Center Drive 734-936-4000
Ann Arbor, MI 48109 Fax: 734-763-2535
www.med.umich.edu/mgpc
Research into gastroenterology, including chemistry of gut hormones, is studied.
*Chung Owyang, MD, Director*
*Juanita Merc, MD, PhD, Associate Director*

1463 **University of Pennsylvania: Harrison Department of Surgical Research**
3400 Spruce Street 215-662-4000
Philadelphia, PA 19104 800-789-PENN
Fax: 215-615-0471
www.uphs.upenn.edu/surgery/res/harrisonr
Offers research and studies on surgical transplantations and gastrointestinal physiology.
*Julie Hagan Koehler MBA, Business Director*
*Georgina Suarez, Administrative Assistant*

## Support Groups & Hotlines

1464 **National Health Information Center**
Office of Disease Prevention & Health Promotion
1101 Wootton Pkwy Fax: 240-453-8281
Rockville, MD 20852 odphpinfo@hhs.gov
www.health.gov/nhic
Supports public health education by maintaining a calendar of National Health Observances; helps connect consumers and health professionals to organizations that can best answer questions and provide up-to-date contact information from reliable sources; updates on a yearly basis toll-free numbers for health information, Federal health clearinghouses and info centers.
*Don Wright, MD, MPH, Director*

1465 **Pull-thru Network**
2312 Savoy Street 205-978-2930
Hoover, AL 35226 www.pullthrough.org
Dedicated to the needs of those born wutith anorectal malformation or colon disease and any of the associated diagnoses.

## Print Resources

1466 **ASAP Forum**
ASAP International Corporate Headquarters
19 Carroll Road 781-935-9776
Woburn, MA 01801 Fax: 781-933-4151
asapgi@sprynet.com
Educates the general public and medical community about chronic intestinal pseudo-obstruction (CIP) and other related digestive motility disorders; serves as an integral source of information for patients of all ages with CIP and related disorders, their families, and members of the medical community.

1467 **American Journal of Gastroenterology**
American College of Gastroenterology
6400 Goldsboro Rd 301-263-9000
Bethesda, MD 20817 gi.org/journals-publications
Serves clinical and scientific information needs of member physicians and surgeons, who specialize in digestive and related disorders. Emphasis is on scholarly practice, teaching, and research.
*Jasmohan Bajaj, MD, MS, FACG, Co-Editor-in-Chief*
*Millie Long, MD, MPH, FACG, Co-Editor-in-Chief*

1468 **Clinical Perspectives in Gastroenterology and Hepatology**
American Gastroenterological Association
4930 Del Ray Avenue 301-654-2055
Bethesda, MD 20814 Fax: 301-654-5920
member@gastro.org
www.gastro.org
Focuses on research, medical and professional developments in the science of gastroenterology.
*Charles J. Kahi, Editor-in-Chief*
*Siddharth Singh, Senior Associate Editor*

1469 **Food & Nutrition**
120 South Riverside Plaza 312-899-0040
Chicago, IL 60606 800-877-1600
foodandnutrition@eatright.org
www.eatright.org
Formerly the ADA Times, Food & Nutrition is the member and professional magazine of the Academy of Nutrition & Dietetics.

1470 **Gastroenterology**
American Gastroenterological Association
4930 Del Ray Avenue 301-654-2055
Bethesda, MD 20814 Fax: 301-654-5920
member@gastro.org
www.gastro.org
Focuses on research, medical, and professional developments in the science of gastroenterology.
*Paul Moayyedi, Co-Editor-in-Chief*
*David S. Weinberg, Co-Editor-in-Chief*

1471 **Gastroenterology Nursing**
Society of Gastroenterology Nurses and Associates
330 N. Wabash Ave. 312-321-5165
Chicago, IL 60611 Fax: 312-673-6694
www.sgna.org

Provides members with information about trends and developments in the field of gastroenterology nursing.
*Kathy A. Baker, Editor-in-Chief*
*Rhoda Redulla, Associate Editor*

1472 **Gastrointestinal Endoscopy**
American Society for Gastrointestinal Endoscopy
3300 Woodcreek Dr. 630-573-0600
Downers Grove, IL 60515 866-353-2743
Fax: 630-963-8332
info@asge.org
www.asge.org
Offers information, training, and practice guidelines about gastrointestinal endoscopic techniques.
*Michael B. Wallace, MD, MPH, FASGE, Editor*

1473 **Journal of Gastrointestinal Surgery (JOGS)**
Society for Surgery of the Alimentary Tract
500 Cummings Center 978-927-8330
Beverly, MA 01915 Fax: 978-524-0461
www.ssat.com
Provides information for physicians specializing in gastrointestinal surgery.
*Richard Hodin, Co-Editor-in-Chief*
*Timothy M. Pawlik, Co-Editor-in-Chief*

1474 **Journal of Parenteral and Enteral Nutrition**
ASPEN
8630 Fenton Street 301-587-6315
Silver Spring, MD 20910 Fax: 301-587-2365
aspen@nutr.org
www.nutritioncare.org
Publishes original, peer-reviewed research on nutrition for healthcare professionals. Published eight times a year.
*100 pages*

1475 **Journal of Pediatric Gastroenterology and Nutrition**
N American Society for Pediatric Gastroenterology
6900 Grove Road 609-848-1000
Thorofare, NJ 08086 Fax: 609-848-5274
www.jpgn.org/
Provides information for professionals in the areas of pediatric GI liver disease, gastroenterology, and nutrition.

1476 **Journal of the Academy of Nutrition and Dietetics**
120 South Riverside Plaza 312-899-4831
Chicago, IL 60606 journal@eatright.org
www.eatright.org
Official research publication of the Academy of Nutrition and Dietetics.

1477 **Nutrition in Clinical Practice**
ASPEN
8630 Fenton Street 301-587-6315
Silver Spring, MD 20910 Fax: 301-587-2365
aspen@nutr.org
www.nutritioncare.org
A peer-reviewed, interdisciplinary publication that offers specialized nutrition support. Published six times a year.
*100 pages*

1478 **Pancreas**
American Pancreatic Association
3 Bethesda Metro Center 301-961-1508
Bethesda, MD 20814 866-726-2737
Fax: 301-657-9776
info@pancreasfoundation.org
pancreasfoundation.org
Provides information on scientific research related to the pancreas.
*Joseph M. Titlebaum, Chair*
*Jessica Kruse, Secretary*

1479 **Phoenix Magazine**
United Ostomy Association of America
P.O. Box 512 800-826-0826
Northfield, MN 55057 Fax: 507-645-5168
info@uoaa.org
www.uoa.org
America's leading ostomy patient magazine providing colostomy, ileostomy, urostomy and continent diversion information, management techniques, new products and much more.
*David Rudzin, President*

## Web Sites

1480 **Academy of Nutrition & Dietetics**
www.eatright.org
Offers information and support to allergy sufferers. Serves the public through the promotion of optimal nutrition, health, and well-being. Formerly the American Dietetic Association.

1481 **American College of Gastroenterology**
www.gi.org
ACG serves clinical and scientific information needs of member physicians and surgeons, who specialize in digestive and related disorders. Emphasis is on scholarly practice, teaching, and research.

1482 **American Gastroenterological Association**
www.gastro.org
AGA fosters the development and application of the science of gastroenterology by providing leadership and aid including patient care, research, teaching, continuing education, scientific communication and matters of national health policy.

1483 **American Hemochromatosis Society**
www.americanhs.org
Educates the public, the medical community, and the media by distributing the most current information available on hereditary hemochromatosis (HH), including DNA screening for HH and pediatric HH; also facilitates patient empowerment through an online network.

1484 **American Porphyria Foundation**
www.porphyriafoundation.com
Advances awareness, research, and treatment of the porphyrias; provides self-help services for members; and provides referrals to porphyria treatment specialists.

1485 **American Pseudo-Obstruction and Hirschsprung's Disease Society**
Promotes public awareness of gastrointestinal motility disorders, in particular intestinal pseudo-obstruction and Hirschsprung's Disease; provides education and support to individuals and families of children who have been diagnosed with these disorders through parent-to-parent contact, publications, and educational symposia; and encourages and supports medical research in the area of gastrointestinal motility disorders.

1486 **American Society for Gastrointestinal Endoscopy**
www.asge.org
ASGE provides information, training, and practice guidelines about gastrointestinal endoscopic techniques.

1487 **American Society of Abdominal Surgeons**
www.abdominalsurg.org
ASAS sponsors extensive continuing education program for physicians in the field of abdominal surgery and maintains library.

1488 **Background on Functional Gastrointestinal Disorders**
www.med.unc.edu
Statistical background information on gastrointestinal disorders.

1489 **Children's Motility Disorder Foundation**
www.motility.org
CMDF works to increase awareness of pediatric motility disorders in the general public and among the physicians most likely to encounter children suffering from these conditions, such as pediatricians and family practice doctors. Supports medical research regarding the causes, treatment, and potentially life-threatening disorders.

1490 **Cyclic Vomiting Syndrome Association**
www.cvsaonline.org
CVSA provides opportunities for patients, families and professionals to offer and receive support and share knowledge about cyclic vomiting syndrome; actively promotes and facilitates medical research about nausea and vomiting.

1491 **Gastrointestinal Research Foundation**

www.giresearchfoundation.org

Founded to help combat gastrointestinal diseases. Raises funds to support research at the Center for the study of the Digestive Diseases at the University of Chicago Medical Center and to support advanced training for scientists. Sponsors educational activities for the public.

1492 **Healing Well**

www.healingwell.com

An online health resource guide to medical news, chat, information and articles, newsgroups and message boards, books, disease-related web sites, medical directories, and more for patients, friends, and family coping with disabling diseases, disorders, or chronic illnesses.

1493 **Healthlink USA**

www.healthlinkusa.com

Health information concerning treatment, cures, prevention, diagnosis, risk factors, research, support groups, email lists, personal stories and much more. Updated regularly.

1494 **Hemochromatosis Foundation**

www.hemochromatosis.org

Provides information to the public, families, and professionals about hereditary hemochromatosis (HH); conducts and raises funds for research; encourages early screening for HH; holds symposiums and meetings; and offers genetic counseling along with support for patients, families, and professionals.

1495 **Inside Tract**

theinsidetract.sgna.org

Content brand of the Society of Gastroenterology Nurses and Associates, with an online portal featuring analysis, editorials, behind the scenes, education, and more.

1496 **International Foundation for Functional Gastrointestinal Disorders (IFFGD)**

www.iffgd.org

Non-profit education, support, and research organization devoted to increasing awareness and understanding of functional gastrointestinal disorders, including irritable bowel syndrome (IBS), constipation, diarrhea, pain, and incontinence. Mission is to inform, assist and support people affected by these disorders.

1497 **MedicineNet**

www.medicinenet.com

An online resource for consumers providing easy-to-read, authoritative medical and health information.

1498 **Medscape**

www.medscape.com

Medscape offers specialists, primary care physicians, and other health professionals the Web's most robust and integrated medical information and educational tools.

1499 **MyHealthfinder**

www.healthfinder.gov

Searchable, carefully developed web site offering information on over 1000 topics. Developed by the US Department of Health and Human Services, the site can be used in both English and Spanish.

1500 **National Kidney and Urologic Diseases Information Clearinghouse**

www.niddk.nih.gov

Offers various educational information, resources and reprints focusing on ulcerative colitis and Crohn's disease.

1501 **North American Society for Pediatric Gastroenterology, Hepatology & Nutrition**

www.naspghan.org

NASPGHAN strives to improve the care of infants, children and adolescents with digestive disorders by promoting advances in clinical care, research and education.

1502 **Nutrition in Clinical Practice**

www.nutritioncare.org

NCP is indexed by PubMed (MEDLINE), Cumulative Index to Nursing and Allied Health Literature, International Nursing Index, International Pharmaceutical Index, Reference Update, Silver Platter, TOXLINE and UMI.

1503 **Oley Foundation**

www.oley.org

Enriches the lives of those requiring home IV & tube feeding through education, outreach, & networking.

1504 **Pull-thru Network**

www.pullthrunetwork.org

Pull-thru Network (PTN) was founded in 1988 and has grown to be one of the largest organizations in the world dedicated to the needs of those born with an anorectal malformation or colon disease and any of the associated diagnoses

1505 **Society for Surgery of the Alimentary Tract**

www.ssat.com

SSAT provides a forum for exchange of information among physicians specializing in alimentary tract surgery.

1506 **Society of American Gastrointestinal Endoscopic Surgeons**

www.sages.org

SAGES encourages the study and practice of gastrointestinal endoscopy, laparoscopy, and minimal access surgery.

1507 **United Ostomy Associations of America, Inc.**

www.ostomy.org

A national network for bowel and urinary diversion support groups in the United States. Its goal is to provide a non-profit association that will serve to unify and strengthen its member support groups, which are organized for the benefit of people who have, or will have intestinal or urinary diversions and their caregivers.

1508 **WebMD**

www.webmd.com

Provides credible information, supportive communities, and in-depth reference material about health subjects. A source for original and timely health information, as well as material from well-known content providers.

# HEPATITIS

*Hepatitis is an inflammation of the liver resulting in swelling that happens when tissues of the body are injured or infected. This swelling interferes with liver function that is essential to life. People with substance use disorders or engage in high-risk behaviors increase their risk of getting a variety of viral infections including hepatitis. Viruses spread through blood and body fluids generally when sharing needles or drug paraphernalia, or when drugs impair judgement, such as leading to unprotected sex. Transmission from an infected mother to the baby at birth is possible. Poor hygiene, such as not washing hands after using the toilet, may also transmit the virus. Poor farming practices may also lead to contaminated food entering the food supply such as recent outbreaks due to organic strawberries, lettuce and scallops.*

There are different types of hepatitis with different causes, including:

- Viral hepatitis, the most common, caused by one of several viruses: A, B, C, and E with A, B, and C the most common in the U.S.
- Alcoholic hepatitis caused by heavy alcohol use and abuse
- Toxic hepatitis caused by certain poisons, medicines, chemicals or supplements
- Autoimmune hepatitis, a chronic hepatitis, when the body's immune system attacks the liver. While the cause is unknown, genetics and environment may play a role.

Hepatitis A and hepatitis E are spread through contact with water or food contaminated with an infected person's stool (feces). Not washing hands after going to the toilet is usually what causes exposure, as the viruses are spread from hands to food. Hepatitis E may be contracted by eating undercooked pork, deer or shellfish. Hepatitis B, C and D are spread through contact with an infected person's blood. Healthcare providers wear gloves to prevent exposure to blood and body fluids. Hepatitis B and D may also be spread by infected bodily fluids, such as when sharing needles or having unprotected sex. Excessive drinking and unprotected sex are two of the most common contributing factors to developing the disease.

Individuals who use or inject drugs should be vaccinated against hepatitis A, and individuals who inject drugs should also be vaccinated against hepatitis B. Testing for hepatitis B and C should occur in all individuals who inject drugs. There is no vaccine for hepatitis C, but prevention includes avoiding behaviors that spread the disease, such as injecting drugs and getting prompt treatment, as cure can occur in 8-12 weeks after testing.

In substance use disorder, drug and alcohol use can directly damage the liver, increasing the risk for chronic liver disease and cancer. To decrease risks, stop using drugs and sharing drug paraphernalia, get tested and treated for viral infections, practice safe sex every time and get treatment for substance use disorder.

While some people infected with hepatitis may not exhibit symptoms, if you do have symptoms of hepatitis they may include:

- Fatigue
- Fever

- Loss of appetite
- Nausea and/or vomiting
- Dark urine
- Abdominal pain
- Clay-colored bowel movements
- Joint pain
- Yellowing of skin and eyes, known as jaundice

Acute infections may cause symptoms at 2 weeks to 6 months after infection. Some chronic forms of hepatitis may not exhibit symptoms until many years later.

Hepatitis infections may lead to scarring of the liver, called cirrhosis, liver failure and liver cancer. Early diagnosis and treatment may help.

An individual can lower the hepatitis risk or even prevent the disease depending on the type of hepatitis exposure. Limiting alcohol prevents alcoholic hepatitis. Safe sex and not sharing needles prevents transmission. Proper hygiene can limit exposure risks. Vaccines are available for prevention of hepatitis A and B. Autoimmune hepatitis can not be prevented. Testing for hepatitis is important for early intervention and treatment.

## Agencies & Associations

1509 **Autoimmune Hepatitis Association**
P.O. Box 844 info@aihep.org
Wayzata, MN 55391-0844 www.aihep.org
Offers support and hope to individuals living with autoimmune hepatitis, and their families. Provides national conferences, virtual support groups, education and research opportunities.
*Craig Lammert, M.D., Executive Director*
*Lisa Devereaux, Executive Member, Secretary/Treasurer*

1510 **Centers for Disease Control & Prevention Hepatitis Branch**
1600 Clifton Road NE 800-232-4636
Atlanta, GA 30329 TTY: 888-232-6348
www.cdc.gov/hepatitis
Monitors the rates of viral hepatitis in the United States, provides epidemiologic assistance for outbreaks of viral hepatitis and coordinates studies to define the risk factors for acute and chronic viral hepatitis.

1511 **HepCoalition**
contact@hepcoalition.org
hepcoalition.org
hepCoalition is a global advocacy network focused on improving access to hepatitis C (HCV) diagnostics, treatments, and care in low-and middle-income countries for people who are most affected, particularly people who use drugs.

1512 **Hepatitis C Association, Inc.**
1351 Cooper Road 908-769-8479
Scotch Plains, NJ 07076-2844 Dennis@hepcassoc.org
hepcassoc.org
Mission is to educate the public about hepatitis C virus through educational programs and materials.
*Susan Simon, President*
*Dennis Simon, Treasurer/Secretary*

1513 **Immunization Action Coalition**
2136 Ford Parkway 651-647-9009
St. Paul, MN 55116 Fax: 651-647-9131
admin@immunize.org
www.immunize.org
The mission of the Immunization Action Coalition is to boost immunization rates and prevent disease. The coalition promotes physician, community and family awareness of and responsibility for appropriate immunization of all children and adults against all diseases.
*Kelly L. Moore, MD, MPH, President & CEO*
*Julie Murphy, MA, Director, Development*

## Foundations

1514 **Hepatitis B Foundation**
3805 Old Easton Road 215-489-4900
Doylestown, PA 18902 Fax: 215-489-4920
info@hepb.org
www.hepb.org
Dedicated to finding a cure and improving the quality of life for those affected by hepatitis B worldwide. Funds research; promotes disease awareness; supports immunization and treatment initiatives; and serves as the primary source of information for patients and their families, the medical and scientific community, and the general public.
*Chari A. Cohen, DrPH, MPH, President*
*Jean Holmes, MBA, VP, Institutional Advancement*

1515 **National Foundation for Infectious Diseases (NFID)**
7201 Wisconsin Avenue 301-656-0003
Bethesda, MD 20814 nfid.org/infectious-diseases/hepatitis/
NFID is a non-profit organization that provides education to the public and healthcare professionals about infectious diseases.
*Marla Dalton, PE, CAE, Executive Director & CEO*
*Joanna Colbourne, CAE, Deputy Executive Director*

## Libraries & Resource Centers

1516 **Hepatitis Education Project**
911 Western Avenue 206-732-0311
Seattle, WA 98104 Fax: 206-732-0312
hep@scn.org
www.hepeducation.org
The mission of the Hepatitis Education Project is to help raise awareness among patients, medical personnel and the public of the facts concerning hepatitis patients and the resources available to help those who live with the disease.
*Steve Graham, President*
*Michael Ninburg, Executive Director*

## Support Groups & Hotlines

1517 **Christ Hospital Hepatitis C Support Group**
Christ Hospital
176 Palisade Avenue 201-795-1230
Jersey City, NJ 07306 dkatz65717@aol.com
For anyone interested in becoming advocates for increasing awareness of this illness.

1518 **Hepatitis Education Project**
911 Western Avenue 206-732-0311
Seattle, WA 98104 hepinfo@hepeducation.org
www.hepeducation.org
Helps raise awareness among patients, medical personeel and the public of the facts concerning hepatitis patients and the resources available to help those who live with the disease
*Steve Graham, President*
*Michael Ninburg, Executive Director*

1519 **National Health Information Center**
Office of Disease Prevention & Health Promotion
1101 Wootton Pkwy Fax: 240-453-8281
Rockville, MD 20852 odphpinfo@hhs.gov
www.health.gov/nhic
Supports public health education by maintaining a calendar of National Health Observances; helps connect consumers and health professionals to organizations that can best answer questions and provide up-to-date contact information from reliable sources; updates on a yearly basis toll-free numbers for health information, Federal health clearinghouses and info centers.
*Don Wright, MD, MPH, Director*

## Print Resources

1520 **Hepatitis Magazine**
Smart + Strong Publishing
157 Columbus Avenue 212-242-2163
New York, NY 10023-6082 Fax: 212-675-8505
www.hepmag.com
Magazine for those with hepatitis. Price listed is for a one year subscription.
*Oriol Gutierrez, Editor-in-Chief*
*Jennifer Morton, Managing Editor*

1521 **Journal of Viral Hepatitis**
Blackwell Science Ltd.
JVH@wiley.com
onlinelibrary.wiley.com/journal/13652893
This international peer-reviewed journal covers reviews and research in the field of viral hepatitis.
*Graham Foster, Editor-in-Chief*
*Divya Udayakumar, Production Editor*

## Web Sites

1522 **Healing Well**
www.healingwell.com
An online health resource guide to medical news, chat, information and articles, newsgroups and message boards, books, disease-related web sites, medical directories, and more for patients, friends, and family coping with disabling diseases, disorders, or chronic illnesses.

1523 **Healthlink USA**

www.healthlinkusa.com

Health information concerning treatment, cures, prevention, diagnosis, risk factors, research, support groups, email lists, personal stories and much more. Updated regularly.

1524 **Healthy Lives**

www.healthylives.com/hepatitis

1525 **HepCoalition**

hepcoalition.org

hepCoalition is a global advocacy network focused on improving access to hepatitis C (HCV) diagnostics, treatments, and care in low- and middle-income countries for people who are most affected, particularly people who use drugs.

1526 **Hepatitis B Coalition**

www.immunize.org

The Immunization Action Coalition (IAC) works to increase immunization rates and prevent disease by creating and distributing educational materials for health professionals and the public that enhance the delivery of safe and effective immunization services.

1527 **Hepatitis Information Network**

www.hepnet.com

1528 **MedicineNet**

www.medicinenet.com

An online resource for consumers providing easy-to-read, authoritative medical and health information.

1529 **Medscape**

www.medscape.com

Medscape offers specialists, primary care physicians, and other health professionals the Web's most robust and integrated medical information and educational tools.

1530 **MyHealthfinder**

www.healthfinder.gov

Searchable, carefully developed web site offering information on over 1000 topics. Developed by the US Department of Health and Human Services, the site can be used in both English and Spanish.

1531 **WebMD**

www.webmd.com

Provides credible information, supportive communities, and in-depth reference material about health subjects. A source for original and timely health information, as well as material from well-known content providers.

# IMPOTENCE

*There is a significant relationship between substance use disorders and sexual dysfunction, particularly impotence. Impotence, also referred to as erectile dysfunction, is the inability to get and keep an erection sufficient for having sex. Substance use disorder may create a lack of libido, or decrease the interest in sex in both men and women.*

As many as 30 million men may suffer from ED. Substance use disorder (SUD) may increase the risk of impotence and can interfere with sexual performance, even years after stopping drug use. Comorbid sexual dysfunction further complicates the clinical burden of substance abuse. SUD can also negatively impact the reproductive system of both men and women. Sexual dysfunction is said to occur in up to 75 percent of individuals abusing alcohol and in approximately 60 percent of individuals with opioid abuse. Whether a young adult or an older individual, SUD has a detrimental effect on sexual performance.

Erectile dysfunction (ED) is the most common dysfunction linked to substance use. Recreational drugs, alcohol, prescription drugs and over-the-counter drugs affect the body in varying ways and may contribute to ED. Recreational drugs include illegal drugs such as cocaine, but also prescription drugs that are misused. Any recreational substance use has the potential to cause serious damage as they alter the way the body functions. Examples of recreational drugs that contribute to ED and their action include:

- Amphetamines, which cause narrowing of blood vessels and decrease blood flow to the penis, limiting erection
- Barbiturates may decrease interest in sex
- Cannabis may increase sexual desire, but prevents the smooth muscles in the penis from relaxing to allow sufficient blood flow to achieve an erection
- Cocaine, like amphetamines, restricts blood flow to the penis
- Heroin decreases the levels of testosterone and decreases the interest in sex
- Nicotine may decrease sexual desire

Consuming alcohol can affect all body parts responsible for creating an erection and may cause symptoms of ED. Alcohol also lowers testosterone and may damage cells in the testes, preventing the individual from achieving an erection.

Prescription drugs, even when prescribed for a needed diagnosis, may interfere with sexual function. Discussing ED with the physician and the potential to change medications is important. Abusing or misusing prescription drugs may contribute to ED. Common medications that may interfere with sexual performance include:

- Antidepressants that alter chemicals in the brain
- Chemotherapy drugs with the potential to damage the nervous system, including nerves in the penis that control erections
- Blood pressure drugs may prevent smooth muscles in the penis from relaxing and not allowing the individual to maintain an erection

- Drugs that decrease or block testosterone such as older antihistamines, heart drugs, corticosteroids, opioids, and older antipsychotics

Over-the-counter drugs may also contribute to ED. H2 receptor blockers, or heartburn medications, may cause ED in rare cases. At higher doses, these drugs may block testosterone from working leading to a decreased interest in sex.

While there are medications for treating ED, they are not always effective with co-occurring drug use. Stopping substance use and abuse may not "cure" erectile dysfunction. At the first sign of ED, the individual needs to talk with his physician about a treatment plan. If a prescription drug is thought to be the cause, the physician may be able to substitute another drug or change the dose. It may take several days to several weeks after changing or stopping a drug for ED to go away. If substance use disorder is present, the physician should be consulted about treatment options. Stopping recreational drug use "cold turkey" is not recommended as withdrawal symptoms may occur. If substance abuse is significant or long term in nature, permanent ED may result.

## Agencies & Associations

1532 **American Urological Association (AUA)**
1000 Corporate Boulevard
Linthicum, MD 21090
410-689-3700
800-828-7866
Fax: 410-689-3800
aua@auanet.org
www.auanet.org
Supports urological research through funding and advocacy; offers educational opportunities for urologists; and advocates for quality patient care on a federal level. Provides information on impotence and erectile dysfunction to the general public.
*Edward M. Messing, MD, FACS, President*
*Mike Sheppard, CPA, CAE, CEO*

1533 **Canadian Urological Association (CUA)**
185 Dorval Avenue
Dorval, QC, H9S-SJ9
514-395-0376
Fax: 514-395-1664
corporate.office@cua.org
www.cua.org
A member-based organization that represents the Canadian urologic community; provides professional development for urologists; and offers advocacy, education, and research in the field of urologic care.
*Tiffany Pizioli, CEO*
*Dr. Armen Aprikian, President*

1534 **Center for Reconstructive Urology**
333 City Boulevard West
Orange, CA 92868
714-456-2951
Fax: 714-456-7263
www.centerforreconstructiveurology.org
A regional, national, and international tertiary referral center committed to the treatment of male urethra disorders.
*Joel Gelman, MD, Director*

1535 **National Institute of Diabetes & Digestive & Kidney Diseases**
31 Center Drive
Bethesda, MD 20892
800-860-8747
TTY: 866-569-1162
healthinfo@niddk.nih.gov
www.niddk.nih.gov
Research areas include diabetes, digestive diseases, endocrine and metabolic diseases, hematologic diseases, kidney disease, liver disease, urologic diseases, as well as matters relating to nutrition and obesity.
*Griffin P. Rodgers, Director*
*Gregory Germino, Deputy Director*

## Foundations

1536 **Canadian Men's Health Foundation**
609 W. Hastings St.
Vancouver, BC V6B-4W4
604-737-2990
info@menshealthfoundation.ca
menshealthfoundation.ca
Offers e-health resources to reduce men's risk for chronic diseases. Provides medically reviewed information on erectile dysfunction, including causes, symptoms, prevention, and treatment.
*Dr. S. Larry Goldenberg, Founder*
*TC Carling, President & CEO*

1537 **Urology Care Foundation**
100 Corporate Blvd.
Linthicum, MD 21090
410-689-3700
800-828-7866
info@UrologyCareFoundation.org
www.urologyhealth.org
The Urology Care Foundation is committed to promoting urology research and education. They work with researchers, healthcare professionals, patients and caregivers to improve patients' lives.
*Harris M. Nagler, MD, FACS, President*
*Gopal H. Badlani, MD, Secretary*

## Research Centers

1538 **Male Sexual Dysfunction Clinic**
3401 N Central Avenue
Chicago, IL 60634
800-788-2873
800-788-2873
Fax: 847-231-4130
www.msdclinic.com
Helping men overcome male sexual dysfunctions such as impotence since 1981.

1539 **New York Male Reproductive Center: Sexual Dysfunction Unit**
161 Fort Washington Avenue
New York, NY 10032
212-305-0123
Fax: 212-305-0126
The New York Male Reproductive Center at Columbia-Presbyterian Medical Center offers state-of-the-art diagnosis and treatment for impotence. Treatments include surgical and non-surgical procedures.

## Support Groups & Hotlines

1540 **Impotents Anonymous**
8630 Fenton Street
Silver Spring, MD 20910
301-588-5777
Serves as an educational organization providing concerned individuals with information regarding impotence.

1541 **National Health Information Center**
Office of Disease Prevention & Health Promotion
1101 Wootton Pkwy
Rockville, MD 20852
Fax: 240-453-8281
odphpinfo@hhs.gov
www.health.gov/nhic
Supports public health education by maintaining a calendar of National Health Observances; helps connect consumers and health professionals to organizations that can best answer questions and provide up-to-date contact information from reliable sources; updates on a yearly basis toll-free numbers for health information, Federal health clearinghouses and info centers.
*Don Wright, MD, MPH, Director*

## Print Resources

1542 **Journal of Urology**
American Urological Association
1000 Corporate Boulevard
Linthicum, MD 21090
410-689-3700
800-828-7866
Fax: 410-689-3800
www.auajournals.org
Cited as the most widely read and highly cited journal in the field, The Journal of Urology is accessible to members of the American Urological Association. Topics covered include male infertility and erectile dysfunction or impotence.
*D. Robert Siemens, Editor*
*Toby C. Chai, Associate Editor*

## Web Sites

1543 **Healing Well**
www.healingwell.com
An online health resource guide to medical news, chat, information and articles, newsgroups and message boards, books, disease-related web sites, medical directories, and more for patients, friends, and family coping with disabling diseases, disorders, or chronic illnesses.

1544 **Healthlink USA**
www.healthlinkusa.com
Health information concerning treatment, cures, prevention, diagnosis, risk factors, research, support groups, email lists, personal stories and much more. Updated regularly.

1545 **MedicineNet**
www.medicinenet.com
An online resource for consumers providing easy-to-read, authoritative medical and health information.

1546 **Medscape**
www.medscape.com
Medscape offers specialists, primary care physicians, and other health professionals the Web's most robust and integrated medical information and educational tools.

1547 **MyHealthfinder**
www.healthfinder.gov

Searchable, carefully developed web site offering information on over 1000 topics. Developed by the US Department of Health and Human Services, the site can be used in both English and Spanish.

1548 **WebMD**

www.webmd.com

Provides credible information, supportive communities, and in-depth reference material about health subjects. A source for original and timely health information, as well as material from well-known content providers.

# INFERTILITY & PREGNANCY

*A decline in human fertility over the past few decades has occurred. Recent research studies are focused on identifying environmental and lifestyle factors that may be modified to slow the fertility decline. There is a direct correlation between unhealthy habits and poor lifestyle choices on fertility and other diseases. Infertility is defined as 12 months with regular, unprotected sex without being able to conceive. Both legal and illegal substances may play a role in the inability to achieve a pregnancy.*

Unhealthy habits such as tobacco and alcohol use and abuse, and substance use disorders have a negative effect on both male and female fertility and reduce the chance of having a baby. In individuals of reproductive age, more than 30 percent are said to smoke tobacco. Smoking has been documented to have a negative effect on the reproductive system and sexual function. Active and passive smoking have a significant association with female infertility and in utero exposure is related to multiple adverse pregnancy outcomes. Smoking and alcohol consumption during pregnancy have both been linked to increased risks of poor pregnancy outcomes and fetal alcohol syndrome. Smoking and alcohol use may also cause epigenetic changes, or changing the way genes work due to behavior and environment. Epigenetic changes are reversible once the stimulus is removed.

In both men and women, the use of recreational drugs can interfere with fertility and reduce the chance of pregnancy with a healthy baby. All drugs pass into the blood stream and some may directly impact sperm or eggs and reduce fertility. Using marijuana can lower men's sperm count, decrease the amount of semen and reduce the ability of sperm to swim (sperm motility) necessary to fertilize an egg, making pregnancy more difficult to achieve. Heavy cannabis use in women may cause hormonal changes in ovulation, negatively impacting the chance of a pregnancy and may lead to stillbirth.

Using anabolic steroids in body building or competitive sports may cause the testes to shrink, and stops sperm production. After stopping steroids, it may take two years for sperm production to return to normal.

Use of cocaine, heroin and ecstasy over a longer period may lead to permanent reproductive issues for both men and women. More frightening is that recreational drugs may pass directly into the baby's blood stream through the placenta, causing health issues for the baby, should a pregnancy be achieved. If abuse is significant and ongoing, the baby may be born addicted. In pregnant women, heroin use and cocaine use may cause a variety of problems. Placental abruption, when the placenta detaches from the wall of the uterus, premature birth and low birth weight and stillbirth or neonatal death (death around the time of birth) are all ways drug use can affect pregnancy.

Smoking, alcohol use and recreational drug use may impair both male and female fertility. Disruptions in normal production of sperm, semen production and motility in males make achieving pregnancy difficult. Studies in current smokers and prenatally smoke-exposed women suggest a decrease in natural fertility. Alcohol use in men may contribute to a decline in fertility but in women, alcohol use seems to have a minimal impact on fertility. Alcohol use in pregnancy to excess may cause damage to the fetus. Smoking in pregnant women may create a higher chance of ectopic pregnancy, creating a non-viable fetus and putting the woman's life at risk. Marijuana use may cause interruption of the menstrual cycle leading to ovulatory infertility. Amenorrhea, or lack of a menstrual cycle, often occurs in addicted women.

Stopping smoking, severely limiting alcohol use and seeking help for substance use disorders may restore fertility over time. Do not suddenly stop recreational drug use without consulting with a physician or treatment center as withdrawal may occur.

### Substance Use Disorder and Pregnancy

Pregnant women with substance use disorder create severe health consequences for infants. Use of tobacco and alcohol, misuse of prescription drugs or illicit drug use by pregnant women triple the risk of stillbirth. Approximately five percent of pregnant women use one or more addictive substances. Many substances easily pass through the placenta from the mother to child, leading to the potential for birth defects and even addiction in the fetus. After birth, substances travel to the infant via the mother's breast milk.

When the mother is regularly using and abusing substances, it may cause neonatal abstinence syndrome, or NAS, causing the baby to be born addicted and forcing them to go through withdrawal at birth. Depending on the substance abused, the type and severity of the withdrawal varies. For example, alcohol, prescription pain relievers such as opioids, benzodiazepines and even caffeine may cause the infant to show withdrawal symptoms at birth. Substance use may also cause the infant to be born prematurely.

Tobacco use during pregnancy increases the risk of stillbirth by 1.8 to 2.8, with higher risks related to heavier smoking. Even passive exposure to tobacco has a 2.1 times greater risk of stillbirth. Marijuana use creates a 2.3 greater risk of stillbirth and evidence of any stimulant, marijuana or prescription pain reliever use, causes a 2.2 greater risk of stillbirth.

Withdrawal symptoms in the newborn can develop immediately or up to two weeks after birth and may include:

- Skin discoloration including blotches
- Diarrhea and vomiting
- High-pitched, excessive crying
- Fever
- Abnormal sucking reflex and poor feeding
- Hyperactive movement to stimuli and irritability, trembling
- Rapid breathing and seizures, stuffy nose and sneezing
- Failure to thrive, indicated by slow weight gain
- Sweating
- Sleep problems

Long term and possibly fatal effects of using some drugs include birth defects, premature birth and low birth weight, small head circumference and sudden infant death syndrome (SIDS), including maternal mortality.

There are a variety of commonly abused substances in addition to alcohol and tobacco. Opioid use disorder in pregnant women is a significant concern in the United States and the number of pregnant women abusing opioids at delivery quadrupled from 1999 to present according to the Centers for Disease Control (CDC). Discuss the need to stop all unnecessary drugs with the physician prior to getting pregnant. Marijuana use during pregnancy should be stopped. Getting high may result in unsafe behavioral choices putting the mother and fetus at risk. There is no safe amount of alcohol to use while trying to get pregnant or during pregnancy. All types are equally harmful.

The American College of Obstetrics and Gynecology (ACOG), the American Academy of Pediatrics (AAP), the American Society of Addiction Medicine (ASAM), the March of Dimes and other organizations have come out in support of evidence-based, compassionate care in the case of substance use disorder in pregnancy. Since about 50 percent of pregnancies in the U.S. are not planned, early prenatal care is important including an assessment for substance abuse and substance use disorder.

## Agencies & Associations

1549 **American Pregnancy Association**
800-672-2296
info@americanpregnancy.org
www.americanpregnancy.org
Provides the public with information about reproductive disease and supports families during struggles with pregnancy, infertility, and adoption. Exists to serve the unique needs of men and women confronting infertility issues.

1550 **American Society for Reproductive Medicine**
J. Benjamin Younger Office of Public Affairs
726 7th St. SE 202-863-4985
Washington, DC 20003 asrm@asrm.org
www.asrm.org
A private, non-profit medical organization devoted to advancing the knowledge, understanding, and expertise in all phases of reproductive medicine and biology. Offers patient education brochures, recommended readings and support. Publishes professional journal and consumer publications.
*Michael A. Thomas, MD, President*
*Jared C. Robins, MD, MBA, Executive Director*

1551 **Canadian Society of Nephrology**
P.O. Box 25255 RDP 514-643-4985
Montreal, QC, H1E-7P9 info@csnscn.ca
www.csnscn.ca
Mission is to support Canadian Nephrologists by offering professional development and educational opportunities; advancing the care of individuals living with, or at risk for, kidney disease; and fostering scholarly advancement in the field of kidney health in Canada.
*Dr. Claudio Rigatto, President*
*Dr. Manish Sood, Secretary/Treasurer*

1552 **HealthyWomen**
P.O. Box 336 732-530-3425
Middletown, NJ 07748 877-986-9472
info@healthywomen.org
www.healthywomen.org
Independent, non-profit organization seeking to educate women in all areas of health, to allow them to make informed choices. The HealthyWomen website features numerous tools and health calculators, plus other media.
*Beth Battaglino, CEO*
*Julia M. Amadio, Chair*

1553 **International Council on Infertility Information Dissemination**
5765 F. Burke Centre Parkway 703-379-9178
Burke, VA 22015 Fax: 703-379-1593
INCIIDinfo@inciid.org
www.inciid.org
Provides information on infertility, pregnancy loss, adoption, high risk pregnancy and parenting.

1554 **National Women's Health Network**
1413 K. Street NW 202-682-2640
Washington, DC 20005 Fax: 202-682-2648
nwhn@nwhn.org
www.nwhn.org
Non-profit organization advocating for national policies that protect and promote all women's health, and providing evidence-based independent information.
*Teri Bordenave, Interim Executive Director*
*Adele Costa, Director, Communications*

1555 **RESOLVE: New England**
395 Totten Pond Road 781-890-2225
Waltham, MA 02451 admin@resolvenewengland.org
resolvenewengland.org
Resolve New England (RNE) provides support for all those struggling with fertility and family building in Connecticut, Maine, Massachusetts, New Hampshire, Rhode Island, and Vermont.
*Jennifer Redmond, President*
*Kate Weldon LeBlanc, Executive Director*

1556 **RESOLVE: The National Infertility Association**
7918 Jones Branch Drive 703-556-7172
McLean, VA 22102 Fax: 703-506-3266
info@resolve.org
www.resolve.org
A nationwide non-profit organization serving the unique needs of those striving to build a family. Provides informed help to people who are experiencing infertility.
*Barbara Collura, President & CEO*
*Betsy Campbell, Chief Engagement Officer*

1557 **Society for the Study of Reproduction**
11130 Sunrise Valley Drive 703-885-3502
Reston, VA 20191 Fax: 703-234-4147
www.ssr.org
International scientific society promotes the study of reproductive biology by fostering interdisciplinary communication within the science by holding conferences and by publishing meritorious studies.
*Julie Utano, Executive Director*
*Erika Martin, Membership Manager*

1558 **Wayfinder Family Services**
8391 Auburn Boulevard 916-923-5444
Citrus Heights, CA 95610 800-325-5359
info@lilliput.org
www.lilliput.org
Formerly known as Lilliput, Wayfinder Family Serivces is an adoption agency that bridges the gap between the public and private sectors of foster care.
*Miki Jordan, CEO*
*Elworth A.E. Williams, Jr., Chair*

## Foundations

1559 **Fertility Friends Foundation**
2225 Sheppard Ave. E. info@fertilityfriendsfoundation.com
Toronto, ON, M2J-5C2 fertilityfriendsfoundation.com
A registered charity that offers support to Canadians struggling with infertility through educational resources, fundraising, and grants.
*Chloe Roumain, Founder & President*
*Frederick Dzineku, Founder & Board Member*

1560 **Fertility Matters Canada (FMC)**
P.O. Box 25077 info@fertilitymatters.ca
Moncton, NB, E1C-9M9 fertilitymatters.ca
A national charitable organization that helps Canadians access fertility treatments through awareness, information, and education.
*Carolynn Dube, Executive Director*
*Dr. Ari Baratz, President*

1561 **Hope for Fertility Foundation**
info@hopeforfertility.org
www.hopeforfertility.org
A non-profit organization that offers financial support to couples struggling with infertility treatments, surrogacy, and/or adoption costs.
*Angela Williams, President*
*McCall Weekes, Vice President, Fundraising*

1562 **Hysterectomy Educational Resources & Services (HERS) Foundation**
610-667-7757
Fax: 610-667-8096
hers@hersfoundation.org
www.hersfoundation.com
A nonprofit foundation which provides information about the alternatives to hysterectomy, the risks of the alternatives, and the consequences of the surgery. HERS provides copies of a medical journals, a quarterly newsletter, and a free lending library of books, videos and audio tapes.

## Research Centers

1563 **Fertility Clinic at the Shepherd Spinal Center**
Shepherd Spinal Center

2020 Peachtree Road NW 404-352-2020
Atlanta, GA 30309 www.shepherd.org
This clinic makes it possible for paralyzed men to father children.
*Gary Ulicny, Chief Executive Officer*

1564 **Fertility and Women's Health Care Center**
130 Maple Street 413-781-8220
Springfield, MA 01103 Fax: 413-732-9088
Conducts basic and clinical studies of male and female infertility.
*Ronald K. Burke, MD, Head*

1565 **Melpomene Institute for Women's Health Research**
550 Rice Street 651-789-0140
Saint Paul, MN 55103 Fax: 651-292-9417
www.melpomene.org
Focuses on women's health including fertility issues.
*Judy Mahle Lutter, President*

1566 **University of California: UCLA Population Research Center**
4284 Public Affairs Building 310-206-7566
Los Angeles, CA 90095 Fax: 310-825-8762
stats@ccpr.ucla.edu
www.ccpr.ucla.edu
Clinical investigations of overpopulation and infertility.
*Judith A. Seltzer, Director*
*Jennie Brand, Associate Director*

1567 **University of Michigan Reproductive Sciences Program**
1500 East Medical Center Drive 734-764-8123
Ann Arbor, MI 48109 Fax: 734-763-5992
juckno@umich.edu
www.med.umich.edu/OBGYN/research/rsp/
Research done into reproductive medicine and infertility treatments.
*Timothy R. Johnson, Chair*
*Janet Hall, Clinical Department Administrator*

1568 **Vanderbilt University: Center for Fertility and Reproductive Research**
Nashville, TN 37232 615-322-6576
Fax: 615-343-4902
Reproductive biology and fertility research.

1569 **Wayne State University: University Women's Care**
26400 W 12 Mile Road 248-352-8200
Southfield, MI 48034 Fax: 248-356-8224
wayne.edu
Reproductive endocrine infertility and gynecologic surgery research. The research spans the woman's life cycle. Research projects include: endometriosis, polycystic ovary syndrome, sexual dysfunction, fibroids and menopause. Additional studies pertaining to women's health and male infertility.

## Support Groups & Hotlines

1570 **National Health Information Center**
Office of Disease Prevention & Health Promotion
1101 Wootton Pkwy Fax: 240-453-8281
Rockville, MD 20852 odphpinfo@hhs.gov
www.health.gov/nhic
Supports public health education by maintaining a calendar of National Health Observances; helps connect consumers and health professionals to organizations that can best answer questions and provide up-to-date contact information from reliable sources; updates on a yearly basis toll-free numbers for health information, Federal health clearinghouses and info centers.
*Don Wright, MD, MPH, Director*

1571 **National Infertility Network Exchange**
P.O. Box 204 516-794-5772
East Meadow, NY 11554 Fax: 516-794-0008
www.nine-infertility.org/
The National Infertility Network Exchange (NINE) is a national, notfor profit organization for persons and couples with impaired fertility. NINE supportes the decision of legal and medical means to build families as well as the decision to remain childfree.

## Print Resources

1572 **Biology of Reproduction**
Society for the Study of Reproduction
11130 Sunrise Valley Drive 703-885-3502
Reston, VA 20191 Fax: 703-234-4147
info@ssr.org
academic.oup.com/biolreprod
This peer-reviewed journal is the official journal of the Society for the Study of Reproduction.
*250 pages Monthly*
*Romana Nowak, PhD, Editor-In-Chief*
*Mary Zelinski, PhD, Co-Editor-in-Chief*

1573 **Family Building Magazine**
RESOLVE: National Infertility Association
1310 Broadway 617-623-1156
Somerville, MA 02144 888-623-0744
Fax: 617-623-0252
info@resolve.org
www.resolve.org
Offers various information on the newest technology and advances in infertility treatments, support groups, helplines, centers and in depth articles written by professionals in the field.
*15-18 pages*
*Bonny Gilbert, Executive Director*

1574 **Fertility and Sterility**
American Society for Reproductive Medicine
726 7th St. S.E. 202-863-4985
Washington, DC 20003 asrm@asrm.org
www.asrm.org
A journal for health professionals who treat infertility, sterility and the physiology of reproduction.
*Kurt Barnhart, M.D., M.S.C.E., Editor-in-Chief*
*Micah J. Hill, D.O., Media Editor*

1575 **Fertility and Sterility Journal**
American Society for Reproductive Medicine
726 7th St. SE 202-863-4985
Washington, DC 20003 asrm@asrm.org
www.asrm.org
Publishes original research on reproductive endocrinology, physiology, immunology, genetics, and menopause.
*Kurt Barnhart, M.D., M.S.C.E., Editor-in-Chief*

1576 **Infertility and Adoption**
RESOLVE: National Infertility Association
1310 Broadway 617-623-1156
Somerville, MA 02144 888-623-0744
Fax: 617-623-0252
info@resolve.org
www.resolve.org
Published by RESOLVE: The National Infertility Association.
*Bonny Gilbert, Executive Director*
*Roy Sokol, Author*

## Web Sites

1577 **Adopt-A-Special-Kid America**
www.adoptaspecialkid.org
Adopt-A-Special-Kid provides information on adoption of children with special needs.

1578 **American Society for Reproductive Medicine**
www.reproductivefacts.org
A private, non-profit medical organization devoted to advancing the knowledge, understanding and expertise in all phases of reproductive medicine and biology. Offers patient education brochures, recommended readings and support. Publishes professional journal and consumer publications, and runs the ReproductiveFacts.org website for patients.

1579 **Center for Disease Control**
cdc.gov/reproductivehealth/infertility
Reproductive health information source. Also a resource for the Society of Reproductive Technology. Invitro fertilization data reports and men's reproductive health.

1580 **Healing Well**
www.healingwell.com
An online health resource guide to medical news, chat, information and articles, newsgroups and message boards, books, disease-related web sites, medical directories, and more for patients, friends, and family coping with disabling diseases, disorders, or chronic illnesses.

1581 **Healthlink USA**
www.healthlinkusa.com
Health information concerning treatment, cures, prevention, diagnosis, risk factors, research, support groups, email lists, personal stories and much more. Updated regularly.

1582 **HealthyWomen**
www.healthywomen.org
Independent, non-profit organization seeking to educate women in all areas of health, to allow them to make informed choices. The HealthyWomen website features numerous tools and health calculators, plus other media.

1583 **Infertility Books**
www.infertilitybooks.com
Nonprofit site includes book titles regarding infertility and a short explanation of each book and how to get it.

1584 **International Council on Infertility Information Dissemination**
www.inciid.org
A nonprofit organization that helps individuals and couples explore their family-building options.

1585 **Internet Health Resources**
www.ihr.com/infertility
This web site provides extensive information about IVF, ICSI, infertility clinics, donor egg and surrogacy services, sperm banks, pharmacies, infertility books and videotapes, sperm testing, infertility newsgroups and support organizations, and drugs and medications.

1586 **MedicineNet**
www.medicinenet.com
An online resource for consumers providing easy-to-read, authoritative medical and health information.

1587 **Medscape**
www.medscape.com
Medscape offers specialists, primary care physicians, and other health professionals the Web's most robust and integrated medical information and educational tools.

1588 **MyHealthfinder**
www.healthfinder.gov
Searchable, carefully developed web site offering information on over 1000 topics. Developed by the US Department of Health and Human Services, the site can be used in both English and Spanish.

1589 **National Institutes of Health**
www.medlineplus.gov
Information regarding all aspects of infertility. Some of the topics include: Latest news, overview of anatomy and physiology, clinical trails, diagnoses and symptoms, treatment, genetics, plus lots of links to other sites. Type infertility into the search engine.

1590 **Progyny**
progyny.com
A support sytem concerned with helping reach a goal of finding the perfect doctor, the diagnosis, as well as the treatment.

1591 **RESOLVE**
www.resolve.org
Provides help to people who are experiencing the infertility crisis and strives to increase the visibility of infertility issues via concerted advocacy and public education.

1592 **Uterine Artery Embolization**
www.uterinearteryembolization.com
Provides information on Uterine Artery Embolization, or Uterine Fibroid Embolization as an alternative to hysterectomy or myomectomy as a treatment for uterine fibroids.

1593 **WebMD**
www.webmd.com
Provides credible information, supportive communities, and in-depth reference material about health subjects. A source for original and timely health information, as well as material from well-known content providers.

# KIDNEY DISEASE

*Substance use disorder (SUD) is a major social problem throughout the world. These abused substances or their metabolites are excreted through the kidneys leading to a variety of renal complications. The most commonly abused drugs are alcohol, cocaine, heroin, morphine and nicotine, and their use is associated with renal toxicity that may lead to acute or chronic kidney failure. Alcohol is considered one of the top five greatest risk factors for disease. Almost half of the worldwide population has used alcohol, tobacco or drugs at some point in their lives. Alcohol is the primary drug of abuse, followed by opioids in the U.S. Cocaine use is considered an epidemic with 15 percent of the population in the U.S. having tried the drug. Almost 10 percent of the general population in the U.S. has a substance use disorder of some type.*

The kidneys are responsible for filtering blood and detoxifying and removing excess waste from the body. This waste is excreted by the kidneys in the urine that moves to the bladder. The kidneys are also responsible for maintaining the fluid and electrolyte balance of sodium, calcium, potassium, acid and magnesium, while preventing waste buildup in the blood. Kidneys also produce hormones to keep blood pressure stable, and assist the body with making red blood cells and keeping bones strong.

All drugs and alcohol are processed by the kidneys as if they were a toxin. Long-term, chronic use may affect the kidney's ability to filter blood and delete waste. Legal and illegal substances that contribute to kidney disease include:

- Tobacco use that speeds up the progression of kidney disease and contributes to renal lupus, kidney inflammation and narrowing of kidney arteries. Tobacco use may increase blood pressure and increase the risk of kidney failure for people with diabetes.
- Over-use and long-term use of painkillers, including acetaminophen (Tylenol) alone, or in combination with opioid painkillers, can cause both chronic kidney failure and analgesic nephropathy, requiring a kidney transplant or dialysis.
- Heroin use that causes decreased breathing rates and lowered heart rates leading to overdose, coma and death. Additionally, dehydration, acidosis, low blood pressure and oxygen deficiencies cause kidney problems leading to renal failure.
- Cocaine abuse causes rhabdomyolysis, or muscle tissue breakdown. One-third of people admitted to the hospital due to cocaine related complaints have kidney failure.
- Alcohol aggravates the liver resulting in direct harm to the kidneys, including electrolyte and fluid imbalances and alcoholic ketoacidosis.

Renal complications of drug abuse are common and may be acute and reversible, or chronic leading to end-stage renal failure. Drugs being eliminated through the kidneys have a nephrotoxic effect in many instances.

SUDs can directly cause acute kidney injury and ultimately lead to end-stage renal disease (ESRD). Intravenous drug use and skin popping—injecting drugs directly under the skin—may cause AA-amyloidosis, which may lead to chronic kidney disease. Heroin may crystallize in the renal tubules with resultant acute kidney injury. Heavy marijuana use in kidney transplant patients may lead to renal failure. Cocaine use results in increased hypertension (high blood pressure) severity leading to both acute kidney injury and ESRD. Patients with hepatitis C that consume alcohol and drugs are likely to develop ESRD. It is recommended that all adolescent patients with chronic kidney disease be screened for SUDs.

Individuals with ESRD and SUDs may be significantly more likely to commit suicide than individuals with ESRD alone. A history of chronic opioid use prior to kidney transplantation may cause a higher mortality risk after transplantation. Almost 20 percent of dialysis patients have been diagnosed with a current SUD, with almost 30 percent of those involving alcohol abuse. Alcohol use negatively impacts survival and kidney graft survival in transplant patients with alcohol dependency.

To prevent kidney disease, seek help for substance use disorders before the kidneys are damaged. If kidney disease is already present, do not seek out substances of abuse. Seek help for any mental health disorders as there is a defined relationship between mental health disorders and SUDs. Talk with a physician or other healthcare team member about any dependency that may negatively impact health and wellness and develop a plan of care.

## Agencies & Associations

1594 **American Association of Kidney Patients**
14440 Bruce B. Downs Blvd.
Tampa, FL 33613
813-636-8100
800-749-2257
Fax: 813-636-8122
info@aakp.org
www.aakp.org
Offers support and information for kidney patients and their families.
*Diana Clynes, Executive Director*

1595 **American Kidney Fund**
11921 Rockville Pike
Rockville, MD 20852
800-638-8299
866-300-2900
helpline@kidneyfund.org
www.kidneyfund.org
A non-profit national health organization providing direct financial assistance to thousands of Americans who suffer from kidney disease.
*LaVarne A. Burton, President & CEO*
*Tara Bunch, EVP & Chief Operating Officer*

1596 **American Society of Nephrology (ASN)**
1401 H St. N.W.
Washington, DC 20005
202-640-4660
Fax: 202-637-9793
email@asn-online.org
www.asn-online.org
Represents over 21,000 kidney health professionals working to advance the treatment of kidney diseases.
*Michelle A. Josephson, MD, FASN, President*
*Prabir Roy-Chaudhury, MD, PhD, Secretary*

1597 **National Institute of Diabetes & Digestive & Kidney Diseases**
31 Center Drive
Bethesda, MD 20892
800-860-8747
TTY: 866-569-1162
healthinfo@niddk.nih.gov
www.niddk.nih.gov
Research areas include diabetes, digestive diseases, endocrine and metabolic diseases, hematologic diseases, kidney disease, liver disease, urologic diseases, as well as matters relating to nutrition and obesity.
*Griffin P. Rodgers, Director*
*Gregory Germino, Deputy Director*

1598 **Nebraska Kidney Association**
212 S. 74th Street
Omaha, NE 68144
402-932-7200
www.chadnebraska.org/kidney
Mission is to improve the lives of all Nebraskans through advocacy, education, early disease detection, and patient services.

## Foundations

1599 **Alabama Kidney Foundation (AFK)**
265 Riverchase Parkway East
Hovoer, AL 35244
205-900-7250
Fax: 205-848-2006
www.alkidney.org
Offers financial assistance, education and support services to assist low-income kidney patients in Alabama.
*Peter C. Martin, Sr., President*
*David Reeves, Executive Director*

1600 **Kidney & Urology Foundation of America (KUFA)**
104 West 40th Street
New York, NY 10018
www.kidneyurology.org
A not-for-profit organization that offers support to patients with kidney and urologic diseases.

1601 **National Kidney Foundation**
30 E 33rd Street
New York, NY 10016
800-622-9010
855-653-2273
Fax: 212-689-9261
info@kidney.org
www.kidney.org
A health organization dedicated to preventing kidney and urinary tract diseases, improving the health and well-being of individuals and families affected, and increasing the availability of all organs for transplantation.
*Sylvia Rosas, MD, MSCE, President*
*Tracy McKibben, Chair*

1602 **National Kidney Foundation of Eastern Pennsylvania and New Jersey**
1900 Market St.
Philadelphia, PA 19103
215-923-8611
800-697-7007
Fax: 215-923-2199
nkfdv@kidney.org
www.kidney.org/offices
*Michele Toy, Executive Director*
*Andrea M. Giannini, Development Manager*

1603 **National Kidney Foundation of Alabama, Georgia and Mississippi**
830 Glenwood Ave.
Atlanta, GA 30316
770-452-1539
800-633-2339
Fax: 770-452-7564
nkfga@kidney.org
www.kidney.org/offices
*Barbara McDowell, President*

1604 **National Kidney Foundation of Arizona**
360 E. Coronado Rd. #180
Phoenix, AZ 85004
602-840-1644
Fax: 602-840-2360
www.kidney.org/offices
*Randy Cooper, MD, Chair*
*Lynne Boschee, Vice Chair*

1605 **National Kidney Foundation of Central Ohio**
1491 Polaris Pkwy.
Columbus, OH 43240
614-882-6184
800-242-2133
Fax: 614-882-6564
Tisha.reynolds@kidney.org
www.nkfofohio.org
*Tisha Reynolds, Executive Director*
*Kari Blackburn, Program Manager*

1606 **National Kidney Foundation of Colorado, Idaho, Montana and Wyoming**
2000 S. Colorado Blvd.
Denver, CO 80222
720-748-9991
800-596-7943
Fax: 720-748-1273
nkfconm@kidney.org
www.kidney.org/offices
*Kendra Burrell, Executive Director*
*Danielle Otsuka, Development Director*

1607 **National Kidney Foundation of Connecticut**
3000 Whitney Avenue
Hamden, CT 06518
203-439-7912
nkfct@kidney.org
www.kidney.org/offices
*Saskia Thomson, Executive Director*
*Marcia Hilditch, Sr. Community Outreach Manager*

1608 **National Kidney Foundation of East Tennessee**
5923 Kingston Pike
Knoxville, TN 37919
865-221-2121
800-242-2133
nkfetn@kidney.org
www.kidney.org/offices
*Michelle Dicken, Executive Director*
*Beau Trussell, Community Outreach Manager*

1609 **National Kidney Foundation of Eastern Missouri, Metro East and Arkansas**
1001 Craig Road
St. Louis, MO 63146
314-961-2828
800-489-9585
Fax: 314-961-0888
nkfemo@kidney.org
www.kidney.org/offices
*Kathleen Davis, Executive Director*
*Kourtney Ilbery, Senior Development Manager*

1610 **National Kidney Foundation of Florida**
5756 S. Semoran Blvd.
Orlando, FL 32822
407-894-7325
800-927-9659
kidneyfl.org
*Savanna Lanza, CEO*
*Jason McKean, CTO*

1611 **National Kidney Foundation of Greater New York**
30 East 33rd Street
New York, NY 10016
212-889-2210
800-622-9010
Fax: 212-686-8916
nkfgny@kidney.org
www.kidney.org/offices
*Saskia Thomas, Executive Director*
*Monique Hardin-Cordero, Director, Programs*

1612 **National Kidney Foundation of Hawaii**
1314 S King Street
Honolulu, HI 96814
808-593-1515
info@kidneyhi.org
kidneyhi.org

1613 **National Kidney Foundation of Illinois**
215 W Illinois
Chicago, IL 60654
312-321-1500
Fax: 312-321-1505
kidney@nkfi.org
www.nkfi.org
*Jill M. Schaaf, President*
*Brian O'Dea, Vice President*

1614 **National Kidney Foundation of Indiana**
911 E 86th Street
Indianapolis, IN 46240-1848
317-722-5640
www.kidney.org/offices
*Margie Evans Fort, Chief Executive Officer*
*Janine Moore, Deputy Director*

1615 **National Kidney Foundation of Kansas, Oklahoma and Western Missouri**
6405 Metcalf Avenue
Overland Park, KS 66212
913-262-1551
800-444-8113
nkfkswmo@kidney.org
www.kidney.org/offices
*Sherri Denny, Regional Administrative Assistant*
*Alexandra Wilson, Special Events Manager*

1616 **National Kidney Foundation of Kentucky**
12468 Lagrange Road
Louisville, KY 40245
502-585-5433
800-737-5433
infonkfk@kidney.org
www.nkfk.org
*Tasha Burks, Program Manager*
*Brittany Statts, Senior Development Manager*

1617 **National Kidney Foundation of Louisiana**
8200 Hampson Street
New Orleans, LA 70118
504-861-4500
800-462-3694
Fax: 504-861-1976
www.kidneyla.org
*Torie Kranze, Chief Executive Officer*
*Tracey Eldridge, Community Dev. and Programs Manager*

1618 **National Kidney Foundation of Maryland and Delaware**
11307 York Road
Cockeysville, MD 21030
410-494-8545
Fax: 410-494-8549
www.kidneymd.org
*Patricia A. Dash, Executive Director*
*Kristin Brooks, Development Director*

1619 **National Kidney Foundation of Michigan**
1169 Oak Valley Drive
Ann Arbor, MI 48108
800-482-1455
www.nkfk.org
*Linda Smith-Wheelock, President & CEO*
*Charlene Cole, Vice Preisdent*

1620 **National Kidney Foundation of Minnesota**
1970 Oakcrest Avenue
Saint Paul, MN 55113
651-636-7300
800-596-7943
Fax: 651-636-9700
nkfmn@kidney.org
www.kidney.org/offices
*Mallory Olson, Executive Director*
*Carly Hodes, Senior Development Manager*

1621 **National Kidney Foundation of New England**
209 West Central Street
Natick, MA 01760
508-907-6030
800-542-4001
Fax: 508-907-6035
nkfne@kidney.org
www.kidney.org/offices
*Donna Nickerson, Executive Director*
*Stacey Senat, Program Director*

1622 **National Kidney Foundation of New Mexico, Montana and Wyoming**
2000 S. Colorado Blvd.
Denver, CO 80222
720-748-9991
800-596-7943
Fax: 720-748-1273
nkfconm@kidney.org
www.kidney.org/offices
*Kendra Burrell, Executive Director*
*Danielle Otsuka, Development Director*

1623 **National Kidney Foundation of North Carolina**
7413 Six Forks Rd.
Raleigh, NC 27615
704-519-0020
800-819-8682
www.nkfnc.org
*Susan Ketron, Regional Vice President*
*Ashby Andrews, Executive Director*

1624 **National Kidney Foundation of North Ohio**
P.O. Box 40544
Bay Village, OH 44140
440-241-6780
www.nkfofohio.org
*Anna S. Tzinis, Executive Director*
*Leah Adams, Program Manager*

1625 **National Kidney Foundation of Northern California**
220 Montgomery Street
San Francisco, CA 94104
415-543-3303
888-427-5653
Fax: 415-543-3331
eventsnca@kidney.org
www.kidney.org/offices
*Amy Hewitt, Executive Director*
*Patty McCormac, RN, Senior Director, Programs*

1626 **National Kidney Foundation of South Carolina**
701 Gervais Street
Columbia, SC 29201
803-799-3870
888-848-5277
www.kidney.org/offices
*Susan Ketron, Regional Vice President*
*Blakely Chikhliker, Executive Director*

1627 **National Kidney Foundation of Southeast Texas**
1333 Old Spanish Trail
Houston, TX 77054
214-351-2393
877-543-6397
Fax: 214-351-3797
texasinfo@kidney.org
www.kidney.org/offices
*Lorna Hankins, Executive Director*
*Amanda Crowley-Rios, Program Director*

1628 **National Kidney Foundation of Southern California and Nevada**
20929 Ventura Blvd.
Woordlands Hills, CA 91364
818-783-8153
800-747-5527
nkfsca@kidney.org
www.kidney.org/offices
*Susan Ketron, Interim Executive Director*
*Julie Himot, Associate Executive Director*

1629 **National Kidney Foundation of Texas**
5429 LBJ Freeway
Dallas, TX 75240
214-351-2393
877-543-6397
Fax: 214-351-3797
texasinfo@kidney.org
www.kidney.org/offices
*Lorna Hankins, Executive Director*
*Amanda Crowley-Rios, Program Director*

1630 **National Kidney Foundation of Upstate and Western New York**
1344 University Avenue
Rochester, NY 14607
585-598-3963
Fax: 585-319-3997
infoupny@kidney.org
www.kidney.org/offices
*Ellen Scalzo, Executive Director*
*Susan Brayer, M.S., Ed., Community Outreach Manager*

1631 **National Kidney Foundation of Utah**
3707 N Canyon Road
Provo, UT 84604
801-226-5111
800-869-5277
Fax: 801-226-8278
NKFU@KidneyUT.org
www.kidneyut.org
*Deen Vetterli, Founder & CEO*
*Luz Lewis-Perez, Director of Development*

1632 **National Kidney Foundation of Virginia**
10286 Staples Mill Rd.
Glen Allen, VA 23060
804-288-8342
Fax: 804-282-7835
Nancy.Castrina@kidney.org
www.kidney.org/offices
*Michele Anthony, Executive Director*
*Ashwani Jain, Program Director*

1633 **National Kidney Foundation of West Tennessee**
4728 Spottswood Avenue
Memphis, TN 38117-4817
901-683-6185
800-273-3869
Fax: 901-683-6189
info@nkfwtn.org
www.kidney.org/offices
*Mabel Barringer, Executive Director*

1634 **National Kidney Foundation of Wisconsin**
10909 W. Greenfield Avenue
West Allis, WI 53314
414-897-8669
800-543-6393
Fax: 414-930-0337
info@kidneywi.org
www.kidneywi.org
*Ahmed Malik, Chair*
*Alyse Bailey, Vice Chair*

1635 **National Kidney Foundation of the National Capital Area & Virginia**
1600 Tysons Blvd.
McLean, VA 22102
202-244-7900
Fax: 202-244-7405
infowdc@kidney.org
www.kidney.org/offices

1636 **PKD Foundation**
1001 E. 101st Terrace
Kansas City, MO 64131
816-931-2600
pkdcure@pkdcure.org
www.pkdcure.org
Helps patients with polycystic kidney disease (PKD) by raising financial support for peer-approved biomedical research projects and fostering public awareness among medical professionals, patients, and the general public.
*Chris Rusconi, PhD, Interim CEO/Chief Research Officer*
*Carmen Gleason, Chief Operating Officer*

1637 **Tennessee Kidney Foundation**
P.O. Box 330989
Nashville, TN 37203
615-383-3887
Fax: 615-383-2647
www.tennesseekidneyfoundation.org
An independent, Tennessee-based organization that raises awareness for kidney disease and invests 100% of funds locally.
*Heather Corum Powell, CEO*
*Chelsey S. Wells, Director, Development*

## Research Centers

1638 **Georgetown University Center for Hypertension and Renal Disease Research**
3800 Reservoir Road NW
Washington, DC 20007
202-687-9183
Fax: 202-687-7893
www.georgetown.edu/research/hrdrc
International institute for basic and clinical investigation, education and clinical practice in hypertension and renal disease.
*Christopher Englert, Jr. CAE, President/CEO*

1639 **Kidney Disease Institute**
Wadsworth Center for Laboratories and Research
Empire State Plaza
Albany, NY 12237
518-474-7354
Fax: 518-737-71
dohweb@health.state.ny.us
www.nyhealth.gov
An information and referral organization for polycystic kidney disease, autoimmune kidney disease and transplantation.
*Andrew M. Cuomo, Governor*
*Nirav R. Shah, Commissioner*

1640 **Lovelace Respiratory Research Institute**
615 S. Preston Street
Louisville, KY 40202
502-852-7350
Fax: 502-852-7643
kdpnet.kdp.louisville.edu
Educates residents and patients regarding kidney diseases and offers a dialysis clinic for people afflicted with kidney disease.
*George R. Ottensmeyer, President*

1641 **Nevada Kidney Disease & Hypertension Centers**
210 S. Desplaines Street
Chicago, IL 60661
312-654-2720
Fax: 312-654-0118
charlotte.chapple@ainmd.com
www.ainmd.com/
A medical group practicing nephrology in the Chicago metropolitan area and it suburbs. Includes 21 nephrologists with expertise in many areas in the field of nephrology including hypertension chronic and acute renal failure hemodialysis and peritoneal dialysis glomerulonephritis acid base disturbances fluid and electrolytes management. Provides personal high quality care to patients with kidney diseases.
*Eduardo Kantor, MD, Founder*

1642 **Polycystic Kidney Research Foundation**
1001 E. 101st Terrace
Kansas City, MO 64131
816-931-2600
pkdcure@pkdcure.org
www.pkdcure.org
Provides information on the cause, treatment, and cure of polycystic kidney disease by raising financial support for peer-approved biomedical research projects and fostering public awareness among medical professionals, patients, and the general public.
*Chris Rusconi, PhD, Interim CEO/Chief Research Officer*
*Carmen Gleason, Chief Operating Officer*

1643 **University of Kansas Kidney and Urology Research Center**
3901 Rainbow Boulevard
Kansas City, KS 66160
913-588-5000
Fax: 913-588-3995
TTY: 913-588-7963
www.kumc.edu
*Jared J. Brosius, Chief*
*Joseph Messana, Professor/Service Chief*

1644 **University of Michigan Nephrology Division**
University of Michigan Health System
1500 E. Medical Center Drive
Ann Arbor, MI 48109
734-936-5645
Fax: 734-763-4151
www.med.umich.edu/intmed/nephrology
*Eric Mullen, Division Administrator*
*Susan Geisser, Financial Consultant*

1645 **University of Rochester: Nephrology Research Program**
601 Elmwood Avenue
Rochester, NY 14642
585-275-3660
Fax: 716-442-9201
www.urmc.rochester.edu
*David A. Bushinsky, MD, Division Chief*

1646 **Warren Grant Magnuson Clinical Center**
National Institute of Health
10 Center Drive MSC 1078
Bethesda, MD 20892
301-496-3311
800-411-1222
Fax: 301-496-2390
TTY: 866-411-1010
mmichael@cc.nih.gov
www.dnrc.nih.gov/reports/programs/ncc.as
Established in 1953 as the research hospital of the National Institutes of Health. Designed so that patient care facilities are close to research laboratories so new findings of basic and clinical scientists can be quickly applied to the treatment of patients. Upon referral by physicians, patients are admitted to NIH clinical studies.
*John Slatopolsky, Director*

1647 **Washington University Chromalloy American Kidney Center**
One Barnes-Jewish Hospital Plaza
Saint Louis, MO 63110
314-362-7209
Fax: 314-747-3743
renal.wustl.edu

Offers a dialysis unit for people afflicted with kidney disease.
*Dr. Eduardo Lanning, RN, JD, President Board of Directors*
*Sean Tully, Vice President Board of Directors*

## Support Groups & Hotlines

1648 **Kidneeds**
Greater Cedar Rapids Community Foundation
200 First Street Southwest 319-366-2862
Cedar Rapids, IA 52404 Fax: 319-386-0431
kidneedsmpgn@yahoo.com
www.medicine.uiowa.edu/kidneeds/
Primary mission of Kidneeds is to fund research on membranoproliferative giomerulonephritis type 2 (MPON type 2, aka, dense deposit disease). Phone support and annual newsletter availiable. No computerized version availiable. No mailing list availble.

1649 **National Health Information Center**
Office of Disease Prevention & Health Promotion
1101 Wootton Pkwy Fax: 240-453-8281
Rockville, MD 20852 odphpinfo@hhs.gov
www.health.gov/nhic
Supports public health education by maintaining a calendar of National Health Observances; helps connect consumers and health professionals to organizations that can best answer questions and provide up-to-date contact information from reliable sources; updates on a yearly basis toll-free numbers for health information, Federal health clearinghouses and info centers.
*Don Wright, MD, MPH, Director*

## Print Resources

1650 **Clinical Journal of the American Society of Nephrology (CJASN)**
American Society of Nephrology
1401 H St., N.W. nngo@asn-online.org
Washington, DC 20005 journals.lww.com/CJASN/
This peer-reviewed journal covers the latest research in clinical nephrology.
*Monthly*
*Rajnish Mehrotra, MD, MS, FASN, Editor-in-Chief*
*Natalie Ngo, Managing Editor*

1651 **Kidney Beginnings: The Magazine**
American Association of Kidney Patients
14440 Bruce B. Downs Boulevard 813-636-8100
Tampa, FL 33613 800-749-2257
Fax: 813-636-8122
info@aakp.org
www.aakp.org
This quarterly member magazine provides articles, news items, and information of interest to those at risk or recently diagnosed with kidney disease, their famliy, and healthcare professionals.
*Diana Clynes, Executive Director*
*Jennifer Rate, Marketing & Communications Manager*

1652 **aakpRENALIFE**
American Association of Kidney Patients
35052 E Frantage Road 813-636-8100
Tampa, FL 33607 800-749-2257
Fax: 813-636-8122
info@aakp.org
www.aakp.org
The official publication for AAKP members, offering articles, news and healthcare information for kidney patients and health care professionals. Published six times a year (January, March, May, July, September and November).
*Kim Buettner, Executive Director*
*Jennifer Rate, Marketing & Communications Manager*

## Web Sites

1653 **American Association of Kidney Patients**
www.aakp.org
This association helps patients and their families cope with the emotional, physical and social impact of kidney disease.

1654 **American Kidney Fund**
www.akfinc.org/
A nonprofit, national health organization providing direct financial assistance to thousands of Americans who suffer from kidney disease.

1655 **Healing Well**
www.healingwell.com
An online health resource guide to medical news, chat, information and articles, newsgroups and message boards, books, disease-related web sites, medical directories, and more for patients, friends, and family coping with disabling diseases, disorders, or chronic illnesses.

1656 **Healthlink USA**
www.healthlinkusa.com
Links to websites which may include treatment, cures, diagnosis, prevention, support groups, email lists, messageboards, personal stories, risk factors, statistics, research and more.

1657 **MedicineNet**
www.medicinenet.com
An online resource for consumers providing easy-to-read, authoritative medical and health information.

1658 **Medscape**
www.medscape.com
Medscape offers specialists, primary care physicians, and other health professionals the Web's most robust and integrated medical information and educational tools.

1659 **MyHealthfinder**
www.healthfinder.gov
Searchable, carefully developed web site offering information on over 1000 topics. Developed by the US Department of Health and Human Services, the site can be used in both English and Spanish.

1660 **WebMD**
www.webmd.com
Provides credible information, supportive communities, and in-depth reference material about health subjects. A source for original and timely health information, as well as material from well-known content providers.

# LIVER DISEASE

*The liver is responsible for digesting food, metabolizing substances and processing and distributing nutrients. The liver makes a digestive juice called bile to digest fats and some vitamins. Bile may be stored in the gallbladder or moved to the small intestine for use. Appropriate liver function is vital to life. In the presence of substance use disorder, related liver disease remains a major medical problem as drug-induced liver injury creates a higher risk for liver failure and increases the need for liver transplant. Illicit drugs, prescription drugs, alcohol and even some over-the-counter drugs such as acetaminophen, herbs and dietary supplements can cause liver dysfunction.*

Drug induced liver injury may occur in the range from significant to asymptomatic in nature. Drugs damage the liver by directly causing damage at the hepatocellular level (in the liver cells) or by blocking the flow of bile. For example, an overdose of acetaminophen (Tylenol) can destroy half of an individual's liver in less than a week. Without complications, the liver can repair itself completely in some cases. Because substance use disorder remains highly prevalent, it poses significant dangers.

Liver disease has complex effects on metabolizing drugs and other substances in the liver. Clearing drugs from the body and interference with the pharmacokinetic actions (how the drug works) of the drug may lead to too much or too little drug being available in the body. Both the liver and the kidneys are at high risk. Alterations in liver function may increase the level of drug bioavailability, in other words, the dose may be within appropriate range, but the liver may restrict how much is available for use or the normal dose may be too potent. For example, with chronic liver disease, a heightened sensitivity to opioids and sedatives may occur. The drug that has the potential to cause liver failure is acetaminophen. If the metabolism of drugs in the liver is negatively impacted by liver disease, the possibility of drug overdoses increases.

How the liver processes drugs and alcohol are unpredictable in the presence of liver disease. In the presence of alcohol abuse, the following may occur: simple steatosis (fat accumulation in the liver with mild inflammation); steatohepatitis (fat buildup in the liver caused by high cholesterol, high blood pressure, high blood sugar, insulin resistance and diabetes) that may occur even absent alcohol use; alcoholic hepatitis (caused by drinking more alcohol than the liver can process); and liver cirrhosis (scarring or fibrosis of the liver caused by long-term liver damage). When the liver is negatively impacted by any of these conditions, it prevents the liver from working properly. If cirrhosis is present, it is considered end-stage liver disease and eventually causes death. Symptoms of liver injury include a change in liver function tests, jaundice, abdominal pain, and itching. Occasionally, blood clotting issues occur.

There is no way to correlate the type of liver injury and its severity with liver function testing results. There are no general guidelines to prescribing medications in the presence of liver disease. Acute liver failure occurs quickly and is commonly caused by a virus or drugs such as acetaminophen. It requires immediate hospitalization because of the serious complications of bleeding and pressure in the brain. It may be reversed with prompt treatment, but many situations require a liver transplant. With illicit drug use, the damage may begin with initial use and continue throughout the course of abuse.

Stopping substance use may reverse the damage to the liver. If exposure to drugs and alcohol is not stopped, eventually the liver damage will be so severe as to warrant a liver transplant or death will occur, as the liver is a vital component of body function. Depending on the cause of the liver toxicity, the following steps may aid in liver recovery:

- Changing prescription medications following a doctor's recommendation
- Stop drinking all alcohol
- Do not use recreational drugs or herbal or nutritional supplements
- Using only the recommended doses of prescription and over-the-counter drugs, especially acetaminophen
- Avoiding exposure to toxic substances at home or in the workplace where possible

Always discuss all substances prescribed, over-the-counter including herbs, and illicit substances used with the doctor before stopping any substance. Seek help if substance use disorder is present. Professional assistance with detoxification is often critical to successfully becoming clean and sober and preventing or reversing liver damage.

## Agencies & Associations

1661 **Administration for Children and Families**
330 C Street, S.W. 877-696-6775
Washington, DC 20201 www.acf.hhs.gov
The Administration for Children & Families (ACF) is a division of the U.S. Department of Health & Human Services (HHS). ACF promotes the economic and social well-being of families, children, individuals and communities.
*Lauren Supplee, Deputy Assistant Secretary*
*Emily Schmitt, Deputy Director*

1662 **Agency for Healthcare Research and Quality**
5600 Fishers Lane 301-427-1364
Rockville, MD 20857 www.ahrq.gov
The Agency for Healthcare Research and Quality's (AHRQ) mission is to produce evidence to make health care safer, higher quality, more accessible, equitable, and affordable, and to work within the U.S. Department of Health and Human Services and with other partners to make sure that the evidence is understood and used.
*Robert Otto Valdez, PhD, MHSA, Director*
*Howard E. Holland, Director, Office of Communications*

1663 **Agency for Toxic Substances and Disease Registry**
1200 Pennsylvania Ave., N.W. 202-566-0844
Washington, DC 20460 800-232-4636
TTY: 888-232-6348
sxj6@cdc.gov
www.atsdr.cdc.gov
The Agency for Toxic Substances and Disease Registry (ATSDR), based in Atlanta, Georgia, is a federal public health agency of the U.S. Department of Health and Human Services. ATSDR serves the public by using the best science, taking responsive public health actions, and providing trusted health information to prevent harmful exposures and diseases related to toxic substances.
*Steve Jones, MS, Director*

1664 **American Association for the Study of Liver Diseases**
P.O. Box 25407 703-299-9766
Alexandria, VA 22313-5407 Fax: 703-299-9622
www.aasld.org
Physicians, researchers, and allied hepatology health professionals dedicated to preventing and curing liver disease by fostering research on liver diseases.
*Matthew R. D'Uva, FASAE, CAE, Chief Executive Officer*

1665 **Association for Glycogen Storage Disease**
info@agsdus.org
www.agsdus.org
Organization for parents of and individuals with glycogen storage disease (GSD) to communicate, share useful information, provide support, create awareness of GSD, and to foster research on glycogen storage diseases.
*Kim Burney, President*
*Rebecca Lichucki, Vice President*

1666 **Centers for Medicare & Medicaid Services**
7500 Security Boulevard 410-786-3000
Baltimore, MD 21244 877-267-2323
TTY: 866-226-1819
www.cms.gov
U.S. federal agency which administers Medicare, Medicaid, and the State Children's Health Insurance Program.
*Chiquita Brooks-LaSure, Administrator*
*Jonathan Blum, Principal Deputy Administrator & COO*

1667 **Children's Liver Association For Support Services (CLASS)**
P.O. Box 186 724-581-5527
Monaca, PA 15061 classkidscares@gmail.com
www.classkids.org
An organization dedicated to addressing the emotional, educational and financial needs of families with children affected by liver disease and transplantation.
*Aimee Seningen, MD, Treasurer*
*Scott Hand, Secretary*

1668 **National Center for Complementary and Integrative Health**
9000 Rockville Pike 888-644-6226
Bethesda, MD 20892 TTY: 866-464-3615
info@nccih.nih.gov
nccih.nih.gov
The National Center for Complementary and Integrative Health (NCCIH) is the Federal Government's lead agency for scientific research on the diverse medical and health care systems, practices, and products that are not generally considered part of conventional medicine.
*Helene M. Langevin, MD, Director*
*David Shurtleff, PhD, Deputy Director*

1669 **National Human Genome Research Institute**
Building 31, Room 4B09 301-402-0911
Bethesda, MD 20892 Fax: 301-402-2218
nhgripressoffice@mail.nih.gov
www.genome.gov
The National Human Genome Research Institute began as the National Center for Human Genome Research (NCHGR), which was established in 1989 to carry out the role of the National Institutes of Health (NIH) in the International Human Genome Project (HGP).
*Eric D. Green, MD, PhD, Director*
*Lawrence Brody, PhD, Director, Division of Genomics & Society*

1670 **National Institute for Occupational Safety and Health**
Centers for Disease Control and Prevention
1600 Clifton Rd. 800-232-4636
Atlanta, GA 30333 www.cdc.gov/niosh
The National Institute for Occupational Safety and Health (NIOSH) is the U.S. federal agency that conducts research and makes recommendations to prevent worker injury and illness.
*John Howard, Director*
*Frank Hearl, Chief of Staff*

1671 **National Institute of Biomedical Imaging and Bioengineering**
9000 Rockville Pike 301-496-8859
Bethesda, MD 20892 info@nibib.nih.gov
www.nibib.nih.gov
The mission of the National Institute of Biomedical Imaging and Bioengineering (NIBIB) is to improve health by leading the development and accelerating the application of biomedical technologies.
*Bruce J. Tromberg, PhD, Director*
*Jill Heemskerk, PhD, Deputy Director*

1672 **National Institute of Diabetes & Digestive & Kidney Diseases**
31 Center Drive 800-860-8747
Bethesda, MD 20892 TTY: 866-569-1162
healthinfo@niddk.nih.gov
www.niddk.nih.gov
Research areas include diabetes, digestive diseases, endocrine and metabolic diseases, hematologic diseases, kidney disease, liver disease, urologic diseases, as well as matters relating to nutrition and obesity.
*Griffin P. Rodgers, Director*
*Gregory Germino, Deputy Director*

1673 **National Institute of Environmental Health Sciences**
P.O. Box 12233 919-541-3345
Research Triangle Park, NC 27709 Fax: 919-541-4395
www.niehs.nih.gov
The mission of the NIEHS is to discover how the environment affects people in order to promote healthier lives.
*Rick Woychik, PhD, Director*
*Trevor K. Archer, PhD, Deputy Director*

1674 **National Institute of General Medical Sciences**
45 Center Drive 301-496-7301
Bethesda, MD 20892 www.nigms.nih.gov
The National Institute of General Medical Sciences (NIGMS) supports basic research that increases understanding of biological processes and lays the foundation for advances in disease diagnosis, treatment and prevention.
*Jon R. Lorsch, PhD, Director*
*Dorit Zuk, PhD, Deputy Director*

1675 **National Institute on Alcohol Abuse and Alcoholism**
National Institute on Health

9000 Rockville Pike
Bethesda, MD 20892
301-443-3860
niaaaweb-r@exchange.nih.gov
www.niaaa.nih.gov

NIAAA supports and conducts research on the impact of alcohol use on human health and well-being. It is the largest funder of alcohol research in the world.
*George F. Koob, PhD, Director*
*Patricia A. Powell, PhD, Deputy Director*

1676 **National Institute on Drug Abuse**
251 Bayview Blvd.
Baltimore, MD 21224
443-740-2463
800-535-8254
www.irp.drugabuse.gov

NIDA's mission is to lead the Nation in bringing the power of science to bear on drug abuse and addiction.
*Amy H. Newman, PhD, Scientific Director*
*Lorenzo Leggio, MD, PhD, Deputy Scientific Director*

1677 **U.S. Food and Drug Administration**
10903 New Hampshire Avenue
Silver Spring, MD 20993
888-463-6332
www.fda.gov

FDA is responsible for protecting the public health by assuring the safety, efficacy and security of human and veterinary drugs, biological products, medical devices, the nation's food supply, cosmetics, and products that emit radiation.
*Robert M. Califf, MD, Commissioner*

1678 **Wilson's Disease Association**
1732 First Avenue
New York, NY 10128
414-961-0533
866-961-0533
info@wilsonsdisease.org
www.wilsonsdisease.org

Serves as a communications support network for individuals affected by Wilson's disease; distributes information to professionals and the public; makes referrals; and holds meetings.
*8 pages*
*Jean Perog, President*
*Rachel Albert, Vice President*

## Foundations

1679 **American Liver Foundation**
P.O. Box 299
West Orange, NJ 07052
800-465-4837
www.liverfoundation.org

ALF raises awareness of liver disease through education, advocacy, and research for the prevention, treatment, and cure of liver disease, and provides support services to those affected.
*Heidi Daniels, Vice President, Development*
*Julie Kimbrough, Chief Marketing & Communications Officer*

1680 **Canadian Liver Foundation**
101-3100 Steeles Ave Est
Markham, ON, L3R-8T3
416-491-3353
800-563-5483
Fax: 905-752-1540
clf@liver.ca
www.liver.ca

Funds research for the prevention, diagnosis, treatment, and cure of liver disease.
*Jennifer Nebesky, President & CEO*
*Nem Maksimovic, Director, Support & Education*

1681 **National Gaucher Foundation**
5410 Edson Lane
Rockville, MD 20852
800-504-3189
www.gaucherdisease.org

National foundation providing information and assistance for those affected by Gaucher disease, as well as education and outreach to increase public awareness.
*Brian Berman, President & CEO*
*Rovin Ely, Clinical Director*

1682 **National Reye's Syndrome Foundation**
426 N Lewis St.
Bryan, OH 43506
800-233-7393
nrsf@reyessyndrome.org
www.reyessyndrome.org

Devoted to conquering Reye's syndrome, primarily a children's disease affecting the liver and brain, but can affect all ages. Provides support, information and referrals. Encourages research.

1683 **National Science Foundation**
2415 Eisenhower Avenue
Alexandria, VA 22314
703-292-5111
800-877-8339
TTY: 800-281-8749
info@nsf.gov
www.nsf.gov

NSF is the only federal agency whose mission includes support for all fields of fundamental science and engineering, except for medical sciences.
*Sethuraman Panchanathan, Director*
*Teresa A. Grancorvitz, Deputy Chief Operating Officer*

## Research Centers

1684 **Clinical Research Center: Pediatrics Children's Hospital Research Foundation**
Children's Hospital Research Foundation
Elland & Bethesda Avenues
Cincinnati, OH 45229
513-559-4412
Fax: 513-559-7431

Studies of pediatric acquired diseases including liver disease and Reye's Syndrome.
*Dr. James G. Redeker, Director*

1685 **University of California Liver Research Unit**
7601 E Imperial Highway
Downey, CA 90242
562-940-8961
Fax: 562-940-6628
*Dr. Allan Lee, MD, FACP, Director*

1686 **University of Texas Southwestern Medical Center**
5323 Harry Hines Boulevard
Dallas, TX 75390
214-645-8300
Fax: 214-645-7999
www.utsouthwestern.edu
*Daniel K. Podolsky, MD, President*
*J. Gregory Fitz, Executive Vice President*

1687 **Yeshiva University Marion Bessin Liver Research Center**
Albert Einstein College of Medicine
1300 Morris Park Avenue
Bronx, NY 10461
718-430-2000
Fax: 718-918-0857
www.einstein.yu.edu/centers/liver-resear

Liver disease research and therapy.
*Allan W. Wolkoff, MD, Director*
*David A. Shafritz, MD, Associate Director*

## Support Groups & Hotlines

1688 **Children's Liver Association for Support Services**
P.O. Box 186
Monaca, PA 15061
724-581-5527
classkidscares@gmail.com
www.classkids.org

Dedicated to addressing the emotional, educational, and financial needs of families with children with liver disease or liver transplantation. Telephone hotline, newsletter, parent matching, literature and financial assistance. Supports research and educates public about organ donations.
*Aimee Seningen, MD, Treasurer*
*Scott Hand, Secretary*

1689 **National Health Information Center**
Office of Disease Prevention & Health Promotion
1101 Wootton Pkwy
Rockville, MD 20852
Fax: 240-453-8281
odphpinfo@hhs.gov
www.health.gov/nhic

Supports public health education by maintaining a calendar of National Health Observances; helps connect consumers and health professionals to organizations that can best answer questions and provide up-to-date contact information from reliable sources; updates on a yearly basis toll-free numbers for health information, Federal health clearinghouses and info centers.
*Don Wright, MD, MPH, Director*

## Print Resources

1690 **Hepatology**
American Assoc. for the Study of Liver Disease

1001 North Fairfax Street 703-299-9766
Alexandria, VA 22314 Fax: 703-299-9622
aasld@aasld.org
www.aasld.org

Information for professionals interested in disease of the liver and biliary tract.

*Gregory J. Gores, Editor*
*Harmeet Malhi, MBBS, FAASLD, Deputy Editor*

1691 **Liver Transplantation**
American Assoc. for the Study of Liver Disease
1001 North Fairfax Street 703-299-9766
Alexandria, VA 22314 Fax: 703-299-9622
aasld@aasld.org
www.aasld.org

Publishes peer-reviewed articles on liver transplantation, liver surgery, and chronic liver disease.

*Robert S. Brown, Jr., MD, MPH, Editor*
*Emili Malatesta, Managing Editor*

## Digital Resources

1692 **Hepatology Communications**
American Assoc. for the Study of Liver Disease
1001 North Fairfax Street 703-299-9766
Alexandria, VA 22314 Fax: 703-299-9622
aasld@aasld.org
www.aasld.org

A peer-reviewed, online-only journal that publishes clinical research in hepatology. All articles are available to read and share.

*Gyongyi Szabo, MD, PhD, Editor-in-Chief*
*Ariel E. Feldstein, MD, Associate Editor*

## Web Sites

1693 **American Association for the Study of Liver Diseases**
www.aasld.org

Conducts symposia and educational courses for professionals interested in disease of the liver and biliary tract. The leading organization for advancing the science and practice of hepatology.

1694 **Children's Liver Alliance**
www.liverkids.org.au/

Empowering the hearts and minds of children with liver disease, their families and the medical professionals who care for them.

1695 **Healing Well**
www.healingwell.com

An online health resource guide to medical news, chat, information and articles, newsgroups and message boards, books, disease-related web sites, medical directories, and more for patients, friends, and family coping with disabling diseases, disorders, or chronic illnesses.

1696 **Healthlink USA**
www.healthlinkusa.com

Health information concerning treatment, cures, prevention, diagnosis, risk factors, research, support groups, email lists, personal stories and much more. Updated regularly.

1697 **Liver Support**
www.liversupport.com

Information about the world's safest, most powerful liver-protecting supplement, milk thistle. Specifically facts about the safe, yet highly potent, Phytosome form.

1698 **MedicineNet**
www.medicinenet.com

An online resource for consumers providing easy-to-read, authoritative medical and health information.

1699 **Medscape**
www.medscape.com

Medscape offers specialists, primary care physicians, and other health professionals the Web's most robust and integrated medical information and educational tools.

1700 **MyHealthfinder**
www.healthfinder.gov

Searchable, carefully developed web site offering information on over 1000 topics. Developed by the US Department of Health and Human Services, the site can be used in both English and Spanish.

1701 **National Institute On Drug Abuse (NIDA)**
251 Bayview Blvd. 443-740-2463
Baltimore, MD 21224 800-535-8254
www.irp.drugabuse.gov

NIDA's mission is to lead the Nation in bringing the power of science to bear on drug abuse and addiction.

1702 **WebMD**
www.webmd.com

Provides credible information, supportive communities, and in-depth reference material about health subjects. A source for original and timely health information, as well as material from well-known content providers.

# NEUROCOGNITIVE DISORDERS

*Substance use disorder is associated with changes in brain function and cognitive deficits. A cognitive deficit is defined as a problem with mental function ranging from perception to memory, managing emotions, or planning activities of daily life. Neurocognitive disorder is a general term describing decreased mental function due to medical disease other than a psychiatric illness. The three subcategories of neurocognitive disorders are delirium, mild neurocognitive disorder (some decreased mental function but able to stay independent), and major neurocognitive disorder (also called dementia) where decreased mental function causes a loss in ability to do daily tasks.*

When an individual has a history of substance use disorder that has been controlled, a cognitive deficit may cause a relapse. Addiction related neurocognitive disorders are often associated with specific drugs, including alcohol, opioids, cannabis, stimulants and depressants. Mild neurocognitive disorders and major neurocognitive disorders are due to alcohol and/or drug induced disorders. As recreational drug use transitions to substance use disorder, changes to neural processing evolves. Neurocognitive disorders caused by substance use disorder are said to exist when impairments persist beyond intoxication and acute withdrawal.

Neurocognitive disorders can develop quickly after taking a drug or medication and may last after stopping the substance. Approximately 30-40 percent of heavy drinkers have some type of alcohol-induced neurocognitive disorder. One-third of cocaine users experience mild neurocognitive disorders after quitting use. Opioid use causes neurocognitive problems in almost 40 percent of users. Substance use disorders including drug and alcohol withdrawal, effects from prescription or illicit substance abuse and effects from required drugs such as antihistamines and corticosteroids all contribute to neurocognitive disorders. Mental skills may improve within a few days of stopping drinking or taking drugs and as detoxification occurs, mental skills also may improve. It may take an extended time, months or years, to recapture normal function if at all.

Determining causes of neurocognitive disorders other than substance use disorders is necessary. Other causes may include:

- Brain injury caused by trauma
- Low blood oxygen (hypoxia)
- Cardiovascular disorders including repeated strokes, heart infections, stroke and transient ischemic attack (TIA)
- Degenerative disorders such as Alzheimer disease, Multiple Sclerosis or Parkinson disease
- Dementia due to metabolic changes such as liver and kidney disease, thyroid disease and vitamin deficiencies
- Infections including septicemia (blood poisoning), sudden onset or long-term infections, or meningitis
- Complications of cancer including programs with chemotherapy treatments

Depression, neurosis and psychosis may mimic neurocognitive issues. Physicians must determine if the cognitive deficit was present before the person abused alcohol, medications or illicit drugs thought to be contributing to the neurocognitive deficit. Mental function is necessary for controlling body movements, coordination, balance, speech and communication of all kinds. When cognitive deficits occur, regardless of cause, life may become difficult and problems with activities of daily activities develop. Neurocognitive deficits caused by substance use disorder may include:

- Lack of concentration and difficulty paying attention to activities
- Difficulty with "executive functioning" or using skills like planning, controlling impulses (including those with long-term implications), and decision-making, ranging from daily life to the future
- Difficulty learning everyday things such as a new technology, learning in school, or learning life skills such as driving
- A loss of memory, including remembering information such as a personal phone number, address and where you are going
- Difficulty communicating with others, including forgetting words and phrases
- Decreased social awareness including using courtesy with others, recognizing scams in person or on social media
- A lack of perception and motor skills, including body control and movements, even with things like walking

Treatment of neurocognitive disorders depend on the cause. Substance use disorder treatment and rehabilitation and supportive care is recommended. Medicines to control aggressive behaviors may be needed. Some disorders are reversible, but in the presence of long-term or repeated abuse, disorders may get worse over time.

## Agencies & Associations

1703 **Alzheimer's Association National Office**
225 N. Michigan Avenue
Chicago, IL 60601 alz.org
Headquarters for Alzheimer's Association, an organization dedicated to helping all those with Alzheimer's disease and dementia, and their families. Funds Alzheimer's research, engages in Alzheimer's advocacy, and offers referrals, support groups, educational sessions, safety services, and publications.
*Sarah Lorance, Chair*
*Harry Johns, Chief Executive Officer*

1704 **Brain Research Through Advancing Innovative Neurotechnologies (BRAIN)**
National Institutes of Health (NIH)
9000 Rockville Pike 301-496-4000
Bethesda, MD 20892 braininfo@ninds.nih.gov
braininitiative.nih.gov
Federal agency focused on supporting neuroscience research and working towards reducing the burdens associated with neurological disease.

1705 **Caregiver Action Network**
1150 Connecticut Ave, NW 202-454-3970
Washington, DC 20036-3904 855-227-3640
info@caregiveraction.org
caregiveraction.org
Caregiver Action Network is a nonprofit organization that acts as a support and an advocate for family caregivers of individuals with chronic conditions, diabilities, diseases, or old age. CAN provides education, peer support, and resources free of charge.
*Melissa Rowley, Chair*
*John Schall, Chief Executive Officer*

1706 **Center for Family Support (CFS)**
333 Seventh Avenue 888-813-5014
New York, NY 10001 svernikoff@cfsny.org
www.cfsny.org
The Center for Family Support offers assistance to individuals with developmental and related disabilities, as well as their families, and provides support services and programs that are designed to accommodate individual needs. Offers services throughout New York City, Westchester County, Long Island, and New Jersey.
*Steven Vernikoff, Executive Director*
*Barbara Greenwald, Chief Operating Officer*

1707 **Center for Mental Health Services (CMHS)**
Substance Abuse and Mental Health Services Admin.
5600 Fishers Lane 240-276-1310
Rockville, MD 20857 samhsa.gov
Promotes the treatment of mental illness and emotional disorders by increasing accessibility to mental health programs; supporting outreach, treatment, rehabilitation, and support programs and networks; and encouraging the use of scientifically-based information when treating mental disorders. CMHS provides information about mental health via a toll-free number and numerous publications.
*Anita Everett, M.D., DFAPA, Director*

1708 **Federation of Associations in Behavioral & Brain Sciences (FABBS)**
1200 New York Ave. NW 202-769-1074
Washington, DC 20005 info@fabbs.org
fabbs.org
FABBS is a coalition of scientific societies focused on expanding scientific knowledge on the brain, mind, and behavior. FABBS educates the public and policymakers on the importance of brain, mind, and behavior sciences research; provides quality sources to federal agencies and the media; advocates for research-focused policy and legislation; and promotes exchange of information among scientific organizations.
*Philip Rubin, Ph.D., President*
*Rae Silver, Ph.D., Vice President*

1709 **National Association for the Dually Diagnosed (NADD)**
321 Wall Street 845-331-4336
Kingston, NY 12401 info@thenadd.org
thenadd.org
NADD is a nonprofit organization designed to increase awareness of, and provide services for, individuals with developmental disabilities and mental illness. NADD emphasizes the importance of quality mental healthcare for people with mental health needs and offers conferences, information resources, educational programs, and training materials to professionals, parents, and organizations.
*Jeanne M. Farr, MA, Chief Executive Officer*
*Robert J. Fletcher, DSW, Founder & CEO Emeritus*

1710 **National Association of Councils on Developmental Disabilities**
1825 K Street Northwest 202-506-5813
Washington, DC 20006 info@nacdd.org
nacdd.org
A national membership association representing the 56 State and Territorial Councils on Developmental Disabilities. An organization with the purpose of promoting the programs and policies that its member councils advocate, as well as ensuring inclusion for Americans with developmental disabilities.
*Donna A. Meltzer, Chief Executie Officer*
*Robin Troutman, Deputy Director*

## Foundations

1711 **BrightFocus Foundation**
22512 Gateway Center Drive 800-437-2423
Clarksburg, MD 20871 Fax: 301-258-9454
researchgrants@brightfocus.org
brightfocus.org
Raises awareness of Alzheimer's disease, macular degeneration, and glaucoma and supports research and programs to cure brain and eye diseases.
*Diane Bovenkamp, PhD, Vice President, Scientific Affairs*
*Sharyn Rossi, PhD, Dir., Scientific Programs, Neuroscience*

1712 **NCI Clinical Research Foundation, Inc.**
111 Howard Blvd. 973-398-2900
Mt. Arlington, NJ 07856 Fax: 973-712-9142
ncifoundation@neuroci.com
neuroci.com
A non-profit organization comprised of neuroscientists committed to better discovering and treating neurocognitive and neuropsychiatric disorders.
*Gerald Tramontano, Ph.D., Executive Director*
*Lillian F. Lewis, M.D., Consultant*

1713 **National Niemann-Pick Disease Foundation**
P.O. Box 49 877-287-3672
Fort Atkinson, WI 53538-0049 nnpdf@nnpdf.org
nnpdf.org
The Foundation promotes research and offers support and funding for individuals with Niemann-Pick Disease and their support network.
*Joslyn Crowe, MSW, MA, Executive Director*
*Laurie Turner, Family Services Manager*

## Libraries & Resource Centers

1714 **Alzheimer's Disease & Related Dementias**
National Institute on Aging
P.O. Box 8057 800-438-4380
Gaithersburg, MD 20898 adear@nia.nih.gov
www.nia.nih.gov/health/alzheimers
The ADEAR Center provides information about Alzheimer's Disease and related disorders to health professionals, patients and their families, and the public.
*Nina Silverberg, Program Director, Alzheimer's*

1715 **National Mental Health Consumers' Self-Help Clearinghouse**
selfhelpclearinghouse@gmail.com
mhselfhelp.org
The Clearinghouse is a peer-run national technical assistance center focused on achieving respect and equality of opportunity for those with mental illnesses. The Clearinghouse helps with the growth of the mental health consumer movement by evaluating mental health services, advocating for mental health reform, and

providing consumers with news, information, publications, and consultation services.
*Joseph Rogers, Founder & Executive Director*
*Susan Rogers, Director*

## Print Resources

**1716 American Journal on Intellectual and Developmental Disabilities (AJIDD)**
American Ass. on Intellectual & Dev. Disabilities
8403 Colesville Road 202-387-1968
Silver Spring, MD 20910 meridian.allenpress.com/ajidd
A scientific, scholarly journal that publishes research on intellectual disability for institutions, libraries, researchers, clinicians, students, and health professionals.
*Bimonthly*
*Frank Symons, PhD, FAAIDD, Editor*
*Breanne Byiers, Assistant Editor*

**1717 The Journal of Neuropsychiatry and Clinical Neurosciences**
American Neuropsychiatric Association
P.O. Box 97 anpaoffice@gmail.com
Abilene, KS 67410-1707 neuro.psychiatryonline.org
Publishes peer-reviewed articles on neuroscience and behavioral disorders, and addresses subjects like Alzheimer's disease, traumatic brain injury, Parkinson's disease, epilepsy, and seizure disorders.
*David B. Arciniegas, M.D., Editor*
*C. Alan Anderson, M.D., Deputy Editor*

## Digital Resources

**1718 PsychiatryOnline.org**
American Psychiatric Association Publishing
800 Maine Avenue, S.W. 202-459-9722
Washington, DC 20024 800-368-5777
Fax: 202-403-3094
appi@psych.org
psychiatryonline.org
Hosts numerous psychiatry and mental health publications, including The American Journal of Psychiatry, FOCUS, The Journal of Neuropsychiatry and Clinical Neurosciences, Psychiatric Services, Psychiatric Research and Clinical Practice, and The American Journal of Psychotherapy.

## Web Sites

**1719 Alzforum**
www.alzforum.org
Information in layman's terms, plus many references and resources listed.

**1720 Alzheimer's Disease International**
www.alzint.org
Umbrella organization of associations that support people with dementia.

**1721 Alzheimersupport.com**
Information and products for people dealing with Alzheimer's Disease.

**1722 American Academy of Neurology**
www.aan.com
Provides information for both professionals and the public on neurology subjects, covering Alzheimer's and Parkinson's diseases to stroke and migraine, includes comprehensive fact sheets.

**1723 American Psychiatric Association**
www.psych.org
Practice guidelines for the treatment of patients with Alzheimer's.

**1724 BrightFocus Foundation - Alzheimer's Disease Research**
www.brightfocus.org/alzheimers
Alzheimer's resource for patients and caregivers.

**1725 CyberPsych**
www.cyberpsych.org
Hosts the American Psychoanalyists Foundation, American Association of Suicideology, Society for the Exploration of Psychotherapy Intergration, and Anxiety Disorders Association of America. Also subcategories of the anxiety disorders, as well as general information, including panic disorder, phobias, obsessive compulsive disorder (OCD), social phobia, generalized anxiety disorder, post traumatic stress disorder, and phobias of childhood. Book reviews and links to web pages sharing the topics.

**1726 Mayo Clinic**
www.mayoclinic.org
Information for dealing with Alzheimer's Disease.

**1727 MentalHealth.com**
Online information and a virtual encyclopedia related to mental disorders, possible causes and treatments. News, articles, on-line diagnostic programs and related links. Designed to improve understanding, diagnosis and treatment of mental illness throughout the world. Awarded the Top Site Award and the NetPsych Cutting Edge Site Award.

**1728 National Institute of Neurological Disorders and Stroke**
www.ninds.nih.gov
Neuroscience updates and articles.

**1729 National Institute on Aging - Alzheimer's Disease & Related Dementias**
www.nia.nih.gov/health/alzheimers
A division of the National Institute on Aging of the National Institute of Health. Solid information and a list of federally funded centers for evaluation, referral, treatment.

**1730 Psych Central**
www.psychcentral.com
Personalized one-stop index for psychology, support, and mental health issues, resources, and people on the Internet.

**1731 Substance Abuse And Mental Health Services Administration (SAMHSA)**
www.store.samhsa.gov
Resources on mental disorders as well as treatment and recovery.

# RESPIRATORY ILLNESSES

*The respiratory system is responsible for moving oxygen throughout the body and removing waste gases like carbon dioxide. The organs that help you breathe and get sufficient oxygen for organ health include the airway, lungs and blood vessels. The airways include the mouth, nose, sinuses, throat, trachea (passage between throat and lungs), bronchial tubes (tubes at the end of the trachea that connect to each lung), and the lungs that collect oxygen from the air and move it into the bloodstream. Allergies such as to pet dander, dust and mold; asthma, a chronic inflammatory disorder in the airways that can make breathing difficult; infections leading to pneumonia, bronchitis or the flu; respiratory disorders (lung diseases) such as lung cancer and COPD (chronic obstructive pulmonary disease); aging; and damage to the respiratory system, such as seen with some substance use disorders or inhaling smoke can all affect the respiratory system.*

There are three main types of lung disease:

- Airway diseases such as asthma, chronic obstructive pulmonary disease (COPD) and cystic fibrosis
- Lung tissue diseases caused by scarring or inflammation restricting lung expansion
- Lung circulation diseases affecting the blood vessels of the lung.

Damage to the respiratory system can come from a variety of factors observable in substance use disorder. Smoking is the number one cause of death in those with substance use disorders. Inhaling or injecting any substance are potentially damaging. Asthma and lung disease are a real issue in individuals with a substance use disorder. Smoking is the most-abused substance and causes lung damage, including damaged airways leading to COPD, including emphysema and chronic bronchitis, and tissue damage in the lungs decreasing oxygen exchange capability. Cigarette smoking also causes most cases of lung cancer, up to 85 percent.

The cause of asthma is still unknown, but certain factors play a role in development. They are:

- Family history
- Allergies
- Viral infections of the respiratory tract
- Smoking
- Occupational exposures and air pollution
- Obesity

Asthma makes breathing difficult and while there is no cure, it can be treated to insure a healthier life. Developing a treatment plan with the physician and strictly following the plan can control asthma. Substance use disorder, especially tobacco use and smoke exposure, and abusing recreational drugs, can trigger asthma symptoms that increase the risk of an asthma attack. At each visit with the physician, list all drugs, both prescribed and illicit, taken and be honest about smoking. If working in an area where smoking is permitted or being around heavy smokers at home, be sure to share that with the physician. During an asthma attack, the airways become swollen and inflamed causing the bronchial tubes to narrow. It becomes difficult to take in sufficient air leading to wheezing, coughing and trouble breathing. An asthma attack may be life-threatening if not treated promptly. If symptoms do not improve after using a rescue (quick-acting) inhaler, emergency treatment may be indicated.

Illicit drug use may worsen asthma symptoms. Smoking crack cocaine and heroin increases the risk of an emergency department visit. Cannabis or marijuana, once used as an alternative medicine to dilate the bronchi, will cause wheezing, coughing, excess sputum production, chest tightness and an acute exacerbation of asthma. Too often, physicians directly question tobacco use but neglect to probe about substance use disorders, or individuals do not disclose illicit drug use. In both cases, treatment for asthma may be insufficient or emergencies requiring hospitalization may occur. The opioid crisis, both the use of heroin and opioids, created a respiratory crisis as well, as these substances induce respiratory depression. Snorting heroin causes direct damage to the lungs, including constricting the bronchi. Cocaine snorting or smoking can also trigger near-fatal asthma attacks. Death from an asthma attack is a real possibility if the attack is severe or prompt treatment is not available.

Damage to the lungs caused by smoking or inhaling substances causes damage to the 500 or so alveoli (air sacs) responsible for pulling in oxygen and releasing carbon dioxide. Unlike other structures in the body, lungs cannot repair themselves. Lung tissue will not grow back once destroyed. Lung damage over time from substance use disorder makes it difficult to take in sufficient breath with each inhalation. Shortness of breath is the hallmark sign of lung damage but it often develops slowly over time. Stopping prescription drug abuse or illicit drug use is an easy to grasp concept, but understanding the effects of smoking on lung tissue is often more difficult. Quitting smoking may not reverse the damage but it may still benefit an individual's health and prevent additional problems such as lung cancer. Smoking can shorten life by 10-15 years.

The respiratory system is a complex system that is critical to life. Both legal and illicit substances may cause substance-induced lung disease, trigger asthma attacks, and contribute to potential morbidity and mortality. Substance use disorder creates significant risks of respiratory diseases as well as other issues, including cardiovascular diseases. Getting help to stop smoking and to detoxify from other substance use disorders is critical to respiratory health.

## Agencies & Associations

1732 **Administration for Children and Families**
330 C Street, S.W. 877-696-6775
Washington, DC 20201 www.acf.hhs.gov
The Administration for Children & Families (ACF) is a division of the U.S. Department of Health & Human Services (HHS). ACF promotes the economic and social well-being of families, children, individuals and communities.
*Lauren Supplee, Deputy Assistant Secretary*
*Emily Schmitt, Deputy Director*

1733 **Agency for Healthcare Research and Quality**
5600 Fishers Lane 301-427-1364
Rockville, MD 20857 www.ahrq.gov
The Agency for Healthcare Research and Quality's (AHRQ) mission is to produce evidence to make health care safer, higher quality, more accessible, equitable, and affordable, and to work within the U.S. Department of Health and Human Services and with other partners to make sure that the evidence is understood and used.
*Robert Otto Valdez, PhD, MHSA, Director*
*Howard E. Holland, Director, Office of Communications*

1734 **Agency for Toxic Substances and Disease Registry**
1200 Pennsylvania Ave., N.W. 202-566-0844
Washington, DC 20460 800-232-4636
TTY: 888-232-6348
sxj6@cdc.gov
www.atsdr.cdc.gov
The Agency for Toxic Substances and Disease Registry (ATSDR), based in Atlanta, Georgia, is a federal public health agency of the U.S. Department of Health and Human Services. ATSDR serves the public by using the best science, taking responsive public health actions, and providing trusted health information to prevent harmful exposures and diseases related to toxic substances.
*Steve Jones, MS, Director*

1735 **Allergy & Asthma Network**
8229 Boone Boulevard 800-878-4403
Vienna, VA 22182 Fax: 703-288-5271
info@allergyasthmanetwork.org
www.allergyasthmanetwork.org
Non-profit membership organization dedicated to eliminating suffering and death due to asthma, allergies and related conditions through education, advocacy, community outreach, and research.
*Tonya Winders, MBA, President & CEO*
*Gary Fitzgerald, Senior Editor & Comms. Strategist*

1736 **American Academy of Allergy, Asthma & Immunology**
555 East Wells Street 414-272-6071
Milwaukee, WI 53202-3823 info@aaaai.org
www.aaaai.org
Strives to serve the public through information on asthma and allergies, as well as referrals to allergists.
*David A. Khan, MD, FAAAAI, President*
*Paul V. Williams, MD, FAAAAI, Secretary-Treasurer*

1737 **American Association for Respiratory Care**
9425 N. MacArthur Boulevard 972-243-2272
Irving, TX 75063-4706 Fax: 972-484-2720
info@aarc.org
www.aarc.org
The national and international professional association for respiratory care.
*Daniel Garrett, Executive Director*
*Doug Laher, Chief Operating Officer*

1738 **American College of Allergy, Asthma & Immunology**
85 West Algonquin Road 847-427-1200
Arlington Heights, IL 60005 Fax: 847-427-9656
mail@acaai.org
www.acaai.org
Focuses on research and public awareness of allergies, asthma, and immunology. Distributes informational brochures and pamphlets, offers referrals and counseling services, as well as patient care.
*Rick Slawny, Executive Director*
*Kevin Bragaw, Chief Financial Officer*

1739 **American Lung Association**
55 W. Wacker Drive 800-586-4872
Chicago, IL 60601 info@lung.org
www.lung.org
The mission of the American Lung Association is to prevent lung disease and promote lung health by fighting disease in all its forms, with special emphasis on asthma, tobacco control and environmental health.
*Harold Wimmer, National President & CEO*
*Neil Ballentine, Chief Technical Officer*

1740 **Asthma Canada**
124 Merton Street 866-787-4050
Toronto, Ontario, M4S-2Z2 info@asthma.ca
www.asthma.ca
National, volunteer-led organization devoted to enhancing the quality of life for individuals with athsma and respiratory allergies.
*Jenna Reynolds, Interim CEO/Dir., Programs & Services*
*Zhen Liu, Dir., Operations & Administration*

1741 **Birth Defect Research for Children, Inc.**
976 Lake Baldwin Lane 407-895-0802
Celebration, FL 32814 staff@birthdefects.org
www.birthdefects.org/allergies
A non-profit organization providing parents and soon-to-be parents with information resources about birth defects, and support services for their children. Offers fact sheets on allergies.

1742 **Canadian Lung Association**
885 Meadowlands Dr. 613-569-6411
Ottawa, ON, K2C-3N2 888-566-5864
info@lung.ca
www.lung.ca
The leading organization in Canada that promotes lung health and funds treatments for lung disease.
*Nora Lacey, Chairperson*
*Deborah Harri, Treasurer*

1743 **Canadian Society of Allergy and Clinical Immunology**
207 Bank St. 613-265-7571
Ottawa, Ontario, K2P-2N2 info@csaci.ca
www.csaci.ca
Promotes the advancement of the knowledge and practice of allergy, clinical immunology, and asthma for optimal patient care.
*Anne Ellis, MD, MSc, FRCPC, President*
*Edmond Chan, MD, MSc, FRCPC, Vice President*

1744 **Centers for Disease Control & Prevention: Division of Adolescent & School Health**
1600 Clifton Road 800-232-4636
Atlanta, GA 30333 TTY: 888-232-6348
www.cdc.gov/HealthyYouth
CDC promotes the health and well-being of children and adolescents to enable them to become healthy and productive adults.

1745 **Centers for Medicare & Medicaid Services**
7500 Security Boulevard 410-786-3000
Baltimore, MD 21244 877-267-2323
TTY: 866-226-1819
www.cms.gov
U.S. federal agency which administers Medicare, Medicaid, and the State Children's Health Insurance Program.
*Chiquita Brooks-LaSure, Administrator*
*Jonathan Blum, Principal Deputy Administrator & COO*

1746 **National Center for Complementary and Integrative Health**
9000 Rockville Pike 888-644-6226
Bethesda, MD 20892 TTY: 866-464-3615
info@nccih.nih.gov
nccih.nih.gov
The National Center for Complementary and Integrative Health (NCCIH) is the Federal Government's lead agency for scientific research on the diverse medical and health care systems, practices, and products that are not generally considered part of conventional medicine.
*Helene M. Langevin, MD, Director*
*David Shurtleff, PhD, Deputy Director*

1747 **National Human Genome Research Institute**
Building 31, Room 4B09 301-402-0911
Bethesda, MD 20892 Fax: 301-402-2218
nhgripressoffice@mail.nih.gov
www.genome.gov
The National Human Genome Research Institute began as the National Center for Human Genome Research (NCHGR), which was established in 1989 to carry out the role of the National Institutes of Health (NIH) in the International Human Genome Project (HGP).
*Eric D. Green, MD, PhD, Director*
*Lawrence Brody, PhD, Director, Division of Genomics & Society*

1748 **National Institute for Occupational Safety and Health**
Centers for Disease Control and Prevention
1600 Clifton Rd. 800-232-4636
Atlanta, GA 30333 www.cdc.gov/niosh
The National Institute for Occupational Safety and Health (NIOSH) is the U.S. federal agency that conducts research and makes recommendations to prevent worker injury and illness.
*John Howard, Director*
*Frank Hearl, Chief of Staff*

1749 **National Institute of Allergy and Infectious Diseases**
NIAID Office of Communications & Govt Relations
5601 Fishers Lane 301-496-5717
Bethesda, MD 20892 866-284-4107
Fax: 301-402-3573
TDD: 800-877-8339
ocpostoffice@niaid.nih.gov
www.niaid.nih.gov
Conducts and supports research on allergies; focused on understanding what happens to the body during the allergic process. Educates patients and health care workers in controlling allergic disease; offers various research centers that conduct and evaluate educational programs focused on methods to control allergic diseases.
*Anthony S. Fauci, MD, Director*

1750 **National Institute of Biomedical Imaging and Bioengineering**
9000 Rockville Pike 301-496-8859
Bethesda, MD 20892 info@nibib.nih.gov
www.nibib.nih.gov
The mission of the National Institute of Biomedical Imaging and Bioengineering (NIBIB) is to improve health by leading the development and accelerating the application of biomedical technologies.
*Bruce J. Tromberg, PhD, Director*
*Jill Heemskerk, PhD, Deputy Director*

1751 **National Institute of Environmental Health Sciences**
P.O. Box 12233 919-541-3345
Research Triangle Park, NC 27709 Fax: 919-541-4395
www.niehs.nih.gov
The mission of the NIEHS is to discover how the environment affects people in order to promote healthier lives.
*Rick Woychik, PhD, Director*
*Trevor K. Archer, PhD, Deputy Director*

1752 **National Institute of General Medical Sciences**
45 Center Drive 301-496-7301
Bethesda, MD 20892 www.nigms.nih.gov
The National Institute of General Medical Sciences (NIGMS) supports basic research that increases understanding of biological processes and lays the foundation for advances in disease diagnosis, treatment and prevention.
*Jon R. Lorsch, PhD, Director*
*Dorit Zuk, PhD, Deputy Director*

1753 **National Institute of Nursing Research**
31 Center Drive 301-496-0207
Bethesda, MD 20892-2178 info@ninr.nih.gov
www.ninr.nih.gov
The mission of the National Institute of Nursing Research (NINR) is to promote and improve the health of individuals, families, communities, and populations.
*Shannon N. Zenk, PhD, MPH, RN, FAAN, Director*
*John Grason, PhD, Acting Deputy Director*

1754 **National Jewish Health**
1400 Jackson Street 800-652-9555
Denver, CO 80206 877-225-5654
physicianline@njhealth.org
www.nationaljewish.org
Leading respiratory hospital in the nation offering comprehensive diagnosis, treatment and rehabilitation of people with chronic obstructive pulmonary disease, asthma, allergies and other respiratory and immune diseases.
*Michael Salem, MD, President & CEO*
*Steven D. Kris, Chair*

1755 **Pulmonary Hypertension Association (PHA)**
1629 K. St. 301-565-3004
Washington, DC 20006 800-748-7274
www.PHAssociation.org
A non-profit organization for pulmonary hypertension patients, families, caregivers and PH-treating medical professionals. PHA works to provide support, education, and find a cure for pulmonary hypertension.
*Matt Granato, President & CEO*
*Elizabeth Joseloff, VP, Quality Care & Research*

1756 **US Environmental Protection Agency: Indoor Environments Division**
1200 Pennsylvania Avenue NW 800-424-8802
Washington, DC 20460 www.epa.gov/indoor-air-quality-iaq
Responsible for implementing EPA's Indoor Environments Program, a voluntary program to address indoor air pollution.

1757 **White Lung Association**
info@whitelung.org
www.whitelung.org
A national non-profit organization dedicated to the education of the public to the hazards of asbestos exposure. The association developed programs of public education and consults with victims of asbestos exposure, school boards, building owners and government representatives.
*Jim Perry, Director of Development*

## Foundations

1758 **American Academy of Allergy, Asthma & Immunology Foundation**
555 East Wells Street 414-272-6071
Milwaukee, WI 53202 Fax: 414-272-6070
www.aaaaifoundation.org
Funds research in an effort to prevent and cure asthma and allergic/immunologic diseases.
*Karen Michaels, M.Ed., Director*
*Michael Clothier, Development Manager*

1759 **American College of Allergy, Asthma & Immunology Foundation**
85 West Algonquin Road 847-427-1200
Arlington Heights, IL 60005 Fax: 847-427-9656
mail@acaai.org
college.acaai.org
Funds faculty research grants and travel scholarships for the education and development of allergies, asthma, and immunology.
*Rick Slawny, Executive Director*

1760 **American Respiratory Care Foundation (ARCF)**
9425 North Macarthur Blvd. 972-243-2272
Irving, TX 75063-4706 Fax: 972-484-2720
arcfoundation.org
The American Respiratory Care Foundation promotes respiratory health by supporting research and education.
*Tonya A. Winders, MBA, Chair*
*Neil MacIntyre, MD, FAARC, Vice Chair*

1761 **Asthma and Allergy Foundation of America**
8201 Corporate Drive 202-466-7643
Landover, MD 20785 800-727-8462
Fax: 202-466-8940
info@aafa.org
www.aafa.org
The AAFA is a non-profit patient organization dedicated to improving the quality of life for people with asthma and allergies and

their caregivers, through education, advocacy, funding, and research.
*Kenneth Mendez, President & CEO*
*Melanie Carver, Chief Mission Officer*

1762 **Asthma and Allergy Foundation of America: St. Louis**
5501 Delmar Blvd.
St. Louis, MO 63112
314-645-2422
Fax: 314-692-2022
admin@aafastl.org
www.aafastl.org
Serves patients of all ages in St. Louis and surrounding counties who are affected by asthma and allergies, and also provides resources to healthcare professionals, caregivers and childcare providers. Offers the BREATH asthma and allergy management program for children.
*Chris Martinez, MIB, CFRE, Executive Director*

1763 **National Science Foundation**
2415 Eisenhower Avenue
Alexandria, VA 22314
703-292-5111
800-877-8339
TTY: 800-281-8749
info@nsf.gov
www.nsf.gov
NSF is the only federal agency whose mission includes support for all fields of fundamental science and engineering, except for medical sciences.
*Sethuraman Panchanathan, Director*
*Teresa A. Grancorvitz, Deputy Chief Operating Officer*

1764 **Ontario Lung Association**
18 Wynford Drive
Toronto, ON, M3C-0K8
416-864-9911
info@lunghealth.ca
hcp.lunghealth.ca
Invests in research that improves lung health, focusing on asthma, chronic obstructive pulmonary disease, lung cancer, infectious respiratory disease, and smoking/vaping prevention.
*Jessica Buckley, President & CEO*
*Peter Glazier, Executive Vice President*

1765 **Pulmonary Fibrosis Foundation**
230 E. Ohio Street
Chicago, IL 60611
888-733-6741
844-825-5733
Fax: 866-587-9158
development@pulmonaryfibrosis.org
www.pulmonaryfibrosis.org
Dedicated to finding a cure for and raising awareness of pulmonary fibrosis.
*William T. Schmidt, President & CEO*
*Scott Staszak, Chief Operating Officer*

## Research Centers

1766 **Brigham and Women's Hospital: Rheumatology Immunology, and Allergy Division**
75 Francis Street
Boston, MA 02115
61 -73 -550
Fax: 617-525-1001
TTY: 617-732-6458
www.brighamandwomens.org
Internationally renowned for excellence in clinical care, clinical investigation and basic research. A faculty of 36 board certified rheumatologists and allergists provide urgent and emergency consultations as necessary.
*Michael B. Brenner, MD, Division Chief*
*Jonathan S. Coblyn, Clinical Director Rheumatology*

1767 **Childrens Hospital Immunology Division**
Children's Hospital
300 Longwood Avenue
Boston, MA 02115
www.childrenshospital.org
Organizational research unit of the Children's Hospital that focuses on the causes, prevention and treatments of asthma, infections and allergies.
*Dr. James Mandell, CEO*
*Sandra Fenwick, President & COO*

1768 **Clinical Immunology, Allergy, and Rheumatology**
Tulane Medical School
1700 Perdido Street
New Orleans, LA 70112
504-988-5187
Fax: 504-988-3686
medsch@tulane.edu
www.som.tulane.edu/medciar
*Mauel Lopez, MD, Director*

1769 **Duke Asthma, Allergy and Airway Center**
4309 Medical Park Drive
Durham, NC 27704
919-620-7300
www.aaac.duhs.duke.edu/
*Raffeal Rau, President*
*Dr. Monica Kraft, Director*

1770 **Enzymology Research Laboratory**
Dept. of Veterans Affairs Medical Center
150 Muir Road
Martinez, CA 94553
925-228-6800
Studies affecting emphysema in mankind.
*Michael C. Gaussig, President*

1771 **Johns Hopkins University: Asthma and Allergy Center**
5501 Hopkins Bayview Circle
Baltimore, MD 21224
410-550-2101
Fax: 410-550-3256
jhuallergy@jhmi.edu
www.hopkinsmedicine.org/allergy
Studies of allergic diseases and individuals with allergic disease pulmonary diseases and diseases involving inflammation and immunological processes.
*Bruce S. Bochner, Director*
*Peter S. Creticos, Clinical Director*

1772 **National Jewish Division of Immunology**
National Jewish Medical and Research Center
1400 Jackson Street
Denver, CO 80206
303-398-1337
80 -42 -889
Fax: 303-270-2125
harbeckr@njc.org
www.njc.org
The only medical center in the country whose research and patient care resources are dedicated to respiratory and immunologic diseases.
*John Cambier, Chairman*
*Ronald J. Harbeck, Medical Director*

1773 **Northwestern University: Division of Allergy and Immunology**
The Feinberg School of Medicine
251 East Huron Street
Chicago, IL 60611
312-926-6895
Fax: 312-926-6905
rpschleimer@northwestern.edu
www.medicine.northwestern.edu
A referral center of local, regional, and national stature. Areas of clinical excellence include asthma, allergic bronchopulmonary aspergillosis, idiopathic anaphylaxis, drug allergy, occupational immunologic lung disease, and allergen immunotherapy.
*Douglas E. Vaughan, MD, Chair*
*James Foody, MD, Vice Chair Clinical Affairs*

1774 **University of Utah Rocky Mountain Center for Occupational & Environmental Health**
University of Utah
391 Chipeta Way
Salt Lake City, UT 84108
801-581-4800
Fax: 801-817-24
TTY: 801-581-7224
rmoser@rmcoeh.utah.edu
medicine.utah.edu/rmcoeh/
Provides graduate and continuing education programs in occupational medicine, occupational health nursing, ergonomics and safety, industrial hygiene, and hazardous materials. Additionally provides clinical evaluations and consultations in the listed areas.
*Dennis Lloyd, Chair*
*Sen Karen Mayne, Advisory Member*

1775 **University of Virginia: General Clinical Research Center**
University of Virginia Health System
2515 Lee Street
Charlottesville, VA 22908
434-924-2394
Fax: 434-924-9960
www.healthsystem.virginia.edu/
Focuses on asthmatic disorders.
*Eugene J. Barrett, Program Director*

1776 **University of Wisconsin: Asthma, Allergy and Pulmonary Research Center**
600 Highland Avenue 608-263-6400
Madison, WI 53792 Fax: 608-263-6401
www.medicine.wisc.edu
*Sheri L. Lawrence, MBA, Administrator*
*Sharon Gehl, MBA, Associate Administrator*

1777 **Warren Grant Magnuson Clinical Center**
National Institute of Health
10 Center Drive MSC 1078 301-496-3311
Bethesda, MD 20892 800-411-1222
Fax: 301-496-2390
TTY: 866-411-1010
mmichael@cc.nih.gov
www.clinicalcenter.nih.gov
Established in 1953 as the research hospital of the National Institutes of Health. Designed so that patient care facilities are close to research laboratories so new findings of basic and clinical scientists can be quickly applied to the treatment of patients. Upon referral by physicians, patients are admitted to NIH clinical studies.
*John Mark, Lung Help Line Director*

## Support Groups & Hotlines

1778 **American Lung Association HelpLine**
55 W. Wacker Drive 800-586-4872
Chicago, IL 60601 info@lung.org
www.lung.org
Provides state-by-state association information, and offers support group referrals.

1779 **National Health Information Center**
Office of Disease Prevention & Health Promotion
1101 Wootton Pkwy Fax: 240-453-8281
Rockville, MD 20852 odphpinfo@hhs.gov
www.health.gov/nhic
Supports public health education by maintaining a calendar of National Health Observances; helps connect consumers and health professionals to organizations that can best answer questions and provide up-to-date contact information from reliable sources; updates on a yearly basis toll-free numbers for health information, Federal health clearinghouses and info centers.
*Don Wright, MD, MPH, Director*

1780 **Support for Asthmatic Youth**
Asthma and Allergy Foundation of America
1080 Glen Cove Avenue 516-625-5735
Glen Head, NY 11545 Fax: 516-625-2976
A network of educational/support groups for adolescents between the ages of 9 and 17. All meetings are free and feature guest speakers, informational programs, games and other fun activities.
*Renee Theodorakis, MA, Director, Adolescent Services*

## Print Resources

1781 **AllergyWatch**
American College of Allergy, Asthma & Immunology
85 West Algonquin Road 847-427-1200
Arlington Heights, IL 60005 Fax: 847-427-9656
mail@acaai.org
college.acaai.org
Published six times per year in one volume, this publication provides a synopsis of allergy and asthma literature from 19 major medical journals.
*Bimonthly*
*Stanley M. Fineman, MD, Editor-in-Chief*

1782 **Annals of Allergy, Asthma & Immunology**
American College of Allergy, Asthma & Immunology
85 West Algonquin Road 847-427-1200
Arlington Heights, IL 60005 Fax: 847-427-9656
mail@acaai.org
www.annallergy.org
A scholarly medical journal that publishes materials on the fields of allergy, asthma, and immunology.
*Monthly*
*Mitchell H. Grayson, MD, FACAAI, Editor-in-Chief*
*Jonthan Spergel, MD, PhD, FACAAI, Deputy Editor*

1783 **Respiratory Care**
American Association for Respiratory Care
9425 N. Macarthur Boulevard 972-514-7710
Irving, TX 75063-4706 info@aarc.org
www.aarc.org/resources/publications/
Publishes original research on the monitoring, prevention, and management of respiratory illnesses.
*Monthly*
*Richard D. Branson, MSC, RRT, FAARC, Editor-in-Chief*
*Dean R. Hess, PhD, RRT, FAARC, Managing Editor*

## Web Sites

1784 **Allergy & Asthma Network**
www.allergyasthmanetwork.org
Non-profit membership organization dedicated to eliminating suffering and death due to asthma, allergies, and related conditions through education, advocacy, community outreach, and research.

1785 **American Academy of Allergy, Asthma & Immunology**
www.aaaai.org
Strives to serve the public through information on asthma and allergies, as well as referrals to allergists.

1786 **American College of Allergy, Asthma & Immunology**
www.acaai.org
Focuses on research and public awareness of allergies, asthma, and immunology. Distributes informational brochures and pamphlets, offers referrals and counseling services, as well as patient care.

1787 **American Lung Association**
www.lung.org
Offers research, medical updates, fund-raising, educational materials and public awareness campaigns relating to lung disease causes.

1788 **Asthma and Allergy Foundation of America**
www.aafa.org
The AAFA is a non-profit patient organization dedicated to improving the quality of life for people with asthma and allergies and their caregivers, through education, advocacy, funding, and research.

1789 **Gazoontite**
www.gazoontite.com
Provides links to websites involving asthma and also asthma-related products, such as books and guides.

1790 **Healing Well**
www.healingwell.com
An online health resource guide to medical news, chat, information and articles, newsgroups and message boards, books, disease-related web sites, medical directories, and more for patients, friends, and family coping with disabling diseases, disorders, or chronic illnesses.

1791 **Health Central**
www.healthcenter.com
Provides support group and diagnostic information regarding lung disease.

1792 **Healthlink USA**
www.healthlinkusa.com
Health information concerning treatment, cures, prevention, diagnosis, risk factors, research, support groups, email lists, personal stories and much more. Updated regularly.

1793 **Lung Disease**
www.lungusa.org
The American Lung Association's website, including information on diseases A to Z, living with lung disease, tobacco control, air quality, data, statistics, research, and more.

1794 **MedicineNet**

www.medicinenet.com

An online resource for consumers providing easy-to-read, authoritative medical and health information.

1795 **Medscape**

www.medscape.com

Medscape offers specialists, primary care physicians, and other health professionals the Web's most robust and integrated medical information and educational tools.

1796 **MyHealthfinder**

www.healthfinder.gov

Searchable, carefully developed web site offering information on over 1000 topics. Developed by the US Department of Health and Human Services, the site can be used in both English and Spanish.

1797 **National Heart, Lung & Blood Institute**

www.nhlbi.nih.gov

A website maintained by the National Institute of Health offering general information regarding the heart, lungs, and blood.

1798 **WebMD**

www.webmd.com

Provides credible information, supportive communities, and in-depth reference material about health subjects. A source for original and timely health information, as well as material from well-known content providers.

# SEXUALLY TRANSMITTED DISEASES

*The misuse of substances such as alcohol and drugs continue to grow in the United States. Changes in sexual thoughts, feelings and behavior have been reported when substance use disorder exists. More than half of individuals in one study reported enhancement in sex but also reported an increase in risky behavior related to sex. The positive effects between substance use and sexual behavior causes individuals to be hesitant to stop substance use when it has a positive effect in their sexual satisfaction.*

Individuals in teenage and early adult years are particularly critical periods of risk for substance use disorder. Sexual risk behaviors, often as a result of substance use disorders, put the individual at risk for HIV and sexually transmitted diseases (STDs). Substance use disorders are closely related to sexually transmitted diseases, including HIV, as substances may cause interference in judgement. Studies have shown that there is a correlation between substance use and sexual risk behaviors in teens such as having unprotected sex and having multiple partners. Sexual risk behaviors increase with alcohol, marijuana, and cocaine use and other illicit drugs but also when prescription drug misuse or abuse occurs. In a survey, teens who are currently sexually active drank alcohol (19%) before their last sexual encounter. Teens reporting no substance use are least likely to engage in risky sexual behaviors.

Common risk factors for substance use and risky sexual behaviors in teenage students include:

- Poverty
- Family history and family problems
- Lack of positive parenting or parental approvable of the behavior, such as drinking alcohol or smoking allowed at home
- Association with substance abusing peers
- Lack of school connectedness, alienation and rebelliousness

Adults with substance use disorder are also at risk for poor judgment related to sexual risk behaviors and about 10 percent of adults with SUD report their sexual behavior is influenced by their primary substance of choice and increased their cravings. Drug users are consistently identified as a population at risk for STIs. The use of crack cocaine is associated with higher levels of risky behaviors including more sex partners and decreased use of condoms. Drug use such as opiates is less associated with risky sexual behavior. Certain substances may more directly cause risky behaviors than others. Small amounts of alcohol and cannabis can enhance sexual arousal but high doses can inhibit sexual function. Both alcohol and other substances may interfere with judgment, leading individuals to act in ways inconsistent with their behavior when sober. There appears to be a clear difference in behaviors between recreational substance use and substance abuse disorder.

Sexually transmitted infection (STI) refers to a disease pathogen that causes infection by sexual contact or exchange of bodily fluids. Prevention and control of STIs depend on:

- Accurate risk assessment and education of individuals in changing risky sexual behaviors

- Use of vaccines for pre-exposure, preventable STIs
- Identification of the individual exhibiting symptoms of an STI and their partners
- Effective diagnosis, treatment, counseling and follow-up
- Evaluation, treatment and counseling of sex partners exposed to STIs

After obtaining a sexual history from the individual, the healthcare provider should discuss strategies designed to encourage risk reduction through prevention counseling.

Sexually transmitted diseases are directly related to unprotected sex and poor judgement in terms of selected partners. Casual, random sex poses a greater risk of inappropriate sexual behaviors, especially when under the influence of illicit substances. Just as sharing needles is an incredibly risky behavior related to HIV and other infections, unprotected sex causes similar health issues as HIV, and a variety of STDs may be transmitted during intercourse.

Substance use disorders are perceived as leading to behaviors not generally seen in individuals with no substance use, including risky sexual behaviors. Unless substance use disorder is treated, the individual remains at risk for STDs.

## Agencies & Associations

1799 **American Sexual Health Association (ASHA)**
P.O. Box 13827 919-361-8400
Research Triangle Park, NC 27709 Fax: 919-361-8425
info@ashasexualhealth.org
www.ashasexualhealth.org
Provides resources to local communities to improve STD control programs through citizen action.
*Lynn Barclay, President & CEO*
*Deborah Arrindell, VP, Health Policy*

1800 **American Sexually Transmitted Diseases Association (ASTDA)**
P.O. Box 12665 919-861-9399
Research Triangle Park, NC 27709 astda@astda.org
www.astda.org
ASTDA is a membership organization representing physicians, research scientists, nurses, public health professionals, and other STD investigators.
*Khalil Ghanem, MD, PhD, President*
*Abby Norris Turner, PhD, VP & President-Elect*

1801 **Centers for Disease Control & Prevention: Division of Adolescent & School Health**
1600 Clifton Road 800-232-4636
Atlanta, GA 30333 TTY: 888-232-6348
www.cdc.gov/HealthyYouth
CDC promotes the health and well-being of children and adolescents to enable them to become healthy and productive adults.

1802 **National Coalition of STD Directors (NCSD)**
1029 Vermont Ave., N.W. 202-842-4660
Washington, DC 20005 Fax: 202-842-4542
dharvey@ncsddc.org
www.ncsddc.org
NCSD is a national public health membership organization representing over 1,000 health department STD directors. Dedicated to promoting STD prevention through various initiatives and projects.
*David C. Harvey, Executive Director*
*Lakita McNeil, Senior Manager, Operations*

1803 **National Institute of Allergy and Infectious Diseases**
NIAID Office of Communications & Govt Relations
5601 Fishers Lane 301-496-5717
Bethesda, MD 20892 866-284-4107
Fax: 301-402-3573
TDD: 800-877-8339
ocpostoffice@niaid.nih.gov
www.niaid.nih.gov
Conducts and supports research on allergies; focused on understanding what happens to the body during the allergic process. Educates patients and health care workers in controlling allergic disease; offers various research centers that conduct and evaluate educational programs focused on methods to control allergic diseases.
*Anthony S. Fauci, MD, Director*

## Research Centers

1804 **Herpes Resource Center**
P.O. Box 13827 919-361-8400
Research Triangle Park, NC 27709 ashasexualhealth.org/herpes
Offers information and referrals for persons affected by herpes and other sexually transmitted disease prevention.
*Deborah Arrindell, VP, Health Policy*

1805 **International Union Against Venereal Diseases**
New York Hospital - Cornell Medical Center
1153 York Avenue 212-746-1200
New York, NY 10021 Fax: 212-746-1202
Encourages campaigns medical and social against venereal disease.
*Lewis Drusin MD, Director*

1806 **University of Chicago Committee on Virology**
Marjorie B Kovler Viral Oncology Laboratories
910 E 58th Street 773-702-1620
Chicago, IL 60637 Fax: 773-702-1631
mgcb.bsd.uchicago.edu
Focuses research into the area of sexually transmitted disease.
*Bernard Roizman, Chairman*
*Olaf Schneewind, Professor and Chairman*

## Support Groups & Hotlines

1807 **National Health Information Center**
Office of Disease Prevention & Health Promotion
1101 Wootton Pkwy Fax: 240-453-8281
Rockville, MD 20852 odphpinfo@hhs.gov
www.health.gov/nhic
Supports public health education by maintaining a calendar of National Health Observances; helps connect consumers and health professionals to organizations that can best answer questions and provide up-to-date contact information from reliable sources; updates on a yearly basis toll-free numbers for health information, Federal health clearinghouses and info centers.
*Don Wright, MD, MPH, Director*

## Print Resources

1808 **Sexually Transmitted Diseases**
American Sexually Transmitted Diseases Association
P.O. Box 12665 919-861-9399
Research Triangle Park, NC 27709 astda@astda.org
astda.org
A peer-reviewed journal that publishes original articles, case reports, reviews, and editorials on sexually transmitted diseases and related fields.
*William C. Miller, MD, PhD, MPH, Editor-in-Chief*
*H. Hunter Handsfield, MD, Associate Editor Emeritus*

## Web Sites

1809 **American Social Health Association**
www.ashasexualhealth.org
The American Sexual Health Association promotes the sexual health of individuals, families and communities by advocating sound policies and practices and educating the public, professionals and policy makers, in order to foster healthy sexual behaviors and relationships and prevent adverse health outcomes.

1810 **Centers for Disease Control**
www.cdc.gov
Offers reprints, reports, public awareness and educational materials and research on sexually transmitted diseases.

1811 **Healing Well**
www.healingwell.com
An online health resource guide to medical news, chat, information and articles, newsgroups and message boards, books, disease-related web sites, medical directories, and more for patients, friends, and family coping with disabling diseases, disorders, or chronic illnesses.

1812 **Healthlink USA**
www.healthlinkusa.com
Health information concerning treatment, cures, prevention, diagnosis, risk factors, research, support groups, email lists, personal stories and much more. Updated regularly.

1813 **MedicineNet**
www.medicinenet.com
An online resource for consumers providing easy-to-read, authoritative medical and health information.

1814 **Medscape**
www.medscape.com
Medscape offers specialists, primary care physicians, and other health professionals the Web's most robust and integrated medical information and educational tools.

1815 **MyHealthfinder**
www.healthfinder.gov

Searchable, carefully developed web site offering information on over 1000 topics. Developed by the US Department of Health and Human Services, the site can be used in both English and Spanish.

1816 **WebMD**

www.webmd.com

Provides credible information, supportive communities, and in-depth reference material about health subjects. A source for original and timely health information, as well as material from well-known content providers.

# SLEEP DISORDERS

*Many common mental disorders are associated with disturbed sleep, including depression and anxiety. Substance use disorders may cause sleep disorders, but insomnia and insufficient sleep may also increase the risk of drug use and addiction. Sleep and sleep disturbances in substance use disorder require prevention and careful management where possible. Both substance use and withdrawal negatively impact sleep. An inability to fall asleep, sleep quality once asleep, and how long an individual sleeps are all influenced by substance use disorder. Insomnia also occurs during withdrawal, fueling drug cravings. Sleep disruptions have an impact on performance the next day. A real issue with sleep disorders and substance use disorders, is the likelihood that an individual will self-medicate in order to achieve sleep.*

Sleep disorders are thought to contribute to initiating and maintaining drug and alcohol abuse and as factors that increase the risk of relapse after treatment. While some drugs of abuse disrupt sleep or daytime alertness, each individual responds differently. Drug-seeking behaviors may initially be used to try to get to sleep. For example, pre-sleep alcohol use may be effective at first in encouraging sleep onset but later becomes less effective. As effectiveness diminishes, the individual may increase the amount of alcohol consumed in an attempt to achieve sleep. Mood-altering drugs or seeking drugs for a euphoric feeling may initially begin in an attempt to sleep. Self-medication is dangerous. Asking the physician about sleep aids is important to preventing increasing dependence on addictive substances.

Dopamine is a neurotransmitter responsible for allowing feelings of pleasure, satisfaction and motivation. When an individual feels good after accomplishing a task, it is because a surge of dopamine has occurred in the brain. Dopamine can be triggered by shopping, sex, and basically any "feel-good" situation. When a drug directly or indirectly stimulates the excretion of dopamine, the dopamine reward pathways may encourage dependence on the substance to continue the "feel-good" situation, leading to addiction. Dopamine also is responsible for the level of alertness in an individual and may influence the sleep-wake cycle. Too much dopamine results in anxiety, difficulty sleeping, mania, stress and an improved ability to focus.

Drugs like cocaine, nicotine and opioids cause dopamine to flood the reward pathway in amounts 10 times a natural reward. The brain remembers the feeling of this dopamine flood and associates it with the addictive substance. Initially substances may aid in getting to sleep, but over time this effect declines and the risk of addiction increases.

Sleep disturbances contribute to substance use disorders, but the direct cause is not understood. Insomnia has been validated as a risk factor for substance abuse. Treatment for substance use disorder will ultimately enhance the ability to sleep as it is understood that chronic alcohol and drug use alters the neurobiology of sleep. All drugs of abuse and alcohol disrupt sleep and next-day alertness. Sleep disturbances may contribute to the development and continuation of substance use disorders and eventual relapses after therapy.

## Agencies & Associations

1817 **American Chronic Pain Association**
11936 W. 119th Street
Overland Park, KS 66213-2216
ACPA@theacpa.org
www.theacpa.org
The ACPA facilitates peer support and education for individuals with chronic pain in its many forms, in order to increase quality of life. Also raises awareness among the healthcare community, and with policy makers.
*Trupti Gokani, MD, President*
*Kathy Sapp, Chief Executive Officer*

1818 **American Sleep Apnea Association**
1414 NE 42nd St.
Seattle, WA 98105
contact@sleepapnea.org
www.sleepapnea.org
Offers help and information to persons with sleep apnea and their families.
*Martinique Edwards, Staff Writer*
*Tochukwu Ikpeze, Staff Writer*

1819 **Canadian Sleep Society**
info@css-scs.ca
css-scs.ca
A national organization that advocates for sleep health through funding research, offering patient information brochures in French and English, and providing training/educational oppportunities to members.
*Celyne Bastien, PhD, President*
*Najib Ayas, MD, MPH, Secretary/Treasurer*

1820 **Narcolepsy Network**
3242 NE 3rd Avenue #1101
Camas, WA 98607
401-667-2523
888-292-6522
info@narcolepsynetwork.org
narcolepsynetwork.org
Offers help and information to persons with narcolepsy and their families.
*Keith Harper, President*
*Paul Reynolds, Vice President*

1821 **National Institute of Neurological Disorders and Stroke**
P.O. Box 5801
Bethesda, MD 20824
800-352-9424
www.ninds.nih.gov
Seeks to reduce the burden of neurological disease affecting individuals from all walks of life.
*Walter Koroshetz, MD, Director*
*Amy Bany Adams, PhD, Acting Principal Deputy Director*

1822 **Sleep Research Society (SRS)**
2510 N Frontage Road
Darien, IL 60561
630-737-9702
coordinator@srsnet.org
www.sleepresearchsociety.org
Facilitates communication among research workers in the field of sleep medicine.
*Namni Goel, PhD, President*
*Stephanie J. Crowley, PhD, Secretary & Treasurer*

## Foundations

1823 **National Sleep Foundation**
2001 Massachusetts Ave., N.W.
Washington, DC 20036
703-243-1697
www.thensf.org
The National Sleep Foundation promotes sleep health as a "crucial measure of overall health" through education and advocacy.
*Temitayo O. Oyegbile-Chidi, MD, PhD, Chair*
*Thomas C. DiSalvi, CDS, Vice Chair*

1824 **Sleep Research Society Foundation**
2510 North Frontage Road
Darien, IL 60561
630-737-9702
coordinator@srsnet.org
sleepresearchsociety.org/foundation/
The Sleep Research Society Foundation funds research and education opportunities in the field of sleep.
*Sairam Parthasarathy, MD, President*
*Stephanie J. Crowley, PhD, Secretary & Treasurer*

## Libraries & Resource Centers

1825 **SleepFoundation.org**
1414 NE 42nd St.
Seattle, WA 98105
877-672-8966
www.sleepfoundation.org
Information for millions of Americans who suffer from sleep disorders, and to prevent the catastrophic accidents that are related to poor or disordered sleep through research, education and the dissemination of information.
*Keith Cushner, Executive Director, Product*
*Logan Foley, Managing Editor, Health & Product*

## Research Centers

1826 **Baylor College of Medicine: Sleep Disorder and Research Center**
6620 Main St
Houston, TX 77030
713-798-1000
800-229-5671
Fax: 713-796-9718
baylorclinicweb@bcm.edu
www.baylorclinic.com
Internal unit of the College that focuses on research into sleep and sexual dysfunction in males.
*Shyam Subramanian, Medical Director*
*Charlie Lan, Assistant Professor of Medicine*

1827 **Capital Regional Sleep-Wake Disorders Center**
St. Peter's Hospital and Albany Medical Center
25 Hackett Boulevard
Albany, NY 12208
518-436-9253

1828 **Center for Narcolepsy Research at the University of Illinois at Chicago**
University of Illinois
845 S Damen Avenue
Chicago, IL 60612
312-996-5176
Fax: 312-996-7008
CNSHR@listserv.uic.edu
www.uic.edu/depts/cnr
Provides information to health professionals and people with sleep disorders regarding diagnosis and treatment.
*6-8 pages*
*David W. Carley, Director*
*Julie Law, Center Administrator*

1829 **Center for Research in Sleep Disorders Affiliated with Mercy Hospital**
Mercy Hospital of Hamilton/Fairfield
1275 E Kemper Road
Cincinnati, OH 45246
513-671-3101

1830 **Center for Sleep & Wake Disorders: Miami Valley Hospital**
One Wyoming Street
Dayton, OH 45409
937-208-8000
www.miamivalleyhospital.org
Offering the largest variety of sleep disorder testing available in the area, it also offers comprehensive sleep care and care of related issues with a sleep lab, clinical treatment, pulmonary treatment, and behavioral treatment in the same facility.
*Kevin Huban, Director*
*Amy Cline, Administrative Director*

1831 **Center for Sleep Medicine of the Mount Sinai Medical Center**
One Gustave L.Levy Place
New York, NY 10029
212-241-6500
Fax: 212-875-84
www.mountsinai.org
The Center for Sleep Medicine at The Mount Sinai Medical Center is a comprehensive program dedicated to the diagnosis and treatment of all aspects of sleep pathology including breathing-related sleep disorders, periodic limb movements in sleep, insomnia. and narcolepsy. Mechanical (CPAP BiPAP ventilator), surgical, dental, and pharmacologic therapies are available.
*E. Neil Schachter, Professor*
*Gwen S. Skloot, Associates Professor*

1832 **Geisinger Wyoming Valley Medical Center: Sleep Disorders Center**
1000 E Mountain Drive
Wilkes-Barre, PA 18711
570-819-5770
www.geisinger.org
Sleep team operates service sleep centers and laboratories to diagnose and treat a broad range of sleep disorders. Geisinger sleep

centers are conveniently located in Danville, Bloomsburg, Shamokin, Wilkes-Barre and Mt. Pocono.
*Andrew Paul Matragrano, Director*
*Stephanie Schaefer, Nurse Practitioner*

1833 **Johns Hopkins University: Sleep Disorders Francis Scott Key Medical Center**
Francis Scott Key Medical Center
601 N Caroline Street 410-550-0545
Baltimore, MD 21287 www.hopkinshospital.org
The Johns Hopkins University Sleep Disorders Center is a tertiary care center for patients with sleep/wake disorders and medical disorders associated with sleep.
*Phillip L. Smith, Director*

1834 **Knollwoodpark Hospital Sleep Disorders Center**
5600 Girby Road 251-660-5120
Mobile, AL 36693 Fax: 251-660-5245
71054.2530@compuserve.com
www.southalabama.edu/usakph

1835 **Loma Linda University Sleep Disorders Clinic**
VA Hospital Medical Services Center
11201 Benton Street 909-825-7084
Loma Linda, CA 92357 800-741-8387
Fax: 909-963-64
www.lom.med.va.gov
*Ralph Downey III, M.D., Director*

1836 **Methodist Hospital Sleep Center Winona Memorial Hospital**
Rehab Centers
6565 Fannin Street 713-441-7854
Houston, TX 77030 Fax: 713-790-2612
www.methodisthealth.com
*Marc L. Boom, President & CEO*
*David M. Underwood, Vice Chairman*

1837 **MidWest Medical Center: Sleep Disorders Center**
Winona Memorial Hospital
Indianapolis, IN 46208 317-927-2100
Fax: 317-927-2914

1838 **Northwest Ohio Sleep Disorders Center Toledo Hospital**
Toledo Hospital
2142 N Cove Boulevard 419-471-5629
Toledo, OH 43606
*Frank O. Horton III, M.D., Director*

1839 **Ohio Sleep Medicine Institute**
4220 Bradenton Avenue 614-766-0773
Dublin, OH 43017 Fax: 614-766-2599
info@sleepmedicine.com
www.sleepmedicine.com
A comprehensive accredited sleep disorders center that is dedicated to excellence in sleep medicine care. Offers evaluation, diagnosis and treatment for adults and children with sleep apnea, insomnia, restless legs syndrome, narcolepsy, parasomnias, circadian rhythms disorders, shift work, fatigue and other sleep problems.
*Betty Palmer, Director*

1840 **Penn Center for Sleep Disorders: Hospital of the University of Pennsylvania**
3400 Spruce Street 215-662-7772
Philadelphia, PA 19104 Fax: 215-349-8038
*Joanne Getsy, M.D., Director*

1841 **Presbyterian-University Hospital: Pulmonary Sleep Evaluation Center**
DeSoto At O'Hara Street 412-647-3475
Pittsburgh, PA 15213
*Mark Sanders, M.D., Director*

1842 **Scripps Clinic Sleep Disorders Center Scripps Clinic**
Scripps Clinic
10666 N Torrey Pines Road 858-455-9100
La Jolla, CA 92037 Fax: 858-828-64
malcoRN@scrippsclinic.com
www.scripps.org
The Scripps Clinic Sleep Center provides evaluation diagnosis and treatment of a full range of sleep disorders such as Circadian rhythm disorders, insomnia, narcolepsy, night terror, nightmares, restless legs syndrome, sleep apnea, sleepwalking, and snoring.
*Dan Dworsky, M.D., Medical Director*
*Merrill M. Mitle, M.D., Scientific Director*

1843 **Sleep Alertness Center: Lafayette Home Hospital**
2400 S Street 765-447-6811
Lafayette, IN 47904

1844 **Sleep Center: Community General Hospital**
750 East Adams Street 315-464-5540
Syracuse, NY 13210 www.cgh.org
The Sleep Center at Community General Hospital is a specialized facility providing accurate diagnosis and recommending treatment of sleep-related problems.

1845 **Sleep Disorders Center Bethesda Oak Hospital**
619 Oak Street 513-569-5400
Cincinnati, OH 45206 www.trihealth.com

1846 **Sleep Disorders Center Columbia Presbyterian Medical Center**
The University Hospital of Columbia & Cornell
161 Fort Washington Avenue 212-305-1860
New York, NY 10032 Fax: 212-305-5496
www.sleepnyp.com
A highly specialized outpatient facility for the evaluation and treatment of patients with problems related to sleep and wakefulness.
*Neil B. Kavey, Medical Director*
*Andrew Tucker, Director*

1847 **Sleep Disorders Center Dartmouth Hitchcock Medical Center**
Darthmouth Hitchcock medical Center
One Rope Ferry Road 603-650-1200
Hanover, NH 03755 877-367-1797
Fax: 603-650-1202
Joanne.MacQuarrie@dartmouth.edu
dms.dartmouth.edu
Provides consultation and testing for all varieties of sleep-related disturbances, including snoring, sleep apnea, narcolepsy, restless legs syndrome, periodic limb movement disorder, insomnia, parasomnias and circadian rhythm disorders.
*Glen Greenough, Fellowship Director*

1848 **Sleep Disorders Center Lankenau Hospital**
100 E Lancaster Avenue 610-645-3400
Wynnewood, PA 19096 Fax: 610-645-2291

1849 **Sleep Disorders Center Ohio State University Medical Center**
410 W.10th Ave 614-257-2500
Columbus, OH 43210 800-293-5123
Fax: 614-257-2551
webmaster@osumc.edu
medicalcenter.osu.edu
*Ulysses J. Magalang, M.D., Medical Director*

1850 **Sleep Disorders Center at California: Pacific Medical Center**
2340 Clay Street 415-923-3336
San Francisco, CA 94115 Fax: 415-923-3584
76307.2221@compuserve.com

1851 **Sleep Disorders Center of Metropolitan Toronto**
500 Alden Road 905-475-5155
Markham Ontario, CA M6B 888-401-5155
Fax: 647-436-7607
sleep@compuserve.com
www.sdc.ca
*Jeffrey Lips, M.D., Director*

1852 **Sleep Disorders Center of Rochester: St. Mary's Hospital**
2110 Clinton Avenue S 716-442-4141
Rochester, NY 14618
*Donald Green, M.D.*

1853 **Sleep Disorders Center of Western New York Millard Fillmore Hospital**
726 Exchange Street 716-859-5600
Buffalo, NY 14210 Fax: 716-887-5332
gates.kaleidahealth.org
*Daniel Rifkin, Director*

1854 **Sleep Disorders Center: Cleveland Clinic Foundation**
9500 Euclid Avenue 216-636-5860
Cleveland, OH 44195 800-223-2273
Fax: 216-445-1022
TTY: 216-444-0261
my.clevelandclinic.org
Accredited by the American Academy of Sleep Medicine, the Cleveland Clinic Sleep Disorders Center is staffed by physicians specializing in sleep disorders from a variety of disciplines, including adult and child neurology, pulmonary and critical care medicine, psychology, psychiatry, otolaryngology and dentistry.

1855 **Sleep Disorders Center: Community Medical Center**
1822 Mulberry Street 717-969-8931
Scranton, PA 18510
*John Goodnow, Director*

1856 **Sleep Disorders Center: Crozer-Chester Medical Center**
Sleep Disorders Center
175 E Chester Pike 610-447-2689
Ridley Park, PA 19078 www.crozer.org
A multidisciplinary facility for the investigation and treatment of sleep problems

1857 **Sleep Disorders Center: Good Samaritan Medical Center**
1020 Franklin Street 814-533-1661
Johnstown, PA 15905

1858 **Sleep Disorders Center: Kettering Medical Center**
3935 Southern Boulevard 937-395-8805
Kettering, OH 45439 Fax: 937-395-8821
www.kmcnetwork.org
*Donna Arand, Ph.D., Clinical Director*
*George G. Burton, M.D., Medical Director*

1859 **Sleep Disorders Center: Medical College of Pennsylvania**
3200 Henry Avenue 215-842-4250
Philadelphia, PA 19129
*June M. Fry, M.D., Ph.D., Director*

1860 **Sleep Disorders Center: Newark Beth Israel Medical Center**
201 Lyons Avenue at Osborne Terrace 973-926-2973
Newark, NJ 07112 www.sbhcs.com
Evaluates a wide range of disorders, including sleep apnea, snoring, insomnia, narcolepsy, sleep-wake schedule disorders, and male impotency. The center also provides board-certified consultants in sleep medicine, neurology, urology, endocrinology, psychiatry, cardiology, and ear, nose, and throat surgery, in addition to certified sleep technologists.
*Monroe S. Karetzky, M.D.*

1861 **Sleep Disorders Center: Rhode Island Hospital**
70 Catamore Boulevard 401-431-5420
E Providence, RI 02914 Fax: 401-431-5429
www.lifespan.org

1862 **Sleep Disorders Center: St. Vincent Medical Center**
2213 Cherry Street 419-321-4980
Toledo, OH 43608

1863 **Sleep Disorders Center: University Hospital, SUNY at Stony Brook**
240 Middle Country Road 631-444-2500
Smithtown, NY 11787 Fax: 631-444-2580
uhmc-xweb1.uhmc.sunysb.edu/sleepdisorder

1864 **Sleep Disorders Center: Winthrop, University Hospital**
259 First Street 516-663-0333
Mineola, NY 11501 www.winthrop.org
*Steven H. Feinsilver, M.D.*

1865 **Sleep Disorders Unit Beth Israel Deaconess Medical Center**
330 Brookline Avenue 617-667-3237
Boston, MA 02215 www.bidmc.org
*Jean K. Matheson, M.D.*

1866 **Sleep Laboratory**
St Joseph's Hospital
301 Prospect Ave 315-703-2138
Syracuse, NY 13203 888-785-6371
Fax: 315-755-77
www.sjhsyr.org
The Sleep Lab focuses on diagnosing and treating Obstructive Sleep Apnea and sleep-related breathing disorders, and has the largest number of sleep-credentialed physicians and registered sleep technologists of any sleep lab in the area.
*Edward T. Downing, Director*

1867 **Sleep Laboratory, Maine Medical Center**
22 Bramhall Street 207-871-2279
Portland, ME 04102

1868 **Sleep Medicine Associates of Texas**
5477 Glen Lakes Drive 214-750-7776
Dallas, TX 13210 Fax: 214-750-4621
www.sleepmed.com
First, largest and longest-standing accredited sleep center in North Texas.
*Philipp Becker, President/Founding Partner*
*Andrew O. Jamieson, M.D., Chair/Co-Founding Partner*

1869 **Sleep and Chronobiology Center: Western Psychiatric Institute and Clinic**
3811 Ohara Street 412-624-2246
Pittsburgh, PA 15213
*Charles F. Reynolds III, M.D., Director*

1870 **Sleep/Wake Disorders Center Montefiore Sleep Disorders Center**
111 E 210th Street 718-920-4321
Bronx, NY 10467 Fax: 718-798-4352
www.montefiore.org
Provides outstanding clinical care for patients with disorders that affect the sleep-wake cycle and are committed to performing high quality research and to making outstanding contributions to the areas of clinical research that includes the entire spectrum of sleep medicine.
*Michael J. Thorpy, M.D., Director*
*Karen Ballab, M.D., Associate Director*

1871 **Sleep/Wake Disorders Center: Community Hospitals of Indianapolis**
1500 N Ritter Avenue 317-355-4275
Indianapolis, IN 46219 Fax: 317-351-2785
*Marvin E. Vollmer, M.D.*

1872 **Sleep/Wake Disorders Center: Hampstead Hospital**
218 East Road 603-329-5311
Hampstead, NH 03841 info@hampsteadhospital.com
*Kathi Collins, CEO*
*Steven Finnegan, COO*

1873 **Sleep/Wake Disorders Center: New York Hospital-Cornell Medical Center**
520 E 70th Street 212-746-2623
New York, NY 10021 Fax: 212-746-5509
www.weillcornell.org
*Charles Poll, M.D., Director*

1874 **Stanford University Center for Narcolepsy**
Dept. of Psychiatry & Behavioral Sciences
450 Broadway Street 650-725-6517
Redwood City, CA 94063 Fax: 650-498-7761
med.stanford.edu
*Dr. Emanuel Mignot, Director*
*Marlene Iry, Admin Associate*

1875 **Thomas Jefferson University: Sleep Disorders Center**
Jefferson Medical College
1020 Walnut Street 215-955-6000
Philadelphia, PA 19107 800-JEF-FNOW
Fax: 215-955-9783
www.jefferson.edu
A comprehensive clinical, research and educational program in sleep and sleep disorders medicine.
*Karl Doghram, M.D., Medical Director*

## Support Groups & Hotlines

1876 **Narcolepsy Institute/Montefiore Medical Center**
111 E 210th Street 718-920-6799
Bronx, NY 10467 Fax: 718-654-9580
MGoswami@aol.com
www.narcolepsyinstitute.org
The Narcolepsy Institute provides psychosocial support services for narcolepsy.
*Dr. Meeta Goswami, Director*

1877 **Narcolepsy Network**
3242 NE 3rd Avenue #1101 401-667-2523
Camas, WA 98607 888-292-6522
info@narcolepsynetwork.org
www.narcolepsynetwork.org
Provides advocacy and education, supports research. Newsletter, conferences, phone support, and group development guidelines.
*Keith Harper, President*
*Paul Reynolds, Vice President*

1878 **National Health Information Center**
Office of Disease Prevention & Health Promotion
1101 Wootton Pkwy Fax: 240-453-8281
Rockville, MD 20852 odphpinfo@hhs.gov
www.health.gov/nhic
Supports public health education by maintaining a calendar of National Health Observances; helps connect consumers and health professionals to organizations that can best answer questions and provide up-to-date contact information from reliable sources; updates on a yearly basis toll-free numbers for health information, Federal health clearinghouses and info centers.
*Don Wright, MD, MPH, Director*

## Print Resources

1879 **Sleep Health: Journal of the National Sleep Foundation**
National Sleep Foundation
2001 Massachusetts Ave., N.W. 703-243-1697
Washington, DC 20036 www.sleephealthjournal.org
This multidisciplinary journal publishes original, evidence-based research, review articles, reports, and commentaries on sleep-related topics.
*Orfeu M. Buxton, PhD, Editor-in-Chief*
*Kelly Baron, PhD, MPH, Senior Associate Editor*

## Web Sites

1880 **American Sleep Apnea Association**
www.sleeppapnea.org
The American Sleep Apnea Association, founded in 1990, is a 501(c)(3) nonprofit organization that promotes awareness of sleep apnea, works for continuing improvements in treatments for this serious disorder, and advocates for the interests of sleep apnea patients.

1881 **American Sleep Disorders Association**
Provides full diagnostic and treatment services to improve the quality of care for patients with all types of sleep disorders.

1882 **Healing Well**
www.healingwell.com
An online health resource guide to medical news, chat, information and articles, newsgroups and message boards, books, disease-related web sites, medical directories, and more for patients, friends, and family coping with disabling diseases, disorders, or chronic illnesses.

1883 **Healthlink USA**
www.healthlinkusa.com
Health information concerning treatment, cures, prevention, diagnosis, risk factors, research, support groups, email lists, personal stories and much more. Updated regularly.

1884 **MGH Neurology WebForums**
Online. Provides both unmoderated message boards and chat rooms for specific neurological disorders.

1885 **MedicineNet**
www.medicinenet.com
An online resource for consumers providing easy-to-read, authoritative medical and health information.

1886 **Medscape**
www.medscape.com
Medscape offers specialists, primary care physicians, and other health professionals the Web's most robust and integrated medical information and educational tools.

1887 **MyHealthfinder**
www.healthfinder.gov
Searchable, carefully developed web site offering information on over 1000 topics. Developed by the US Department of Health and Human Services, the site can be used in both English and Spanish.

1888 **Neurology Channel**
www.healthcommunities.com
Find clearly explained, medically accurate information regarding conditions, including an overview, symptoms, causes, diagnostic procedures and treatment options. On this site it is possible to ask questions and get information from a neurologist and connect to people who have similar health interests.

1889 **Sleep Research Society (SRS)**
www.sleepresearchsociety.org
Facilitates communication among research workers in this field, but does not sponsor research investigations on its own.

1890 **SleepFoundation.org**
www.sleepfoundation.org
Information for millions of Americans who suffer from sleep disorders, and to prevent the catastrophic accidents that are related to poor or disordered sleep through research, education and the dissemination of information.

1891 **WebMD**
www.webmd.com
Provides credible information, supportive communities, and in-depth reference material about health subjects. A source for original and timely health information, as well as material from well-known content providers.

# STROKE

*Substance use disorder is a significant risk factor leading to cerebrovascular conditions, including stroke. There is morbidity and disability associated with illicit drug use, including prescription drug abuse. Illicit drug use is a frequent cause of stroke in the young adult. Substance use disorder in the older population, coupled with an unhealthy lifestyle, also increases stroke risk. While illicit drug use generally declines as individuals age, it is still an issue that must be considered, as is prescription drug abuse, whether intentional or accidental, as memory issues evolve with age.*

If the blood supply to the brain is suddenly interrupted, a stroke is said to occur and brain tissue is damaged. Usually, this damage is caused by a blood clot blocking a blood vessel in the head or neck, known as an ischemic stroke. Ischemic strokes account for about 85% of all strokes. Fatty deposits lining the blood vessels (atherosclerosis) are the main cause of ischemic strokes. Clots form at the site of the fatty plaque within the blood vessel of the brain or neck or may form elsewhere such as the heart and break loose and travel to the brain. Strokes may also be hemorrhagic in nature, meaning a blood vessel breaks and bleeds into the brain causing brain cells to die. Causes may be a bleeding aneurysm, an artery wall that breaks or a congenital malformation known as an arteriovenous malformation (AVM). The most common cause of hemorrhagic stroke is uncontrolled blood pressure.

Alcohol use in adults 65 and older is increasing over previous years. While red wine consumption is considered protective, too much can lead to problems. Heavy alcohol intake increases the risk of stroke, particularly hemorrhagic stroke which is more destructive to the body. The cause of stroke brought on by excessive alcohol consumption is generally related to high blood pressure and impaired blood clotting. Alcohol, specifically, can interact with prescribed medications and can exacerbate medical conditions such as stroke, high blood pressure, memory loss and other diseases. Stroke may be the most potentially damaging to the individual if early intervention does not occur. Significant paralysis, loss of speech and vision, and death may occur.

Substance use disorder increases the risk of both ischemic stroke and intracerebral hemorrhage or hemorrhagic stroke. Stimulants such as cocaine, amphetamines and others can cause elevated blood pressure and vasospasm. Illicit drugs are more often associated with stroke, especially cocaine and amphetamines. Less commonly, causative agents are opioids and cannabis. Toxicology screening for illicit drugs in young people with stroke is recommended.

Stroke damage may include movement problems including paralysis of an extremity, pain, numbness and problems with speaking, thinking and remembering. Depression may also occur post-stroke. An American adult is hospitalized every two minutes with a stroke. Treatments are available if the stroke is managed promptly.

Using the F.A.S.T. warning signs is one way to save a life from a stroke. If you notice any of the F.A.S.T. warning signs take action:

## Agencies & Associations

1892 **American Heart Association**
7272 Greenville Avenue 214-570-5943
Dallas, TX 75231 800-242-8721
www.heart.org
The American Heart Association is the nation's oldest, largest voluntary organization devoted to fighting cardiovascular diseases and stroke. Funds research and raises public awareness of heart diseases.
*Michelle A. Albert, President*
*Nancy Brown, Chief Executive Officer*

1893 **American Stroke Association**
7272 Greenville Avenue 800-242-8721
Dallas, TX 75231 www.stroke.org
Dedicated to the prevention, diagnosis, and treatment of stroke. Funds research on stroke and advises the public on how to detect and avoid stroke.
*Nancy Brown, Chief Executive Officer*

1894 **March of Dimes Canada**
10 Overlea Blvd. 416-425-3463
Toronto, Ontario, M4H-1A4 800-263-3463
Fax: 416-425-1920
www.marchofdimes.ca
A national service offering support, education and community programs for stroke survivors, their caregivers and families.
*Leonard Baker, President & CEO*
*Tim Alcock, Vice President & COO*

1895 **National Heart, Lung & Blood Institute**
31 Center Drive nhlbiinfo@nhlbi.nih.gov
Bethesda, MD 20892 www.nhlbi.nih.gov
Trains, conducts research, and educates in order to promote the prevention and treatment of heart, lung, and blood disorders.
*Gary H. Gibbons, MD, Director*

1896 **National Institute of Neurological Disorders and Stroke**
P.O. Box 5801 800-352-9424
Bethesda, MD 20824 www.ninds.nih.gov
Seeks to reduce the burden of neurological disease affecting individuals from all walks of life.
*Walter Koroshetz, MD, Director*
*Amy Bany Adams, PhD, Acting Principal Deputy Director*

## Foundations

1897 **American Stroke Foundation**
6405 Metcalf Ave. 913-649-1776
Overland Park, KS 66202 www.americanstroke.org
The vision of the American Stroke Foundation is to reach out to stroke survivors and their families across America and empower them to reclaim hope for life after stroke.
*Jane Savidge, Executive Director*

1898 **Heart and Stroke Foundation of Canada**
2300 Yonge St. 888-473-4636
Toronto, Ontario, M4P-1E4 www.heartandstroke.ca
Leading authority on cardiovascular disease, providing resources for individuals and funding scientific research on heart disease and stroke.
*Doug Roth, Chief Executive Officer*

## Research Centers

1899 **Cerebral Blood Flow Laboratories Veterans Administration Medical Center**
Veterans Administration Medical Center
2002 Holcombe Boulevard 713-795-5807
Houston, TX 77030 Fax: 713-957-01
Offers research in cerebrovascular disorders and risk factors for stroke.
*John S. Meyer, M.D., Director*

1900 **Comprehensive Stroke Center of Oregon**
University of Oregon Health Sciences Center
3181 SW Sam Jackson Park Road 503-494-7225
Portland, OR 97239 www.ohsu.edu
The Oregon Stroke Center (OSC) was established over 20 years ago to provide comprehensive treatment and prevention services to stroke patients throughout the Northwest. Recognized as a national leader in acute stroke treatment, the OSC mobile stroke team provides novel stroke treatments to multiple Portland hospitals. In addition to clinical care, the OSC is actively involved in clinical and basic research and provides extensive stroke related education to the public and providers.
*Wayne Clark, M.D., Professor*
*Helmi Lutsep, M.D., Professor*

1901 **Departments of Neurology & Neurosurgery: University of California, San Francisco**
UCSF Medical Center
505 Parnassus Avenue 415-476-1537
San Francisco, CA 94143 Fax: 415-476-0616
bill.dillon@radiology.ucsf.edu
www.radiology.ucsf.edu
The Department of Radiology & Biomedical Imaging at the University of California, San Francisco combines clinical excellence, trailblazing research, and outstanding education in a leading academic health sciences institution. The faculty includes some of the foremost names in diagnostic and interventional radiology today.
*Dr. Ronald Arenson, Chairman*
*Catherine Garzio, Director of Administration*

1902 **Hospital of the University of Pennsylvania**
3400 Spruce Street 215-662-4000
Philadelphia, PA 19104 800-789-PENN
Fax: 215-903-09
pleasure@email.chop.edu
www.pennmedicine.org
The Hospital of the University of Pennsylvania (HUP) is world-renowned for its clinical and research excellence, forging the way for newer and better ways to diagnose and treat illnesses and disorders. The world-class faculty and staff of the Hospital of the University of Pennsylvania are dedicated to superior patient care, education and research for a better, healthier future. Their significant and groundbreaking contributions to medicine are recognized both nationally and internationally.
*David E. Pleasure, M.D., Director*

1903 **Massachusetts General Departments of Neurology and Neurosurgery**
Massachusetts General Hospital
55 Fruit Street 617-726-2000
Boston, MA 02114 www.massgeneral.org
Mission is to be the preeminent academic neurology department in the US by: providing outstanding clinical care while rapidly discovering new treatments to reduce and eliminate the devastating impact of neurological disorders; training the very best neurologists and scientists of the future, and improving the health and well-being of the diverse communities they serve.
*Peter Slavin, Director*
*Robert Ackerman, Doctor*

1904 **Stroke Research and Treatment Center UAB Medical Center**
Medical Center
1530 3rd Ave S 205-934-9999
Birmingham, AL 35294 800-822-6478
Fax: 205-996-4039
www.main.uab.edu/neurology
The nationally-ranked UAB Department of Neurology is home to eight comprehensive divisions and seven centers offering an array of clinical activities. Over 26,000 patients are cared for annually through state-of-the-art subspecialty care and innovative treatments. Residents have the opportunity to work in various neurology fields with 50 clinical and research faculty members.
*Andrei V. Alexandrov, M.D., Director, Comprehensive Stroke Research*

1905 **University of Iowa College of Medicine**
451 Newton Road 319-335-6707
Iowa City, IA 52242 www.medicine.uiowa.edu
The Roy J. and Lucille A. Carver College of Medicine is a highly ranked medical school where students learn to become accomplished clinicians and top-flight researchers and educators. Students come to Iowa to study medicine in a program that uses

case-based learning as the basis of their education. With its emphasis on problem-solving skills, early exposure to patients, and enhanced community-based experiences, UI medical students typically earn impressive scores on Step 1 of the U.S. Medical Li
*Debra A. Schwinn, MD, Dean*
*Donna L. Hammond, PhD, Executive Associate Dean*

1906 **University of Maryland Center for Studies of Cerebrovascular Disease & Stroke**
16 S Utah Street 410-328-4323
Baltimore, MD 21201 Fax: 410-328-1149
*Thomas R Price MD, Principal Investor*

1907 **University of Miami School of Medicine Department of Neurology**
1120 NW 14th Street 305-243-6732
Miami, FL 33136 877-243-4340
Fax: 305-243-1632
RSacco@med.miami.edu
www.med.miami.edu
*Ralph L. Sacco, MD, Chairman-Department of Neurology*
*Myron D. Ginsberg, MD, Professor*

1908 **Wake Forest University: Cerebrovascular Research Center**
Department of Neurology
300 S Hawthorne Road 336-748-2338
Winston-Salem, NC 27103 Fax: 336-748-5477
Cerebrovascular research.
*Dr. James Toole, Director*

1909 **Washington University School of Medicine**
660 S Euclid Avenue 314-362-5000
Saint Louis, MO 63110 www.medicine.wustl.edu
Washington University School of Medicine is a leader in improving human health throughout the world. As noted leaders in patient care, research and education, their faculty members have contributed many discoveries and innovations to the field of science since the founding of the School of Medicine in 1891. The School of Medicine is one of seven schools of Washington University in St. Louis.
*Larry J. Shapiro, M.D, Executive Vice Chancellor*

## Support Groups & Hotlines

1910 **National Health Information Center**
Office of Disease Prevention & Health Promotion
1101 Wootton Pkwy Fax: 240-453-8281
Rockville, MD 20852 odphpinfo@hhs.gov
www.health.gov/nhic
Supports public health education by maintaining a calendar of National Health Observances; helps connect consumers and health professionals to organizations that can best answer questions and provide up-to-date contact information from reliable sources; updates on a yearly basis toll-free numbers for health information, Federal health clearinghouses and info centers.
*Don Wright, MD, MPH, Director*

## Print Resources

1911 **Stroke Connection**
7272 Greenville Ave. 800-242-8721
Dallas, TX 75231 www.americanstroke.org
Official magazine of the American Stroke Foundation. Supports stroke survivors, their families, caregivers and friends by providing resources, services, education and information that improves the quality of life.

## Web Sites

1912 **American Heart Association**
www.heart.org
A national organization whose primary concern is the reduction of death and disability due to cardiovascular diseases and stroke.

1913 **Healing Well**
www.healingwell.com
An online health resource guide to medical news, chat, information and articles, newsgroups and message boards, books, disease related web sites, medical directories, and more for patients, friends, and family coping with disabling diseases, disorders, or chronic illnesses.

1914 **Healthlink USA**
www.healthlinkusa.com
Health information concerning treatment, cures, prevention, diagnosis, risk factors, research, support groups, email lists, personal stories and much more. Updated regularly.

1915 **MedicineNet**
www.medicinenet.com
An online resource for consumers providing easy-to-read, authoritative medical and health information.

1916 **Medscape**
www.medscape.com
Medscape offers specialists, primary care physicians, and other health professionals the Web's most robust and integrated medical information and educational tools.

1917 **MyHealthfinder**
www.healthfinder.gov
Searchable, carefully developed web site offering information on over 1000 topics. Developed by the US Department of Health and Human Services, the site can be used in both English and Spanish.

1918 **National Heart, Lung & Blood Institute**
www.nhlbi.nih.gov
Primary responsibility of this organization is the scientific investigation of heart, blood vessel, lung and blood disorders. Oversees research, demonstration, prevention, education and training activities in these fields and emphasizes the control of stroke.

1919 **National Stroke Association**
www.stroke.org
A national organization whose sole purpose is to reduce the incidence and impact of stroke through prevention, treatment, rehabilitation and research, and support for stroke survivors and their families. Educational resources on all aspects of stroke available on website.

1920 **Neurology Channel**
www.healthcommunities.com
Find clearly explained, medically accurate information regarding conditions, including an overview, symptoms, causes, diagnostic procedures and treatment options. On this site it is possible to ask questions and get information from a neurologist and connect to people who have similar health interests.

1921 **WebMD**
www.webmd.com
Provides credible information, supportive communities, and in-depth reference material about health subjects. A source for original and timely health information, as well as material from well-known content providers.

# SECTION FOUR: APPENDIXES & INDEXES

# GLOSSARY OF TERMS

**12-Step program:** A group providing mutual support and fellowship for people recovering from addictive behaviors. The first 12-step program was Alcoholics Anonymous (AA), founded in 1935; an array of 12-step groups following a similar model have since emerged and are the most widely used mutual aid groups and steps for maintaining recovery from alcohol and drug use disorders. It is not a form of treatment, and it is not to be confused with the treatment modality called Twelve-Step Facilitation.

**Abstinence:** Not using alcohol or drugs.

**Addiction:** The most severe form of substance use disorder, associated with compulsive or uncontrolled use of one or more substances. Addiction is a chronic brain disease that has the potential for both recurrence (relapse) and recovery.

**Agonist:** A chemical substance that binds to and activates certain receptors on cells, causing a biological response. Fentanyl and methadone are examples of opioid receptor agonists.

**Antagonist:** A chemical substance that binds to and blocks the activation of certain receptors on cells, preventing a biological response. Naloxone is an example of an opioid receptor antagonist.

**Binge-drinking:** For men, drinking 5 or more standard alcoholic drinks, and for women, 4 or more standard alcoholic drinks on the same occasion on at least 1 day in the past 30 days.

**Case management:** A coordinated approach to delivering health care, substance use disorder treatment, mental health care, and social services. This approach links clients with appropriate services to address specific needs and goals.

**Clinical decision support:** A system that provides health care professionals, staff, patients, or other individuals with knowledge and person-specific information, intelligently filtered or presented at appropriate times, to enhance health and health care.

**Clinical trial:** Any research study that prospectively assigns human participants or groups of participants to one or more health-related interventions to evaluate the effects on health outcomes.

**Compulsivity:** Repetitive behaviors in the face of adverse consequences, as well as repetitive behaviors that are inappropriate to a particular situation. People suffering from compulsions often recognize that the behaviors are harmful, but they nonetheless feel emotionally compelled to perform them. Doing so reduces tension, stress, or anxiety.

**Continuum of care:** An integrated system of care that guides and tracks a person over time through a comprehensive array of health services appropriate to the individual's need. A continuum of care may include prevention, early intervention, treatment, continuing care, and recovery support.

**Cost-benefit study:** A study that determines the economic worth of an intervention by quantifying its costs in monetary terms and comparing them with the benefits, also expressed in monetary terms. Total benefits divided by total costs is called a cost-benefit ratio. If the ratio is greater than 1, the benefits outweigh the costs.

**Cost-effectiveness study:** A comparative analysis of two or more interventions against their health and economic outcomes. These outcomes could be lives saved, illnesses prevented, or years of life gained.

**Dependence:** A state in which an organism only functions normally in the presence of a substance, experiencing physical disturbance when the substance is removed. A person can be dependent on a substance without being addicted, but dependence sometimes leads to addiction.

**Dissemination:** The active distribution of evidence-based interventions (EBIs) to specific audiences, with the goal of increasing their adoption.

**Drug Diversion:** A medical and legal concept involving the transfer of any legally prescribed controlled substance from the person for whom it was prescribed to another person for any illicit use.

**Fidelity:** The extent to which an intervention is delivered as it was designed and intended to be delivered.

**Gender:** The social, cultural, or community designations of masculinity or femininity.

**Health care system:** The World Health Organization defines a health care system as (1) all the activities whose primary purpose is to promote, restore, and/or maintain health, and (2) the people, institutions, and resources, arranged together in accordance with established policies, to improve the health of the population they serve. The health care system is made up of diverse health care organizations ranging from primary care, specialty substance use disorder treatment (including residential and outpatient settings), mental health care, infectious disease clinics, school clinics, community health centers, hospitals, emergency departments, and others.

**Health disparities:** Preventable differences in the burden of disease or opportunities to achieve optimal health that are experienced by socially disadvantaged populations, defined by factors such as race or ethnicity, gender, education or income, disability, geographic location (e.g., rural or urban), or sexual orientation.

**Heavy drinking:** Defined by the Centers for Disease Control and Prevention (CDC) as consuming 8 or more drinks per week for women, and 15 or more drinks per week for men, and by the Substance Abuse and Mental Health Services Administration (SAMHSA), for research purposes, as binge drinking on 5 or more days in the past 30 days.

**Implementation:** A specified set of activities designed to put policies and programs into practice.

**Impulsivity:** Inability to resist urges, deficits in delaying gratification, and unreflective decision-making. Impulsivity is a tendency to act without foresight or regard for consequences and to prioritize immediate rewards over long-term goals.

**Inpatient treatment:** Intensive, 24-hour-a-day services delivered in a hospital setting.

**Integration:** The systematic coordination of general and behavioral health care. Integrating services for primary care, mental health, and substance use use-related problems together produces the best outcomes and provides the most effective approach for supporting whole-person health and wellness.

**Intervention:** A professionally delivered program, service, or policy designed to prevent substance misuse (prevention intervention) or treat a substance use disorder (treatment intervention).

**Learning health care system:** As described by the IOM, a learning health care system is "designed to generate and apply the best evidence for the collaborative healthcare choices of each patient and provider; to drive the process of discovery as a natural outgrowth of patient care; and to ensure innovation, quality, safety, and value in health care."

**Longitudinal study:** A type of study in which data on a particular group of people are gathered repeatedly over a period of years or even decades.

**Meaningful use:** Using certified EHR technology to improve quality, safety, efficiency, and reduce health disparities; engage patients and family; improve care coordination and population and public health; and maintain privacy and security of patient health information.

**Negative reinforcement:** The process by which removal of a stimulus such as negative feelings or emotions increases the probability of a response like drug taking.

**Net economic benefit:** The value of total benefits minus total costs.

**Neurobiology:** The study of the anatomy, function, and diseases of the brain and nervous system.

**Opioid Treatment Program (OTP):** SAMHSA-certified program, usually comprising a facility, staff, administration, patients, and services, that engages in supervised assessment and treatment, using methadone, buprenorphine, or naltrexone, of individuals who have opioid use disorders. An OTP can exist in a number of settings, including but not limited to intensive outpatient, residential, and hospital settings. Services may include medically supervised withdrawal and/or maintenance treatment, along with various levels of medical, psychiatric, psychosocial, and other types of supportive care.

**Pharmacokinetics:** What the body does to a drug after it has been taken, including how rapidly the drug is absorbed, broken down, and processed by the body.

**Positive reinforcement:** The process by which presentation of a stimulus such as a drug increases the probability of a response like drug taking.

**Prescription drug misuse:** Use of a drug in any way a doctor did not direct an individual to use it.

**Prevalence:** The proportion of a population who have (or had) a specific characteristic—for example, an illness, condition, behavior, or risk factor— in a given time period.

**Protective factors:** Factors that directly decrease the likelihood of substance use and behavioral health problems or reduce the impact of risk factors on behavioral health problems.

**Public health system:** Defined as "all public, private, and voluntary entities that contribute to the delivery of essential public health services within a jurisdiction" and includes state and local public health agencies, public safety agencies, health care providers, human service and charity organizations, recreation and arts-related organizations, economic and philanthropic organizations, education and youth development organizations, and education and youth development organizations.

**Quality-Adjusted Life Year (QALY):** A measure of the burden of disease used in economic evaluations of the value of health care interventions that accounts for both the years of life lived and the quality of life experienced during those years, relative to quality associated with perfect health.

**Randomized Controlled Trial (RCT):** A clinical trial of an intervention in which people are randomly assigned either to a group receiving the intervention being studied or to a control group receiving a standard intervention, a placebo (a medicine with no therapeutic effect), or no intervention. At the end of the study, the results from the different groups are compared.

**Recovery:** A process of change through which individuals improve their health and wellness, live a self-directed life, and strive to reach their full potential. Even individuals with severe and chronic substance use disorders can, with help, overcome their substance use disorder and regain health and social function. This is called remission. When those positive changes and values become part of a voluntarily adopted lifestyle, that is called "being in recovery". Although abstinence from all substance misuse is a cardinal feature of a recovery lifestyle, it is not the only healthy, pro-social feature.

**Relapse:** The return to alcohol or drug use after a significant period of abstinence.

**Remission:** A medical term meaning that major disease symptoms are eliminated or diminished below a pre-determined, harmful level.

**Residential treatment:** Intensive, 24-hour a day services delivered in settings other than a hospital.

**Risk factors:** Factors that increase the likelihood of beginning substance use, of regular and harmful use, and of other behavioral health problems associated with use.

**Sex:** The biological and physiological characteristics that define human beings as female or male.

**Substance:** A psychoactive compound with the potential to cause health and social problems, including substance use disorders (and their most severe manifestation, addiction).

**Substance misuse:** The use of any substance in a manner, situation, amount or frequency that can cause harm to users or to those around them. For some substances or individuals, any use would constitute as misuse (e.g., under-age drinking, injection drug use).

**Substance misuse problems or consequences:** Any health or social problem that results from substance misuse. Substance misuse problems or consequences may affect the substance user or those around them, and they may be acute (e.g., an argument or fight, a motor vehicle crash, an overdose) or chronic (e.g., a long-term substance-related medical, family, or employment problem, or chronic medical condition, such as various cancers, heart disease, and liver disease). These problems may occur at any age and are more likely to occur with greater frequency of substance misuse.

**Substance use:** The use—even one time—of any substance.

**Substance use disorders:** A medical illness caused by repeated misuse of a substance or substances. According to the Fifth Edition of the *Diagnostic and Statistical Manual of Mental Disorders* (DSM-5), substance use disorders are characterized by clinically significant impairments in health, social function, and impaired control over substance use and are diagnosed through assessing cognitive, behavioral, and psychological symptoms. Substance use disorders range from mild to severe and from temporary to chronic. They typically develop gradually over time with repeated misuse, leading to changes in brain circuits governing incentive salience (the ability of substance-associated cues to trigger substance seeking), reward, stress, and executive functions like decision making and self-control. Note: Severe substance use disorders are commonly called *addictions*.

**Substance use disorder treatment:** A service or set of services that may include medication, counseling, and other supportive services designed to enable an individual to reduce or eliminate alcohol and/or other drug use, address associated physical or mental health problems, and restore the patient to maximum functional ability.

**Telehealth:** The use of digital technologies such as electronic health records, mobile applications, telemedicine, and web-based tools to support the delivery of health care, health-related education, or other health-related services and functions.

**Telemedicine:** Two-way, real-time interactive communication between a patient and a physician or other health care professional at a distant site. Telemedicine is a subcategory of *telehealth*.

**Tolerance:** Alteration of the body's responsiveness to alcohol or a drug such that higher doses are required to produce the same effect achieved during initial use.

**Withdrawal:** A set of symptoms that are experienced when discontinuing use of a substance to which a person has become dependent or addicted, which can include negative emotions such as stress, anxiety, or depression, as well as physical effects such as nausea, vomiting, muscle aches, and cramping, among others.

**Wrap-around services:** Non-clinical services that facilitate patient engagement and retention in treatment as well as their ongoing recovery. This can include services to address patient needs related to transportation, employment, childcare, housing, legal and financial problems, among others.

*Source:* "Facing Addiction in America: The Surgeon General's Report on Alcohol, Drugs, and Health." U.S. Department of Health & Human Services, 2016. addiction.surgeongeneral.gov.

### Terms to Avoid, Terms to Use, and Why

Consider using these recommended terms to reduce stigma and negative bias when talking about addiction.

**Addict** → Person with substance use disorder
**User** → Person with OUD or person with opioid addiction (when substance in use is opioids)
**Substance or drug abuser** → Patient
**Junkie** → Person in active use; use the person's name, and then say "is in active use."
**Alcoholic** → Person with alcohol use disorder
**Drunk** → Person who misuses alcohol/engages in unhealthy/hazardous alcohol use
**Former addict** →Person in recovery or long-term recovery
**Reformed addict** → Person who previously used drugs

- Person-first language.
- The change shows that a person "has" a problem, rather than "is" the problem.
- The terms avoid eliciting negative associations, punitive attitudes, and individual blame.

**Habit** → Substance use disorder; drug addiction

- Inaccurately implies that a person is choosing to use substances or can choose to stop.
- "Habit" may undermine the seriousness of the disease.

**Abuse** → Use (for illicit drugs); misuse, or other than prescribed (for prescription medications)

- The term "abuse" was found to have a high association with negative judgments and punishment.
- Legitimate use of prescription medications is limited to their use as prescribed by the person to whom they are prescribed. Consumption outside these parameters is misuse.

**Opioid substitution replacement therapy, or Medication-assisted treatment (MAT) →** Opioid agonist therapy; pharmacotherapy; addiction medication; medication for a substance use disorder; medication for opioid use disorder (MOUD)

- It is a misconception that medications merely "substitute" one drug or "one addiction" for another.
- The term MAT implies that medication should have a supplemental or temporary role in treatment. Using "MOUD" aligns with the way other psychiatric medications are understood (e.g., antidepressants, antipsychotics), as critical tools that are central to a patient's treatment plan.

**Clean →** Testing negative (for toxicology screen results); being in remission or recovery; abstinent from drugs; not drinking or taking drugs; not currently or actively using drugs (for non-toxicology purposes)

- Use clinically accurate, non-stigmatizing terminology the same way it would be used for other medical conditions.
- Set an example with your own language when treating patients who might use stigmatizing slang.
- Use of such terms may evoke negative and punitive implicit cognitions.

**Dirty →** Testing positive (for toxicology screen results); person who uses drugs (for non-toxicology purposes)

- Use clinically accurate, non-stigmatizing terminology the same way it would be used for other medical conditions.
- May decrease patients' sense of hope and self-efficacy for change.

**Addicted baby →** Baby born to mother who used drugs while pregnant; baby with signs of withdrawal from prenatal drug exposure; baby with neonatal opioid withdrawal/neonatal abstinence syndrome; newborn exposed to substances

- Babies cannot be born with addiction because addiction is a behavioral disorder—they are simply born manifesting a withdrawal syndrome.
- Use clinically accurate, non-stigmatizing terminology the same way it would be used for other medical conditions.
- Using person-first language can reduce stigma.

*Source*: "Words Matter - Terms to Use and Avoid When Talking About Addiction." National Institute on Drug Abuse, November 29, 2021.
nida.nih.gov/nidamed-medical-health-professionals/health-professions-education/words-matter-terms-to-use-avoid-when-talking-about-addiction

DEA INTELLIGENCE REPORT

# Slang Terms and Code Words: A Reference for Law Enforcement Personnel

DEA-HOU-DIR-022-18

JULY 2018

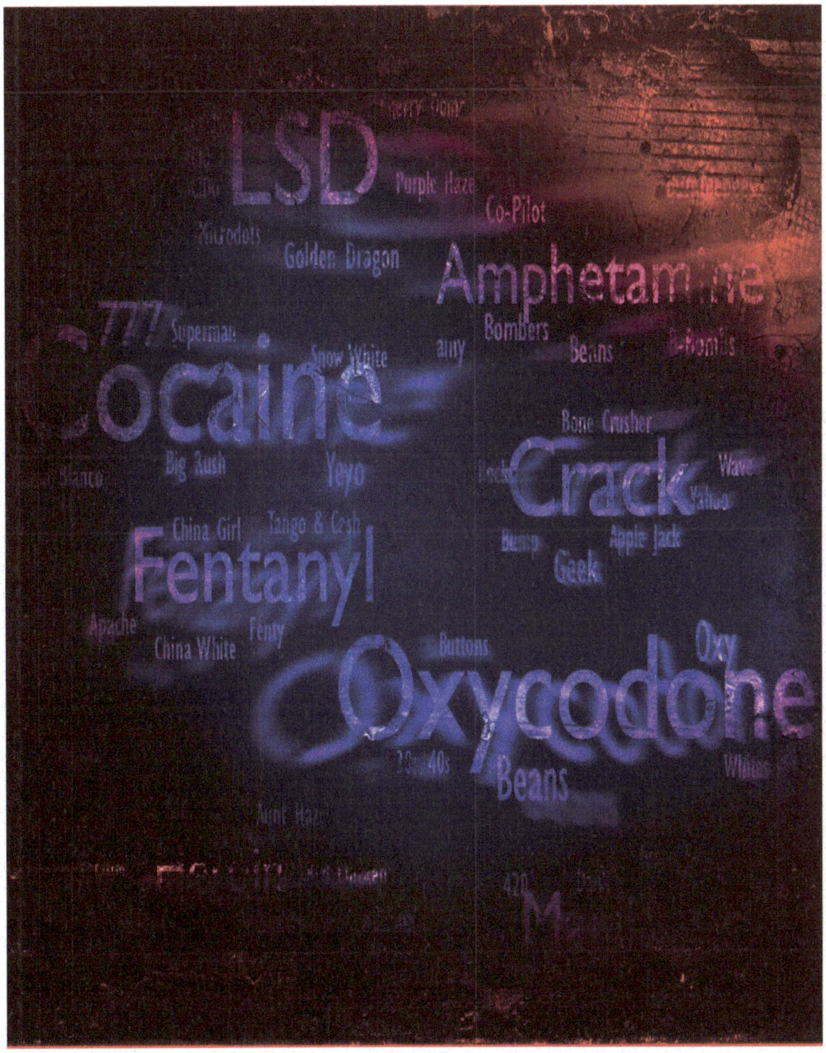

# Executive Summary

This Drug Enforcement Administration (DEA) Intelligence Report contains new and updated information on slang terms and code words from a variety of law enforcement and open sources, and serves as an updated version to the product entitled "Drug Slang Code Words" published by the DEA in May 2017. It is designed as a ready reference for law enforcement personnel who are confronted with hundreds of slang terms and code words used to identify a wide variety of controlled substances, designer drugs, synthetic compounds, measurements, locations, weapons, and other miscellaneous terms relevant to the drug trade. Although every effort was made to ensure the accuracy and completeness of the information presented, due to the dynamics of the ever-changing drug scene, subsequent additions, deletions, and corrections are inevitable. Future addendums and updates to this report will attempt to capture changed terminology to the furthest extent possible. This compendium of slang terms and code words is alphabetically ordered, with new additions presented in *italic text*, and identifies drugs and drug categories in English and foreign language derivations.

## Drug Slang Terms and Code Words[a]

### Acetaminophen and Oxycodone Combination (Percocet®)

512s; Bananas; Blue; *Blue Dynamite;* Blueberries; Buttons; Ercs; Greenies; Hillbilly Heroin; Kickers; M-30s; *Paulas*; Percs; Rims; Tires; Wheels

### Alprazolam (Xanax®)

Bars; *Benzos;* Bicycle Handle Bars; *Bicycle Parts*; *Bricks*; Footballs; *Handlebars*; Hulk; *L7*; Ladders; *Palitroque*; Planks; School Bus; Sticks; *Upjohns*; *White Boys*; *White Girls*; Xanies; *Yellow Boys*; Zanbars; Zannies; Z-Bars

### Amphetamine

*Acelerador*; Amy; Amps; Bam; B-Bombs; Beans; Bennies; Benz; Black and Whites; Black Beauties; Black Birds; Black Bombers; Black Mollies; Blacks; Blue Boys; Bombita; Brain Ticklers; Brownies; Bumblebees; Cartwheels; Chalk; Chicken Powder; Chochos; *Chocolates*; Christina; Chunk; Co-Pilot; Coast-to-Coasts; Crisscross; Cross Roads; Cross Tops; *Crosses*; Debs; Dexies; Diablos; Diamonds; Diet Pills; Dolls; Dominoes; Double Cross; Drivers; *Dulces*; Fives; *Flour*; Footballs; French Blues; *Geeked Up*; Goofballs; Greenies; Head Drugs; Hearts; Horse Heads; In-Betweens; Jelly Babies; Jelly Beans; Jolly Beans; Jugs; *LA Turnaround*; Leapers; Lid Poppers; Lightening; Little Bombs; Marathons; Mini Beans; Mini Bennies; Morning Shot; Nuggets; Oranges; *Pastas*; Pastillas; Peaches; Pep Pills; *Pepper*, *Pingas*; Pink Hearts; Pixies; Pollutants; Purple Hearts; Rhythm; Rippers; Road Dope; Roses; Rueda; Snaps; Snow Pallets; Sparkle Plenty; Sparklers; Speed; Splash; Sweeties; Sweets; Tens; Thrusters; TR-6s; Truck Drivers; Turnabouts; Uppers; Wake Ups; West Coast Turnarounds; Wheels; Whiffle Dust; White Crosses; Whites; Zoomers

### *Amphetamine and Dextroamphetamine Combination (Adderall®)*

*A-Train; Abby; Addy; Amps; Christmas Trees; Co-Pilots; Lid Poppers; Smart Pills; Smarties; Study Buddies; Study Skittles; Truck Drivers; Zing*

### Buprenorphine and Naloxone Combination (Suboxone®)

*Boxes, Bupes; Oranges; Sobos; Stop Signs; Stops; Subs*

a See Appendix A for an alphabetized list of drug slang and code words for common drugs.

## Clonazepam (Klonopin®)

*Benzos;* K; K-Pin; Pin; Super Valium; *Tranks*

## Cocaine

*7*; *62*; *77*; *777*; *921*; A-1; *Adidas*; All-American Drug; *Ancla*; Angel Powder; Angie; Animals; *Apache*; *Apodo*; *Arriba*; Audi; Aunt Nora; Azucar; Baby Powder; Barrato; Basuco; Bazooka (cocaine paste mixed with marijuana); Beach; Belushi (cocaine mixed with heroin); *Bernice*; Bernie's Flakes; Bernie's Gold Dust; *Big Bird*; Big Bloke; Big C; Big Flake; Big Rush; Billie Hoke; Bird; Birdie Powder; Blanca Nieves; Blanco; Blast; Blizzard; Blonde; Blocks; Blow; BMW; *Board*; Bobo; Bolitas; Bolivian Marching Powder; Bombita (cocaine mixed with heroin); *Booger Sugar*, *Bose*; Bouncing Powder; Brisa; *Bump*; C-Dust; *Caballo*; Caca; Cadillac; California Pancakes; Calves; *Canelon*; Candy; Car; Carney; Carrie Nation; Cars; Case; Cebolla; Cecil; Cement; Charlie; Chevy; Cheyenne; *Chica*; *Chicanitas*; Chinos; Chiva; *Cielo*; Clear Kind; Clear Tires; Coca; Coca-Cola; Cocazo; Coconut; Coke; Cola; Colorado; *Comida*; *Comida Dulce*; Connie; Cookie; *Cosa; Coso; Cosos;* Crow; Crusty Treats; Cuadro; Death Valley; Designer Jeans; Devil's Dandruff; *Diamonds*; Diente; Dienton; *Diesel*; *Diosa Blanca*; Dona Blanca; Double Bubble; *Double Letters*; Dove; Dream; Dulces; Duracell; *Durazno*; *Duro*; Dust; Escama; Escorpino; Falopa; *Fef1*; *Fichas*; *Fiesta*; *Fire (cocaine base)*; Fish (liquid cocaine); *Fish Scale*; Flake; Flea Market Jeans; Florida Snow; Flour; Food; Foolish Powder; Fox; Freeze; Friskie Powder; Frula; *Funtime*; Gabacho; Galaxy; Gallos; Gato; Gift of the Sun; Gin; Girl; Girlfriend; Glad Stuff; Gold Dust; Green Gold; Gringa; *Gringito*; Grout; *Guerillo*; Gueros; Guitar; *H1*; *Hai Hit*; Hamburger; Happy Dust; Happy Powder; Happy Trails; Heaven; Heaven Dust; *Heavy One*; *Hen*; Henry VIII; *HH*; *HHJ*; *High Heat*; *HMH*; Hooter; Hundai; Hunter; *Ice Cream*; Icing; Inca Message; Izzy; Jam; *Jaime Blanco*; *Jaula*; Jeep; Jelly; John Deere; Joy Flakes; Joy Powder; *Juguetes*; *Jump Rope*; Junk; *K13*; King's Habit; Kordell; *La Familia*; Lady; Lady Snow; Late Night; Lavada; Leaf; *Libreta*; Line; Loaf; Love Affair; *LV*; Maca Flour; *Madera*; Mama Coca; Mandango; *Manita*; Maradona; *Marbol*; *Material*; *Mayback (62 grams)*; Mayo; Melcocha; *Media Lata*; Mercedes; Milk; Milonga; Mojo; Mona Lisa; *Monte*; *Morro*; Mosquitos; Movie Star Drug; *Muchacha*; *Muebles*; Mujer; Napkin; Nieve; Niña; *Normal*; Nose Candy; Nose Powder; Old Lady; Oyster Stew; Paint; Paloma; *Paleta*; Palomos; Pantalones; Papas; Paradise; Paradise White; Parrot; Pearl; Pedrito; Perico; *Personal*; Peruvian; Peruvian Flake; Peruvian Lady; Pescado; *Peta*; Pez; *Pichicata*; Pillow; Pimp; *Pingas*; *Pingos*; *Pintura Blanca*; *Poli*; Pollo; Polvo; Powder; Powder Diamonds; *Puma*; Puritain; *Quadros*; Queso Blanco; Racehorse Charlie; Rambo; Refresco; Refrescas; *Regular Kind*; *Regular Work*; Reindeer Dust; *Richie*; Rims; Rocky Mountain; Rolex; *Rolex HH*; Rooster; Scale; Schmeck; Schoolboy; Scorpion; Scottie; Seed; Serpico; Sierra; Shirt; Ski Equipment; Sleigh Ride; *Sneeze*; *Sniff*; Snow; Snow Bird; Snow Cone; Snow White; Snowball; Snowflake; Society High; Soda; Soditas; Soft; Space (cocaine mixed with PCP); *Special*; Speedball (cocaine mixed with heroin); Stardust; Star Spangled Powder; Studio Fuel; Suave; Sugar; Superman; Sweet Stuff; *Tabique*; *Tablas*; Talco; Talquito; Tamales; Taxi; Tecate; Teenager; Teeth; Tequila; Thunder; Tire; Tonto; Toot; Tortes; *Tortuga*; Toyota; T-Shirts; *Tubo*; *Tucibi (pink variety)*; Turkey; Tutti-Frutti; Vaquita; Wash; Wet; Whack (cocaine mixed with PCP); White; White Bitch; White Cross; *White Dove*; White Girl; White Goat; White Horse; White Lady; White Mercedes Benz; White Mosquito; White Paint; White Powder; *White Rock*; White Root; White Shirt; White T; *White Wall Tires*; Whitey; Whiz Bang; Wings; Wooly; Work; Yayo; Yeyo; Yoda; *Zapato*; Zip

## Crack Cocaine

51s; 151s; 501s; Apple Jack; Baby T; Base; Baseball; Bazooka; Beam Me Up; Beautiful Boulders; Beemer; Bill Blass; Bings; BJ; Black Rock; Blowcaine; Blowout; Blue; Bobo; Bolo; Bomb; Bone Crusher; Bone; Boo-Boo; Boulder; Boy; Breakfast of Champions; Bubble Gum; Bullion; Bump; Candy; Caps; Casper the Ghost; Caviar; CD; Cheap Basing; Chewies; Chingy; Clicker; Climax; Cloud; Cloud Nine; Cookies; *CRC*; Crib; Crunch and Munch; Devil; Devil Smoke; Dice; Dime Special; Dirty Basing; Dirty Fentanyl (crack cocaine mixed with fentanyl); Double Yoke; Durin; Eastside Player; Egg; Eye Opener; Famous Dimes; Fat Bags; Fifty-One; Fish Scales; Freebase; French Fries; Garbage Rock; Geek; Glo; Gold; Golf Ball; Gravel; Great White Hope; Grit; Groceries; Hail; Hamburger Helper; Hard; Hotcakes; Hubba; Ice; Ice Cubes; Issues; Jelly Beans; Johnson; Kangaroo; Kokoma; Kryptonite; Love; Mixed Jive; Moon Rock; Nickle; Nuggets; One-Fifty-One; Paste; Pebbles; Pee Wee; Piedras; Pile; Pony; Primo; Quarters; Raw; Ready Rock; Red Caps; RIP (Rest in Peace);

Roca; Rock; Rock Attack; Rocks of Hell; Rocky III; Rooster; Rox; Roxanne; Roz; Schoolcraft; Scotty; Scramble; Scruples; Seven-Up; Sherms; Sight Ball; Slab; Sleet; Smoke; Speed Boat; Square Time Bomb; Stone; Sugar Block; Takeover (crack cocaine mixed with fentanyl); Teeth; Tension; Tissue; Top Gun; Troop; Ultimate; *Up*; Uzi; Wave; White Ball; White Ghost; White Sugar; White Tornado; Wrecking Crew; Yahoo; Yale; Yimyom

## Ecstasy/MDMA/Molly

Adam; Baby Slits; Beans; Blue Kisses; *Blue Superman*; *Bombs*; Booty Juice (dissolved in liquid); Candy; Chocolate Chips; Clarity; Dancing Shoes; Decadence; *Disco Biscuits*; Doctor; Domex (ecstasy mixed with PCP); Drop; E; E-Bomb; Essence; Eve; *Go*; *Goog*; *Green Apple*; *Happy Pill; Hug*; *Hug Drug*; Kleenex; Love Doctor; Love Drug; *Love Flip (taken with mescaline)*; Love Potion #9; Love Trip (ecstasy mixed with mescaline); *Lover's Speed*; *Malcolm X*; Moon Rock; *Peace*; *Pingaz*; *Pingers*; Rolls; Rolling; Running; Scooby Snacks; Skittle; *Smacks*; Slits; Smarties; Speed for Lovers; Sweets; *Tacha*; *Thizz*; Vitamin E; *Vowels*; *White Mercedes*; X; XTC; Yokes

## Fentanyl and Fentanyl Derivatives

Apache; Birria (fentanyl mixed with heroin); *Blonde*; *Blue Diamond*; *Blue Dolphin*; *Blues*; Butter; China Girl; China Town; China White; Chinese; *Chinese Buffet*; Chinese Food; Crazy; Crazy One; Dance Fever; Dragon; Dragon's Breath; *F*; *Food*; *Freddy*; *Fuf (furanyl fentanyl)*; Facebook (fentanyl mixed with heroin in pill form); Fent; Fenty; Fire; Friend; Girl; Goodfella; Great Bear; *Gray Stuff*; He-Man; *Heineken*; Huerfanito; *Humid*; Jackpot; King Ivory; Lollipop; Murder 8; *Nal*; *Nil*; *Nyl*; *Opes*; *Pharmacy;* Poison; Shoes; *Snowflake*; Tango and Cash; *TNT*; Toe Tag Dope; White Girl; *White Ladies*

## Flunitrazepam (Rohypnol®)

*542; Circles; Date Rape Drug; Forget Pill; La Rocha; Lunch Money; Mexican Valium; Mind Eraser; Pingus; R2; Reynolds; Roach; Roapies; Rochas; Roofies; Rope; Rophies; Ro-Shay; Trip-and-Fall; Wolfies*

## GHB (Gamma-Hydroxybutyric Acid)

*Blowout*; *Bruno Mars*; *Cherry Meth*; *Easy Lay*; *Everclear*, *Fantasy*; G; *Gamma Oh*; GEEB; Georgia Home Boy; *Goop*; *Great Hormones at Bedtime*; Grievous Bodily Harm; *G-Riffic*; Gina; *Jib*; Liquid E; Liquid X; *Monkey Juice*; *Organic Quaalude*; *Salty Water*, Scoop; *Soap*; *Water*

## Heroin

*Abajo*; A-Bomb (heroin mixed with marijuana); Achivia; Adormidera; *Amarilla*; *Anestesia de Caballo (heroin mixed with the horse anesthetic xylazine)*; Antifreeze; *Apodo*; *Arpon*; Aunt Hazel; Avocado; Azucar; Bad Seed; *Baja Corte (diluted heroin)*; Ballot; Basketball; Basura; Beast; Beyonce; Big Bag; Big H; Big Harry; Bird; Birdie Powder; *Birria*; *Birria Blanca*; Black; Black Bitch; Black Goat; Black Olives; Black Paint; Black Pearl; Black Sheep; *Black Shirt*; Black Tar; Blanco; Blue; Blow Dope; Blue Hero; Bombita (heroin mixed with cocaine); Bombs Away; Bonita; Boy; Bozo; Brea Negra; Brick Gum; Brown; Brown Crystal; Brown Rhine; Brown Sugar; Bubble Gum; Burrito; *Butter*, Caballo; Caballo Negro; Caca; Café; *Cajeta*; Capital H; *Cardio (white heroin)*; Carga; Caro; Cement; *Certificada (pure heroin)*; Chapopote; Charlie; Charlie Horse; *Chavo*; Cheese; Chicle; Chiclosa; China; *China Blanca (white heroin)*; China Cat; China White; *Chinese Buffet (white heroin)*; Chinese Food; Chinese Red; Chip; Chiva; Chiva Blanca; *Chiva Loca (heroin mixed with fentanyl)*; *Chiva Negra*; Chivones; Chocolate; Chocolate Balls; *Chocolate Shake*; Choko; Chorizo; *Churro Negro*; Chutazo; Coco;

Coffee; *Cohete*; Comida; Crown Crap; Curley Hair; Dark; Dark Girl; *Dark Kind*; Dead on Arrival (DOA); Diesel; Dirt; Dog Food; Doggie; Doojee; Dope; Dorado; Down; Downtown; *Dragon*; Dreck; Dynamite; Dyno; El Diablo; Engines; *Enrique Grande*; *Esquina*; *Esquinilla*; Fairy Dust; Flea Powder; *Food (white heroin)*; Foolish Powder; Galloping Horse; Gamot; Gato; George Smack; Girl; *Globo (balloon of heroin)*; *Goat*; Golden Girl; Good and Plenty; Good H; *Goofball (heroin mixed with methamphetamine)*; Goma; Gorda; Gras; Grasin; Gravy; Gum; H; H-Caps; Hairy; Hard Candy; *Hard One*; Harry; Hats; Hazel; Heaven Dust; Heavy; Helen; Helicopter; Hell Dust; Henry; Hercules; Hero; Him; Hombre; Horse; Hot Dope; *Huera*; Hummers; Jojee; Joy Flakes; Joy Powder; Junk; Kabayo; Karachi; Karate; King's Tickets; *La Tierra*; Lemonade; Lenta; Lifesaver; Manteca; Marias; *Marrion*; Mayo; Mazpan; Meal; Menthol; Mexican Brown; *Mexican Food (black tar heroin)*; Mexican Horse; Mexican Mud; Mexican Treat; Modelo Negra; Mojo; Mole; Mongega; Morena; Morenita; Mortal Combat; Motors; Mud; Mujer; *Murcielago*; Muzzle; Nanoo; Negra; Negra Tomasa; Negrita; Nice and Easy; Night; Noise; Obama; Old Steve; Pants; Patty; Peg; P-Funk; Piezas; Plata; Poison; Polvo; *Polvo de Alegria*; *Polvo de Estrellas*; *Polvo Feliz*; Poppy; Powder; Prostituta Negra; Puppy; Pure; Rambo; *Raw (uncut heroin)*; Red Chicken; Red Eagle; Reindeer Dust; Roofing Tar; *Ruby*; Sack; Salt; Sand; Scag; Scat; Schmeck; *Scramble (uncut heroin)*; Sheep; Shirts; Shoes; Skag; *Skunk*; Slime; Smack; Smeck; Snickers; *Soda*; Speedball (heroin mixed with cocaine); Spider Blue; Sticky Kind; Stufa; Sugar; Sweet Jesus; Tan; Tar; Tecata; *Thunder*; Tires; *Tomasa*; Tootsie Roll; Tragic Magic; Trees; Turtle; Vidrio; *Weights*; Whiskey; White; White Boy; White Girl; White Junk; White Lady; White Nurse; White Shirt; White Stuff; Wings; Witch; Witch Hazel; Zapapote

## Hydrocodone (Norco®, Vicodin®, Lorcet®)

357s; Bananas; *Dones*, Dro; *Droco*; Fluff; Hydros; *Idiot Pills*; *Lemonade*; *Lorries*; *Scratch*; Tabs; *Triple V (Vicodin® taken with Valium® and Vodka)*; *Veeks*; Vics; Vikes; Watsons

## *Hydromorphone (Dilaudid®)*

*D; Dillies; K4; Needle Candy*

## Ketamine (Ketalar®)

*Barry Farrell*; Blind Squid; *Cat Food*; Cat Valium; *Donkey*; Green; *Green K*; Honey Oil; Jet; *Jet K*; K; Keller; Kelly's Day; K-Hold; *Kit Kat*; *Kitty Flip*; K-Ways; *Purple*; Special K; *Special La Coke*; Super Acid; *Super C*; Vitamin K; *Wobble*; *Wonky*

## Khat

*Abyssian Tea; African Salad; Catha; Chat; Kat; Oat*

## LSD (Lysergic Acid Diethylamide)

Aceite; *Acelide*; Acid; Acido; Alice; Angels in a Sky; Animal; *Avandaro*; Backbreaker (LSD mixed with strychnine); Barrel; Bart Simpson; Battery Acid; Beast; Big D; Black Acid (LSD mixed with PCP); Black Star; Black Sunshine; Black Tabs; *Blanco de España*; Blotter Acid; Blotter Cube; Blue Acid; Blue Barrel; Blue Chair; Blue Cheer; Blue Heaven; Blue Microdots; Blue Mist; Blue Moon; Blue Sky; Blue Star; Blue Tabs; *Bomba*; Brown Bomber; Brown Dots; California Sunshine; Cherry Dome; Chief; Chinese Dragons; *Cid*; Coffee; *Colorines*; Conductor; Contact Lens; Crackers; Crystal Tea; *Cubo*; Cupcakes; Dental Floss; Dinosaurs; *Divina*; Domes; Dots; Double Dome; El Cid; Electric Kool Aid; *Elefante Blanco*; Ellis Day; Fields; Flash; Flat Blues; Ghost; Golden Dragon; Golf Balls; Goofy; Gota; Grape Parfait; Green Wedge; Grey Shields; Hats; Hawaiian Sunshine; Hawk; Haze; Headlights; Heavenly Blue; Hits; Instant Zen; Jesus Christ Acid; Kaleidoscope; Leary; Lens; *Lentejuela*; Lime Acid; Live, Spit and Die; *Lluvia de Estrellas*; *Looney Tunes*; *Lucy*; *Maje*; Mellow Yellow; Mica; Microdot; *Micropunto Azul (white tablet with drop of blue LSD)*; *Micropunto Morado (white tablet with drop of purple LSD)*; Mighty Quinn; Mind Detergent; Mother of God; *Mureler*; *Nave*; Newspapers; Orange Barrels; Orange Cubes; Orange Haze; Orange Micros; Orange Wedges; Owsley; Paper Acid; Pearly Gates; Pellets; Phoenix; Pink Blotters; Pink Panthers; Pink Robots; Pink Wedges; Pink Witches; Pizza; *Pop*; Potato; Pure Love; Purple Barrels; Purple Haze; Purple Hearts; Purple Flats; Recycle; Royal Blues; Russian Sickles; Sacrament; Sandoz; Smears; Square Dancing Tickets; Sugar Cubes; Sugar Lumps; Sunshine; *Superman*; Tabs; Tacatosa; Tail Lights; Teddy Bears; Ticket; Uncle Sid; Valley Dolls; Vodka Acid; Wedding Bells; Wedge; White Dust; White Fluff; White Lightening; White Owsley; Window Glass; Window Pane; Yellow Dimples; Yellow Sunshine; Zen

## Marijuana

420; *A-Bomb (marijuana mixed with heroin)*; Acapulco Gold; Acapulco Red; Ace; African Black; African Bush; Airplane; *Alfalfa*; Alfombra; Alice B Toklas; All-Star; *Almohada*; Angola; Animal Cookies (hydroponic); Arizona; Ashes; Aunt Mary; *AZ*; Baby; Bale; Bambalachacha; Barbara Jean; Bareta; Bash; *Bazooka (marijuana mixed with cocaine paste)*; BC Budd; Bernie; Bhang; Big Pillows; Biggy; *Bionic (marijuana mixed with PCP)*; Black Bart; Black Gold; Black Maria; Blondie; Blue Cheese; Blue Crush; *Blue Dream*; Blue Jeans; Blue Sage; Blueberry; Bobo Bush; Boo; Boom; *Branches*; Broccoli; Bud; Budda; Burritos Verdes; Bush; Cabbage; *Café*; *Cajita*; Cali; *Camara*; Canadian Black; Catnip; Cheeba; Chernobyl; Cheese; Chicago Black; Chicago Green; Chippie; Chistosa; Christmas Tree; Chronic; Churro; Cigars; Citrol; Cola; Colorado Cocktail; Cookie (hydroponic); Cotorritos; Crazy Weed; Creeper Bud; Crippy; Crying Weed; Culican; Dank; *Devils's Lettuce*; Dew; Diesel; Dimba; Dinkie Dow; *Diosa Verde*; Dirt Grass; Ditch Weed; Dizz; Djamba; Dody; Dojo; Domestic; Donna Juana; Doobie; Downtown Brown; Drag Weed; Dro (hydroponic); Droski (hydroponic); Dry High; *Elefante Pata*; Endo; *Escoba*; *Fattie*; Fine Stuff; Fire; Flower; Flower Tops; Fluffy; Fuzzy Lady; *Gallina*; Gallito; Garden; *Garifa*; Gauge; Gangster; Ganja; Gash; Gato; Ghana; Gigi (hydroponic); Giggle Smoke; Giggle Weed; Girl Scout Cookies (hydroponic); Gloria; Gold; Gold Leaf; Gold Star; Gong; Good Giggles; Gorilla; Gorilla Glue; Grand Daddy Purp; Grass; Grasshopper; Green; *Green Crack*; Green-Eyed Girl; Green Eyes; Green Goblin; Green Goddess; Green Mercedes Benz; Green Paint; Green Skunk; *Greenhouse*; Grenuda; Greta; Guardada; Gummy Bears; Gunga; Hairy Ones; Hash; Hawaiian; Hay; Hemp; Herb; Hierba; Holy Grail; Homegrown; Hooch; *Hoja*; Humo; Hydro; Indian Boy; Indian Hay; Jamaican Gold; Jamaican Red; Jane; Jive; Jolly Green; Jon-Jem; Joy Smoke; Juan Valdez; Juanita; Jungle Juice; Kaff; Kali; Kaya; KB; Kentucky Blue; KGB; Khalifa; Kiff; Killa; Kilter; King Louie; Kona Gold; Kumba; Kush; Laughing Grass; Laughing Weed; Leaf; Lechuga; Lemon-Lime; *Leña*; Liamba; Lime Pillows; Little Green Friends; Little Smoke; *Llesca*; Loaf; Lobo; Loco Weed; *Loud*; Love Nuggets; Love Weed; *Lucas*; M.J.; Machinery; Macoña; Mafafa; Magic Smoke; Manhattan Silver; *Manteca*; Maracachafa; Maria; Marimba; Mariquita; Mary Ann; Mary Jane; Mary Jones; Mary Warner; Mary Weaver; Matchbox; Matraca; Maui Wowie; Meg; Method; *Mersh*; Mexican Brown; *Mexicali Haze*; Mexican Green; Mexican Red; *MMJ*; Mochie (hydroponic); Moña; Monte; Moocah; Mootie; Mora; Morisqueta; Mostaza; Mota; Mother; Mowing the Lawn; Muggie; *My Brother*; Narizona; Northern Lights; *Nug*; O-Boy; *OG*; O.J.; Owl; Paja; Palm; Paloma; *Palomita*; Panama Cut; Panama Gold; Panama Red; Pakalolo; Parsley; *Pasto*; *Pasture*; *Peliroja*; Pelosa; Phoenix; Pine; *Pink Panther*; *Pintura*; *Plant*; Platinum Cookies (hydroponic); Platinum Jack; Pocket Rocket; Popcorn; *Porro*; Pot; Pretendo; *Prop 215*; Puff; Purple Haze; *Purple OG*; Queen Ann's Lace; *Red Hair*; Ragweed; Railroad Weed; Rainy Day Woman; Rasta Weed; Red Cross; Red Dirt; Reefer; Reggie; Repollo; Righteous Bush; Root; Rope; Rosa Maria; Salt and Pepper; Santa Marta; Sasafras; Sativa; *Shoes*; Sinsemilla; Shmagma; Shora; Shrimp; Shwag; Skunk; Skywalker (hydroponic); Smoke; Smoochy Woochy Poochy; Smoke Canada; *Sour OG*; Spliff; Stems; *Sticky*; Stink Weed; Sugar Weed; Sweet Lucy; Tahoe (hydroponic); *Tangy OG*; *Terp*; *Terpenes*; Tex-Mex; Texas Tea; *Tigitty*; Tila; Tims; *Top Shelf*; Tosca; *Train Wreck*; Trees; *Trinity OG*; Tweeds; *Valle*; Wake and Bake; Weed; Weed Tea; Wet (marijuana dipped in PCP); Wheat; White-Haired Lady; Wooz; Yellow Submarine; Yen Pop; Yerba; Yesca; Young Girls; Zacate; Zacatecas; Zambi; *Zip*; Zoom (marijuana mixed with PCP)

## Marijuana Concentrates/Hash Oil

*710*; *BHNO*; BHO; *Black Glass*; *Bubble Hash*; Budder; *Butane Hash Oil*; *Butane Honey Oil*; *Caviar*; *CBD*; *CBD oil*; *Crystalline*; *Crumble*; Dabs; *Dipper*; Ear Wax; *Edibles*; *ENail*; Errl; *Extract*; *Full Melt*; *Glob*; *Gorilla Glue*;

*Heady*; Honey Oil; *IWE*; *Ice Water Hash*; *Klear*; *Live Resin*; *Moon Rocks*; *Rosin*; *Rosin Tech*; SAP; *Sauce*; Shatter; *Solventless*; *Terp Sauce*; *THCA*; *THCA Crystal*; *THCA Crystalline*; *THCA Powder*; *Trichrome*; Wax

## Mescaline/Peyote

Big Chief; Black Button; Blue Caps; Britton; Buttons; Cactus; Green Button; Half Moon; Hikori; Hikuli; Hyatari; *Love Flip (taken with Ecstasy)*; Media Luna; Mescal; *Mescapade*; Mezcakuba; *Microdot*; Moon; Nubs; San Pedro; Seni; Shaman; Topi; Tops

## Methamphetamine

Accordion; *Amp*; Aqua; *Arroz*; *Assembled (crystal meth)*; Batu; *Begok*; *Biker's Coffee*; Blue; Blue Bell Ice Cream; Beers; Bottles; *Bucio*; Bud Light; Bump; Cajitas; Chalk; *Chandelier*; Chavalone; Chicken; *Chicken Feed*; Chicken Powder; *Chris*; Christine; Christy; Clear; Clothing Cleaner; *Cold*; *Cold One*; Colorado Rockies; Crank; Cream; Cri-Cri; Crink; Crisco; *Crissy*; *Christy*; Crypto; Crystal; Cuadro; Day; *Diamond*; *Dunk*; El Gata Diablo; Evil Sister; Eye Glasses; Fire; Fizz; Flowers; *Foco*; Food; Frio; *Fruit*; *Gak*; *Garbage*; G-Funk; Gifts; Girls; Glass; Go-Fast; *Go-Go*; *Goofball (methamphetamine mixed with heroin)*; Groceries; Hard Ones; Hare; Hawaiian Salt; Hielo; *Hiropon*; Hot Ice; *Hubbers*; Ice; Ice Cream; *Ice Water*, *Icehead*; *Jale*; Jug of Water; L.A. Glass; L.A. Ice; Lemons; Lemon Drop; Light; Light Beige; Livianas; Madera; *Mamph*; Meth; *Methlies Quick*; Mexican Crack; Mexican Crank; Miss Girl; Montura; Motor; Muchacha; Nails; One Pot; *No-Doze*; *Paint*; Pantalones; *Patudas*; Peanut Butter Crank; Piñata; Pointy Ones; Pollito; Popsicle; Purple; Raspado; Rims; *Rocket Fuel*; Salt; Shabu; Shards; Shatter; Shaved Ice; Shiny Girl; *Small Girl*; Soap Dope; Soft Ones; *Speed*; *Speed Dog*; Spicy Kind; *Spin*; Stove Top; Stuff; Super Ice; Table; Tina; *Tires*; *Trash*; Truck; Tupperware; *Tweak; Unassembled (powder meth)*; *Uppers*; Ventanas; Vidrio; Walking Zombie; Water; *Wazz*; White; *Whizz*; Windows; Witches Teeth; *Yaba*; Yellow Barn; *Yellow Cake*; Yellow Kind; Zip

## Methylphenidate (Ritalin®, Concerta®, Daytrana®)

*Diet Coke*; *Jif*; *Johnny*; Kibbles and Bits; *Kiddie Cocaine*; *Kiddie Coke*; *MPH*; *Pineapple*; *Poor Man's Cocaine*; *R-Ball*; *R-Pop*; *Rids*; *Rittys*; *Skippy*; *Skittles*; *Smarties*; *Study Buddies*; *Truck Drivers*; *Vitamin R*

## Morphine

*Dreamer*, *First Line*; *God's Drug*; *Joy Juice*; *Miss Emma*; *Monkey*; *Mister Blue*; *Morpho*; *Unkie*; *White Stuff*

## Opium

*Ah-Pen-Yen*; Auntie; Aunt Emma; Big O; Black; *Black Pill*; Black Russian (opium mixed with hashish); Chandoo; China; Chinese Molasses; Chinese Tobacco; Chocolate; Cruz; Dopium; Dover's Powder; Dream Gum; Dream Stick; Dreams; Easing Powder; *Fi-Do-Nie*; *Gee*; God's Medicine; Goma; Gondola; Goric; Great Tobacco; Gum; *Guma*; Hocus; Hops; Incense; Joy Plant; Midnight Oil; *Mira*; *Ope*; Opio; Pen Yan; Pin Gon; Pin Yen; Pox; Skee; Toxy; Toys; When-Shee; Zero

## Oxycodone (Oxycontin®, Roxicodone®, Oxaydo®)

30s; 40s; *512s*; Beans; Blues; Buttons; *Cotton*; Greens; *Hillbilly Heroin*; *Kickers*; *Killers*; *Muchachas*; *Mujeres*; OC; Oxy; *Oxy 80s*; *Roxy*; *Roxy Shorts*; Whites

## PCP (Phencyclidine)

Ace; Alien Sex Fiend (PCP mixed with heroin); Amoeba; Angel; Angel Dust; Angel Hair; Angel Mist; Angel Poke; Animal Tranquilizer; *Ashy Larry*; Aurora Borealis; *Bionic (PCP mixed with marijuana)*; Black Acid (PCP mixed with LSD); Black Whack; Blue Madman; Blue Star; Boat; Busy Bee; Butt Naked; Cadillac; Cliffhanger; Columbo; Cozmos; Crazy Coke; Crazy Eddie; Cucuy; Cyclones; Detroit Pink; Dipper; Domex (PCP mixed with MDMA); Dummy Dust; Dust; Dust Joint; Dust of Angels; Elephant; Elephant Tranquilizer; Embalming

Fluid; Energizer; Fake STP; Flakes; Goon; Gorilla Tab; Gorilla Biscuits; Green Leaves; Green Tea; Heaven and Hell; Hog; Horse Tracks; Horse Tranquilizers; Jet Fuel; Juice; Kaps; K-Blast; Killer; Kools; Leaky Leak; Lemon 714; Lethal Weapon; Love Boat; Mad Dog; Mad Man; Magic Dust; Mean Green; Mint Leaf; Mint Weed; Mist; Monkey Dust; Monkey Tranquilizer; New Acid; New Magic; Orange Crystal; Ozone; Paz; Peace Pill; Peep; Peter Pan; Pig Killer; Puffy; Purple Rain; Red Devil; Rocket Fuel; Rupture; Scuffle; Sheets; Sherms; Shermstick; Space (PCP mixed with cocaine); Spores; Stardust; STP; Super Grass; Super Kools; *Super Weed*; Surfer; Synthetic Cocaine; Taking a Cruise; T-Buzz; Tic Tac; Tish; Trank; Venom; Wack (PCP mixed with cocaine); Water; Wet (marijuana dipped in PCP); White Horizon; Wobble Weed; Wolf; Worm; Yellow Fever; Zombie; Zoom (PCP mixed with marijuana)

## Promethazine

Act; Drank; *Juice*; Lean; *Orange Crush*; Purple; Purple Drank; *Rojo*; Sizurup; Sizzurp; *Skittles*; Syrup; *Velvet*

## Psilocybin Mushrooms

Alice; *Blue Meanies*; Boomers; Buttons; Caps; Champiñones; *Cubes*; *God's Flesh*; Hongos; *Lazers*; *Liberties*; *Liberty Caps*; *Little Smoke*; Magic; Mushies; *Musk*; Pizza Toppings; *Psilly Billy*; *Purple Passion*; *Silly Putty*; *Simple Simon*; *Stemmies*; Tweezes

## Synthetic Cannabinoids

4-20; Abyss; Ace of Spades; AK-47; Amnesia; Atomic Blast; Big Bang; Black Magic Smoke; Black Mamba; Blaze; *Bliss*; Blue Cheese; *Bombay Blue*; Brain Freeze; Buzz Haze; Cherry Bomb; Chill; Chrome; Clockwork Orange; Cloud 10; Cowboy Kush; Crystal Skull; Dead Man; Devil's Venom; Dr. Feel Good; Dragon Eye; Earth Blend; Exodus; Extreme; Fake Bake; *Fire*; Fruit Candy Flavors; Funky Buddha; Funky Monkey; *Garden Salad*; *Genie*; G-Force; GI Joe; Green Dream; Green Peace; Hammer Head; Helix; Hipster; Hysteria; Ice Dragon; *Joker*; Juicy Leaf; Jungle Juice; Just Chill; K2; Kaos; Karma; Kong; Krazy Kandy; Kryp2nite; Kush; Layer Cake; Limitless; Mad Hatter; Mile High; Mystique; Ninja; Odyssey; OMG; Pandora's Box; Phoenix; Pineapple Express; Posh; Potpourri; Pow; Rapture; Red Magic; Rewind; Scooby Snax; Sexy; Sky High; Snake Bite; *Solar Flare*; Spice; Spike Diamond; Storm; Sweet Leaf; Synthetic Marijuana; Terraband; Time Traveler; Top Gear; Train Wreck; Ultimate; Viper; Voodoo Child; Wazabi; Wicked; Wizard; Xtreme; *Yucatan*; *Yucatan Fire*; Zero Gravity; *Zohai*; Zombie

**Synthetic Cathinones**

*Bath Blow*; Bath Salts; Bliss; Bloom; Blow; Blue Silk; *Bubbles*; Cloud 9; *Cosmic Beast*; Drone; Energy-1; Explosion; Flakka (Alpha-PVP); Gravel (Alpha-PVP); Insect Repellent ; Ivory Wave; Jewelry Cleaner; Lunar Wave; M-Cat; Meow-Meow; Ocean Burst; Phone Screen Cleaner; *Plant Feeder*; Plant Food; Pure Ivory; Purple Wave; Recharge; Red Dove; *Salting*; Scarface; Snow Leopard; Stardust; Vanilla Sky; White Dove; White Knight; White Lightening; White Magic; *Wicked X*; Zoom

## Steroids

*Arnolds*; *Gear*; *Gym Candy*; *Juice*; *Pumpers*; *Roids*; *Stackers*; *Weight Gainers*

## U-47700

*Pink*; *Pinky*; *U4*

## A

## B

## C

## I



## J



## K



## L

## M



## N

## O



## P

## Q



## R



## S



## T

## Y

## Alabama



## Alaska



## Arizona



## Arkansas



## California

## Canada



## Colorado



## Connecticut



## Delaware



## District of Columbia

## Florida



## Georgia



## Hawaii



## Idaho



## Illinois



## Indiana

## Massachusetts



## Michigan



## Minnesota



## Mississippi



## Missouri

## Montana



## Nebraska



## Nevada



## New Hampshire



## New Jersey



## New Mexico



## New York

## North Carolina



## North Dakota



## Ohio



## Oklahoma



## Oregon



## Pennsylvania

## Rhode Island



## South Carolina



## South Dakota



## Tennessee



## Texas

## Utah



## Vermont



## Virginia



## Washington



## West Virginia



## Wisconsin



## Wyoming

# Titles from Grey House

Visit www.GreyHouse.com for Product Information, Table of Contents, and Sample Pages.

## Opinions Throughout History

Opinions Throughout History: Church & State
Opinions Throughout History: The Death Penalty
Opinions Throughout History: Diseases & Epidemics
Opinions Throughout History: Drug Use & Abuse
Opinions Throughout History: The Environment
Opinions Throughout History: Free Speech & Censorship
Opinions Throughout History: Gender: Roles & Rights
Opinions Throughout History: Globalization
Opinions Throughout History: Guns in America
Opinions Throughout History: Immigration
Opinions Throughout History: Law Enforcement in America
Opinions Throughout History: National Security vs. Civil & Privacy Rights
Opinions Throughout History: Presidential Authority
Opinions Throughout History: Robotics & Artificial Intelligence
Opinions Throughout History: Social Media Issues
Opinions Throughout History: Voters' Rights
Opinions Throughout History: War & the Military
Opinions Throughout History: Workers Rights & Wages

## This is Who We Were

This is Who We Were: Colonial America (1492-1775)
This is Who We Were: 1880-1899
This is Who We Were: In the 1900s
This is Who We Were: In the 1910s
This is Who We Were: In the 1920s
This is Who We Were: A Companion to the 1940 Census
This is Who We Were: In the 1940s (1940-1949)
This is Who We Were: In the 1950s
This is Who We Were: In the 1960s
This is Who We Were: In the 1970s
This is Who We Were: In the 1980s
This is Who We Were: In the 1990s
This is Who We Were: In the 2000s
This is Who We Were: In the 2010s

## Working Americans

Working Americans—Vol. 1: The Working Class
Working Americans—Vol. 2: The Middle Class
Working Americans—Vol. 3: The Upper Class
Working Americans—Vol. 4: Children
Working Americans—Vol. 5: At War
Working Americans—Vol. 6: Working Women
Working Americans—Vol. 7: Social Movements
Working Americans—Vol. 8: Immigrants
Working Americans—Vol. 9: Revolutionary War to the Civil War
Working Americans—Vol. 10: Sports & Recreation
Working Americans—Vol. 11: Inventors & Entrepreneurs
Working Americans—Vol. 12: Our History through Music
Working Americans—Vol. 13: Education & Educators
Working Americans—Vol. 14: African Americans
Working Americans—Vol. 15: Politics & Politicians
Working Americans—Vol. 16: Farming & Ranching
Working Americans—Vol. 17: Teens in America
Working Americans—Vol. 18: Health Care Workers

## Grey House Health & Wellness Guides

The Autism Spectrum Handbook & Resource Guide
Autoimmune Disorders Handbook & Resource Guide
Cardiovascular Disease Handbook & Resource Guide
Dementia Handbook & Resource Guide
Diabetes Handbook & Resource Guide
Nutrition, Obesity & Eating Disorders Handbook & Resource Guide

## Consumer Health

Complete Mental Health Resource Guide
Complete Resource Guide for Pediatric Disorders
Complete Resource Guide for People with Chronic Illness
Complete Resource Guide for People with Disabilities
Older Americans Information Resource
Parenting: Styles & Strategies

## Education

Complete Learning Disabilities Resource Guide
Educators Resource Guide
The Comparative Guide to Elem. & Secondary Schools
Special Education: A Reference Book for Policy & Curriculum Development

## General Reference

American Environmental Leaders
Constitutional Amendments
Encyclopedia of African-American Writing
Encyclopedia of Invasions & Conquests
Encyclopedia of Prisoners of War & Internment
Encyclopedia of the Continental Congresses
Encyclopedia of the United States Cabinet
Encyclopedia of War Journalism
The Environmental Debate
Financial Literacy Starter Kit
From Suffrage to the Senate
The Gun Debate: Gun Rights & Gun Control in the U.S.
Historical Warrior Peoples & Modern Fighting Groups
Human Rights and the United States
Political Corruption in America
Privacy Rights in the Digital Age
The Religious Right and American Politics
Speakers of the House of Representatives, 1789-2021
US Land & Natural Resources Policy
The Value of a Dollar 1600-1865 Colonial to Civil War
The Value of a Dollar 1860-2019

## Business Information

Business Information Resources
The Complete Broadcasting Industry Guide: Television, Radio, Cable & Streaming
Directory of Mail Order Catalogs
Environmental Resource Handbook
Food & Beverage Market Place
The Grey House Guide to Homeland Security Resources
The Grey House Performing Arts Industry Guide
Guide to Healthcare Group Purchasing Organizations
Guide to U.S. HMOs and PPOs
Guide to Venture Capital & Private Equity Firms
Hudson's Washington News Media Contacts Guide
New York State Directory
Sports Market Place

# Grey House Imprints

Visit www.GreyHouse.com for Product Information, Table of Contents, and Sample Pages.

## Statistics & Demographics

America's Top-Rated Cities
America's Top-Rated Smaller Cities
The Comparative Guide to American Suburbs
Profiles of America
Profiles of California
Profiles of Florida
Profiles of Illinois
Profiles of Indiana
Profiles of Massachusetts
Profiles of Michigan
Profiles of New Jersey
Profiles of New York
Profiles of North Carolina & South Carolina
Profiles of Ohio
Profiles of Pennsylvania
Profiles of Texas
Profiles of Virginia
Profiles of Wisconsin

## Canadian Resources

Associations Canada
Canadian Almanac & Directory
Canadian Environmental Resource Guide
Canadian Parliamentary Guide
Canadian Venture Capital & Private Equity Firms
Canadian Who's Who
Cannabis Canada
Careers & Employment Canada
Financial Post: Directory of Directors
Financial Services Canada
FP Bonds: Corporate
FP Bonds: Government
FP Equities: Preferreds & Derivatives
FP Survey: Industrials
FP Survey: Mines & Energy
FP Survey: Predecessor & Defunct
Health Guide Canada
Libraries Canada

## Weiss Financial Ratings

Financial Literacy Basics
Financial Literacy: How to Become an Investor
Financial Literacy: Planning for the Future
Weiss Ratings Consumer Guides
Weiss Ratings Guide to Banks
Weiss Ratings Guide to Credit Unions
Weiss Ratings Guide to Health Insurers
Weiss Ratings Guide to Life & Annuity Insurers
Weiss Ratings Guide to Property & Casualty Insurers
Weiss Ratings Investment Research Guide to Bond & Money Market Mutual Funds
Weiss Ratings Investment Research Guide to Exchange-Traded Funds
Weiss Ratings Investment Research Guide to Stock Mutual Funds
Weiss Ratings Investment Research Guide to Stocks

## Books in Print Series

American Book Publishing Record® Annual
American Book Publishing Record® Monthly
Books In Print®
Books In Print® Supplement
Books Out Loud™
Bowker's Complete Video Directory™
Children's Books In Print®
El-Hi Textbooks & Serials In Print®
Forthcoming Books®
Law Books & Serials In Print™
Medical & Health Care Books In Print™
Publishers, Distributors & Wholesalers of the US™
Subject Guide to Books In Print®
Subject Guide to Children's Books In Print®

SALEM PRESS

# Titles from Salem Press

SALEM PRESS

Visit www.SalemPress.com for Product Information, Table of Contents, and Sample Pages.

## LITERATURE

### Critical Insights: Authors

Louisa May Alcott
Sherman Alexie
Isabel Allende
Maya Angelou
Isaac Asimov
Margaret Atwood
Jane Austen
James Baldwin
Saul Bellow
Roberto Bolano
Ray Bradbury
The Brontë Sisters
Gwendolyn Brooks
Albert Camus
Raymond Carver
Willa Cather
Geoffrey Chaucer
John Cheever
Joseph Conrad
Charles Dickens
Emily Dickinson
Frederick Douglass
T. S. Eliot
George Eliot
Harlan Ellison
Louise Erdrich
William Faulkner
F. Scott Fitzgerald
Gustave Flaubert
Horton Foote
Benjamin Franklin
Robert Frost
Neil Gaiman
Gabriel Garcia Marquez
Thomas Hardy
Nathaniel Hawthorne
Robert A. Heinlein
Lillian Hellman
Ernest Hemingway
Langston Hughes
Zora Neale Hurston
Henry James
Thomas Jefferson
James Joyce
Jamaica Kincaid
Stephen King
Martin Luther King, Jr.
Barbara Kingsolver
Abraham Lincoln
Mario Vargas Llosa
Jack London
James McBride
Cormac McCarthy
Herman Melville
Arthur Miller
Toni Morrison
Alice Munro
Tim O'Brien
Flannery O'Connor
Eugene O'Neill
George Orwell
Sylvia Plath
Edgar Allan Poe
Philip Roth
Salman Rushdie
J.D. Salinger
Mary Shelley
John Steinbeck
Amy Tan
Leo Tolstoy
Mark Twain
John Updike
Kurt Vonnegut
Alice Walker
David Foster Wallace
Edith Wharton
Walt Whitman
Oscar Wilde
Tennessee Williams
Virginia Woolf
Richard Wright
Malcolm X

### Critical Insights: Works

Absalom, Absalom!
Adventures of Huckleberry Finn
Adventures of Tom Sawyer
Aeneid
All Quiet on the Western Front
Animal Farm
Anna Karenina
The Awakening
The Bell Jar
Beloved
Billy Budd, Sailor
The Book Thief
Brave New World
The Canterbury Tales
Catch-22
The Catcher in the Rye
The Color Purple
The Crucible
Death of a Salesman
The Diary of a Young Girl
Dracula
Fahrenheit 451
The Grapes of Wrath
Great Expectations
The Great Gatsby
Hamlet
The Handmaid's Tale
Harry Potter Series
Heart of Darkness
The Hobbit
The House on Mango Street
How the Garcia Girls Lost Their Accents
The Hunger Games Trilogy
I Know Why the Caged Bird Sings
In Cold Blood
The Inferno
Invisible Man
Jane Eyre
The Joy Luck Club
Julius Caesar
King Lear
The Kite Runner
Life of Pi
Little Women
Lolita
Lord of the Flies
The Lord of the Rings
Macbeth
The Metamorphosis
Midnight's Children
A Midsummer Night's Dream
Moby-Dick
Mrs. Dalloway
Nineteen Eighty-Four
The Odyssey
Of Mice and Men
The Old Man and the Sea
On the Road
One Flew Over the Cuckoo's Nest
One Hundred Years of Solitude
Othello
The Outsiders
Paradise Lost
The Pearl
The Poetry of Baudelaire
The Poetry of Edgar Allan Poe
A Portrait of the Artist as a Young Man
Pride and Prejudice
The Red Badge of Courage
Romeo and Juliet
The Scarlet Letter
Short Fiction of Flannery O'Connor
Slaughterhouse-Five
The Sound and the Fury
A Streetcar Named Desire
The Sun Also Rises
A Tale of Two Cities
The Tales of Edgar Allan Poe
Their Eyes Were Watching God
Things Fall Apart
To Kill a Mockingbird
War and Peace
The Woman Warrior

### Critical Insights: Themes

The American Comic Book
American Creative Non-Fiction
The American Dream
American Multicultural Identity
American Road Literature
American Short Story
American Sports Fiction
The American Thriller
American Writers in Exile
Censored & Banned Literature
Civil Rights Literature, Past & Present
Coming of Age
Conspiracies
Contemporary Canadian Fiction
Contemporary Immigrant Short Fiction
Contemporary Latin American Fiction
Contemporary Speculative Fiction
Crime and Detective Fiction
Crisis of Faith
Cultural Encounters
Dystopia
Family
The Fantastic
Feminism

# Titles from Salem Press



Visit www.SalemPress.com for Product Information, Table of Contents, and Sample Pages.

Flash Fiction
Gender, Sex and Sexuality
Good & Evil
The Graphic Novel
Greed
Harlem Renaissance
The Hero's Quest
Historical Fiction
Holocaust Literature
The Immigrant Experience
Inequality
LGBTQ Literature
Literature in Times of Crisis
Literature of Protest
Love
Magical Realism
Midwestern Literature
Modern Japanese Literature
Nature & the Environment
Paranoia, Fear & Alienation
Patriotism
Political Fiction
Postcolonial Literature
Pulp Fiction of the '20s and '30s
Rebellion
Russia's Golden Age
Satire
The Slave Narrative
Social Justice and American Literature
Southern Gothic Literature
Southwestern Literature
Survival
Technology & Humanity
Truth & Lies
Violence in Literature
Virginia Woolf & 20th Century Women Writers
War

## Critical Insights: Film

Bonnie & Clyde
Casablanca
Alfred Hitchcock
Stanley Kubrick

## Critical Approaches to Literature

Critical Approaches to Literature: Feminist
Critical Approaches to Literature: Moral
Critical Approaches to Literature: Multicultural
Critical Approaches to Literature: Psychological

## Critical Surveys of Literature

Critical Survey of American Literature
Critical Survey of Drama
Critical Survey of Graphic Novels: Heroes & Superheroes
Critical Survey of Graphic Novels: History, Theme, and Technique
Critical Survey of Graphic Novels: Independents & Underground Classics
Critical Survey of Graphic Novels: Manga
Critical Survey of Long Fiction
Critical Survey of Mystery and Detective Fiction
Critical Survey of Mythology & Folklore: Gods & Goddesses
Critical Survey of Mythology & Folklore: Heroes and Heroines
Critical Survey of Mythology & Folklore: Love, Sexuality, and Desire
Critical Survey of Mythology & Folklore: World Mythology
Critical Survey of Poetry
Critical Survey of Poetry: Contemporary Poets
Critical Survey of Science Fiction & Fantasy Literature
Critical Survey of Shakespeare's Plays
Critical Survey of Shakespeare's Sonnets
Critical Survey of Short Fiction
Critical Survey of World Literature
Critical Survey of Young Adult Literature

## Cyclopedia of Literary Characters & Places

Cyclopedia of Literary Characters
Cyclopedia of Literary Places

## Introduction to Literary Context

American Poetry of the 20th Century
American Post-Modernist Novels
American Short Fiction
English Literature
Plays
World Literature

## Magill's Literary Annual

Magill's Literary Annual, 2022
Magill's Literary Annual, 2021
Magill's Literary Annual, 2020
Magill's Literary Annual (Backlist Issues 2019-1977)

## Masterplots

Masterplots, Fourth Edition
Masterplots, 2010-2018 Supplement

## Notable Writers

Notable African American Writers
Notable American Women Writers
Notable Mystery & Detective Fiction Writers
Notable Writers of the American West & the Native American Experience
Novels into Film: Adaptations & Interpretation
Recommended Reading: 600 Classics Reviewed

# Titles from Salem Press



Visit www.SalemPress.com for Product Information, Table of Contents, and Sample Pages.

## CAREERS

Careers: Paths to Entrepreneurship
Careers in Artificial Intelligence
Careers in the Arts: Fine, Performing & Visual
Careers in the Automotive Industry
Careers in Biology
Careers in Building Construction
Careers in Business
Careers in Chemistry
Careers in Communications & Media
Careers in Education & Training
Careers in Engineering
Careers in Environment & Conservation
Careers in Financial Services
Careers in Forensic Science
Careers in Gaming
Careers in Green Energy
Careers in Healthcare
Careers in Hospitality & Tourism
Careers in Human Services
Careers in Information Technology
Careers in Law, Criminal Justice & Emergency Services
Careers in the Music Industry
Careers in Manufacturing & Production
Careers in Nursing
Careers in Physics
Careers in Protective Services
Careers in Psychology & Behavioral Health
Careers in Public Administration
Careers in Sales, Insurance & Real Estate
Careers in Science & Engineering
Careers in Social Media
Careers in Sports & Fitness
Careers in Sports Medicine & Training
Careers in Technical Services & Equipment Repair
Careers in Transportation
Careers in Writing & Editing
Careers Outdoors
Careers Overseas
Careers Working with Infants & Children
Careers Working with Animals

## BUSINESS

Principles of Business: Accounting
Principles of Business: Economics
Principles of Business: Entrepreneurship
Principles of Business: Finance
Principles of Business: Globalization
Principles of Business: Leadership
Principles of Business: Management
Principles of Business: Marketing

# Titles from H.W. Wilson

Visit www.HWWilsonInPrint.com for Product Information, Table of Contents, and Sample Pages.

## Core Collections

Children's Core Collection
Fiction Core Collection
Graphic Novels Core Collection
Middle & Junior High School Core
Public Library Core Collection: Nonfiction
Senior High Core Collection
Young Adult Fiction Core Collection

## The Reference Shelf

Affordable Housing
Aging in America
Alternative Facts, Post-Truth and the Information War
The American Dream
Artificial Intelligence
The Business of Food
Campaign Trends & Election Law
College Sports
Democracy Evolving
The Digital Age
Embracing New Paradigms in Education
Food Insecurity & Hunger in the United States
Future of U.S. Economic Relations: Mexico, Cuba, & Venezuela
Global Climate Change
Guns in America
Hate Crimes
Immigration
Income Inequality
Internet Abuses & Privacy Rights
Internet Law
LGBTQ in the 21st Century
Marijuana Reform
Mental Health Awareness
National Debate Topic 2014/2015: The Ocean
National Debate Topic 2015/2016: Surveillance
National Debate Topic 2016/2017: US/China Relations
National Debate Topic 2017/2018: Education Reform
National Debate Topic 2018/2019: Immigration
National Debate Topic 2019/2021: Arms Sales
National Debate Topic 2020/2021: Criminal Justice Reform
National Debate Topic 2021/2022: Water Resources
National Debate Topic 2022/2023
New Frontiers in Space
Policing in 2020
Pollution
Prescription Drug Abuse
Propaganda and Misinformation
Racial Tension in a Postracial Age
Reality Television
Representative American Speeches, Annual Editions
Rethinking Work
Revisiting Gender
The South China Sea Conflict
Sports in America
The Supreme Court
The Transformation of American Cities
The Two Koreas
UFOs
Vaccinations
Voters' Rights
Whistleblowers

## Current Biography

Current Biography Cumulative Index 1946-2021
Current Biography Monthly Magazine
Current Biography Yearbook

## Readers' Guide to Periodical Literature

Abridged Readers' Guide to Periodical Literature
Readers' Guide to Periodical Literature

## Indexes

Index to Legal Periodicals & Books
Short Story Index
Book Review Digest

## Sears List

Sears List of Subject Headings
Sears: Lista de Encabezamientos de Materia

## History

American Game Changers: Invention, Innovation & Transformation
American Reformers
Speeches of the American Presidents

## Facts About Series

Facts About the 20th Century
Facts About American Immigration
Facts About China
Facts About the Presidents
Facts About the World's Languages

## Nobel Prize Winners

Nobel Prize Winners: 1901-1986
Nobel Prize Winners: 1987-1991
Nobel Prize Winners: 1992-1996
Nobel Prize Winners: 1997-2001
Nobel Prize Winners: 2002-2018

## Famous First Facts

Famous First Facts
Famous First Facts About American Politics
Famous First Facts About Sports
Famous First Facts About the Environment
Famous First Facts: International Edition

## American Book of Days

The American Book of Days
The International Book of Days